VISUALIZING

NUTRITION
EVERYDAY CHOICES

CREDITS

EXECUTIVE VP AND PUBLISHER Kaye Pace
MANAGING DIRECTOR Helen McInnis
EDITOR Kevin Witt
DIRECTOR OF DEVELOPMENT Barbara Heaney
MANAGER, PRODUCT DEVELOPMENT Nancy Perry
DEVELOPMENT EDITORS Irene Nunes, Carolyn Smith
PROJECT EDITOR Lorraina Raccuia
EDITORIAL ASSISTANTS Lauren Morris, Alissa Etrheim, Sean Boda
EXECUTIVE MARKETING MANAGER Clay Stone
SENIOR PRODUCTION MANAGER Micheline Frederick
SENIOR MEDIA EDITOR Linda Muriello
CREATIVE DIRECTOR Harry Nolan
COVER DESIGNER Harry Nolan
INTERIOR DESIGN Vertigo Design
PHOTO EDITORS Hilary Newman, Teri Stratford
PHOTO RESEARCHER Stacy Gold, National Geographic Society
SENIOR ILLUSTRATION EDITOR Sandra Rigby
PRODUCTION SERVICES Furino Production

COVER IMAGE
Top photo: ©Bill Bettencourt
Bottom inset photos (from left to right): ©Justin Guariglia/
NG Image Collection; ©Jean Claude Revy/Phototake;
©Edward Kinsman/Photo Researchers, Inc.; ©James Forte/
NG Image Collection; ©Mediscan/Visuals Unlimited

This book was set in Times New Roman by GGS Higher Education
Resources, a Division of PreMedia Global, Inc., printed and bound
by Quebecor World. The cover was printed by Quebecor World.

ISBN: 978-0-470-19758-5
BRV ISBN: 978-0-470-55652-8

Printed in the United States of America

10 9 8 7 6 5 4 3 2 1

VISUALIZING

NUTRITION
EVERYDAY CHOICES

Mary B. Grosvenor, MS, RD
Lori A. Smolin, PhD
University of Connecticut

WILEY

In collaboration with
THE NATIONAL GEOGRAPHIC SOCIETY

Wiley Nutrition—Right for You!

Wiley is deeply committed to nutrition education. Through our teaching and learning materials, we aspire to excellence in nutrition by providing students with engaging resources that will help them to understand the most difficult concepts in nutrition. Our goal is to provide you and your students with the right resources for your course, such as animations that teach tough topics in nutrition. To ensure that we are producing the highest-quality resources for nutrition, we have assembled an expert advisory board to guide the direction of our materials—to review all data, art, references, and media before publication.

What Is the Nutrition Advisory Board?

The mission of the Wiley Nutrition Advisory Board (NAB) is to provide a voice that helps shape and guide Wiley's vision for nutrition and message to the intended markets.

Selected by the Wiley editorial team, NAB members are called on to participate in the following ways:

- Guide Wiley's vision for nutrition and help develop the message to the market
- Serve as expert reviewers and contributors
- Be available for phone conversations or email exchanges on specific topics
- Contribute ideas and resources for best practices initiative and faculty development
- Oversee the accuracy of our nutrition products, including review of manuscript, scientific art, and supplements
- Align textbook learning objectives with course and discipline objectives
- Assist in the development of animation storyboards

NAB Members

NANCY BERKOFF
California State University–Los Angeles and Los Angeles Trade Technical College

LINDA BROWN
Florida State University and Kaplan

JUDY MYHAND
Louisiana State University

JOHN ORTA
California State University–Los Angeles

JANET PETERSON
Linfield College

DIANA SPILLMAN
University of Ohio–Miami

PRIYA VENKATASEN
Pasadena City College

SHAHLA WUNDERLICH
Montclair State University

PREFACE

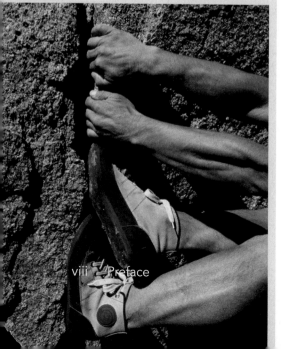

Students can do more than just read about the world; they can experience it through vivid images and creative videos. In writing *Visualizing Nutrition: Everyday Choices*, we wanted to take advantage of this uniquely modern way that students can take in information. Using striking images from the National Geographic Society's photo reservoir, this text integrates photography and illustrations into the learning process while maintaining the rigor needed in the study of science. Information that would be buried in the text of other books is presented within the context of colorful illustrations and vibrant photographs. The images grab students' attention and, along with the text, tell the absorbing story of nutrition. The text captures the interest of college students from every background and engages them by demonstrating the applications of the science of nutrition to everyday choices.

This book is intended to serve as an introductory text for undergraduate students. The accessible format of *Visualizing Nutrition: Everyday Choices*, which assumes that readers have little prior knowledge of nutrition, allows students to easily make the connection between their individual experience with food and nutrition concepts and the science of nutrition. The text uses a critical thinking approach to teaching human nutrition, bringing nutrition out of the classroom by asking students to apply the logic of science to their own nutrition concerns. *Visualizing Nutrition: Everyday Choices* educates students about the functions and sources of individual nutrients and also focuses on the total diet, so students understand that no one food choice determines the healthfulness of their overall dietary pattern. The examples and exercises throughout the book allow students to think critically while exploring the similarities and differences in the diets and health concerns of the diverse ethnic and cultural mix of the population of the United States and the rest of the world. The text presents information using a clear, concise writing style and addresses the most recent advances in nutrition science. Each chapter extensively references the most current literature.

NATIONAL GEOGRAPHIC SOCIETY

Visualizing Nutrition: Everyday Choices offers an array of remarkable photographs, media, and film from the National Geographic Society collections. Students using the book benefit from the long history and rich, fascinating resources of National Geographic.

Fact-Checking: The National Geographic Society has also performed an invaluable service in fact-checking *Visualizing Nutrition: Everyday Choices*. They have verified every fact in the book with two outside sources, to ensure that the text is accurate and up-to-date.

ORGANIZATION

Visualizing Nutrition: Everyday Choices is unique in its integrated approach to the presentation of nutrition science. While the chapter organization follows the traditional format of nutrition books, this book integrates metabolism and health and disease information throughout the text. To make the study of metabolism more accessible, *Visualizing Nutrition: Everyday Choices* provides a simple overview of metabolism in Chapter 3 and then builds on this base with more complex discussions in subsequent chapters. In Chapter 4, the discussion of carbohydrate metabolism presents the basics of intermediary metabolism. Chapters 5 through 10, which cover lipids, proteins, micronutrients, energy balance, and exercise, review and add to this information. The integration throughout the text of discussions of nutrition, health, and disease serves to consistently engage student interest. By incorporating this information, students can see that a nutrient's function in metabolism is related to its role in health and disease. This integration continuously reinforces the applicability of nutrition science to students' lives and helps them appreciate how and why their food choices affect their health.

- ■ The first two chapters of this book introduce nutrition science. **Chapter 1, "Nutrition: Everyday Choices,"** begins by discussing the U.S. diet—how it has changed and how healthy it is—and emphasizing the fact that food choices affect current and future health. This chapter provides an overview of the nutrients and their roles in the body and defines the basic principles of balance, variety, and moderation that are key to a healthy diet. It also introduces the scientific method and the steps students need to follow to sort accurate from inaccurate nutrition information. **Chapter 2, "Guidelines for a Healthy Diet,"** begins with a history of nutrition recommendations and a discussion of how valuable these recommendations are for assessing the nutritional health of populations and individuals. It then takes the science out of the laboratory and shows how advances in nutrition knowledge have been used to develop the Dietary Reference Intakes (DRIs), the *Dietary Guidelines for Americans*, and tools for diet planning, including MyPyramid, food labels, and exchange lists.

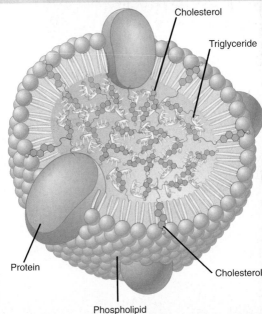

- ■ **Chapter 3, "Digestion: From Meals to Molecules,"** provides the background students need to understand how nutrients are used by their bodies. It discusses how food is digested, how nutrients from foods are absorbed into the body and transported to the cells where metabolism occurs, and how wastes are removed. This chapter provides an overview of metabolism that serves as a launching pad for the more in-depth metabolism information presented in subsequent chapters.

MyPyramid
STEPS TO A HEALTHIER YOU
MyPyramid.gov

■ Chapters 4, 5, and 6 feature the energy-yielding nutrients carbohydrates, lipids, and proteins. Each of these chapters begins with a discussion of the respective macronutrient in the food we eat. The body of each chapter then illustrates the digestion and absorption of these nutrients, their functions, and the impact of each on health and particular disease states. Each chapter ends with a discussion of how to choose a diet that meets recommendations. Emphasis is placed on the types and proportions of these nutrients that are optimal for health. **Chapter 4, "Carbohydrates: Sugars, Starches, and Fibers,"** discusses the health impact of refined grains and added sugar versus whole grains and foods that naturally contain sugars. **Chapter 5, "Lipids: Fats, Phospholipids, and Sterols,"** points out that Americans are not eating too much fat but are often choosing the wrong types of fat for a healthy diet. **Chapter 6, "Proteins and Amino Acids,"** discusses animal and plant sources of protein and points out that both can meet protein needs, but these protein sources contain different combinations of nutrients. In addition to discussing how to meet protein needs, this chapter includes information on how to plan a healthy vegetarian diet.

■ The next two chapters present the micronutrients and water. **Chapter 7, "Vitamins,"** begins with a general overview of vitamins: where vitamins are found in the diet, factors affecting their bioavailability, and how they function. The chapter then discusses each of the vitamins individually, providing information on sources in the diet, functions in the body, impact on health, recommended intakes, and potential for toxicity. The chapter ends with a discussion of dietary supplements, who might benefit from using them, and risks associated with their use. **Chapter 8, "Water and Minerals,"** addresses water, a nutrient often overlooked, and the major and trace minerals. The chapter presents information on the sources of these nutrients in the diet and discusses their functions in the body, relationships to health and disease, and recommended intakes. A discussion of hypertension illustrates the importance of these nutrients in blood pressure regulation and the impact of the total diet on healthy blood pressure. A discussion of nutrients and bone health includes a section on the relationship between nutrition and the development of osteoporosis. Sections on trace minerals engage students with discussions of health concerns related to both deficiencies and excesses.

■ **Chapter 9, "Energy Balance and Weight Management,"** begins with a discussion of the obesity epidemic and the effect of excess body fat on health. The chapter explains energy balance, illustrates the impact of small changes in diet and behavior on long-term weight management, and presents up-to-date information on how body weight is regulated and the role of genetic versus environmental factors in determining body fatness. The chapter includes recommendations for healthy body weight and composition and equations for determining energy needs. It also discusses weight-loss options that range from simple caloric restriction to potentially risky surgical approaches. The chapter also includes a comprehensive discussion of eating disorders and their causes, consequences, and treatment.

■ **Chapter 10, "Nutrition, Fitness, and Physical Activity,"** discusses the relationships among physical activity, nutrition, and health. It emphasizes the importance of exercise for health maintenance as well as the impact nutrition can have on exercise performance. Because nutrients fuel activity, this chapter serves as a review of metabolism. By this point in the text, students have studied all the essential nutrients, so this chapter includes a complete discussion of the macronutrients and micronutrients needed for ATP production. A discussion of ergogenic aids for competitive athletes directs students to use a risk–benefit analysis of these products before deciding whether to use them.

■ **Chapter 11, "Nutrition During Pregnancy and Infancy,"** addresses the role of nutrition in human development and discusses the nutritional needs of a woman during pregnancy and lactation as well as the nutritional needs of an infant. The chapter also discusses the benefits and risks of breast versus bottle feeding.

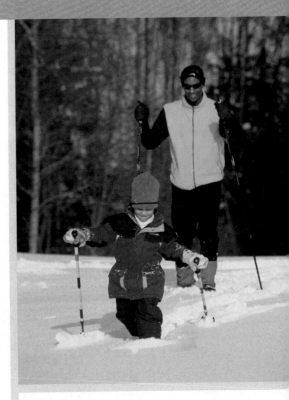

■ **Chapter 12, "Nutrition from 1 to 100,"** travels through the life cycle, discussing the energy and nutrient needs of growing children, adolescents, and adults. The chapter discusses the importance of learning healthy eating habits early in life, particularly in relation to the rising rates of obesity and other chronic diseases in today's youth. The chapter then addresses how nutrition affects aging and how aging affects nutrition. It presents the interrelationships between aging and nutritional status and the impact medications and chronic disease can have on nutritional status. The chapter ends with a discussion of alcohol: how it affects metabolism and impacts health at all stages of life.

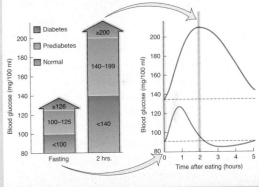

■ **Chapter 13, "How Safe Is Our Food Supply?"** discusses the risks and benefits associated with the U.S. food supply and includes information on the impact of microbial hazards, chemical toxins, food additives, irradiation, and food packaging. It addresses the directives of the Food Safety Initiative, including the use of HACCP (Hazard Analysis Critical Control Point) to ensure safe food and advances in technology that help identify the sources of food-borne illness. The chapter ends with a discussion of biotechnology, including an explanation of how plants are genetically modified and the potential benefits and risks associated with this expanding technology.

■ **Chapter 14, "Feeding the World,"** discusses the coexistence of hunger and malnutrition along with obesity in both developed and developing nations. It examines the causes of world hunger and potential solutions that can affect the amounts and types of food that are available.

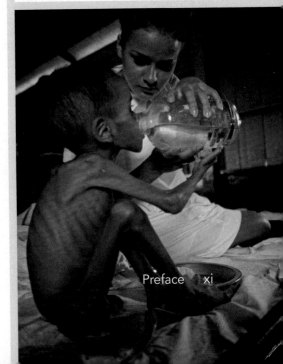

HELPING STUDENTS VISUALIZE NUTRITION

A number of pedagogical features using visuals have been developed specifically for *Visualizing Nutrition: Everyday Choices*. Presenting the highly varied and often technical concepts woven throughout nutrition raises challenges for reader and instructor alike. This **Illustrated Book Tour** on the following pages provides a guide to the diverse features that contribute to the pedagogical plan of *Visualizing Nutrition: Everyday Choices*.

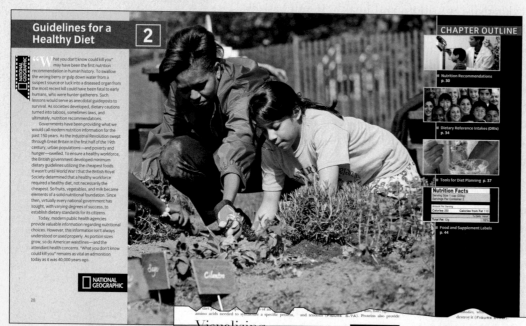

CHAPTER INTRODUCTIONS are intriguing narratives that address nutrition concepts and ideas from popular culture and society. The information provided in the chapter expands on the introductory text to help students better understand the broader issues associated with nutrition science. **CHAPTER OUTLINES** use thumbnails of illustrations from the chapter to show students nutrition concepts and how they are related to the material in the chapter.

VISUALIZING features are a specially designed multipart visual spreads that focus on key concepts or topics in the chapter, exploring them in detail or in broader context using a combination of photos and figures.

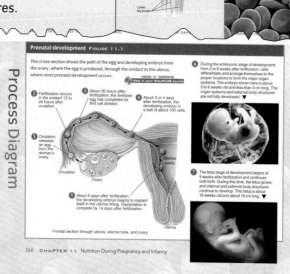

PROCESS DIAGRAMS are designed to help students understand challenging processes. They include a complex illustration or a series of figures and/or photos with numbered steps. Students can use the numbers to follow the process and see changes that occur as they progress to the different parts of the diagram. This approach unburdens the text and lets the images tell the story.

CASE STUDIES use a critical thinking approach to walk students through the thought processes needed to make decisions and solve problems regarding nutrition. These exercises appear in each chapter of the book to help students apply their developing nutrition knowledge to everyday situations. They present a nutrition-related problem and then guide the students through the logical progression of thought needed to collect the appropriate information and solve the problem.

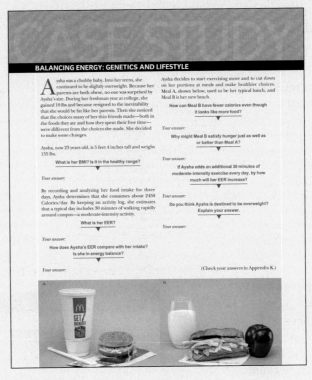

WHAT A SCIENTIST SEES features highlight a nutrition concept or phenomenon that would stand out to a professional in the field. Photos and figures are used to compare how a nonscientist and a scientist see the issue.

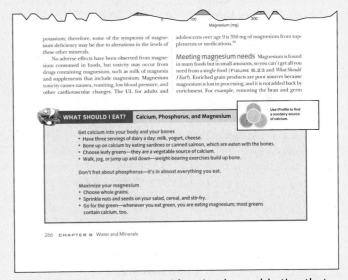

WHAT SHOULD I EAT? provides simple, usable tips that help students translate the nutrition recommendations discussed in each chapter into healthy food choices. The **iProfile icon** appears with suggestions to help students analyze their own diets and apply the information they are learning to their own everyday food choices.

PROVIDING STUDENTS WITH PROVEN LEARNING TOOLS

LEARNING OBJECTIVES at the beginning of each section indicate in behavioral terms the concepts that students are expected to master while reading the section.

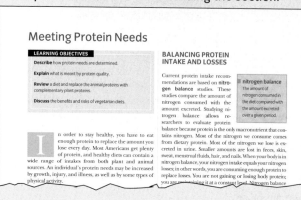

Meeting Protein Needs

LEARNING OBJECTIVES

Describe how protein needs are determined.

Explain what is meant by protein quality.

Review a diet and replace the animal proteins with complementary plant proteins.

Discuss the benefits and risks of vegetarian diets.

I n order to stay healthy, you have to eat enough protein to replace the amount you lose every day. Most Americans get plenty of protein, and healthy diets can contain a wide range of intakes from both plant and animal sources. An individual's protein needs may be increased by growth, injury, and illness, as well as by some types of physical activity.

BALANCING PROTEIN INTAKE AND LOSSES

Current protein intake recommendations are based on **nitrogen balance** studies. These studies compare the amount of nitrogen consumed with the amount excreted. Studying nitrogen balance allows researchers to evaluate protein balance because protein is the only macronutrient that contains nitrogen. Most of the nitrogen we consume comes from dietary protein. Most of the nitrogen we lose is excreted in urine. Smaller amounts are lost in feces, skin, sweat, menstrual fluids, hair, and nails. When your body is in nitrogen balance, your nitrogen intake equals your nitrogen losses; in other words, you are consuming enough protein to replace losses. You are not gaining or losing body protein; you are maintaining it at a constant level. Nitrogen balance

nitrogen balance The amount of nitrogen consumed in the diet compared with the amount excreted over a given period.

---

dren are at particular risk for lead toxicity because they absorb lead much more efficiently than do adults.[50] Once it has been absorbed from the gastrointestinal tract, lead circulates in the bloodstream and then accumulates in the bones and, to a lesser extent, the brain, teeth, and kidneys. Lead disrupts the functioning of neurotransmitters and thus interferes with the functioning of the nervous system.

In young children, lead poisoning can cause learning disabilities and behavior problems.[51,52] There is evidence that even blood lead levels below 10 microgram/100 ml, which were once thought to be safe, may impair IQ in young children.[52] Higher levels of lead can contribute to iron deficiency anemia, changes in kidney function, nervous system changes, and even seizures, coma, and death.

Because of the risks of lead toxicity from environmental contamination, lead is no longer used in house paint, gasoline, or solder. As a result, the number of children ages 1 to 5 with elevated blood lead levels decreased from 77.8% in 1976–1980 to only 1.6% in 1999–2002.[51]

these groups are at greater risk of elevated blood lead levels than others (FIGURE 12.7). The effects of lead poisoning are permanent, but if high levels are detected early, the lead can be removed with medical treatment. Most children in the United States are at sufficient risk of lead exposure that they should have their blood lead concentration measured at least once.[53]

CONCEPT CHECK STOP

HOW do children's energy and protein requirements change as they age?

What factors affect children's food choices?

HOW does television viewing affect eating and exercise patterns?

Why is lead toxicity more common in low-income children than in others?

CONCEPT CHECK questions at the end of each section give students the opportunity to test their comprehension of the section's learning objectives.

ILLUSTRATIONS and **PHOTOS** demonstrate and oftentimes introduce concepts covered in the text, elaborate on relevant issues, and add visual detail. Many of the photos are from National Geographic's abundant sources.

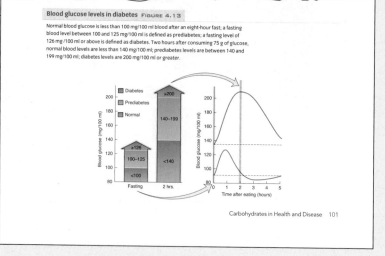

sorption (FIGURE 3.10). Together the features provide . . . from the pancreas and small intestine to function.

Visualizing

The structure of the small intestine FIGURE 3.10

A The wall of the small intestine is arranged in large circular folds, which increase the surface area in contact with nutrients. ▼

SMALL INTESTINE

Large circular folds

Lumen
Microvilli
Mucosal cell
Lacteal

Capillary

Villi

Microvilli

C Each villus is covered with tiny projections of the mucosal cell membrane called **microvilli**, often referred to as the **brush border**. Some of the digestive enzymes produced by the small intestine are located in the membrane, and some are located inside the mucosal cells.

B The entire inner surface of the small intestine is covered with fingerlike projections called **villi** (the singular is *villus*). Each villus contains a **capillary** (small blood vessel) and a **lacteal** (small lymph vessel). Nutrients must cross only the single-cell layer of the mucosa to reach the blood or lymph for delivery to the tissues of the body.

Artery
Vein
Lymph vessel

Digestion and Absorption of Nutrients 67

GRAPHS and **TABLES** summarize and organize important information in an accessible format. The data sources for these illustrations are cited at the end of the book.

---

type 1 diabetes The form of diabetes caused by autoimmune destruction of insulin-producing cells in the pancreas, usually leading to absolute insulin deficiency.

autoimmune disease A disease that results from immune reactions that destroy normal body cells.

MARGIN GLOSSARY TERMS (in green boldface) define each chapter's most important terms. Other important terms appear in **black boldface** and are defined in the text.

Blood glucose levels in diabetes FIGURE 4.13

Normal blood glucose is less than 100 mg/100 ml blood after an eight-hour fast; a fasting blood level between 100 and 125 mg/100 ml is defined as prediabetes; a fasting level of 126 mg /100 ml or above is defined as diabetes. Two hours after consuming 75 g of glucose, normal blood levels are less than 140 mg/100 ml; prediabetes levels are between 140 and 199 mg/100 ml; diabetes levels are 200 mg/100 ml or greater.

Diabetes
Prediabetes
Normal

≥126
100–125
<100

≥200
140–199
<140

Fasting   2 hrs.

Blood glucose (mg/100 ml)

Time after eating (hours)

Carbohydrates in Health and Disease 101

The **SUMMARY** highlights important concepts addressed in the chapter. The glossary terms are featured here, in boldface, and are also included in the **KEY TERMS** list. Students are thus able to study vocabulary words in the context of related concepts. Each portion of the **SUMMARY** is illustrated with a relevant photo or illustration from its respective chapter section.

CRITICAL AND CREATIVE THINKING QUESTIONS appear at the end of each chapter, helping students to think critically and apply key nutrition concepts from the chapter. Some of these exercises feature clinical applications and therefore also help reinforce the importance of nutrition in health promotion and disease prevention. Some of these can be done as collaborative learning exercises that encourage students to work together and learn from each other to solve a problem.

The **SELF-TEST** at the end of each chapter allows students to assess their progress upon completing the chapter. These questions, which test students' understanding of the key points covered, include graphs, diagrams, and other images taken from the text, encouraging students to actively and visually engage with the material.

WHAT IS HAPPENING IN THIS PICTURE? is an end-of-chapter feature that presents a photograph that is relevant to a chapter topic and illustrates a situation students are not likely to have encountered previously. The photograph is paired with questions designed to stimulate creative thinking.

MEDIA AND SUPPLEMENTS

Visualizing Nutrition: Everyday Choices is accompanied by a rich array of media and supplements that incorporate the visuals from the textbook to form a pedagogically cohesive package. For example, a Process Diagram from the book may be the subject of a short video or an animation, and it may also appear with questions in the Test Bank.

WILEYPLUS

WileyPLUS is an online teaching and learning environment that integrates the entire digital textbook with the most effective instructor and student resources to fit every learning style. With **WileyPLUS**:

- Students achieve concept mastery in a rich, structured environment that's available 24/7.
- Instructors can personalize and manage their course more effectively with assessments, assignments, grade tracking, and more.

WileyPLUS can be used with or in place of the textbook.

INSTRUCTOR SUPPLEMENTS

The following supplements are available on the **Instructor Companion Website**, www.wiley.com/college/grosvenor, or through **WileyPLUS**.

VIDEOS

A collection of **videos**, some from the award-winning National Geographic Film Collection, have been selected to accompany and enrich the text. Each chapter includes a video clip, available online as digitized streaming video. Discussion questions that can further develop student understanding are included with each video. The videos are available in **WileyPLUS**.

ANIMATIONS

How It Works animations have been developed specifically to strengthen student understanding of the most difficult topics in nutrition. These animations break difficult processes into understandable steps.

Animated Process Diagrams have been developed for each chapter to allow students to interact with a process diagram to learn important processes in nutrition.

POWERPOINT PRESENTATIONS AND IMAGE GALLERY

A complete set of highly visual **PowerPoint presentations**, prepared by Nancy Berkoff of California State University–Los Angeles and Los Angeles Trade Technical College, is available online to enhance classroom presentations.

All figures from the text are online, in the **Nutrition Visual Library**, and can be used as you wish in the classroom.

TEST BANK (AVAILABLE IN WileyPLUS AND ELECTRONIC FORMAT)

The visuals from *Visualizing Nutrition: Everyday Choices* are also included in the Test Bank, by Brenda Malinauskas of East Carolina University. The Test Bank contains approximately 1,200 test items, at least 25% of which incorporate visuals from the book. The test items include multiple-choice and essay questions that test a variety of comprehension levels. The Test Bank is available as Word files and on the Instructor Companion Website. These test questions are also used in WileyPLUS.

INSTRUCTOR'S RESOURCE GUIDE (AVAILABLE IN ELECTRONIC FORMAT)

The Instructor's Resources Guide begins with the special introduction *Using Visuals in the Classroom*, prepared by Matthew Leavitt of Arizona State University, which provides guidelines and suggestions on how to use the visuals in teaching the course. Teaching resources are provided for every chapter.

iProfile 2.0: ASSESSING YOUR DIET AND ENERGY BALANCE

The new version of this dynamic software has been updated to make it easier to search for foods. iProfile includes nutrient values for more than 34,000 foods.

Students can use a variety of reports in iProfile to analyze their food intakes and activities, including Intake Compared to DRI, Macronutrient Distribution, MyPyramid, Intake Spreadsheet, and more. Distinctive animations and photos help students understand portion sizes and different food measurements.

DEDICATION

To my boys, in appreciation for the time this work takes from them and the inspiration (and in recent years, editorial assistance) they give to me.

MBG

To my sons, Zachary and Max, and to my husband, David Knecht, who help me maintain perspective and recognize and appreciate the important things in life.

LAS

ABOUT THE AUTHORS

Mary B. Grosvenor holds a bachelor of arts in English and a master of science in Nutrition Science, affording her an ideal background for nutrition writing. She is a registered dietitian and has worked in clinical as well as research nutrition, in hospitals and communities large and small in the western United States. She teaches at the community college level and has published articles in peer-reviewed journals in nutritional assessment and nutrition and cancer. Her training and experience provide practical insights into the application and presentation of the science in this text.

Lori A. Smolin received a bachelor of science degree from Cornell University, where she studied human nutrition and food science. She received a doctorate from the University of Wisconsin at Madison, where her doctoral research focused on B vitamins, homocysteine accumulation, and genetic defects in homocysteine metabolism. She completed postdoctoral training both at the Harbor–UCLA Medical Center, where she studied human obesity, and at the University of California—San Diego, where she studied genetic defects in amino acid metabolism. She has published articles in these areas in peer-reviewed journals. Dr. Smolin is currently at the University of Connecticut, where she teaches both in the Department of Nutritional Science and in the Department of Molecular and Cell Biology. Courses she has taught include introductory nutrition, life cycle nutrition, food preparation, nutritional biochemistry, general biochemistry, and introductory biology.

ACKNOWLEDGMENTS

PROFESSIONAL FEEDBACK

Throughout the process of writing and developing this text and the visual pedagogy, we benefited from the comments and constructive criticism provided by the instructors and colleagues listed below. We offer our sincere appreciation to these individuals for their helpful reviews:

Kwaku Addo
University of Kentucky

Giovanni Antunez
St. Cloud State University

Paul Arciero
Skidmore College

Wayne Askew
University of Utah

Dan Benardo
Georgia State University

Valerie Benedix
Clovis Community College

Virginia Bennett
Central Washington University

Claire Berg
Brookdale Community College

Joye Bonds
Minnesota State University, Mankato

Linda Brothers
Indiana University–Purdue University, Indianapolis

Melanie Burns
Eastern Illinois University

Jayne Byrne
College of St. Benedict

Jau-Jiin Chen
University of Nevada, Las Vegas

Sai Chidambaram
Canisius College

Anne Cioffi
Hudson Valley Community College

Rachel Clark
Purdue University

Debbie Cohen
University of New Mexico

Sylvia Crixell
Texas State University, San Marcos

Eileen Daniel
State University of New York, Brockport

Robert Davidson
Brigham Young University, Provo

Lisa Diewald
Montgomery County Community College

Marty DuBois
University of Phoenix

Sarah Ducey
Montgomery College, Rockville

Stephen Duggan
California Culinary Academy

Rachelle Duncan
Oklahoma State University

Gary Fosmire
Pennsylvania State University

Carol Friesen
Ball State University

Bernard Frye
University of Texas, Arlington

Sylvia Giraudo
University of Georgia

Joanne Gould
Keane University

Patricia Grace-Farfaglia
University of Connecticut, Waterbury

Artis Grady
Southern Utah University

Margaret Gunther
Palomar College

Sandra Haggard
University of Maine, Augusta

Theresa Han-Markey
University of Michigan, Ann Arbor

Susan Hawk
Central Washington University

Jeanne Hoff
Clark College

Laura Hutchinson
Holyoke Community College

Dana Jacko
William Paterson University

Mary Beth Kavanagh
Case Western Reserve University

Martin Kelly
Genesee Community College

Younghee Kim
Bowling Green State University

Michael Klecan
Ocean County College

Allen W. Knehans
University of Oklahoma

Jennifer Koslo
Mesa Community College

Elizabeth Kotyla
University of Massachusetts, Lowell

Gina L. Kraft
Oklahoma Baptist University

Darlene Levins
Oakland Community College at Orchard Ridge

Michelle Lewis
Virginia Tech

Brenda Malinauskas
East Carolina University

Rose Martin
Pennsylvania State University

Kathleen J. Melanson
University of Rhode Island

Shireen Merrill
Pensacola Junior College

Molly Michelman
University of Nevada, Las Vegas

Sandra Mimms
Alabama State University

Ryan Morris
Pierce College

Katherine Musgrave
University of Maine, Orono

Judith Myhand
Louisiana State University

Cheryl Neudauer
Minneapolis Community Technical College

Deborah Ocken
Seattle Central Community College

John Orta
California State University, Los Angeles

Peter Pribis
Andrews University

Christian Roberts
University of California–Los Angeles

Alayne Ronnenburg
University of Massachusetts, Amherst

Daniel Rowlson
Oakland Community College, Orchard Ridge

Karen Shinville
Illinois State University

Carol Sloan
Henry Ford Community College

Mollie Smith
California State University–Fresno

Leslie Spencer
Rowan University

Diana Spillman
Miami University

Lydia Steinman
University of Texas at Austin

Maura Stevenson
Community College of Allegheny County

Barbara Troy
Marquette University

Simin Vaghefi
University of North Florida

Elizabeth Vargo
Community College of Allegheny County

Priya Venkatesan
Pasadena City College

Eric Vlahof
University of Tampa

Sally Weerts
University of North Florida

Maureen Zimmerman
Mesa Community College

SPECIAL THANKS

Special thanks to Peter Ambrose for providing a fresh eye by writing the chapter introductions for this project. We appreciate his "non-nutritionist" view of the science we know so well. His ability to help us organize and articulate our thoughts throughout the text is greatly appreciated.

We also appreciate the professors who wrote quizzes for WileyPLUS: Jeanne Hoff, Clark College; Jennifer Koslo, Mesa Community College; and Anne Rogan, SUNY Cobleskill. Sincere thanks also to John Orta for his ongoing contributions and to Carole Sloan for writing the iProfile questions and sample profile.

Special thanks also to Irene Nunes, developmental editor, for thinking about things in ways that no one else does, and to Carolyn Smith, developmental editor, for her careful editing of our book.

We are extremely grateful to the many members of the editorial and production staff at John Wiley and Sons who guided us through the challenging steps of developing this book. Their tireless enthusiasm, professional assistance, and endless patience smoothed the path for us. We thank, in particular, Executive Editor Bonnie Roesch, who expertly launched and directed our process; Editor Kevin Witt, who took up the mantle and lent us his unflagging support; Helen McInnis, managing director, Wiley Visualizing, who oversaw the concept of the project; Nancy Perry, manager, product development, who guided us through the development of the book; and Micheline Frederick, senior production manager, who stepped in whenever we needed expert advice. Our sincere thanks also go to Kaye Pace, vice president and executive publisher, who oversaw the entire project; and Jeffrey Rucker and Clay Stone, executive marketing managers, who, together with Christine Kushner adeptly represent the Visualizing imprint. We appreciate the expertise of Hilary Newman, director of photo research, in managing and researching our photo program; Teri Stratford, who found new or replacement photos at a moment's notice; and Sandra Rigby, senior illustration editor, in managing the extensive illustration program. We also wish to thank Senior Media Editor Linda Muriello and Project Editor Lorraina Raccuia, who worked on the wide assortment of media and ancillary materials. We are grateful to the editorial assistants who helped bring this project to fruition: Sean Boda, Alissa Etrheim, and Lauren Morris.

Next, we would like to offer our thanks to Furino Production—particularly Jeanine Furino, whose dedication and desire for perfection can be seen throughout this book. The careful and professional approach of Jeanine and her staff was critical to the successful production of this edition.

We thank Stacy Gold, research editor and account executive at the National Geographic Image Collection, for her valuable expertise in selecting National Geographic Society photos. Many other individuals at National Geographic offered their expertise and assistance in developing this book: Richard Easby, supervising editor, National Geographic School Division; Mimi Dornack, sales manager, and Lori Franklin, assistant account executive, National Geographic Image Collection; and Jocelyn Shearer, Jim Burch, and Tracey Stewart of National Geographic Digital Media TV. We appreciate their contributions and support.

CONTENTS *in Brief*

CONTENTS

Blood

VISUALIZING FEATURES

Multipart visual presentations that focus on a key concept or topic in the chapter.

PROCESS DIAGRAMS

A series or combination of drawings and photos that describe and depict a complex process.

ALL THE HELP, **RESOURCES**, AND PERSONAL **SUPPORT** YOU AND YOUR STUDENTS NEED!

2-Minute Tutorials and all
of the resources you & your
students need to get started
www.wileyplus.com/firstday

Student support from an
experienced student user
Ask your local representative
for details!

Collaborate with your colleagues,
find a mentor, attend virtual and live
events, and view resources
www.WhereFacultyConnect.com

Pre-loaded, ready-to-use
assignments and presentations
www.wiley.com/college/quickstart

Technical Support 24/7
FAQs, online chat,
and phone support
www.wileyplus.com/support

Your *WileyPLUS*
Account Manager
Training and implementation support
www.wileyplus.com/accountmanager

www.wiley**plus**.com

MAKE IT YOURS!

VISUALIZING

NUTRITION
EVERYDAY CHOICES

Nutrition: Everyday Choices 1

How do you choose what to eat? For most of the world's population, the answer is simple: You eat what you can grow, raise, catch, kill, or afford. Fundamentally, subsistence is the principal motivator of food consumption: If you don't eat, you die. Historically, the game or crops people could kill or cultivate successfully became staples of their diet. As agriculture and food production became more sophisticated, a greater array of food choices became available. Colonization and exploitation of native peoples introduced new foods to the colonizers: Corn became part of the diet of European settlers in North America, for instance, and the potato was brought to the Old World from the New. Today, in a cosmopolitan, global society, one may literally choose from the world's dinner table.

The implications of food choices are significant not only because what you eat affects your health but also because what you like affects what you choose to eat. Hundreds of millions of people enjoy eating insects, raw fish, horses, and even dogs, while hundreds of millions of others abhor pork, beef, shellfish, dairy products, and even chocolate! Most of us enjoy the sweet and avoid the bitter, yet some of us choose the zip of the bitter or the bite of the zesty.

Because the nutrients in the food we eat form and maintain the structure of our bodies, we really are what we eat. The challenge is to find a satisfying balance between what we like and what optimizes our health. The choice is ours.

Food Choices and Nutrient Intake

W hat are you going to eat today? Will breakfast be a vegetable omelet or a bowl of sugar-coated cereal? How about lunch—a burger or a hummus sandwich? The foods we choose determine the **nutrients** we consume. To stay healthy, humans need more than 40 **essential nutrients**. Because the foods we eat vary from day to day, so do the amounts and types of nutrients and the number of **calories** we consume.

nutrients Substances in food that provide energy and structure to the body and regulate body processes.

NUTRIENTS FROM FOODS, FORTIFIED FOODS, AND SUPPLEMENTS

Any food you eat adds some nutrients to your diet, but to make your diet healthy, it is important to choose nutrient-dense foods. Foods with a high **nutrient density** contain more nutrients per calorie than do foods with a lower nutrient density (**FIGURE 1.1**). If a large proportion of your diet consists of foods that are low in nutrient density, such as soft drinks, chips, and candy, you will have a hard time meeting your nutrient needs without exceeding your calorie needs. By choosing nutrient-dense foods, you can meet all your nutrient needs and have calories

essential nutrients Nutrients that a person must consume in order to maintain health.

calorie A unit of measure used to express the amount of energy provided by food.

nutrient density A measure of the nutrients provided by a food relative to its calorie content.

Nutrient density FIGURE 1.1

Low-fat milk
Ice cream

Calories — Calcium (mg) — Vitamin D (IU) — Potassium (mg)

A Nutrient density is important in choosing a healthy diet. For example, a cup of low-fat milk provides fewer calories but more calcium, vitamin D, and potassium than does a cup of ice cream.

Instead of this ...

Low Nutrient Density

Have this ...

High Nutrient Density

B Typically, less processed foods have a higher nutrient density. ▶ For example, a roasted chicken breast is more nutrient dense, providing more nutrients per calorie, than chicken nuggets; a baked potato is more nutrient dense than French fries; and an apple is more nutrient dense than apple pie.

left over for occasional treats that are lower in nutrients and higher in calories.

In addition to nutrients that occur naturally in foods, we obtain nutrients from **fortified foods**. The fortification of foods was begun to help eliminate nutrient deficiencies in the population, with the federal government mandating that certain nutrients be added to certain foods. Foods such as milk with added vitamin D and grain products with added B vitamins and iron are examples of this mandated fortification that have been part of the U.S. food supply for decades.

Recently, however, voluntary fortification of foods has become common practice. Vitamins and minerals are routinely added to breakfast cereals and a variety of snack foods. The amounts and types of nutrients added to these voluntarily fortified foods are at the discretion of the manufacturer. These added nutrients contribute to the diet but are not necessarily designed to address deficiencies and may increase the likelihood of consuming an excess of some nutrients.

Dietary supplements are another source of nutrients, with about half of U.S. adults taking some sort of daily dietary supplement. Supplements provide nutrients but do not offer all the benefits of food.

FOOD PROVIDES MORE THAN NUTRIENTS

In addition to nutrients, food contains substances that, though not essential to life, can be beneficial for health. In plants, these health-promoting substances are called **phytochemicals** (FIGURE 1.2). Although fewer such substances have been identified in animal foods, animal foods also contain substances with health-promoting properties. These are called **zoochemicals**.

Foods that are high in phytochemicals FIGURE 1.2

Fruits, vegetables, and whole grains provide a variety of phytochemicals, such as those highlighted here. Supplements of individual phytochemicals are available, but there is little evidence that they provide the health benefits obtained from foods that are high in phytochemicals.[1] Foods provide mixtures of these chemicals, and we do not yet know what combinations provide the greatest health benefits.

Broccoli, garlic, and onions provide sulfur-containing phytochemicals that protect us from cancer by inactivating carcinogens or stimulating the body's natural defenses.[7,8]

Soybeans are a source of phytoestrogens, hormone-like compounds found in plants that may reduce the risk of certain types of cancer and cause small reductions in blood cholesterol.[4,5,6]

Yellow-orange fruits and vegetables, such as apricots, carrots, and cantaloupe, as well as leafy greens, are rich in carotenoids, which are phytochemicals that may prevent oxygen from damaging our cells.[2]

Berries, purple grapes, and onions provide red, purple, and pale yellow pigments called flavonoids, which prevent oxygen damage and may reduce cancer risk.[3]

Examples of functional foods TABLE 1.1

Food	Potential health benefit
Whole-grain bread	Provides fiber and phytochemicals that may help reduce the risk of cancer and heart disease.[9,10]
Oatmeal	Contains a type of fiber that helps reduce blood cholesterol.
Green and black teas	Contain phytochemicals that may reduce the risk of certain types of cancer.[11]
Leafy green vegetables	Contain phytochemicals that may reduce the risk of age-related blindness (macular degeneration).[12]
Nuts	Contain a type of fat that may reduce the risk of heart disease.
Margarine with added plant sterols	Helps reduce blood cholesterol levels.
Orange juice with added calcium	Helps prevent osteoporosis.
Breakfast cereal with added flaxseed	Helps reduce blood cholesterol levels and the overall risk of heart disease.

functional foods
Foods that have health-promoting and/or disease-preventing properties beyond basic nutritional functions.

Some foods, because of the complex mixtures of nutrients and other chemicals they contain, provide health benefits that extend beyond basic nutrition. Such foods have been termed **functional foods**. The simplest functional foods are unmodified whole foods, such as broccoli and fish, that naturally contain substances that promote health and protect against disease, but some foods fortified with nutrients or enhanced with phytochemicals or other substances are also classified as functional foods (TABLE 1.1). These modified foods, such as water with added vitamins, oatmeal with added soy protein, and orange juice with added calcium, have also been called **designer foods** or **neutraceuticals**. As food manufacturers cash in on the concept that "health sells,"

the line between what is a dietary supplement and what is a food has become blurred (FIGURE 1.3).

WHAT DETERMINES FOOD CHOICES?

Do you eat oranges to boost your vitamin C intake or ice cream to add a little calcium to your diet? Probably not. We need these nutrients to survive, but we generally choose foods for reasons other than the nutrients they contain. Sometimes we choose a food simply because it is put in front of us; often our choices also depend on what we have learned to eat, what is socially acceptable in our cultural heritage or religion, what we think is healthy, or what our personal convictions—such as environmental consciousness or vegetarianism—demand. Tradition and values may dictate what foods we consider appropriate, but individual preferences for taste, smell, appearance, and texture affect which foods we actually consume. All these factors are involved in food choices because food does more than meet our physiological requirements. It also provides sensory pleasure and helps meet our social and emotional needs (FIGURE 1.4).

Are these foods or dietary supplements?

FIGURE 1.3

Energy bars fortified with 23 vitamins and minerals, bottled water with vitamin C, fruit juice with added phytochemicals, soft drinks with vitamins and amino acids—are these foods or are they dietary supplements? Before purchasing these highly fortified products, consider whether they provide the benefits they claim to provide and whether they are safe.

CONCEPT CHECK STOP

Which has a higher nutrient density, a soda or a glass of milk?

Why are foods fortified?

Why is it better to meet your vitamin C needs by eating an orange than by taking a dietary supplement?

What factors determine which foods you eat at a family picnic?

◄ **B** Food can provide comfort and security. "Comfort foods" such as hot tea, chicken soup, and chocolate help us to feel better when we are sick, cold, tired, or lonely.

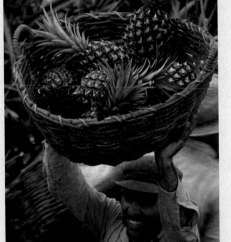

A We use food as reward and punishment. A well-behaved child may be rewarded with an ice cream cone, while a child who misbehaves may be sent to bed without dessert. We also use food to commemorate milestones such as birthdays and anniversaries.

D Food preferences and eating habits are learned as part of an individual's family, cultural, national, and social background. In many parts of the world, insects, such as these palm beetle larvae, are considered a delicacy but in U.S. culture, insects are considered food contaminants, and most people would refuse to eat them. ▼

◄ **C** We can choose only from foods that are available to us. What is available is affected by season, geography, economics, health, and living conditions. In many parts of the world, food choices are limited to foods produced locally, but in more developed regions many nonnative and seasonal foods, such as these pineapples, are available year-round because they can be stored and shipped from distant locations.

E For an adolescent, stopping for pizza after school may be part of being accepted by his or her peers. Food is the centerpiece of everyday social interactions. We meet friends for dinner or a cup of coffee. The family dinner table is a focal point for communication, where experiences of the day are shared.

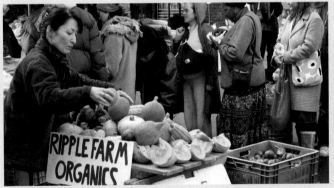

F Often people's attitudes about what foods they think are good for them or good for the environment affect what they choose. For example, you may choose organic produce, because you are concerned about exposure to pesticides, or green tea to increase your intake of cancer-fighting antioxidants.

NATIONAL GEOGRAPHIC

Nutrients and Their Functions

There are six classes of nutrients: carbohydrates, lipids, proteins, water, vitamins, and minerals. Carbohydrates, lipids, proteins, and water are considered **macronutrients** because they are needed in large amounts. Vitamins and minerals are referred to as **micronutrients** because they are needed in small amounts. Together the macronutrients and micronutrients in our diet provide us with energy, contribute to the structure of our bodies, and regulate the biological processes that go on inside us. Each nutrient provides one or more of these functions, but all nutrients together are needed to provide for growth, maintain and repair the body, and support reproduction.

THE SIX CLASSES OF NUTRIENTS

> **organic compounds** Substances that contain carbon bonded to hydrogen.

> **carbohydrates** A class of nutrients that includes sugars, starches, and fibers. Chemically, they all contain carbon, along with hydrogen and oxygen, in the same proportions as in water (H_2O).

> **fiber** A type of carbohydrate that cannot be digested by humans.

Carbohydrates, lipids, and proteins are all **organic compounds** that provide energy to the body. Although we tend to think of each of them as a single nutrient, there are actually many different types of molecules in each of these classes. **Carbohydrates** include starches, sugars, and fiber (FIGURE 1.5A). Several types of **lipids** play important roles in nutrition (FIGURE 1.5B). The most familiar of these are **cholesterol, saturated fats**, and **unsaturated fats**. There are thousands of different **proteins** in our bodies and our diets. All proteins are made up of units called **amino acids** that are linked together in different combinations to form different proteins (FIGURE 1.5C).

Water, unlike the other classes of nutrients, is only a single substance. Water makes up about 60% of an adult's body weight. Because we can't store water, the water the body loses must constantly be replaced by water obtained from the diet. In the body, water acts as a lubricant, a transport fluid, and a regulator of body temperature.

Vitamins are organic molecules that are needed in small amounts to maintain health. There are 13 vitamins, which perform a variety of unique functions in the body, such as regulating energy production, maintaining vision, protecting cell membranes, and helping blood to clot. **Minerals** are **elements** that are essential nutrients needed in small amounts to provide a variety of diverse functions in the body. For example, iron is an element needed for the transport of oxygen in the blood, calcium is an element important in keeping bones strong. We consume vitamins and minerals in almost all the foods we eat. Some are natural sources: Oranges contain vitamin C, milk provides calcium, and carrots give us vitamin A. Other foods are fortified with vitamins and minerals; fortified breakfast cereals often have 100% of the recommended intake of many vitamins and minerals. Dietary supplements are another source of vitamins and minerals for some people.

> **lipids** A class of nutrients that is commonly called fats. Chemically, they contain carbon, hydrogen, and oxygen, and most of them do not dissolve in water.

> **cholesterol** A type of lipid that is found in the diet and in the blood. High blood levels increase the risk of heart disease.

> **saturated fats** Lipids that are most abundant in solid animal fats and are associated with an increased risk of heart disease.

> **unsaturated fats** Lipids that are most abundant in plant oils and are associated with a reduced risk of heart disease.

> **protein** A class of nutrients that includes molecules made up of one or more intertwining chains of amino acids. They contain carbon, hydrogen, oxygen, and nitrogen.

A Some high-carbohydrate foods, such as rice, pasta, and bread, contain mostly starch; some, such as berries, kidney beans, and broccoli, are high in fiber; and others, such as cookies, cakes, and carbonated beverages, are high in added sugar. High-fiber, low-sugar foods have a higher nutrient density than do low-fiber, high-sugar foods.

B High-fat plant foods such as vegetable oils, olives, nuts, and avocados have no cholesterol and are high in unsaturated fat so they don't increase heart disease risk. High-fat animal foods such as butter, meat, and milk are high in saturated fat and cholesterol, which increase the risk of developing heart disease.

C The proteins we obtain from animal foods, such as meat, fish, and eggs, better match our amino acid needs than do individual plant proteins, such as those found in grains, nuts, and beans. However, when plant proteins are combined, they can provide all the amino acids we need.

A Physical activity, whether it consists of gardening, walking to the mailbox, or riding a bike through the Fall foliage, is fueled by the energy in the food we eat.

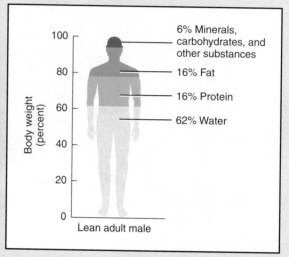

B The shape and structure of our bodies are formed and maintained by proteins, lipids, carbohydrates, minerals, and water.

WHAT NUTRIENTS DO

FIGURE 1.6 illustrates some of the ways in which various nutrients are involved in providing energy, forming body structures, and regulating physiological processes. Carbohydrates, lipids, and proteins are often referred to as **energy-yielding nutrients**; they provide energy that can be measured in calories. The calories people talk about and see listed on food labels are actually **kilocalories**, units of 1000 calories (abbreviated kcalorie or kcal). When spelled with a capital *C*, Calorie means kilocalorie. Carbohydrates provide 4 Calories per gram; they are the most immediate source of energy for the body. Lipids also help fuel our activities and are the major form of

stored energy in the body. One gram of lipid provides 9 Calories. Protein can supply 4 Calories per gram but is not the body's first choice for meeting energy needs because protein has other roles that take priority. Alcohol, although it is not a nutrient because it is not needed for life, provides about 7 Calories per gram. Water, vitamins, and minerals do not provide energy (calories).

With the exception of vitamins, all the classes of nutrients are involved in forming and maintaining the body's structure. Fat deposited under the skin softens our curves, for instance, and proteins form the ligaments and tendons that hold our bones together and attach our muscles to our bones. Minerals harden bone. Protein and water make up the structure of the muscles,

C Water helps regulate body temperature. When body temperature increases, sweat is produced, cooling the body as it evaporates from the skin.

D Lipids, such as the hormone testosterone, shown in the diagram, help regulate body processes. Testosterone is made from cholesterol. In men, it stimulates sperm production and the development of secondary sex characteristics such as body and facial hair, a deep voice, and increased muscle mass.

which help define our body contours, and protein and carbohydrates form the connective tissue that holds us together. On a smaller scale, lipids, proteins, and water form the structure of individual cells. Lipids and proteins make up the membranes that surround each cell, and water and dissolved substances fill the cells and the spaces around them.

All six classes of nutrients play important roles in regulating body processes. Keeping body temperature, blood pressure, blood sugar level, and hundreds of other parameters relatively constant involves thousands of chemical reactions and physiological processes. Proteins, vitamins, and minerals are regulatory nutrients that help control how quickly chemical reactions take place throughout the body. Lipids and proteins are needed to make regulatory molecules called **hormones** that stimulate or inhibit various body processes.

CONCEPT CHECK STOP

Which classes of nutrients provide energy?

What three nutrient functions help ensure normal growth, maintenance of body structure and functions, and reproduction?

Nutrition in Health and Disease

LEARNING OBJECTIVES

Describe the different types of malnutrition.

Explain ways in which nutrient intake can affect health in both the short term and the long term.

Discuss how the genes you inherit affect the amounts of nutrients and food components that optimize your health.

What we eat has an enormous impact on how healthy we are now and how likely we are to develop chronic diseases such as heart disease, obesity, and diabetes. Consuming either too much or too little of one or more nutrients or energy will result in **malnutrition**. Malnutrition can affect your health not just today but 20, 30, or 40 years from now. The impact of your diet on your health is also affected by your genetic background.

malnutrition
A condition resulting from an energy or nutrient intake either above or below that which is optimal.

UNDERNUTRITION AND OVERNUTRITION

Undernutrition occurs when intake doesn't meet the body's needs (**FIGURE 1.7**). The more severe the deficiency, the more dramatic the symptoms. Some nutrient deficiencies occur quickly. Dehydration, a deficiency of water, can cause symptoms in a matter of hours. Drinking water can relieve the headache, fatigue, and dizziness caused by dehydration almost as rapidly as these symptoms appeared. Other nutritional deficiencies may take much longer to become evident. Symptoms of scurvy, a disease caused by a deficiency in vitamin C, appear after months of deficient intake; **osteoporosis**, a condition in which the bones become weak and break easily, occurs after years of consuming a calcium-deficient diet.

We typically think of malnutrition as undernutrition, but **overnutrition,** an excess intake of calories or nutrients, is also a concern. An overdose of iron can cause liver failure, for example, and too much vitamin B_6 can cause nerve damage. These nutrient toxicities usually result from taking large doses of vitamin and mineral supplements because foods generally do not contain high enough concentrations of nutrients to be toxic. However, chronic overconsumption of calories and certain nutrients from foods can cause health problems. The typical U.S. diet, which provides more calories than we need, has resulted in an epidemic of obesity in which more than 65% of adults are overweight or obese (**FIGURE 1.8A**).[13] Diets that are high in sodium contribute to high blood pressure; an excess intake of saturated fat and cholesterol contribute to heart disease; and a dietary pattern that is high in red meat and saturated fat and low in fruits, vegetables, and fiber may increase the risk of colon cancer.[14] It has been estimated that over 16% of all deaths in the United States can be attributed to poor diet and sedentary lifestyle (**FIGURE 1.8B**).[15]

Undernutrition FIGURE 1.7

A Even though this child looks normal and healthy, she has low iron stores. If the iron content of her diet is not increased, she will eventually develop iron deficiency anemia. Mild nutrient deficiencies like hers may go unnoticed because the symptoms either are not immediately apparent or are nonspecific. Two common nonspecific symptoms of iron depletion are fatigue and a decreased ability to fight infection.

B The symptoms of starvation, the most obvious form of undernutrition, occur gradually over time when the energy provided by the diet is too low to meet the body's needs. Body tissues are broken down to provide the energy to support vital functions, resulting in loss of body fat and wasting of muscles.

Overnutrition FIGURE 1.8

A Obesity is a form of overnutrition that occurs when energy intake surpasses energy expenditure over a long period, causing the accumulation of an excessive amount of body fat. Adults are not the only ones who are getting fatter. An estimated 16.3% of U.S. children and adolescents ages 2 to 19 years are obese.[16]

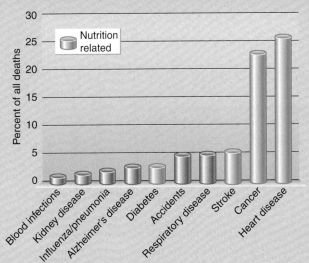

B The top three causes of death in the United States are nutrition related.[17] They are all thought to be exacerbated by obesity.

DIET–GENE INTERACTIONS

Diet affects your health, but diet alone does not determine whether you will develop a particular disease. Each of us inherits a unique combination of **genes**. Some of these genes affect your risk of developing chronic diseases such as heart disease, cancer, high blood pressure, and diabetes, but their impact is affected by what you eat (FIGURE 1.9). Your genetic makeup determines the impact a certain nutrient will have on you. For example, some people inherit a combination of genes that results in a tendency to have high blood pres-

> **genes** Units of a larger molecule called DNA that are responsible for inherited traits.

sure. When these individuals consume even an average amount of sodium, their blood pressure increases (discussed further in Chapter 8). Others inherit genes that allow them to consume more sodium without much of a rise in blood pressure. Those whose genes dictate a significant rise in blood pressure with a high-sodium diet can reduce their blood pressure, and the complications associated with high blood pressure, by eating a diet that is low in sodium.

Our increasing understanding of human genetics has given rise to the discipline of **nutritional genomics** or **nutrigenomics**, which explores the interaction between genetic variation and nutrition.[18] This research has led to the development of the concept of "personalized nutrition," the idea that a diet based on the genes an individual has inherited can be used to prevent, moderate, or cure chronic disease. Although today we do not know enough to take a sample of your DNA and use it to tell you what to eat to optimize your health, we do know that certain dietary patterns can reduce the risk of many chronic diseases.

> **nutritional genomics** or **nutrigenomics**
> The study of how diet affects our genes and how individual genetic variation can affect the impact of nutrients or other food components on health.

Nutritional genomics FIGURE 1.9

Your actual risk of disease results from the interplay between the genes you inherit and the diet and lifestyle choices you make.

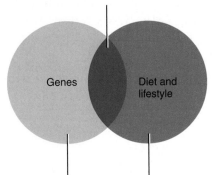

The genes you inherit may give you a greater or lesser tendency to develop conditions like obesity, heart disease, high blood pressure, or diabetes.

The nutrients and food components you consume and the amount of exercise you get can increase or decrease your risk of developing nutrition-related diseases.

CONCEPT CHECK **STOP**

What causes malnutrition?

How can your diet today affect your health 20 years from now?

Why might the diet that optimizes health be different for different people?

Choosing a Healthy Diet

LEARNING OBJECTIVES

Explain why it is important to eat a variety of foods.

Describe how you can eat favorite foods that are low in nutrient density and still have a healthy diet.

Discuss how dietary moderation can reduce the risk of chronic disease.

A healthy diet is one that provides the right number of calories to keep your weight in the desirable range; the proper balance of carbohydrates, proteins, and fat; plenty of water; and sufficient but not excessive amounts of vitamins and minerals. Such a healthy diet is rich in whole grains, fruits, and vegetables; high in fiber; moderate in fat, sugar, and sodium; and low in unhealthy fats (saturated fat, cholesterol, and *trans* fat). In short, a healthy diet is based on variety, balance, and moderation (see the *Case Study*).

CASE STUDY

WHAT'S WRONG WITH THIS DIET?

For many adolescents, freshman year at college is their first chance to make their own decisions about what to eat. The choices they make aren't always the best, however, and many students' food choices lead to the "freshman 15"—the 15 or so pounds gained in the first year away from home. Learning how to choose a healthy diet can prevent this weight gain.

Amad loves fast food. He grabs a doughnut for breakfast, a burger and fries for lunch, and either tacos or pizza for dinner.

What's wrong with Amad's diet?
▼

Amad's diet needs more balance. An occasional fast-food meal is fine, but eating these foods every day results in a diet that is high in calories and fat and low in some vitamins and minerals. Amad needs to balance his fast-food choices, which are low in nutrient density, with meals that are higher in nutrient density. For example, if he plans to eat a doughnut for breakfast, he could balance this with a sandwich on whole-grain bread with lettuce, tomatoes, and peppers for lunch. If his dinner is high in calories, he can balance this by snacking on low-calorie, nutrient-dense fruits and vegetables.

What about Helen? She has cereal with milk for breakfast, a peanut butter sandwich for lunch, and meat with rice and a lettuce salad for dinner every day.

What's wrong with Helen's diet?
▼

Your Answer:

Amy takes advantage of the variety of foods offered at the cafeteria. She often has two types of whole-grain cereals each day for breakfast, selects eight or more ingredients at the salad bar, and includes two or three vegetables with her dinner. Despite these healthy choices, there is a problem with her diet.

Based on this photo, what might be wrong with Amy's diet?
▼

Your Answer:

(Check your answers in Appendix K.)

Balance calories in with calories out FIGURE 1.10

Extra calories you consume during the day can be balanced by increasing the calories you burn in physical activity.

If you have a Big Mac for lunch instead of a smaller plain burger, you will have to increase your energy expenditure by 300 Calories.

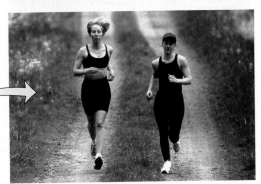

You could do this by playing golf for about an hour, carrying your own clubs.

If you have a grande mocha frappuccino instead of a regular iced coffee, you will have to increase your energy expenditure by 370 Calories.

You could do this by jogging for about 30 minutes.

EAT A VARIETY OF FOODS

In nutrition, choosing a variety of foods is important because no single food can provide all the nutrients the body needs for optimal health. *Variety* means choosing foods from different food groups—vegetables, grains, fruits, dairy products, and meats and beans. Some of these foods are rich in vitamins and phytochemicals, others are rich in protein and minerals, and all are important.

Variety also means choosing diverse foods from within each food group. Different vegetables provide different nutrients. Potatoes, for example, are the only vegetable in many Americans' diets. Potatoes provide vitamin C but are low in vitamin A. If potatoes are your only vegetable, it is unlikely that you will meet your nutrient needs. If instead you have a salad, potatoes, and broccoli, you will be getting plenty of vitamins C and A as well as many other vitamins and minerals. Making varied choices both from the different food groups and from within each food group is also important because nutrients and other food components interact. Such interactions may be positive, enhancing nutrient utilization, or negative, inhibiting nutrient availability. Variety averages out these interactions.

Variety involves choosing different foods not only each day but also each week and throughout the year. If you had apples and grapes today, have blueberries and cantaloupe tomorrow. If you can't find tomatoes in the winter, replace them with a winter vegetable such as squash.

BALANCE YOUR CHOICES

Choosing a healthy diet is a balancing act. Healthy eating doesn't mean giving up your favorite foods. There is no such thing as a good food or a bad food—only healthy diets and unhealthy diets. Any food can be part of a healthy diet, as long as your diet throughout the day or week provides enough of all the nutrients you need without excesses of any. When you choose a food that is lacking in fiber, for example, balance it with one that provides lots of fiber. When you choose a food that is very high in fat, balance that choice with a low-fat one.

A balanced diet also balances the calories you take in with the calories you use up in your daily activities so that your body weight stays in the healthy range (FIGURE 1.10).

Use iProfile to calculate the Calories in your favorite fast-food meal.

Eat a variety of foods
- Snack on something other than chips. Try trail mix that contains fruit and nuts.
- Add almonds and dried cranberries to your salad.
- Try a new vegetable or fruit each week. Tired of carrots? Try jicama.
- Vary your protein sources. Have fish one day and beef the next, or skip the meat and have beans.

Balance your choices
- Going out to dinner? Have a salad for lunch.
- Add a vegetable instead of pepperoni to your pizza.
- When you have cookies for a snack, have fruit for dessert.
- Had soda with lunch? Have milk with dinner.

Practice moderation
- Push back from the table before you are stuffed and go for a walk.
- Reduce your portions by using a smaller bowl.
- Skip the seconds or split your restaurant meal with a friend.
- If you eat some extra fries, take some extra steps.

PRACTICE MODERATION

Moderation means not overdoing it—watching portion sizes and passing up the super sizes. Moderation means not having too many calories, too much fat, too much sugar, too much salt, or too much alcohol. Choosing moderately will help you maintain a healthy weight and prevent some of the chronic diseases, such as heart disease and cancer, that are on the rise in the U.S. population (see *What Should I Eat?*).

The fact that more than 65% of adult Americans are overweight demonstrates that we have not been practicing moderation when it comes to calorie intake.[13]

Moderation makes it easier to balance your diet and allows you to enjoy a greater variety of foods.

CONCEPT CHECK STOP

Why is variety in a diet important?

How might you balance the 400-Calorie cinnamon roll you had for a morning snack with your lunch choice?

What is the connection between obesity and moderation in a diet?

Evaluating Nutrition Information

LEARNING OBJECTIVES

Explain how the scientific method is used in nutrition.

Discuss three different types of experiments used to study nutrition.

Describe the components of a sound scientific experiment.

Distinguish between reliable and unreliable nutrition information.

We are bombarded with nutrition information almost every day. The evening news, the morning papers, and the World Wide Web continually offer us tantalizing tidbits of nutrition advice. Food and nutrition information that used to take professionals years to disseminate now travels with lightning speed, reaching millions of people within hours or days. Much of this information is reliable, but some can be misleading. In order to choose a healthy diet, we need to be able to sort out the useful material in this flood of information.

THE SCIENCE BEHIND NUTRITION

Like all other sciences, the science of nutrition is constantly evolving. As new discoveries provide clues to the right combination of nutrients needed for optimal health, new nutritional principles and recommendations are developed. Sometimes established beliefs and concepts give way to new information. Understanding the process of science can help consumers understand the nutrition information they encounter.

The systematic, unbiased approach that allows any science to acquire new knowledge and correct and update previous knowledge is the **scientific method**.

The scientific method involves making observations of natural events, formulating **hypotheses** to explain these events, designing and performing experiments to test these hypotheses, and developing **theories** that explain the observed phenomenon based on the results (**FIGURE 1.11**). In nutrition, the scientific method is used to develop nutrient recommendations, understand the functions of nutrients, and learn about the role of nutrition in promoting health and preventing disease.

■ hypothesis
A proposed explanation for an observation or a scientific problem that can be tested through experimentation.

■ theory
A formal explanation of an observed phenomenon made after a hypothesis has been supported and tested through experimentation.

The scientific method FIGURE 1.11

The scientific method is a process used to ask and answer scientific questions through observation and experimentation.

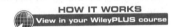
HOW IT WORKS
View in your WileyPLUS course

① The first step of the scientific method is to make an observation and ask questions about that observation.

② The next step is to propose an explanation for this observation. This proposed explanation is called a *hypothesis*.

③ Once a hypothesis has been proposed, experiments like this one are designed to test it. To generate reliable theories, the experiments done to test hypotheses must produce reliable results and be interpreted accurately.

④ If the results from repeated experiments support the hypothesis, a scientific theory can be developed. A single experiment is not enough to develop a theory; rather, repeated experiments showing the same conclusion are needed to develop a sound theory. Even then, a theory can be challenged. As new information becomes available, even a theory that has been accepted by the scientific community for years can be proved wrong.

Observation
People who skip breakfast weigh more than people who don't.

Hypothesis
Skipping breakfast makes people eat more calories during the rest of the day.

Experiment
Compare total calorie intake of groups of breakfast skippers and breakfast eaters. Result: Those who skip breakfast eat more calories, supporting the hypothesis.

Theory
Skipping breakfast makes you eat more at other times of the day.

Process Diagram

HOW SCIENTISTS STUDY NUTRITION

Many different types of experiments are used to expand our knowledge of nutrition. Some make observations about relationships between diet and health; these are based on the science of **epidemiology**. Other types of experiments evaluate the affect of a particular dietary change on health. Some of these experiments study humans, others use animals; some look at whole populations, others study just a few individuals, and some use just cells or molecules (FIGURE 1.12). For any nutrition study to provide reliable information, it must collect quantifiable data from the right experimental population, use proper experimental controls, and be interpreted accurately.

Reliable data can be quantified, meaning that they include parameters that can be measured reliably and repeatedly, such as body weight or blood pressure. Individual testimonies or opinions alone are not quantifiable objective measures.

For an experiment to answer the right question, scientists must study the appropriate group of people and include enough subjects. For example, if a dietary supplement claims to increase bone strength in older women, it must be tested in older women and include enough subjects to demonstrate that the supplement causes the effect to occur more frequently than it would by chance. The number of subjects needed depends on what is being studied. Fewer subjects are needed to demonstrate an effect that rarely occurs by chance. For example, if only one man in a million can increase his muscle mass by weight training for four weeks, then an experiment to test whether a supplement increases muscle mass in men who weight train for four weeks would require only a few subjects to demonstrate an effect. If many men can increase muscle mass by weight training for four weeks, then more experimental subjects would be needed to demonstrate that the increase in muscle mass was due to the supplement rather than the weight training alone.

In order to know whether what is being tested has an effect, one must compare it with something. A control group acts as a standard of comparison for the factor, or **variable**, being studied. A control group is treated in the same way as the **experimental group** except that the control group does not receive the treatment being tested. For example, in a study examining the effect of a dietary supplement on muscle strength, the control group would consist of individuals of similar age, gender, and ability, eating similar diets and following similar workout regimens as individuals in the experimental group. Instead of the supplement, the control subjects would consume a **placebo**, a fake product that is identical in appearance to the dietary supplement.

When an experiment has been completed, the results must be interpreted. Accurate interpretation is just as important as conducting a study carefully. If a study conducted on a large group of men indicates that a change in diet reduces cancer risk, the results of that study cannot be used to claim the same effect in women. Likewise, if the study looks only at the connection between a change in diet and colon cancer, the findings can't be used to claim a reduced risk for other cancers. One way to ensure that the results of experiments are interpreted correctly is to have them reviewed by experts in the field who did not take part in the study being evaluated. This **peer-review process** is used in determining whether experimental results should be published in scientific journals. The reviewing scientists must agree that the experiments were conducted properly and that the results were interpreted fairly. Nutrition articles that have undergone peer review can be found in journals such as *The American Journal of Clinical Nutrition*, *The Journal of Nutrition*, *The Journal of the American Dietetic Association*, *The New England Journal of Medicine*, and *The International Journal of Sport Nutrition*. Newsletters from reputable institutions, such as the *Tufts Health and Nutrition Letter* and the *Harvard Health Letter*, are also reliable sources of nutrition and health information. The information in these newsletters comes from peer-reviewed articles but is written for a consumer audience.

> **epidemiology**
> The branch of science that studies health and disease trends and patterns in populations.

> **control group**
> In a scientific experiment, the group of participants used as a basis of comparison. They are similar to the participants in the experimental group but do not receive the treatment being tested.

> **experimental group** In a scientific experiment, the group of participants who undergo the treatment being tested.

Types of nutrition studies FIGURE 1.12

◀ A Epidemiological studies

Epidemiological studies of populations around the world explore the impact of nutrition on health. This graph shows that a high intake of saturated fat in a population is associated with an increased incidence of coronary heart disease. However, epidemiology does not determine cause-and-effect relationships—it just identifies patterns. Therefore, it cannot determine whether the higher incidence of heart disease is *caused* by the high intake of saturated fat.

(Reprinted by permission of the publisher from SEVEN COUNTRIES: A MULTIVARIATE ANALYSIS OF DEATH AND CORONARY HEART DISEASE by Ancel Keys, p. 253, Cambridge, Mass.: Harvard University Press, Copyright © 1980 by the President and Fellows of Harvard College.)

B Clinical trials ▶

The observations and hypotheses that arise from epidemiology can be tested using clinical trials. Nutrition clinical trials are studies planned to explore the health effects of altering people's diets—for instance, the possible effects of eliminating meat on blood cholesterol levels.

C Animal studies ▲

Ideally, studies of human nutrition should be done with human subjects. However, because studying humans is costly, time-consuming, inconvenient for the subjects, and in some cases impossible for ethical reasons, many studies are done using animals. Guinea pigs are a good model for studying heart disease, but even the best animal model is not the same as a human, and care must be taken when extrapolating animal results to humans.

D Biochemistry and molecular biology ▶

These techniques can be used to study nutrient functions in the body. For example, biochemists can study the chemical reactions that generate energy and synthesize molecules, such as cholesterol, and molecular biology can be used to study how nutrients regulate our genes.

Behind the Claims

This product must be amazing! It will increase your muscle strength, decrease your body fat, and boost your drive and motivation. This is what consumers see. The claims sound great, but a scientist looking at the same ad may have some concerns.

First of all, the claims about muscle strength and motivation are testimonials based on individuals' feelings and impressions, and these are not objective measures.

A scientist would also question whether the research evidence supports the claim that the product increases lean body mass and decreases body fat. The study measured the amount of lean tissue and fat tissue in weightlifters before and four weeks after they began consuming the Power Boost drink. The measures used provide quantifiable, repeatable data. The results report a gain of 5.2 pounds of lean tissue and a loss of 4.5 lbs of fat tissue in weightlifters taking Power Boost. This looks convincing, but the results for the control group are not reported in the ad. When the results for the experimental group are compared to those for the control group, a different picture emerges. This comparison (see graph) shows that the control group gained almost as much lean mass and lost slightly more fat mass than those taking Power Boost. Given this new information, explain why you would or would not recommend this product.

POWER BOOST

BOOST your STRENGTH • POWER up your DRIVE • MAXIMIZE your MASS

4 out of 5 users report:

"It increased my muscle strength."

"It pumped up my drive and motivation!"

Years of research have developed this special nutritional formulation. Just mix with water and drink one shake with every meal or snack.

University Study Shows: 25 experienced weight lifters added one POWER BOOST shake at meals and snacks 5 times a day for 4 weeks.
Lean body mass and fat mass were measured by underwater weighing before POWER BOOST was added and after 4 weeks of training with POWER BOOST.

RESULTS
The weight lifters gained an average of 5.2 pounds of lean muscle and lost 4.5 pounds of unwanted fat.

Individual testimonies are not proof FIGURE 1.13

Weight-loss products commonly show before and after photos of people who have successfully lost weight using a particular product. The success of such individuals is not a guarantee that the product they used will produce the same results for you or anyone else. These individuals' results are not compared to those for a control group or subjected to scientific evaluation. Therefore, it cannot be assumed that similar results will occur in other people.

JUDGING FOR YOURSELF

Not everything you hear is accurate. Because much of the nutrition information we encounter is intended to sell products, that information may be embellished to make it more appealing. Understanding the principles scientists use to perform nutrition studies can help consumers judge the nutrition information they encounter in their daily lives (see *What a Scientist Sees*). Some things that may tip you off to misinformation are claims that sound too good to be true, information from unreliable sources, information intended to sell a product, and information that is new or untested.

Here are four questions that can help you evaluate any piece of nutrition information you encounter:

1. **Does it make sense?** Some claims are too outrageous to be true. For example, if a product claims to increase your muscle size without any exercise or decrease your weight without a change in diet, common sense should tell you that the claim is too good to be true. In contrast, an article that tells you that adding exercise to your daily routine will help you lose weight and increase your stamina is not so outrageous.

2. **What's the source?** If a claim seems reasonable, look to see where it came from. Personal testimonies are not a reliable source (FIGURE 1.13), but government recommendations regarding healthy dietary practices and information disseminated by universities generally are. Government recommendations are developed by committees of scientists who interpret the latest well-conducted research studies and use their conclusions to develop recommendations for the population as a whole. The information is designed to improve the health of the population. Information that comes from universities is supported by research studies that are well scrutinized and published in peer-reviewed journals. Many universities also provide information that targets the general public. Nonprofit organizations such as the American Dietetic Association and the American Medical Association are also reliable sources of nutrition information.

These rats, which were given large doses of vitamin E, lived longer than rats that consumed less vitamin E. Does this mean that dietary supplements of vitamin E would increase longevity in people? Not necessarily. The results of animal studies can't always be extrapolated to humans, but they are often the basis of claims in ads for dietary supplements.

VITAMIN E SUPPLEMENTS INCREASE LONGEVITY

If you are looking at an article in a printed medium or posted on a Web site, checking the author's credentials can help you evaluate the credibility of the information. Where does the author work? Does this person have a degree in nutrition or medicine? Although "nutritionists" and "nutrition counselors" may provide accurate information, the term *nutritionist* is not legally defined and is used by a wide range of people, from college professors with doctoral degrees from reputable universities to health food store clerks with no formal training.

One reliable source of nutrition information is registered dietitians (RDs). An RD is a nutrition professional who has earned a four-year college degree in a nutrition-related field and has met established criteria for certification to provide nutrition education and counseling.

3. **Is it selling something?** If a person or company will profit from the information presented, be wary. Advertisements from such companies are designed to increase sales, and the company stands to profit if you believe the claims it makes. Even information presented in newspapers and magazines and on television may be biased or exaggerated because it is designed to help sell magazines or boost ratings, not necessarily to promote health and well-being. Even a well-designed, carefully executed study published in a peer-reviewed journal can be a source of misinformation if its results have been interpreted incorrectly or exaggerated (**FIGURE 1.14**).

4. **Has it stood the test of time?** Often the results of a new scientific study are on the morning news the same day they are presented at a meeting or published in a peer-reviewed journal. However, a single study cannot serve as a basis for a reliable theory. Results need to be reproduced and supported numerous times before they can be used as a basis for nutrition recommendations.

Headlines based on a single study should therefore be viewed skeptically. The information may be accurate, but there is no way to know because there has not been enough time to repeat the work and reaffirm the conclusions. If, for example, someone has found the secret to easy weight loss, you will undoubtedly encounter this information again at some later time if the finding is valid. If the finding is not valid, it will fade away with all the other weight-loss concoctions that have come and gone.

CONCEPT CHECK STOP

What is the difference between a hypothesis and a theory?

How is epidemiology used to study nutrition?

Why are control groups important in any scientific experiment?

Why is information in advertisements likely to be exaggerated or inaccurate?

SUMMARY

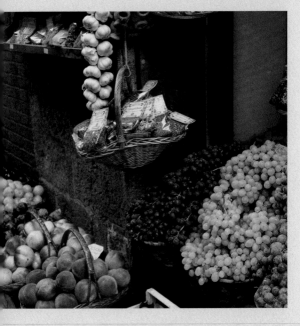

1 Food Choices and Nutrient Intake

1. The foods you choose determine which **nutrients** you consume. Choosing foods that are high in **nutrient density** allows you to obtain more nutrients in fewer calories. **Fortified foods**, or foods to which nutrients have been added, and **dietary supplements** can also contribute nutrients to the diet.

2. Food contains not only nutrients but also nonnutritive substances, such as **phytochemicals**, that may provide additional health benefits. Foods that provide health benefits beyond basic nutrition are called **functional foods**. Some foods are naturally functional and others are created through fortification.

3. The food choices we make are affected by many factors other than nutrition, including food availability; what we learn to eat from family, culture, and traditions; personal tastes; and what we think we should eat to maintain health.

2 Nutrients and Their Functions

1. Nutrients are grouped into six classes. **Carbohydrates**, **lipids**, **proteins**, and **water** are referred to as **macronutrients** because they are needed in large amounts. **Vitamins** and **minerals** are **micronutrients** because they are needed in small amounts to maintain health.

2. Carbohydrates, lipids, and proteins are nutrients that provide energy, typically measured in **calories**. Lipids, proteins, carbohydrates, minerals, and water perform structural roles, forming and maintaining the structure of our bodies. All six classes of nutrients help regulate body processes. The energy, structure, and regulation provided by nutrients are needed for growth, maintenance and repair of the body, and reproduction.

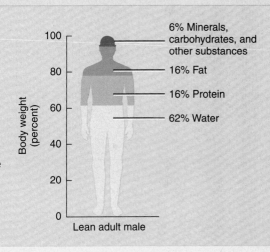

3 Nutrition in Health and Disease

1. Your diet affects your health. The foods you choose contain the nutrients needed to keep you alive and healthy and prevent **malnutrition**. **Undernutrition** results from consuming too few calories and/or too few nutrients. **Overnutrition** can result from a toxic dose of a nutrient or from a chronic excess of nutrients or calories, which over time contributes to chronic diseases.

2. The diet you consume can affect your genetic predisposition for developing a variety of chronic diseases.

4 Choosing a Healthy Diet

1. A healthy diet includes a variety of nutrient-dense foods from the different food groups as well as a variety of foods from within each group. Variety is important because different foods provide different nutrients and health-promoting substances as well as a variety of tastes.

2. Balance means mixing and matching foods and meals in order to obtain enough of the nutrients you need and not too much of the ones that can potentially harm your health.

3. Moderation means not ingesting too many calories or too much fat, sugar, salt, or alcohol. Eating moderate portions helps you maintain a healthy weight and helps prevent chronic diseases such as heart disease and cancer.

Observation
People who skip breakfast weigh more than people who don't.

⇩

Hypothesis
Skipping breakfast makes people eat more calories during the rest of the day.

⇩

Experiment
Compare total calorie intake of groups of breakfast skippers and breakfast eaters. Result: Those who skip breakfast eat more calories, supporting the hypothesis.

⇩

Theory
Skipping breakfast makes you eat more at other times of the day.

5 Evaluating Nutrition Information

1. Nutrition uses the **scientific method** to study the relationships among food, nutrients, and health. The scientific method involves observing and questioning natural events, formulating **hypotheses** to explain these events, designing and performing experiments to test the hypotheses, and developing **theories** that explain the observed phenomena based on the experimental results.

2. To be valid, a nutrition experiment must provide quantifiable measurements, study the right type and number of subjects, and use appropriate **control groups**. When a study has been completed, the results must be interpreted fairly and accurately. The **peer-review process** ensures that studies published in professional journals adhere to a high standard of experimental design and interpretation of results.

3. Not all the nutrition information we encounter is accurate. The first step in deciding whether a nutritional claim is valid is to ask whether the claim makes sense. If it sounds too good to be true, it probably is. It is also important to determine whether the information came from a reliable source, whether it is trying to sell a product, and whether it has been confirmed by multiple studies.

KEY TERMS

- **nutrients** p. 4
- **essential nutrients** p. 4
- **calorie** p. 4
- **nutrient density** p. 4
- **fortified foods** p. 5
- **dietary supplements** p. 5
- **phytochemicals** p. 5
- **zoochemicals** p. 5
- **functional foods** p. 6
- **designer foods** or **neutraceuticals** p. 6
- **macronutrients** p. 8

- **micronutrients** p. 8
- **organic compounds** p. 8
- **carbohydrates** p. 8
- **fiber** p. 8
- **lipids** p. 8
- **cholesterol** p. 8
- **saturated fats** p. 8
- **unsaturated fats** p. 8
- **protein** p. 8
- **amino acids** p. 8
- **vitamins** p. 8

- **minerals** p. 8
- **elements** p. 8
- **energy-yielding nutrients** p. 10
- **kilocalories** p. 10
- **hormones** p. 11
- **malnutrition** p. 12
- **undernutrition** p. 12
- **osteoporosis** p. 12
- **overnutrition** p. 12
- **genes** p. 13

- **nutritional genomics** or **nutrigenomics** p. 13
- **scientific method** p. 17
- **hypothesis** p. 17
- **theory** p. 17
- **epidemiology** p. 18
- **control group** p. 18
- **variable** p. 18
- **experimental group** p. 18
- **placebo** p. 18
- **peer-review process** p. 18

CRITICAL AND CREATIVE THINKING QUESTIONS

1. Which type of malnutrition—overnutrition or undernutrition—is most common in the United States today? Why?

2. Nutrients provide energy, structure, and regulation in our bodies. Based on the fact that about 50% of the calories we consume are from carbohydrates, yet less than 1% of our body weight is carbohydrates, which of these three functions do you think carbohydrates provide in the body? How about the function of a nutrient that is present in small amounts in the diet but in large amounts in the body?

3. A typical fast-food meal consists of a cheeseburger, French fries, and a soft drink. Use iProfile to calculate the calories in this meal. For each food in this meal, suggest a more nutrient-dense alternative.

4. Zach has a banana and a glass of orange juice for breakfast and potatoes or corn for dinner every day at the dorm cafeteria, but he doesn't eat any other fruits or vegetables. How could his choices be improved? Why is such an improvement important?

5. Moderation and balance are important in choosing a healthy diet. Explain how these principles help a person maintain a healthy weight.

6. A scientist observes that colon cancer is rare in Japan but common in the United States. He hypothesizes that this difference is due to differences in diet. Propose an experiment that might be used to test this hypothesis.

7. Look up an advertisement for a dietary supplement on the Internet. What nutrients does the supplement contain? Does it contain substances that are not nutrients? Do you think this dietary supplement is worth the money? Why or why not?

What is happening in this picture ?

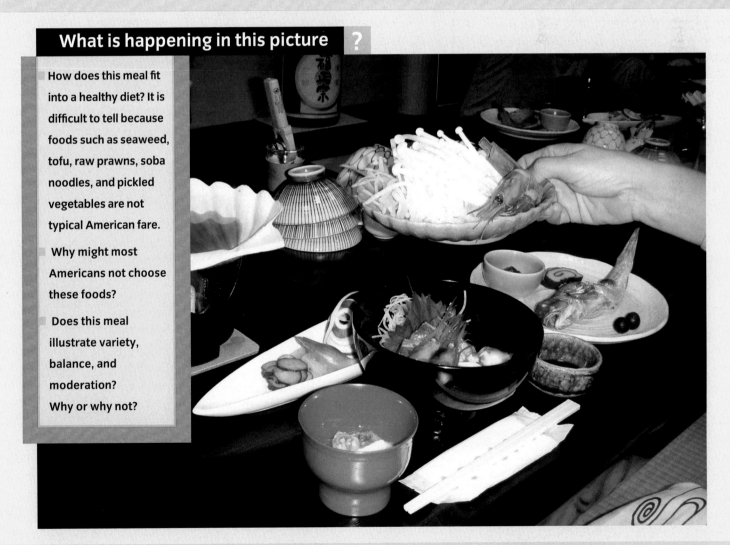

How does this meal fit into a healthy diet? It is difficult to tell because foods such as seaweed, tofu, raw prawns, soba noodles, and pickled vegetables are not typical American fare.

Why might most Americans not choose these foods?

Does this meal illustrate variety, balance, and moderation? Why or why not?

SELF-TEST

(Check your answers in Appendix L.)

1. True or false: If you choose a high-fat, high-salt, fast-food lunch, your nutrient intake for the day cannot meet the recommendations for a healthy diet.

   a. True
   b. False

2. Which of these foods has the lowest nutrient density?

   a. an orange
   b. strawberry yogurt
   c. whole-wheat bread
   d. orange soda

3. This graph indicates that _____.

   a. low-fat milk contains more calcium per calorie than ice cream
   b. ice cream is a poor source of calcium
   c. ice cream is more nutrient dense than milk
   d. low-fat milk has less vitamin D per calorie than ice cream

4. Which group consists only of nutrients that are classified as energy-yielding nutrients?

   a. vitamins and minerals
   b. carbohydrates, lipids, and proteins
   c. lipids, carbohydrates, proteins, and water
   d. carbohydrates and vitamins

5. Which group consists only of nutrients that are considered micronutrients?

   a. protein and water
   b. carbohydrates, lipids, and proteins
   c. vitamins and minerals
   d. minerals and water

6. Which nutrient class provides the most Calories per gram?

   a. carbohydrates
   b. proteins
   c. lipids
   d. vitamins

7. Based on this illustration, which nutrient class makes up the greatest proportion of body weight?

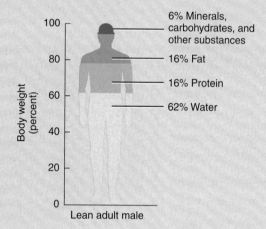

   a. protein
   b. carbohydrate
   c. fat
   d. water

8. Which of these statements about essential nutrients is false?

   a. If you do not get enough of them in your diet, your body will synthesize enough to meet its needs.
   b. If you do not get enough of them in your diet, deficiency symptoms will eventually appear.
   c. Some of them provide energy.
   d. Some of them provide structure.

9. Why it is better to obtain your nutrients from foods than from dietary supplements?

   a. Dietary supplements are more likely to contain toxic amounts of nutrients.
   b. Foods provide phytochemicals and zoochemicals.
   c. Foods provide pleasurable tastes and aromas.
   d. All of the above are correct.

10. Which of these factors can limit the availability of food?

   a. socioeconomic status
   b. health status
   c. living conditions
   d. All of the above are correct.

11. A diet that follows the principles of variety, balance, and moderation _____.

   a. can include all kinds of foods
   b. includes only foods that have high nutrient density
   c. includes exactly the right amount of each nutrient each day
   d. includes only unprocessed foods

12. Which of these sources would be most likely to exaggerate the beneficial effects of a dietary supplement?

   a. a government publication
   b. a dietitian's recommendations
   c. a pamphlet published by the manufacturer
   d. a peer-reviewed article in a scientific journal

13. When the scientific method is used, a hypothesis is first proposed and then tested through experimentation. Which of the following hypotheses can be tested by means of experiments that use a quantifiable measure?

   a. Iron supplements increase feelings of vitality.
   b. A high vitamin E intake makes you feel younger.
   c. Eating an apple a day will lower blood cholesterol.
   d. B vitamin supplements give you an energy boost.

14. The information in this graph was collected in an epidemiological study. Which of the following statements is true? *

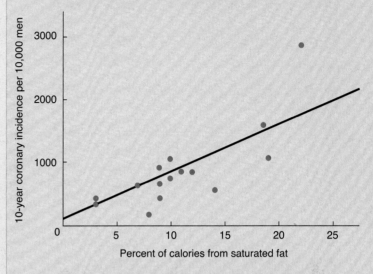

   a. A diet that is high in saturated fat causes heart disease.
   b. A higher incidence of coronary heart disease is associated with a higher intake of saturated fat.
   c. People who lower their intake of saturated fat will have fewer heart attacks.
   d. Moving to a country with less coronary heart disease will lower your intake of saturated fat.

15. In a scientific experiment, a group that is identical to the experimental group in every way except that its members do not receive the treatment being tested is called

   _____.

   a. a control group
   b. a placebo
   c. a variable
   d. an alternative group

Guidelines for a Healthy Diet

"What you don't know could kill you" may have been the first nutrition recommendation in human history. To swallow the wrong berry or gulp down water from a suspect source or tuck into a diseased organ from the most recent kill could have been fatal to early humans, who were hunter-gatherers. Such lessons would serve as anecdotal guideposts to survival. As societies developed, dietary cautions turned into taboos, sometimes laws, and ultimately, nutrition recommendations.

Governments have been providing what we would call modern nutrition information for the past 150 years. As the Industrial Revolution swept through Great Britain in the first half of the 19th century, urban populations—and poverty and hunger—swelled. To ensure a healthy workforce, the British government developed minimum dietary guidelines utilizing the cheapest foods. It wasn't until World War I that the British Royal Society determined that a healthy workforce required a healthy diet, not necessarily the cheapest. So fruits, vegetables, and milk became elements of a solid nutritional foundation. Since then, virtually every national government has sought, with varying degrees of success, to establish dietary standards for its citizens.

Today, modern public health agencies provide valuable information regarding nutritional choices. However, this information isn't always understood or used properly. As portion sizes grow, so do American waistlines—and the attendant health concerns. "What you don't know could kill you" remains as vital an admonition today as it was 40,000 years ago.

Nutrition Recommendations

What should we be eating if we want to satisfy our nutrient needs? Our taste buds, food marketers and advertisers, and magazine and newspaper headlines all influence our choices. These choices may not always be healthy ones, however. Our taste buds respond to flavor and sensation, not necessarily to sensible nutrition; manufacturers want to sell products; and magazines want to sell subscriptions. Government recommendations, on the other hand, are designed with individual health as well as public health in mind. They can be used to plan diets and to evaluate what we are eating, both as individuals and as a nation.

A World War II nutrition poster FIGURE 2.1

Food shortage was a national concern in the United States during World War II. People were expected to cooperate with rationing efforts and to plant home gardens, called victory gardens. The food that could be produced from a plot of land was too valuable to waste. Not to grow a garden or care for fruiting shrubs and trees was considered unpatriotic.

PAST AND PRESENT U.S. RECOMMENDATIONS

The federal government has been in the business of making nutritional recommendations for over 100 years. These recommendations have changed over time as our food intake patterns have changed and our knowledge of what constitutes a healthy diet has evolved.

The first dietary recommendations in the United States, published in 1894 by the U.S. Department of Agriculture (USDA), suggested amounts of protein, carbohydrate, fat, and "mineral matter" needed to keep Americans healthy.[1] At the time, specific vitamins and minerals essential for health had not been identified; nevertheless, this work set the stage for the development of the first **food guides**. Food guides translate nutrient-intake recommendations into recommended food choices. The food guide *How to Select Foods*, released in 1917, was designed to help people choose a healthy diet based on five food groups: meat and milk, cereals, vegetables and fruit, fats and fatty foods, and sugars and sugary foods. In the 1930s, as food became scarce for many Americans because of the Depression, the USDA began to publish low-cost food plans to help people meet their nutritional needs on a limited income.

In the early 1940s, as the United States entered World War II, the Food and Nutrition Board was established to advise the Army and other federal agencies regarding problems related to food and the nutritional health of the armed forces and the general population (FIGURE 2.1). The Food and Nutrition Board developed the first set of recommendations for specific amounts of nutrients. These came to be known as the Recommended Dietary Allowances (RDAs). The original RDAs made recommendations on amounts of energy and on specific nutrients that were most likely to be deficient in people's diets—protein, iron, calcium, vitamins A and D, thiamin, riboflavin, niacin, and vitamin C. Recommended intakes were based on amounts that would prevent nutrient deficiencies.

Over the years since those first standards were developed, dietary habits and disease patterns have changed, and dietary recommendations have had to change along with them. Overt nutrient deficiencies are now rare in the United States, but the incidence of diet-related chronic diseases, such as heart disease, diabetes, and obesity, has increased. To combat these more recent health concerns, recommendations are now intended to promote health as well as prevent deficiencies. The original RDAs have been expanded into the Dietary Reference Intakes; the *Dietary Guidelines for Americans*, a set of diet and lifestyle recommendations first published in 1980, have been updated to better promote health and reduce chronic disease risk in the population; early food guides have evolved into *MyPyramid: Steps to a Healthier You*, which suggests servings from five food group to meet the recommendations of the

Dietary Guidelines; and standardized food labels have been developed to help consumers choose foods that meet these recommendations.

HOW WE USE NUTRITION RECOMMENDATIONS

Nutrition recommendations are developed to address the nutritional concerns of the population and help individuals meet their nutrient needs. These recommendations can also be used to evaluate the nutrient intake of populations and of individuals within populations. Determining what people eat and how their nutrient intake compares to nutrition recommendations is important for assessing their **nutritional status**.

When evaluating the nutritional status of a population, food intake can be assessed by having individuals track their food intake or by using information about the amounts and types of food that is available to the population to identify trends in the diet (see *What a Scientist Sees*).

> ■ **nutritional status**
> An individual's health, as it is influenced by the intake and utilization of nutrients.

What a Scientist Sees

Trends in Milk Consumption

The graph shows estimates of milk consumption in the United States from 1909 to 1999, based on the amount of milk available for human consumption during that period. Anyone looking at the graph can tell that overall milk consumption and consumption of whole milk both declined, while consumption of lower-fat milks increased. A nutrition scientist looking at this graph, however, would see not just changes in the amounts and types of milk consumed but the nutritional and public health implications of these changes as well.

Because whole milk is high in saturated fat, replacing whole milk with lower-fat milk decreases saturated fat intake. This is good from the standpoint of heart health, but the decline in total milk consumption may be bad for bone health. Milk is one of the most important sources of calcium in the North American diet. The scientist will be alerted to the fact that calcium intake from milk has been declining. Unless more calcium from other sources is being consumed, this drop in milk consumption may indicate that the population is at risk for fragile bones and an increase in fractures.

Based on this analysis, what kinds of measures would you suggest to increase the population's calcium intake?

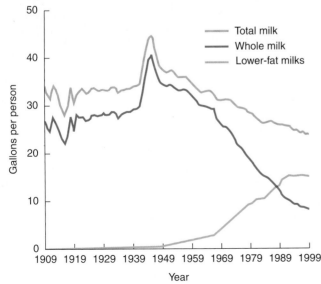

Source: U.S. Department of Agriculture, Economic Research Service. Major trends in the U.S. food supply. 1909–1999. Food Review 23:12, 2000.

Bone fracture due to osteoporosis

Process Diagram

A complete assessment of an individual's nutritional status includes a diet analysis, a physical exam, a medical history, and an evaluation of nutrient levels in the body. An interpretation of this information can determine whether an individual is well nourished, malnourished, or at risk of malnutrition.

1 Determine typical food intake. People's typical food intake can be evaluated by having them record their food as they consume it or recall what they have eaten during the past day or so. Because food intake varies from day to day, to obtain a realistic picture, an individual's intake should be monitored for more than one day. An accurate food record includes all food and beverages consumed, along with descriptions of cooking methods and brand names of products. It is often difficult to obtain an accurate record because people may change what they are eating rather than record it, or they may forget what they ate when recalling it.

FOOD DIARY

Record all the food and beverages you eat. Include the food, how it was prepared, the amount you ate and the brand name. Don't forget to list all fats used in cooking and all spreads and sauces added.

Time	Food	Kind and how prepared	Amount
7:00 A.M.	Eggs	scrambled	2
	Butter	in eggs	1 tsp.
	toast	whole wheat	2 slices
	Butter	on toast	2 tsp.
	Milk	non-fat	8 oz.
	Orange juice	from frozen concentrate	8 oz.
12:00 P.M.	Big Mac	McDonald's	1

2 Analyze nutrient intake. A computer analysis of an individual's food intake can calculate nutrient intake and compare it with the appropriate nutrition recommendations. In this example, which shows only a few nutrients, intake of vitamin A, iron, and calcium is below the recommended amounts, and intake of vitamin C and saturated fat is above the recommended amounts.

Nutrient	Percent of recommendation 0% 50% 100%
Vitamin A	75%
Vitamin C	115%
Iron	54%
Calcium	75%
Saturated fat	134%

3 Evaluate physical health. A physical examination can detect signs of nutrient deficiencies or excesses. Measures of body dimensions such as height and weight can be monitored over time or compared with standards for a given population. Drastic changes in measurements or measurements that are significantly above or below the standards could indicate a nutritional deficiency or excess.

When food intake data are evaluated in conjunction with information about the health and nutritional status of individuals in the population (FIGURE 2.2), relationships between dietary intake and health and disease can be identified. This is important for developing public health measures that address nutritional problems. For example, population surveys such as the National Health and Nutrition Examination Survey (NHANES) helped public health officials recognize that low iron levels are a problem for many people, including young women, preschool children, and the elderly. This information led to the fortification of grain products with iron, beginning in the 1940s. Recent NHANES data have also shown that the number of calories Americans consume per day has increased over the past few decades and that the incidence of obesity has increased dramatically during the same period. This has led public health experts to develop programs to improve both the diet and the fitness of Americans.

4 **Consider medical history.** Personal and family medical histories are important because genetic risk factors affect an individual's risk of developing a nutrition-related disease. For example, if you have high cholesterol and your father died of a heart attack at age 50, you have a higher-than-average risk of developing heart disease and may need to modify your diet to reduce your risk.

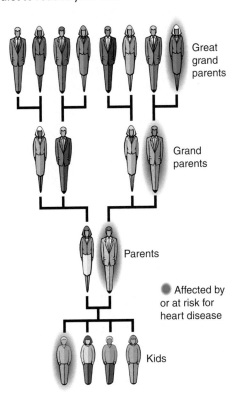

Great grand parents

Grand parents

Parents

● Affected by or at risk for heart disease

Kids

5 **Assess with laboratory tests.** Measures of nutrients, their by-products, or their functions in the blood, urine, and body cells can help detect nutrient deficiencies and excesses (Appendix B). For instance, levels of iron and iron-carrying proteins in the blood can be used to determine whether a person has iron-deficiency anemia, and levels of blood cholesterol such as those shown here can provide information about an individual's risk of heart disease.

Blood Lipid Panel

Test	Result	Healthy range[2]
Cholesterol, total	185 mg/dL	<200
Triglycerides	56 mg/dL	<150
HDL cholesterol	59 mg/dL	>40
LDL cholesterol, calculated	90 mg/dL	<100

The information obtained from population health and nutrition surveys is also used to determine whether the nation is meeting health and nutrition goals, such as those established by *Healthy People*. This set of health-promotion and disease-prevention objectives is revised every 10 years, with the goal of increasing the quality and length of healthy lives for the population as a whole and eliminating health disparities among different segments of the population. The newest version of these objectives, *Healthy People 2020*, will be released in 2010 (see Appendix D).[3]

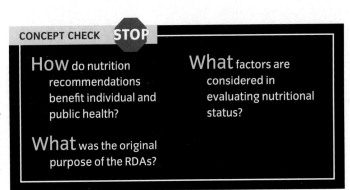

CONCEPT CHECK **STOP**

How do nutrition recommendations benefit individual and public health?

What was the original purpose of the RDAs?

What factors are considered in evaluating nutritional status?

Dietary Reference Intakes (DRIs)

The **Dietary Reference Intakes (DRIs)** are recommendations for the amounts of energy, nutrients, and other food components that healthy people should consume in order to stay healthy, reduce the risk of chronic disease, and prevent deficiencies.[4] The DRIs can be used to evaluate whether a person's diet provides all the essential nutrients in adequate amounts. They include several types of recommendations that address both nutrient intake and energy intake and include values that are appropriate for people of different genders and stages of life (**FIGURE 2.3**).

DRIs for different groups FIGURE 2.3

Because gender and life stage affect nutrient needs, Dietary Reference Intake values have been set for each gender and for various life-stage groups. These values take into account the physiological differences that affect the nutrient needs of men and women, infants, children, adolescents, adults, older adults, and pregnant and lactating women.

RECOMMENDATIONS FOR NUTRIENT INTAKE

The DRI recommendations for nutrient intake include four sets of values. The **Estimated Average Requirements (EARs)** are average amounts of nutrients or other dietary components required by healthy individuals in a population (**FIGURE 2.4**). They are determined using experimental data on nutrient needs and are used in assessing the adequacy of a population's food supply or typical intake. They are not appropriate for evaluating an individual's intake but are used to calculate the **Recommended Dietary Allowances (RDAs)**. The RDAs recommend specific amounts of nutrients and other dietary components to meet the needs of most healthy people (Figure 2.4). When there aren't enough data about nutrient requirements to establish EARs and RDAs, **Adequate Intakes (AIs)** are set, based on what healthy people typically eat. RDA or AI values can be used as goals for individual intake and to plan and evaluate individual diets (Appendix A and inside covers). They are meant to represent the amounts that most healthy people should consume, on average, over several days or even weeks, not each

Estimated Average Requirements (EARs) Nutrient intakes estimated to meet the needs of 50% of the healthy individuals in a given gender and life-stage group.

Recommended Dietary Allowances (RDAs) Nutrient intakes that are sufficient to meet the needs of almost all healthy people in a specific gender and life-stage group.

Adequate Intakes (AIs) Nutrient intakes that should be used as a goal when no RDA exists. AI values are an approximation of the nutrient intake that sustains health.

EARs and RDAs are determined by measuring the different amounts of nutrients required by different individuals in a population group and plotting the resulting values. Because a few individuals in the group need only a small amount, a few need a large amount, and most need an amount that falls between the extremes, the result is a bell-shaped curve like the one shown here.

The RDA is set by adding a safety factor to the EAR. About 97% of the population meets its needs by consuming this amount (shown as yellow shading). If nutrient intake meets the RDA, the risk of deficiency is very low. As intake falls, the risk of a deficiency increases.

An EAR is the average amount of a nutrient required for good health. If everyone in the population consumed this amount, only 50% would obtain enough of the nutrient to meet their requirements (shown as diagonal lines).

The UL is set well above the needs of everyone in the population and represents the highest amount of the nutrient that will not cause toxicity symptoms in the majority of healthy people. As intake rises above the UL, the likelihood of toxicity increases.

EAR   RDA   UL

Number of people →

Daily nutrient requirement →

and every day. Because they are set high enough to meet the needs of almost all healthy people, intake below the RDA or AI does not necessarily mean that an individual is deficient, but the risk of deficiency is greater than if the individual consumed the recommended amount.

The fourth set of values, **Tolerable Upper Intake Levels (ULs)**, specifies the maximum amount of a nutrient that most people can consume on a daily basis without some adverse effect (Figure 2.4). For most nutrients, it is difficult to exceed the UL by consuming food. Most foods do not contain enough of any one nutrient to cause toxicity; however, some dietary supplements may. For some nutrients, the UL is set for total intake from all sources, including food, fortified foods, and dietary

■ **Tolerable Upper Intake Levels (ULs)** Maximum daily intake levels that are unlikely to pose risks of adverse health effects to almost all individuals in a given gender and life-stage group.

■ **Estimated Energy Requirements (EERs)** Average energy intake values predicted to maintain body weight in healthy individuals.

supplements. For other nutrients, the UL refers to intake from supplements alone or from supplements and fortified foods. For many nutrients, there is no UL because too little information is available to determine it.

RECOMMENDATIONS FOR ENERGY INTAKE

The DRIs make two types of recommendations about energy intake. The first, called **Estimated Energy Requirements (EERs)**, provides an estimate of how many calories are needed to keep body weight stable. EER calculations take into account a person's age, gender, weight, height, and level of physical activity. A change in any of these variables

◄ A A 17-year-old girl who is 5'4" tall, weighs 127 pounds, and gets no exercise has an EER of about 1730 Calories a day. If she adds an hour of moderate activity to her daily routine, her EER will increase to 2380 Calories, so she must eat 650 Calories more per day to maintain her current weight and support growth.[4] If she grows taller or gains weight, her EER will also increase.

B A healthy diet can include different proportions of carbohydrate, protein, and fat. These two plates show very different food combinations, but both are within the AMDRs for protein, carbohydrate, and fat. ▼

This meal contains approximately 480 Calories, of which 55% is from carbohydrate, 20% is from protein, and 25% is from fat.

This meal contains approximately 740 Calories, of which 30% is from carbohydrate, 35% is from protein, and 35% is from fat.

■ **Acceptable Macronutrient Distribution Ranges (AMDRs)** Healthy ranges of intake for carbohydrate, fat, and protein, expressed as percentages of total energy intake.

changes the person's energy needs (FIGURE 2.5A).

The second type of energy recommendation, called **Acceptable Macronutrient Distribution Ranges (AMDRs)**, makes recommendations about the proportions of calories that should come from carbohydrate, fat, and protein in a healthy diet. AMDRs are ranges—10 to 35% of calories from protein, 45 to 65% of calories from carbohydrate, and 10 to 35% of calories from fat—not exact values; they are intended to promote

diets that minimize disease risk while allowing flexibility in food intake patterns (FIGURE 2.5B).

CONCEPT CHECK **STOP**

What are RDAs and AIs used for?

How might you use ULs?

What are three variables that affect your energy needs?

Why are AMDR values given as ranges rather than as single numbers?

Tools for Diet Planning

Explain how the Dietary Guidelines and MyPyramid are related.

Discuss how following the recommendations of the Dietary Guidelines can help prevent chronic disease.

Determine your individualized MyPyramid recommendations.

Identify foods that are high in discretionary calories.

The DRIs tell you how much of each nutrient you need, but they do not help you choose foods that will meet these needs. To help consumers choose diets that will meet their needs, the U.S. government has developed the *Dietary Guidelines for Americans* and *MyPyramid: Steps to a Healthier You*. The Dietary Guidelines are a set of diet and lifestyle recommendations designed to promote health and reduce the risk of chronic diseases in the U.S. population.[5] The USDA's MyPyramid is the most recent pyramid-shaped food guide. It divides foods into groups based on the nutrients they supply most abundantly and recommends appropriate amounts from each food group. MyPyramid was developed to help Americans put the recommendations of the 2005 Dietary Guidelines into practice.

RECOMMENDATIONS OF THE *DIETARY GUIDELINES FOR AMERICANS*

The *Dietary Guidelines for Americans 2005* include recommendations that promote nutrient-dense food choices, a balance between food intake and exercise (intended to support a healthy body weight), limited intake of dietary components that contribute to chronic disease, and prevention of food-borne illness (**TABLE 2.1**). These recommendations are designed for all healthy Americans 2 years of age and older. Additional recommendations target specific subpopulations (see Appendix D).

Make nutrient-dense choices Despite the great variety of foods available to most Americans, many of us do not make the most nutritious choices. To address this problem, the Dietary Guidelines recommend choosing a variety of nutrient-dense foods. They encourage Americans to improve their nutrient intakes by eating more vegetables, fruits, whole grains, low-fat dairy products, lean meats, beans, and nuts and seeds. Whole grains, fruits, vegetables, and beans are rich in fiber, micronutrients, and phytochemicals. Low-fat dairy products provide calcium and protein without too much saturated fat. Beans, peas, nuts, seeds, and lean meats and fish are nutrient-dense protein sources.

Key recommendations of the *Dietary Guidelines for Americans 2005*[5] TABLE 2.1

1. Consume a variety of foods within and among the various food groups.
2. Balance calorie intake with expenditure to manage body weight.
3. Be physically active every day.
4. Choose more fruits and vegetables, whole grains, and low-fat dairy products.
5. Choose fats wisely.
6. Choose fiber-rich carbohydrates and limit added sugars.
7. Choose and prepare foods with little salt.
8. If you drink alcoholic beverages, do so in moderation.
9. Prepare, handle, and store food safely.

Balance food intake with physical activity

More Americans are overweight than ever before, and the numbers continue to grow. To address this problem, the Dietary Guidelines recommend that Americans balance the calories they consume in food and beverages with the calories they expend through physical activity in order to achieve and maintain a healthy weight. Weight maintenance requires consuming the same number of calories as you burn; this means that if you eat more, you need to exercise more (discussed in Chapter 9). Losing weight requires consuming fewer calories than you burn. This can be accomplished by reducing energy intake and increasing energy expenditure through exercise (**FIGURE 2.6**).

Limit nutrients that increase health risks

The Dietary Guidelines recommend reducing intake of saturated fat, *trans* fat, and cholesterol—the types of lipids that increase the risk of heart disease (discussed in Chapter 5). Most of the fats in our diet should come from vegetable oils and fish, which promote heart health. The Dietary Guidelines also recommend limiting salt intake in order to prevent high blood pressure and minimizing intake of foods to which refined sugar has been added because such foods provide calories but contribute few nutrients.

The Dietary Guidelines also make recommendations regarding alcohol consumption. Those who drink alcohol should do so in moderation. Excess alcohol consumption can alter judgment, lead to addiction, and cause serious

---

Healthy weight and exercise recommendations FIGURE 2.6

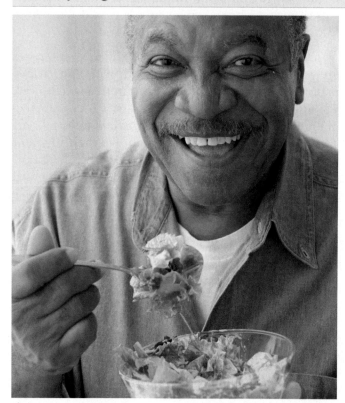

▲ A To promote a healthy weight, the *Dietary Guidelines for Americans* recommend moderating calorie intake by limiting portion sizes and reducing consumption of added sugars, fats, and alcohol, which provide calories but few essential nutrients. The Dietary Guidelines emphasize that the key to weight management is consuming the appropriate number of calories rather than the relative proportions of carbohydrate, fat, and protein in the diet.

B To reduce the risk of chronic disease, the Dietary Guidelines recommend 30 minutes of moderate activity most days. Ideally, this activity should include aerobic exercise to strengthen the heart, stretching exercises for flexibility, and weight lifting for muscle strength and endurance. Greater health benefits can be obtained by engaging in more vigorous activity or being active longer. Sixty minutes of moderate to vigorous activity on most days is recommended to help manage weight and prevent weight gain. For those who have lost weight and want to keep it off, 60 to 90 minutes of moderate activity per day is recommended. **▼**

Moderate alcohol consumption FIGURE 2.7

Having a glass of wine with dinner is considered moderate drinking (one drink per day for women and two for men) and is the amount of alcohol associated with the lowest overall mortality as well as the lowest mortality from coronary heart disease. Alcohol consumption is not recommended for people who cannot restrict their intake; women who are or may become pregnant; lactating women; children and adolescents; people with conditions or taking medications that interact with alcohol; and people who are engaging in activities that require attention, skill, or coordination.

health and societal problems (discussed in Chapter 12). Moderate alcohol consumption may have some beneficial effects in middle-aged and older adults, but it is not recommended that anyone who does not drink begin drinking for the sake of its potential health benefits (FIGURE 2.7) (see also *What Should I Eat?*).

Keep food safe Paying attention to food safety is part of healthful eating. To reduce the risk of food-borne illness, the Dietary Guidelines encourage Americans to choose and prepare foods with safety in mind and to cook and store foods at the recommended temperatures (discussed in Chapter 13).

 WHAT SHOULD I EAT? **Following the Dietary Guidelines**

 Use iProfile to look up the saturated fat and sugar content in your breakfast cereal.

Increase nutrient density
- Add more vegetables and less mayo to your turkey sandwich.
- Snack on fruit and nuts rather than on chips and cookies.
- Have a whole grain such as bulgur, quinoa, or brown rice rather than packaged, flavored white rice with dinner.
- Stir-fry a variety of vegetables.
- Have strawberries rather than strawberry shortcake for dessert.

Balance intake with activity
- Don't skip breakfast; if you do, you're more likely to overeat later in the day.
- Pass on that second helping. When you eat out, split an entrée with a friend.
- Walk an extra 1000 steps; the more you exercise, the easier it is to keep your weight at a healthy level.
- Ride your bike to work or when running errands.
- Lift some weights or walk on a treadmill while watching the news.

Limit nutrients that increase health risks
- Look at product labels for sodium and saturated and *trans* fat content before making a choice.
- Choose lean meat, fish, and low-fat dairy products in order to limit saturated fat.
- Have water and skip the soft drink—it adds nothing but sugar to your diet.
- Pass on the salt; instead, try lemon juice or some basil and oregano.
- If you drink alcohol, stop after one drink.

Physical activity reduces the risk of chronic disease, improves physical fitness, and increases energy needs, making weight management easier.

Moderation is represented by the triangle shapes. The wide base of each triangle includes the most nutrient-dense choices, which should be selected more often. The narrower tip includes foods within the group that should be selected only infrequently because they contain more added sugars and solid fats.

Proportionality is demonstrated by the widths of the colored triangles. The widest triangles are groups from which we should make most of our choices – grains, vegetables, fruits, and milk. The narrower the triangle, the smaller the amounts we need; the meat and beans triangle is narrower, and the oils triangle is the narrowest.

Variety is symbolized by the six colored triangles representing the five food groups plus oils. Foods from all the groups are needed each day for good health.

MyPyramid

STEPS TO A HEALTHIER YOU
MyPyramid.gov

GRAINS	VEGETABLES	FRUITS	MILK	MEAT & BEANS
Make half your grains whole	**Vary your veggies**	**Focus on fruits**	**Get your calcium rich foods**	**Go lean with protein**
Eat at least 3 oz. of whole-grain cereals, breads, crackers, rice, or pasta every day	Eat more dark-green veggies like broccoli, spinach, and other dark leafy greens	Eat a variety of fruit	Go low-fat or free-fat when you choose milk, yogurt, and other milk products	Choose low-fat or lean meats and poultry
1 oz. is about 1 slice of bread, about 1 cup of breakfast cereal, or ½ up of cooked rice, cereal, or pasta	Eat more orange vegetables like carrots and sweet potatoes	Choose fresh, frozen, canned, or dried fruit	If you don't or can't consume milk, choose lactose-free products or other calcium sources such as fortified foods and beverages	Bake it, broil it, or grill it
	Eat more dry beans and peas like pinto beans, kidney beans, and lentils	Go easy on fruit juices		Vary your protein routine—choose more fish, beans, peas, nuts, and seeds

MyPyramid messages and symbolism FIGURE 2.8

Simple messages guide our choices from each food group. We are advised to select whole grains for half of our grain choices, vary our vegetables, focus on fruits, choose calcium-rich foods, and go lean with protein.

MYPYRAMID: PUTTING THE GUIDELINES INTO PRACTICE

The recommendations of the Dietary Guidelines are made more usable by *MyPyramid: Steps to a Healthier You*. This food guide is built around five main food groups—grains, vegetables, fruits, milk, and meat and beans—represented by the colored triangles that make up the pyramid (FIGURE 2.8). Oils, though not a food group, provide essential nutrients that are needed in small amounts, so they are represented by a sixth thin triangle.

Activity, variety, proportionality, and moderation

The MyPyramid icon emphasizes the key messages of the Dietary Guidelines: activity, variety, proportionality, and moderation (see Figure 2.8). Physical activity is represented by the steps and the person climbing them, a reminder of the importance of daily exercise. Variety, illustrated by the different-colored triangles, is important for a healthy diet because no one type of food provides all the nutrients and food components the body needs.

Proportionality means eating more of some types of foods than others. The widths of the triangles show us that the proportions of grains, fruits, and vegetables in your diet should be larger than the proportion of meat and beans.

Moderation means avoiding excesses of saturated fat, *trans* fat, cholesterol, added sugars, salt, and alcohol, all of which can increase health risks. Practicing moderation means choosing more of the nutrient-dense foods at the wide base of each triangle and fewer from the less-nutrient-dense foods in the tips of the triangles.

A personalized approach
The colored triangles of MyPyramid indicate different food groups, but the pyramid icon does not show a recommended number of servings from each group. The reason for this is that people's needs vary. You can obtain your own personalized eating plan by going to the Web site www.MyPyramid.gov, clicking on MyPyramid Plan, and entering your age, gender, and activity level. After you enter this information, the site provides recommendations from each food group, based on your individual calorie needs (FIGURE 2.9). The amounts recommended from the vegetables, fruits, and milk groups are given in cups, and oil recommendations are given in teaspoons. The amounts from the grains group and the meat and beans group are expressed in ounces. Some examples of 1 ounce of grains are; 1 cup of cold cereal, 1/2 cup of cooked cereal or grains, or a slice of bread. In the meat and beans group; one egg, a tablespoon of peanut butter, a quarter-cup of cooked dry beans, and 1/2 ounce of nuts or seeds are equivalent to 1 ounce of cooked meat, poultry, or fish.

Individual MyPyramid recommendations FIGURE 2.9

This individualized MyPyramid plan for a person who requires about 2000 Calories per day shows the recommended amounts from each food group and advises nutrient-dense choices from within each group.

MyPyramid
STEPS TO A HEALTHIER YOU

Based on the information you provided, this is your daily recommended amount from each food group.

GRAINS 6 ounces	VEGETABLES 2 1/2 cups	FRUITS 2 cups	MILK 3 cups	MEAT & BEANS 5 1/2 ounces
Make half your grains whole Aim for at least **3 ounces** of whole grains a day	**Vary your veggies** Aim for these amounts each week: **Dark green veggies** = 3 cups **Orange veggies** = 2 cups **Dry beans & peas** = 3 cups **Starchy veggies** = 3 cups **Other veggies** = 6 1/2 cups	**Focus on fruits** Eat a variety of fruit Go easy on fruit juices	**Get your calcium-rich foods** Go low-fat or fat-free when you choose milk, yogurt, or cheese	**Go lean with protein** Choose low-fat or lean meats and poultry Vary your protein routine—choose more fish, beans, peas, nuts, and seeds

Find your balance between food and physical activity

Be physically active for at least **30 minutes** most days of the week.

Know your limits on fats, sugars, and sodium

Your allowance for oils is **6 teaspoons a day.**

Limit extras—solid fats and sugars—to **265 calories a day.**

Your results are based on a 2000 calorie pattern.

Name: _____

This calorie level is only an estimate of your needs. Monitor your body weight to see if you need to adjust your calorie intake.

Discretionary calories

discretionary
calories

The calories remaining
after an individual has
met recommended
intake levels with
healthy choices from
all the food groups.

In addition to the food group recommendations of MyPyramid, your personalized pyramid plan tells you to limit extras to a certain number of Calories (see Figure 2.9). These "extras," called **discretionary calories**, come from dietary components that should be consumed in limited amounts, such as added sugars, alcohol, and solid fats, which are high in saturated or *trans* fat (FIGURE 2.10). If you imagine your energy intake as a calorie "budget," discretionary calories are the calories you have left over after making nutrient-dense choices, according to your MyPyramid recommendations. The more

active you are, the more calories you need and the more of these discretionary, or "splurge," calories you can consume while meeting nutrient needs without exceeding your calorie needs.

Based on your individual MyPyramid recommendations, you can choose foods that suit your food preferences. It is easy to see how some foods in your diet fit into a MyPyramid plan. For example, a chicken breast is 3 ounces from the meat and beans group; a scoop of rice is 2 oz from the grains group. It is more difficult to see how much mixed foods such as pizza, stews, and casseroles contribute to each food group. Often individual ingredients must be considered. For example, a slice of pizza provides 1 ounce of grains, 1/8 cup of vegetables, and 1/2 cup of milk. Having meat on your pizza adds about 1/4 oz from that group. One way to see how your

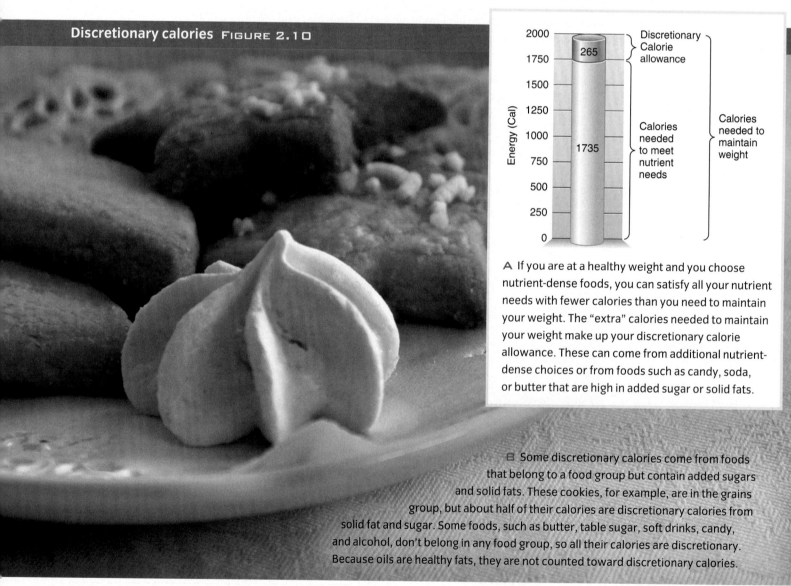

Discretionary calories FIGURE 2.10

A If you are at a healthy weight and you choose nutrient-dense foods, you can satisfy all your nutrient needs with fewer calories than you need to maintain your weight. The "extra" calories needed to maintain your weight make up your discretionary calorie allowance. These can come from additional nutrient-dense choices or from foods such as candy, soda, or butter that are high in added sugar or solid fats.

B Some discretionary calories come from foods that belong to a food group but contain added sugars and solid fats. These cookies, for example, are in the grains group, but about half of their calories are discretionary calories from solid fat and sugar. Some foods, such as butter, table sugar, soft drinks, candy, and alcohol, don't belong in any food group, so all their calories are discretionary. Because oils are healthy fats, they are not counted toward discretionary calories.

The MyPyramid Menu Planner (at www.mypyramid.gov) helps you visualize each food's contribution to your diet. It shows you whether your diet includes enough food from each group and whether you are meeting or exceeding calorie recommendations. It can be used to evaluate up to a week's worth of meals and snacks.

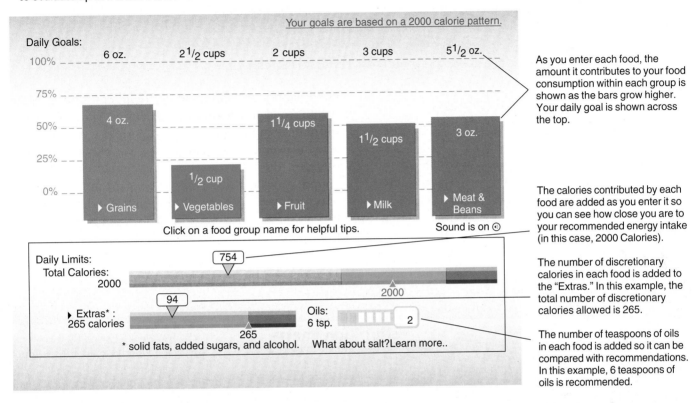

As you enter each food, the amount it contributes to your food consumption within each group is shown as the bars grow higher. Your daily goal is shown across the top.

The calories contributed by each food are added as you enter it so you can see how close you are to your recommended energy intake (in this case, 2000 Calories).

The number of discretionary calories in each food is added to the "Extras." In this example, the total number of discretionary calories allowed is 265.

The number of teaspoons of oils in each food is added so it can be compared with recommendations. In this example, 6 teaspoons of oils is recommended.

daily intake matches the MyPyramid recommendations is to use the interactive tools on the MyPyramid Web site to help track your progress toward choosing a healthy diet (FIGURE 2.11).

EXCHANGE LISTS

The **Exchange Lists** are a set of food-group recommendations developed in the 1950s to plan diets for people with diabetes. Since then, their use has been expanded to planning diets for anyone who has to monitor calorie intake. They group foods based on the amounts of energy, carbohydrate, protein, and fat they provide per serving. Foods in the same exchange list each contain approximately the same amounts of energy, carbohydrate, protein, and fat. Therefore, any one of the foods on a list can be exchanged with any other food on the list without altering the calories or percentages of carbohydrate, protein, or fat in the diet.

Exchange Lists provide a useful tool whether you are controlling calorie intake for purposes of weight loss or carbohydrate intake for purposes of diabetes management. Appendix E provides more information about exchange lists.

CONCEPT CHECK STOP

How does MyPyramid help you follow the recommendations of the Dietary Guidelines?

How many ounces from the grains group are recommended each day for you?

What is the significance of the size and shape used to represent each food group in the MyPyramid graphic.

Which contains more discretionary calories— a bagel or a doughnut?

Food and Supplement Labels

The Dietary Guidelines and MyPyramid recommend appropriate amounts of nutritious foods, but sometimes it is difficult to tell how nutritious a particular food is. How do you know whether your frozen entree is a good source of vitamin C, how much fiber your breakfast cereal provides, or how much calcium is in your daily vitamin/mineral supplement? You can find this information on food and supplement labels.

FOOD LABELS

Food labels are designed to help consumers make healthy food choices by providing information about the nutrient composition of a food and how that food fits into the overall diet (**FIGURE 2.12**).[6] Knowing how to interpret the information on these labels can help you choose a healthy diet. This doesn't mean that you can never choose high-calorie, low-nutrient-density foods, but rather that you should balance your choices. It is your total diet—not each choice—that counts.

Visualizing

Food labels FIGURE 2.12

Standard serving sizes are required to allow consumers to compare products. For example, the number of calories in one serving of this macaroni and cheese can be compared to the number of calories in one serving of packaged rice because the values for both are for a standard 1-cup serving.

Food labels must list the "% Daily Value" for total fat, saturated fat, cholesterol, sodium, total carbohydrate, and dietary fiber, as well as for vitamins A and C, calcium, and iron. A daily value of 5% or less is considered low, and one of 20% or more is considered high.

The label provides information about the amounts of total fat, saturated fat, *trans* fat, cholesterol, and sodium, nutrients whose intake should be limited.

The label provides information about the amounts of fiber, vitamins A and C, calcium, and iron, nutrients that tend to be low in the American diet.

The footnote gives the "Daily Values" for a 2,000 and a 2,500 Calorie diet to illustrate that for some nutrients the daily value increases with increasing caloric intake.

A Food labels must appear on all packaged foods except those produced by small businesses and those in packages too small to accommodate the information. This label from a macaroni-and-cheese package illustrates how the Nutrition Facts panel and the ingredient list can help you evaluate the nutritional contribution this food will make to your diet.

Nutrition Facts

Serving Size 1 cup (228g)
Servings Per Container 2

Amount Per Serving

Calories 250	Calories from Fat 110

	% Daily Value*
Total Fat 12g	18%
Saturated Fat 3g	15%
Trans Fat 1.5g	
Cholesterol 30mg	10%
Sodium 470mg	20%
Total Carbohydrate 31g	10%
Dietary Fiber 0g	0%
Sugars 5g	
Protein 5g	

Vitamin A	4%
Vitamin C	2%
Calcium	20%
Iron	4%

* Percent Daily Values are based on a 2,000 calorie diet. Your daily values may be higher or lower depending on your calorie needs:

		Calories:	2,000	2,500
Total Fat	Less than		65g	80g
Sat. Fat	Less than		20g	25g
Cholesterol	Less than		300mg	300mg
Sodium	Less than		2,400mg	2,400mg
Total Carbohydrate			300g	375g
Dietary Fiber			25g	30g

Ingredients
Enriched macaroni product (wheat flour, niacin, ferrous sulfate [iron], thiamine mononitrate, riboflavin, folic acid); cheese sauce mix (whey, modified food starch, milk fat, salt, milk protein concentrate, contains less tha 2% of sodium tripolyphosphate, cellulose gel, cellulose gum, citric acid, sodium phosphate, lactic acid, calcium phosphate, milk, yellow 5, yellow 6, enzymes, cheese culture)

The ingredients are listed in descending order by weight, from the most abundant to the least abundant. The enriched white flour in the macaroni is the most abundant ingredient in this product.

Labels must contain basic product information, such as the name of the product, the weight or volume of the contents, and the name and place of business of the manufacturer, packager, or distributor.

Nutrition Facts All food labels must contain a **Nutrition Facts** panel (**FIGURE 2.12A**).[8] This section of the label presents information about the amounts of specific nutrients in a standard serving. The serving size on the label is followed by the number of servings per container, the total Calories, and the Calories from fat in each serving. If a person eats twice the standard serving, he or she is consuming twice the number of Calories listed.

The next section of the Nutrition Facts panel lists the amounts of nutrients contained in a serving and, for most, the amount they provide as a percentage of the **Daily Value**. The % Daily Value is the amount of a nutrient in a food as a percentage of the Daily Value recommended for a 2000-Calorie diet. For example, if a food provides 10% of the Daily Value for vitamin C, it provides 10% of the recommended daily intake for vitamin C in a 2000-Calorie diet (see Appendix F). Because a Daily Value is a single standard for all consumers, it may overestimate the amount of a nutrient needed for some population groups, but it does not underestimate the requirement for any group except pregnant and lactating women.

> **Daily Value**
> A reference value for the intake of nutrients used on food labels to help consumers see how a given food fits into their overall diet.

Ingredient List

Do you want to know exactly what goes into your food? The ingredient list is the place to look. The ingredient list presents the contents of the product in order of their prominence by weight. This information can be very helpful to consumers who are allergic to nuts, trying to avoid animal products, or just curious about what is in the food they eat.

An ingredient list is required on all products containing more than one ingredient and optional on products that contain a single ingredient. Food additives, including food colors and flavorings, must be listed among the ingredients.

B Raw fruits, vegetables, fish, meat, and poultry are not required to carry individual labels. However, grocery stores are asked to provide nutrition information voluntarily for the raw foods most frequently eaten in the United States. The information can appear on large placards or in consumer pamphlets or brochures. ▼

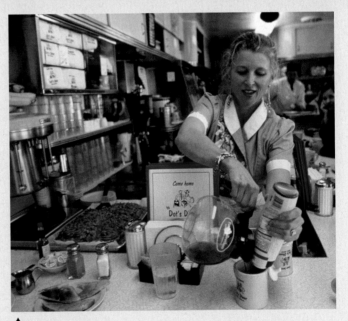

▲

C Food served in restaurants and other eating establishments, such as delicatessens and bakeries, is not required to carry labels. However, if a claim is made about a food's nutritional content or health benefits, such as "low-fat" or "heart healthy," the eating establishment must provide nutritional information about that food, if requested.[7]

Nutrient content and health claims

Looking for low-fat or high-fiber foods (see the *Case Study*)? You may not even need to look at the Nutrition Facts. Food labels often contain **nutrient content claims**. These are statements that highlight specific characteristics of a product that might be of interest to consumers, such as "fat free" or "low sodium." Standard definitions for these descriptors have been established by the Food and Drug Administration (FDA) (see TABLE 2.2 and Appendix F).

Because of the importance of many types of foods in disease prevention, food labels are permitted to include a number of **health claims**. Health claims refer to a relationship between a nutrient, food, food component, or dietary supplement and reduced risk of a disease or health-related condition. All health claims are reviewed by the FDA. To carry a health claim, a food must be a naturally good source of one of six nutrients (vitamin A, vitamin C, protein, calcium, iron, or fiber) and must not

Nutrient content claims[8] TABLE 2.2	
Claim	**Description**
Free	Used on products that contain no amount of, or a trivial amount of, fat, saturated fat, cholesterol, sodium, sugars, or calories. For example, "sugar free" and "fat free" both mean <0.5 g per serving. Synonyms for *free* include *without*, *no*, and *zero*.
Low	Used for foods that can be eaten frequently without exceeding the Daily Value for fat, saturated fat, cholesterol, sodium, or calories. Specific definitions have been established for each of these nutrients. For example, *low-fat* means that the food contains ≤3 g of fat per serving, and *low cholesterol* means that the food contains ≤20 mg of cholesterol per serving. Synonyms for *low* include *little*, *few*, and *low source of*.
Lean and extra lean	Used to describe the fat content of meat, poultry, seafood, and game meats. *Lean* means that the food contains <10 g fat, ≤4.5 g saturated fat, and <95 mg of cholesterol per serving and per 100 g. *Extra lean* is defined as containing <5 g fat, <2 g saturated fat, and <95 mg of cholesterol per serving and per 100 g.
High	Used for foods that contain 20% or more of the Daily Value for a particular nutrient. Synonyms for *high* include *rich in* and *excellent source of*.
Good source	Used for foods that contain 10 to 19% of the Daily Value for a particular nutrient per serving.
Reduced	Used on nutritionally altered products that contain 25% less of a nutrient or energy than the regular or reference product.
Less	Used on foods, whether altered or not, that contain 25% less of a nutrient or energy than the reference food. For example, pretzels may claim to have "less fat" than potato chips. *Fewer* may be used as a synonym for *less*.
Light	Used in different ways. First, it can be used on a nutritionally altered product that contains one-third fewer calories or half the fat of a reference food. Second, it can be used when the sodium content of a low-calorie, low-fat food has been reduced by 50%. The term *light* can be used to describe properties such as texture and color as long as the label explains the intent—for example, "light and fluffy."
More	Used when a serving of food, whether altered or not, contains a nutrient in an amount that is at least 10% of the Daily Value more than the reference food. Synonyms for *more* are *fortified*, *enriched*, and *added*.
Healthy	Used to describe foods that are low in fat and saturated fat, contain limited amounts of sodium and cholesterol, and provide at least 10% of the Daily Value for vitamins A or C, or iron, calcium, protein, or fiber.
Fresh	Used on foods that are raw and have never been frozen or heated and contain no preservatives.

USING FOOD LABELS TO MAKE HEALTHY CHOICES

Scott is trying to improve his nutritional health. He has visited the MyPyramid Web site and now knows how much food he should choose from each food group, but he sometimes has trouble making decisions when shopping for food.

For breakfast he likes hot or cold cereal. Whether he eats oatmeal or granola, it is a serving from the grains group.

Use the labels shown here to determine whether they are equivalent in terms of the amounts of saturated fat and added sugar.

Old Fashioned Oats

Nutrition Facts

Serving Size 1/2 cup (40g) dry
Servings Per Container about 13

Amount Per Serving	Dry	Cereal with 1/2 cup Skim Milk
Calories	150	190
Calories from Fat	25	30

	% Daily Value**	
Total Fat 3g	5%	5%
Saturated Fat 0.5g	3%	3%
Trans Fat 0g		
Cholesterol 0mg	0%	0%
Sodium 0mg	0%	3%
Total Carbohydrate 27g	9%	11%
Dietary Fiber 4g	16%	16%
Sugars 0g		
Protein 5g		

Natural Granola

Nutrition Facts

Serving Size 1/2 cup (51g)
Servings Per Container about 16

Amount Per Serving
Calories 230   Calories from Fat 80

	% Daily Value*
Total Fat 9g	13%
Saturated Fat 3.5g	18%
Trans Fat 1g	
Polyunsaturated Fat 1g	
Monounsaturated Fat 4g	
Cholesterol 0mg	0%
Sodium 20mg	1%
Potassium 250mg	7%
Total Carbohydrate 34g	11%
Other Carbohydrate 15g	
Dietary Fiber 3g	13%
Sugars 16g	
Protein 5g	

Your answer:

Scott likes to have juice with his breakfast. He is deciding between plain orange juice and the less expensive juice drink, which claims to be an excellent source of vitamin C.

How much of the sugar in the orange juice is added?

Your answer:

The only ingredients in the ingredient list are water and concentrated orange juice. This tells Scott that no sugar has been added. The 22 grams of sugars listed in the Nutrition Facts panel all come from the sugar found naturally in oranges.

Orange Juice

Nutrition Facts

Serving Size 8 fl oz (240.0 g)

Amount Per Serving
Calories 110

	% Daily Value*
Sodium 0mg	0%
Total Carbohydrates 26.0g	9%
Sugars 22.0g	

Vitamin A 0%	•	Vitamin C 120%
Calcium 2%	•	Iron 0%

* Based on a 2000 calorie diet

Ingredients: Water, concentrated orange juice

Juice Drink

Nutrition Facts

Serving Size 8 fl oz (240.0 g)

Amount Per Serving
Calories 120

	% Daily Value*
Sodium 160mg	7%
Total Carbohydrates 29.0g	10%
Sugars 28.0g	

Vitamin A 0%	•	Vitamin C 100%
Calcium 0%	•	Iron 0%

* Based on a 2000 calorie diet

Ingredients: Water, high-fructose corn syrup, pear and grape juice concentrates, citric acid, water extracted orange and pineapple juice concentrates, ascorbic acid (vitamin C), natural flavor

Which choice provides more vitamin C?

Your answer:

Other than water, what is the most abundant ingredient, by weight, in the juice drink? in the orange juice?

Your answer:

The added vitamin C increases the nutrient density of the juice drink, but does that make it a better choice than the orange juice?

Your answer:

When Scott is choosing between more- and less-processed products, what advice would you give him?

Your answer:

(Check your answers in Appendix K.)

contain more than 20% of the Daily Value for fat, saturated fat, cholesterol, or sodium. Approved health claims are supported by strong scientific evidence (**FIGURE 2.13** and Appendix F). Health claims for which there is emerging but not well-established evidence are called **qualified health claims**, and such a claim must be accompanied by an explanatory statement to avoid misleading consumers.

DIETARY SUPPLEMENT LABELS

Products ranging from multivitamin pills to protein powders and herbal elixirs all meet the definition of a dietary supplement. These products are considered foods, not drugs, and therefore are regulated by the laws that govern food safety and labeling. To help consumers understand what they are choosing when they purchase these products, dietary supplements are required to carry a **Supplement Facts** panel similar to the Nutrition Facts panel found on food labels (**FIGURE 2.14**).[9]

Health claims FIGURE 2.13

Oatmeal helps reduce cholesterol

Old Fashion Oatmeal

Made from 100% rolled oats

4 grams of soluble fiber from oatmeal daily in a diet low in saturated fat and cholesterol may reduce the risk of heart disease

Oatmeal contains enough soluble fiber to be permitted to include this health claim about the relationship between soluble fiber and the risk of heart disease. Other health claims focus on relationships such as those between sodium and high blood pressure, dietary fat and cancer, saturated fat and cholesterol and heart disease, calcium and reduced risk of osteoporosis, and fruits and vegetables and reduced risk of cancer (see Appendix F).[8]

Dietary supplement label FIGURE 2.14

Unlike food labels, dietary supplement labels must provide directions for use and must provide information about ingredients that are not nutrients and for which Daily Values have not been established. For such ingredients, it is difficult to tell from the label whether the amount included in a serving is helpful, is harmful, or has no effect at all.

The serving size tells you the recommended dose.

SUGGESTED USE: Take 3 capsules daily with meals.

Supplement Facts

Serving Size 3 Capsules   Servings Per Container 33

	Amount Per Serving	% Daily Value*
Calories	20	
Calories from Fat	20	
Total Fat	2 g	3%
Total Omega-3 Fatty Acids	1100 mg	
EPA (Eicosapentaenoic Acid)	450 mg	†
DHA (Docosahexaenoic Acid)	500 mg	†
DPA (Docosapentaenoic Acid)	60 mg	†
Stearidonic, Eicosatrienoic, Eicosatetraenoic, Heneicosapentaenoic, and Alpha-Linolenic Acids	90 mg	†

* Percent Daily Values are based on 2,000 calorie diet
† Daily Value not established

INGREDIENTS: Salmon Oil, UHPO3 Omega-3 Fatty Acid Concentrate (Sardines, Tuna, Anchovies), Gelatin, Glycerin and Water.

Each serving of Fish Oil Omega A–C provides the complete spectrum of healthful Omega-3 fatty acids equivalent to approximately one serving of fresh salmon.

Research shows Omega-3 fatty acids play a role in the health and function of the cardiovascular system, central nervous system, vision, connective tissue, and the inflammatory response.

These statements have not been evaluated by the Food and Drug Administration. This product is not intended to diagnose, treat, cure or prevent any disease.

The name, quantity per serving, and % Daily Values for nutrients are listed. You can use these to assess how that amount compares to the recommended intake and UL for each nutrient. Nutrients with Daily Values are listed first, followed by ingredients without Daily Values.

All ingredients must be listed on the label either in the Supplement Facts panel or in the ingredient list below the panel. Ingredients are listed in descending order of prominence.

All these products must include the words *dietary supplement* on the label.

Because structure/function claims are based on the manufacturer's interpretation and are not approved by the FDA, products with these claims must include this disclaimer.

Labels on dietary supplements may also include nutrient content claims and FDA-approved health claims similar to those on food labels. For example, a product can claim to be an excellent source of a particular nutrient. This means that one serving of the product contains at least 20% of the Daily Value for that nutrient. A label that says "high potency" means that one serving provides 100% or more of the Daily Value for the nutrient it contains. For multinutrient products, high potency means that a serving provides more than 100% of the Daily Value for two-thirds of the vitamins and minerals present.

Dietary supplement labels may also carry **structure/function claims**, which describe the role of a dietary ingredient in maintaining normal structure, function, or general well-being. For example, a structure/function claim about calcium may state that "calcium builds strong bones"; one about fiber may say "fiber maintains bowel regularity." These statements can be misleading. For example, the health claim "lowers cholesterol" requires FDA approval, but the structure/function claim "helps maintain normal cholesterol levels" does not. It would not be unreasonable for consumers with high cholesterol to conclude that a product that "helps maintain normal cholesterol levels" would help lower their elevated blood cholesterol level to within the normal range.

Manufacturers must notify the FDA when including a structure/function claim on a dietary supplement label and are responsible for ensuring the accuracy and truthfulness of these claims. Structure/function claims are not approved by the FDA. For this reason, the law says that if a dietary supplement label includes such a claim, it must state in a disclaimer that the FDA has not evaluated the claim. The disclaimer must also state that the dietary supplement product is not intended to "diagnose, treat, cure or prevent any disease" because only a drug can legally make such a claim (Figure 2.14). Structure/function claims may also appear on food labels, but the FDA does not require conventional food manufactures to notify them about their structure/function claims, and disclaimers are not required.

CONCEPT CHECK STOP

Why are serving sizes standardized on food labels?

Where should you look to see if a food contains nuts?

What food label information helps you find foods that are low in saturated fat and cholesterol?

How can structure/function claims on dietary supplement labels be misleading?

FOOD DIARY

Record all the food and beverages you eat. Include the food, how it was prepared, the amount you ate and the brand name. Don't forget to list all fats used in cooking and all spreads and sauces added.

Time	Food	Kind and how prepared	Amount
7:00 A.M.	Eggs	scrambled	2
	Butter	in eggs	1 tsp.
	toast	whole wheat	2 slices
	Butter	on toast	2 tsp.
	Milk	non-fat	8 oz.
	Orange juice	from frozen concentrate	8 oz.
12:00 P.M.	Big Mac	McDonald's	1

SUMMARY

1 Nutrition Recommendations

1. Nutrition recommendations are designed to encourage consumption of a diet that promotes health and prevents disease. Some of the earliest nutrition recommendations in the United States were in the form of **food guides**, which translate nutrient intake recommendations into food intake recommendations. The first set of Recommended Dietary Allowances, developed during World War II, focused on energy and the nutrients most likely to be deficient in a typical diet. Current recommendations focus on promoting health and preventing chronic disease as well as nutrient deficiencies.

2. Dietary recommendations can be used as a standard for assessing the **nutritional status** of individuals and of populations. Records of dietary intake along with information obtained from a physical examination, a medical history, and laboratory tests can be used to assess an individual's nutritional status.

Collecting information about the food intake and health of individuals in the population or surveying the foods available can help identify potential and actual nutrient deficiencies and excesses within a population and help policymakers develop improved nutrition recommendations.

2 Dietary Reference Intakes (DRIs)

1. **Dietary Reference Intakes (DRIS)** are recommendations for the amounts of energy, nutrients, and other food components that should be consumed by healthy people to promote health, reduce the incidence of chronic disease, and prevent deficiencies. **Estimated Average Requirements (EARs)** can be used to evaluate the adequacy of a population's nutrient intake. **Recommended Dietary Allowances (RDAs)** and **Adequate Intakes (AIs)** can be used by individuals as a goal for nutrient intake, and **Tolerable Upper Intake Levels (ULs)** indicate a safe upper intake limit.

2. The DRIs make two types of energy-intake recommendations. **Estimated Energy Requirements (EERs)** provide an estimate of how many calories are needed to maintain body weight. **Acceptable Macronutrient Distribution Ranges (AMDRs)** make recommendations about the proportion of energy that should come from carbohydrate, fat, and protein in a healthy diet.

3 Tools for Diet Planning

1. The *Dietary Guidelines for Americans* are a set of diet and lifestyle recommendations designed to promote health and reduce the risk of chronic disease in the population. They recommend choosing nutrient-dense foods; balancing calorie intake and exercise; limiting intake of saturated fat, *trans* fat, cholesterol, salt, added sugar, and alcohol; and taking steps to keep food safe.

2. **MyPyramid** is the USDA's current food guide. It recommends amounts from five food groups plus oils, based on individual energy needs. It also makes recommendations about the number of **discretionary calories** allowed in an individual's diet. MyPyramid stresses using variety, proportionality, and moderation in choosing a healthy diet and promotes the physical activity recommendations included in the Dietary Guidelines.

3. **Exchange lists** are a food group system used to plan individual diets that provide specific amounts of energy, carbohydrate, protein, and fat.

4 Food and Supplement Labels

1. Standardized food labels are designed to help consumers make healthy food choices by providing information about the nutrient composition of foods and about how a food fits into the overall diet. The **Nutrition Facts** panel presents information about the amount of various nutrients in a standard serving. For most nutrients, the amount is also given as a percent of the **Daily Value**. A food label's ingredient list lists the contents of the product in order of prominence by weight. Food labels often include FDA defined **nutrient content claims**, such as "low fat" or "high fiber," and **health claims**, which refer to a relationship between a nutrient, food, food component, or dietary supplement and the risk of a particular disease or health-related condition. All health claims are reviewed by the FDA and permitted only when they are supported by scientific evidence, but the level of scientific support for such claims varies.

2. A **Supplement Facts** panel appears on the label of every dietary supplement. When dietary supplement labels include a **structure/function claim**, which describes the role of a nutrient or dietary ingredient in maintaining normal structure or function in humans, it must be accompanied by a disclaimer.

Oatmeal helps reduce cholesterol

Old Fashion Oatmeal

Made from 100% rolled oats

4 grams of soluble fiber from oatmeal daily in a diet low in saturated fat and cholesterol may reduce the risk of heart disease

KEY TERMS

CRITICAL AND CREATIVE THINKING QUESTIONS

1. The Dietary Guidelines recommend reducing serving sizes to keep weight in a healthy range, limiting salt intake to prevent high blood pressure, limiting dietary cholesterol and saturated fat to reduce the risk of heart disease, and limiting added sugar to increase the nutrient density of the diet. Suggest some changes that the food industry could implement to support these nutrition recommendations.

2. Keep a food diary of everything you eat for a day. Go to www.mypyramid.gov and look up the MyPyramid recommendations for a person of your age, gender, and activity level. Now use the MyPyramid Menu Planner to compare your intake with your MyPyramid plan.

3. If a food record indicates that Gina consumes less than the RDA for vitamin C and more than the RDA for vitamin A, what does this mean in terms of her nutritional status? Does she have a vitamin C deficiency? Is she at risk of vitamin A toxicity? What other factors need to be considered before you can draw any conclusions about her nutritional status?

4. If a survey indicates that the consumption of red meat, which is an excellent source of iron, has been declining over the past five years, what can be concluded about the iron intake of the population during that period? How might this decline affect public health? How might it affect public health policy?

5. Select three packaged foods that have food labels. What is the percentage of calories from fat in each product? How many grams of carbohydrate, fat, and fiber are in a serving of each? How does each product fit into your daily diet with regard to total carbohydrate recommended? total fat? dietary fiber? If you consumed a serving of each of these three foods, how much more saturated fat could you consume during the day without exceeding the recommendations? How much more total carbohydrate and fiber should you consume that day to meet recommendations for a 2000-Calorie diet?

6. Maryellen is trying to increase her intake of calcium and vitamin D by taking a dietary supplement. How can she determine whether it contains enough of these nutrients to meet her needs but not so much that it will cause toxicity? If the product claims to build strong bones, does this mean that it will help reverse Maryellen's osteoporosis? Why or why not?

What is happening in this picture ?

This man is snacking on chips while watching television.

Why might he consume a larger portion than he plans to?

The label on the bag says that a serving consists of about 20 chips. The bag contains 11 servings, and each serving provides 150 Calories.

If the man eats half the bag, how many Calories will he have ingested?

How might he moderate his portion size without counting every chip he eats?

SELF-TEST

(Check your answers in Appendix L.)

1. Which DRI standards can be used as goals for individual intake?

    a. AIs
    b. RDAs
    c. EARs
    d. A and B only

2. Based on this graph, showing one day's intake of selected nutrients, which of these statements about this person's nutrient intake is true?

Nutrient	Percent of recommendation 0% 50% 100%
Vitamin A	75%
Vitamin C	115%
Iron	54%
Calcium	75%
Saturated fat	134%

    a. She has an iron deficiency.
    b. She consumes the recommended amount of vitamin A.
    c. If she consumes this amount of iron every day, she is at risk for iron deficiency.
    d. She has osteoporosis.

3. Which DRI standard can help you determine whether a supplement contains a toxic level of a nutrient?

    a. RDA   c. EAR
    b. AI   d. UL

4. Which letter labels the DRI standard that represents the average needs of the population?

    a. A
    b. B
    c. C
    d. None of the above is correct.

5. Which of the following statements is false?

    a. An EER value gives the amount of energy needed to maintain body weight.
    b. Your EER stays the same when you gain weight.
    c. If you consume more calories than your EER, you will gain weight.
    d. Your EER depends on your age, gender, weight, height, and activity level.

6. Use this label to determine which of the following statements about the amount of saturated fat in this product is true.

Nutrition Facts	
Serving Size 1 cup (228g)	
Servings Per Container 2	

Amount Per Serving	
Calories 250	**Calories from Fat** 110

	% Daily Value*
Total Fat 12g	18%
Saturated Fat 3g	15%
Trans Fat 1.5g	
Cholesterol 30mg	10%
Sodium 470mg	20%
Total Carbohydrate 31g	10%
Dietary Fiber 0g	0%
Sugars 5g	
Protein 5g	

Vitamin A	4%
Vitamin C	2%
Calcium	20%
Iron	4%

* Percent Daily Values are based on a 2,000 calorie diet. Your daily values may be higher or lower depending on your calorie needs:

	Calories:	2,000	2,500
Total Fat	Less than	65g	80g
Sat. Fat	Less than	20g	25g
Cholesterol	Less than	300mg	300mg
Sodium	Less than	2,400mg	2,400mg
Total Carbohydrate		300g	375g
Dietary Fiber		25g	30g

    a. This product contains 15% of the maximum daily recommended amount of saturated fat.
    b. This product is high in saturated fat.
    c. To meet nutritional needs, the other foods you consume during the day should provide 17 g of saturated fat.
    d. This product is low in saturated fat.

7. The different colors of the triangles that make up MyPyramid are designed to illustrate that _____.

    a. a variety of foods are needed to make up a healthy diet

    b. we need more of some food groups than others to make up a healthy diet

    c. there are foods within each food group that should be chosen more often than others

    d. exercise is important for a healthy lifestyle

8. Which of these foods is highest in discretionary calories?

    a. an apple

    b. a tablespoon of olive oil

    c. a slice of whole-wheat bread

    d. a doughnut

9. In which order are the ingredients listed on a food label?

    a. alphabetical

    b. from largest to smallest, by volume

    c. from largest to smallest, by weight

    d. dry ingredients first, followed by liquid ingredients

10. Which of the following statements is an invalid interpretation of this graph showing trends in milk consumption?

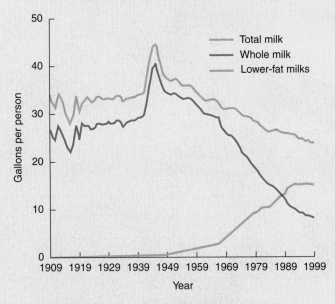

    a. People drank more milk in 1949 than in 1999.

    b. People drank more low-fat milk in 1999 than in 1949.

    c. Children drank less milk in 1999 than in 1949.

    d. Total consumption of whole milk declined between 1949 and 1999

11. Which of the following is stressed by the Dietary Guidelines?

    a. Choose nutrient-dense foods.

    b. Balance food intake with physical activity.

    c. Limit nutrients that are associated with an increased risk of chronic disease.

    d. Handle food safely to prevent food-borne illness.

    e. All of the above

12. Which of the following is used to assess nutritional status?

    a. nutritional analysis of the diet

    b. measurements of body dimensions

    c. medical history and physical examination

    d. laboratory tests

    e. All of the above

13. Which of the following is a structure/function claim?

    a. Fiber maintains bowel regularity.

    b. Soluble fiber helps reduce the risk of heart disease.

    c. Calcium helps reduce the risk of osteoporosis.

    d. Diets that are low in sodium can reduce the risk of high blood pressure.

14. What is meant by nutritional status?

    a. how healthy a person's diet is relative to that of his or her peer group

    b. the measure of a person's health in terms of his or her intake and utilization of nutrients

    c. a person's blood values relative to normal levels

    d. the quality of foods a family is able to afford

15. Which of the following is *not* a food group in MyPyramid?

    a. milk

    b. meat and beans

    c. vegetables

    d. fats and sweets

Digestion: From Meals to Molecules 3

The human body has been compared to a car: We fill the tank of our car with gasoline to get down the highway; we fill our body with food to get on with life. In both "machines," combustion with oxygen releases energy. In a car's engine, the explosion releasing the energy is contained within a cylinder. In a human, the energy is released by reactions within a living cell.

Our bodies are machine-like in another way as well: They are virtually identical to one another. Like cars, we look different on the outside but are the same on the inside. The processes that drive us—like the internal combustion engine, no matter where it's manufactured—are more similar than different because they are based on the same fundamental chemical reactions.

Despite the similarities, however, there are differences between human bodies and machines. An automobile cannot use gasoline to heal itself or to grow, as we do with nutrients. Although a gas tank and a stomach both store fuel, gasoline travels unchanged through the fuel line to the engine, whereas in humans the digestive system must break down the "fuel" into smaller units *before* it can be used by the body. Cars are fueled only by gasoline, but the human digestive system must process fuel from many sources for use by the "high-performance machine" that is the human body.

NATIONAL GEOGRAPHIC

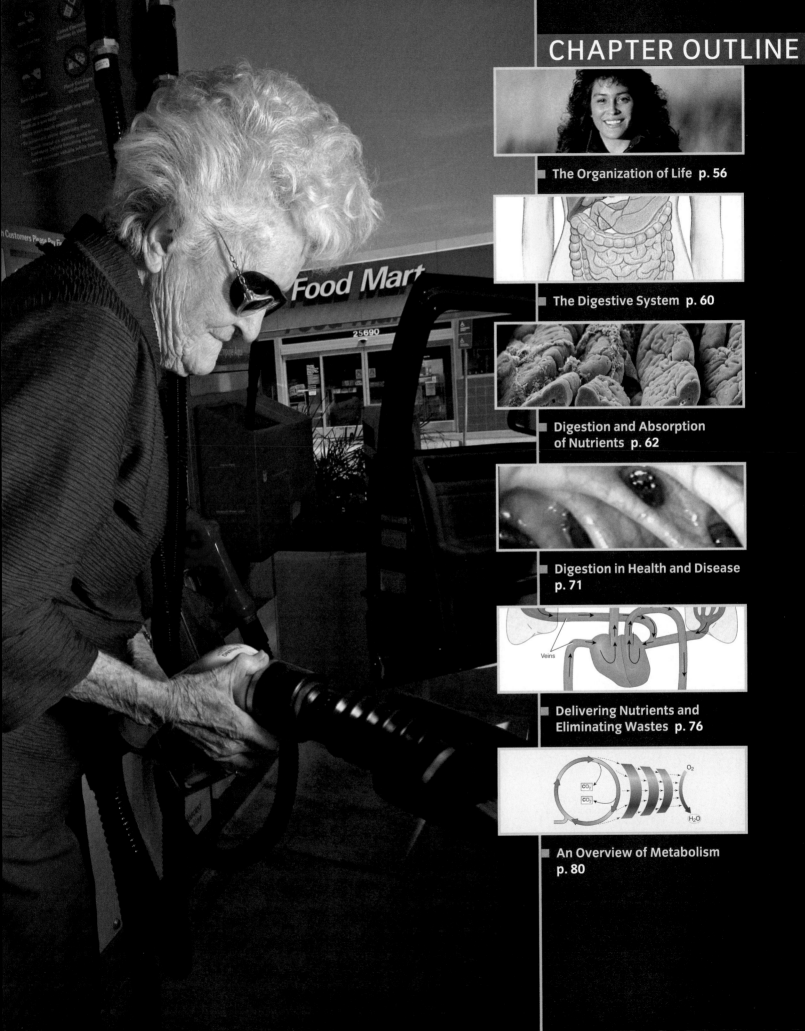

The Organization of Life

LEARNING OBJECTIVES

Describe the organization of living things, from atoms to organisms.

Name the organ systems that work with the digestive system to deliver nutrients and eliminate wastes.

M atter, be it a meal you are about to eat or the plate you are about to eat it from, is made up of **atoms** (FIGURE 3.1). Atoms combine to form **molecules**, which can have different properties from those of the atoms they contain. In any living sys-

atoms The smallest units of an element that retain the properties of the element.

tem, the molecules are organized into **cells**, the smallest units of life. Cells that are similar in structure and function form **tissues**. The human body contains four types of tissue: muscle, nerve, epithelial, and connective. These tissues are organized in vary-

molecules Units of two or more atoms of the same or different elements bonded together.

cells The basic structural and functional units of living things.

Process Diagram

From atoms to organisms FIGURE 3.1

The organization of life begins with atoms that form molecules, which are then organized into cells to form tissues, organs, and whole organisms.

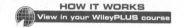
HOW IT WORKS
View in your WileyPLUS course

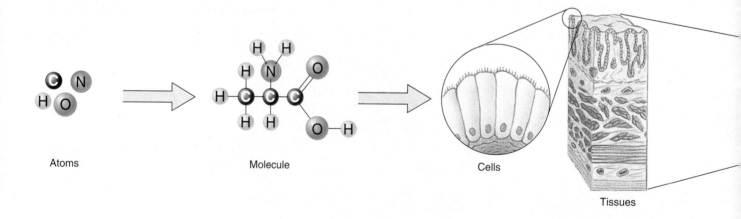

Atoms   Molecule   Cells

Tissues

1 Atoms linked by chemical bonds form molecules.

2 Molecules form the structures that make up cells. Each cell is bounded by a membrane. In multicellular organisms, cells are usually specialized to perform specific functions.

3 Groups of similar cells form tissues. The tissue layers shown here make up the stomach wall.

organs Discrete structures composed of more than one tissue that perform a specialized function.

hormones Chemical messengers that are produced in one location in the body, released into the blood, and travel to other locations, where they elicit responses.

ing combinations to form **organs**. Most organs do not function alone but are part of an **organ system** (FIGURE 3.2 on the next page). Moreover, an organ may be part of more than one organ system. For example, the pancreas is part of the endocrine system and also part of the digestive system.

The body's 11 organ systems interact to perform all the functions necessary for life. For example, the digestive system, which is the primary organ system responsible for moving nutrients into the body, is assisted by the endocrine system, which secretes **hormones** that help regulate how much we eat and how quickly food and nutrients travel through the digestive system. The digestive system is also aided by the nervous system, which sends nerve signals that help control the passage of food through the digestive tract; by the cardiovascular system, which transports nutrients to individual cells in the body; and by the urinary, respiratory, and integumentary systems, which eliminate wastes generated in the body.

CONCEPT CHECK STOP

HOW are atoms, molecules, and cells related to one another?

HOW do the endocrine and nervous systems interact with the digestive system?

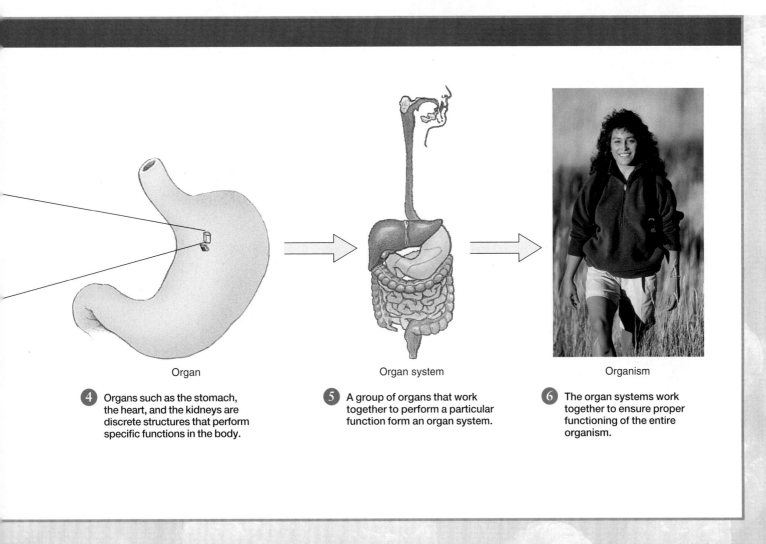

Organ

④ Organs such as the stomach, the heart, and the kidneys are discrete structures that perform specific functions in the body.

Organ system

⑤ A group of organs that work together to perform a particular function form an organ system.

Organism

⑥ The organ systems work together to ensure proper functioning of the entire organism.

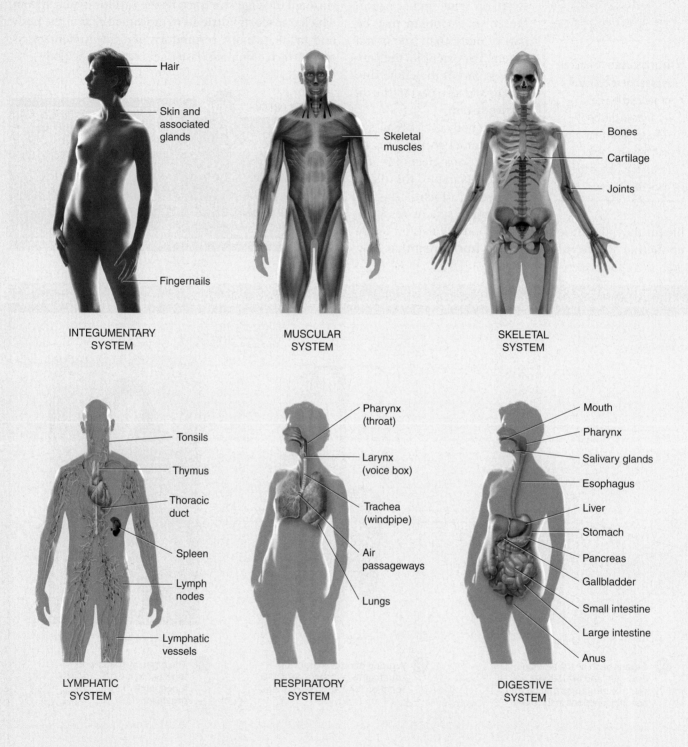

INTEGUMENTARY
SYSTEM

- Hair
- Skin and associated glands
- Fingernails

MUSCULAR
SYSTEM

- Skeletal muscles

SKELETAL
SYSTEM

- Bones
- Cartilage
- Joints

LYMPHATIC
SYSTEM

- Tonsils
- Thymus
- Thoracic duct
- Spleen
- Lymph nodes
- Lymphatic vessels

RESPIRATORY
SYSTEM

- Pharynx (throat)
- Larynx (voice box)
- Trachea (windpipe)
- Air passageways
- Lungs

DIGESTIVE
SYSTEM

- Mouth
- Pharynx
- Salivary glands
- Esophagus
- Liver
- Stomach
- Pancreas
- Gallbladder
- Small intestine
- Large intestine
- Anus

NERVOUS
SYSTEM

- Brain
- Spinal cord
- Nerves

ENDOCRINE
SYSTEM

- Pineal gland
- Pituitary gland
- Thyroid gland
- Thymus
- Pancreas
- Adrenal glands
- Ovaries
- Testes

CIRCULATORY
SYSTEM

- Arteries
- Veins
- Heart

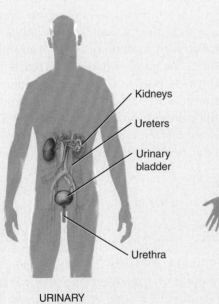

URINARY
SYSTEM

- Kidneys
- Ureters
- Urinary bladder
- Urethra

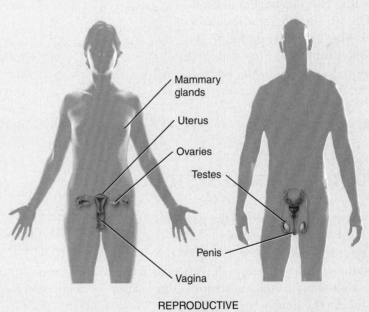

REPRODUCTIVE
SYSTEM

- Mammary glands
- Uterus
- Ovaries
- Testes
- Penis
- Vagina

The Organization of Life   59

The Digestive System

LEARNING OBJECTIVES

Define digestion and absorption.

List the organs that make up the digestive system.

Describe the tissues that make up the wall of the gastrointestinal tract.

Explain the roles of mucus, enzymes, nerves, and hormones in digestion.

The digestive system is the organ system that is primarily responsible for **digestion** and for the **absorption** of nutrients into the body. When you eat a taco, for example, the tortilla, meat, cheese, lettuce, and tomato are broken apart, releasing the nutrients and other food components they contain. Water, vitamins, and minerals are taken into the body without being broken into smaller units, but proteins, carbohydrates, and fats must be digested further. Proteins are broken down into amino acids, most of the carbohydrate is broken down into sugars, and most fats are digested to produce molecules with long carbon chains called **fatty acids**. The sugars, amino acids, and fatty acids can then be absorbed into the body. The fiber in whole grains, fruits, and vegetables cannot be digested and therefore is not absorbed into the body. It and other unabsorbed substances pass through the digestive tract and are eliminated in **feces**.

digestion The process by which food is broken down into components small enough to be absorbed into the body.

absorption The process of taking substances from the gastrointestinal tract into the interior of the body.

feces Body waste, including unabsorbed food residue, bacteria, mucus, and dead cells, which is eliminated from the gastrointestinal tract by way of the anus.

ing your blood or cells. Only after substances have been absorbed into the cells that line the intestine can they be said to be inside the body.

The lumen is lined with a layer of **mucosal cells** called the **mucosa**. Because mucosal cells are in direct contact with churning food and harsh digestive secretions, they live only about two to five days. The dead cells are sloughed off into the lumen, where some components are digested and absorbed and the rest are eliminated in feces. New mucosal cells are formed continuously to replace those that die. To allow for this rapid replacement, the mucosa has high nutrient requirements and is one of the first parts of the body to be affected by nutrient deficiencies.

The time it takes food to travel the length of the GI tract from mouth to anus is called the **transit time**. The shorter the transit time, the more rapidly material is passing through the digestive tract. In a healthy adult, transit time is 24 to 72 hours, depending on the composition of the individual's diet and his or her level of physical activity, emotional state, health status, and use of medications.

ORGANS OF THE DIGESTIVE SYSTEM

The digestive system is composed of the **gastrointestinal tract** and accessory organs (FIGURE 3.3A). The gastrointestinal tract is a hollow tube, about 30 feet long, that runs from the mouth to the anus. It is also called the gut, GI tract, alimentary canal, or digestive tract. The inside of the tube is the **lumen** (FIGURE 3.3B). Food in the lumen is not technically inside the body because it has not been absorbed. When you swallow something that cannot be digested, such as a whole sesame seed or an unpopped kernel of popcorn, it passes through your digestive tract and exits in the feces without ever enter-

DIGESTIVE SYSTEM SECRETIONS

Digestion is aided by substances secreted into the digestive tract from cells in the mucosa and from a number of accessory organs. One of these substances is **mucus**, which moistens, lubricates, and protects the digestive tract.

mucus A viscous fluid secreted by glands in the digestive tract and other parts of the body. It lubricates, moistens, and protects cells from harsh environments.

Structure of the digestive system FIGURE 3.3

A The digestive system consists of the organs of the digestive tract—mouth, pharynx, esophagus, stomach, small intestine, and large intestine—plus four accessory organs—salivary glands, liver, gallbladder, and pancreas. ▼

Mouth: Chews food and mixes it with saliva

Salivary glands: Produce saliva, which contains a starch-digesting enzyme

Pharynx: Swallows chewed food mixed with saliva

Esophagus: Moves food to the stomach

Stomach: Churns and mixes food; secretes acid and a protein-digesting enzyme

Liver: Makes bile, which aids in digestion and absorption of fat

Pancreas: Releases bicarbonate to neutralize intestinal contents; produces enzymes that digest carbohydrate, protein, and fat

Gallbladder: Stores bile and releases it into the small intestine when needed

Small intestine: Absorbs nutrients into blood or lymph; most digestion occurs here

Large intestine: Absorbs water and some vitamins and minerals; home to intestinal bacteria; passes waste material
- Colon
- Rectum

Anus: Opens to allow waste to leave the body

B This cross-section through the wall of the small intestine reveals the four tissue layers that make up the wall of the gastrointestinal tract. ▼

Contraction of the layers of smooth muscle–over which we do not have voluntary control–helps mix food, break it into small particles, and propel it through the digestive tract.

This external layer of connective tissue provides support and protection.

Lumen

This layer of connective tissue contains nerves and blood vessels. It provides support, nourishes the mucosa, and sends the nerve signals that control secretions and muscle contractions.

The mucosa, which lines the GI tract, is a type of epithelial tissue. Nutrients must pass through these mucosal cells before they can reach the blood or lymph.

Smaller carbohydrate molecules   Large carbohydrate molecule

Enzyme activity FIGURE 3.4

Enzymes are needed to break down different food components. The enzyme shown here, called an *amylase*, breaks large carbohydrate molecules, such as those in bread, into smaller ones. Amylases have no effect on fat, whereas enzymes called *lipases* digest fat and have no effect on carbohydrate.

HOW IT WORKS
View in your WileyPLUS course

> **enzymes** Protein molecules that accelerate the rate of specific chemical reactions without themselves being changed.

Enzymes are also present in digestive system secretions. They accelerate the chemical reactions that break down food into units that can be absorbed (FIGURE 3.4).

The gastrointestinal tract is part of the endocrine system as well as the digestive system. It releases hormones that help prepare different parts of the gut for the arrival of food and thus regulate digestion and the rate at which food moves through the digestive system. Some hormonal signals slow digestion, whereas others facilitate it. For example, when the nutrients from your lunch reach your small intestine, they trigger the release of hormones that signal the pancreas and gallbladder to secrete digestive substances into the small intestine.

CONCEPT CHECK STOP

What happens during digestion and absorption?

Which organs make up the gastrointestinal tract?

What are mucosal cells?

How are enzymes important for digestion and absorption?

Digestion and Absorption of Nutrients

LEARNING OBJECTIVES

Describe what happens in each of the organs of the gastrointestinal tract.

Discuss factors that influence how quickly food moves through the GI tract.

Explain how the structure of the small intestine aids in its function.

Distinguish passive diffusion from active transport.

magine warm slices of freshly baked bread smeared with melting butter. Is your mouth watering? You don't even need to put food in your mouth for activity to begin in the digestive tract. Sensory input alone—the sight of the bread being lifted out of the oven, the smell of the bread, the clatter of the butter knife—may make your mouth water and your stomach begin to secrete digestive substances.

This response occurs when the nervous system signals the digestive system to ready itself for a meal. In order for food to be used by the body, however, you need to do more than smell your meal. The food must be consumed and digested, and the nutrients must be absorbed and transported to the body's cells. This involves the combined functions of all the organs of the digestive system, as well as the help of some other organ systems.

THE MOUTH

Digestion involves chemical and mechanical processes, both of which begin in the mouth. The presence of food in the mouth stimulates the flow of **saliva** from the salivary glands. Saliva moistens the food and carries dissolved food molecules to the taste buds, most of which are located on the tongue. Signals from the taste buds, along with the aroma of food, allow us to enjoy the taste of the food we eat. Saliva contains the enzyme **salivary amylase**, which begins the chemical digestion of food by breaking starch molecules into shorter carbohydrate chains (see Figure 3.4). Saliva also helps protect against tooth decay because it washes away food particles and contains substances that inhibit the growth of bacteria that cause tooth decay.

Chewing food begins the mechanical aspect of digestion. Adult humans have 32 teeth, which are specialized for biting, tearing, grinding, and crushing foods. Chewing breaks food into pieces that are small enough to be swallowed and increases the surface area in contact with digestive juices. The tongue helps mix food with saliva and aids chewing by constantly repositioning food between the teeth. Chewing also breaks up fiber, which traps nutrients. If the fiber is not broken up, some of the nutrients in the food cannot be absorbed. For example, if the fibrous skin of a raisin is not broken open by the teeth, the nutrients inside the raisin remain inaccessible, and the raisin travels, undigested, through the intestines for elimination in the feces.

THE PHARYNX

The **pharynx**, the part of the gastrointestinal tract that is responsible for swallowing, is also part of the respiratory tract. Food passes through the pharynx on its way to the stomach, and air passes through the pharynx on its way to and from the lungs. As we prepare to swallow, the mass of chewed food mixed with saliva, called a **bolus**, is directed to the back of the mouth by the tongue. During swallowing, the air passages are blocked by a valvelike flap of tissue called the **epiglottis** so that food goes to the esophagus and not to the lungs (**FIGURE 3.5A**). Sometimes eating too quickly or talking while eating interferes with the closing of the epiglottis, and food passes into an upper air passageway. This food can usually be dislodged with a cough, but if it becomes stuck and causes choking, it can be forced out by means of the Heimlich maneuver (**FIGURE 3.5B**)

Swallowing and choking FIGURE 3.5

A When a bolus is swallowed, it normally pushes the epiglottis down over the opening to the passageway that leads to the lungs.

Bolus
Pharynx
Epiglottis
Esophagus
Passageway to lungs

Bolus forces epiglottis to cover passageway to lungs

Epiglottis returns to its original position once bolus has passed; airway to lungs reopens

B If food becomes lodged in the passageway leading to the lungs, it can block the flow of air into the lungs. The Heimlich maneuver, which involves a series of thrusts directed upward from under the diaphragm (the muscle separating the chest and abdominal cavities), forces air out of the lungs, blowing the lodged food out of the blocked air passageway.

Diaphragm

THE ESOPHAGUS

The esophagus connects the pharynx with the stomach. In the esophagus, the bolus is moved along by rhythmic contractions of the smooth muscles, an action called **peristalsis** (FIGURE 3.6). The contractions of peristalsis are strong enough so that even if you ate while standing on your head, food would reach your stomach. This contractile movement, which is controlled automatically by the nervous system, occurs throughout the gastrointestinal tract, pushing the bolus along from the pharynx through the large intestine.

To leave the esophagus and enter the stomach, food must pass through a **sphincter**, a muscle that encircles the tube of the digestive tract and acts as a valve. When the sphincter contracts, the valve is closed; when it relaxes, the valve is open (Figure 3.6). The sphincter located between the esophagus and the stomach prevents food from moving from the stomach back into the esophagus, but occasionally stomach contents do move in this direction. This is what occurs with heartburn (as discussed later in this chapter): Some of the acidic stomach contents leak up through this sphincter into the esophagus, causing a burning sensation.

Vomiting is the result of reverse peristalsis. A complex series of signals from the brain causes the sphincter to relax and forces stomach contents upward, out of the stomach and toward the mouth.

Moving food through the GI tract FIGURE 3.6

The food we swallow doesn't just fall down the esophagus and into the stomach. It is pushed along by muscular contractions and enters the stomach in response to the opening and closing of the sphincter located where the esophagus meets the stomach.

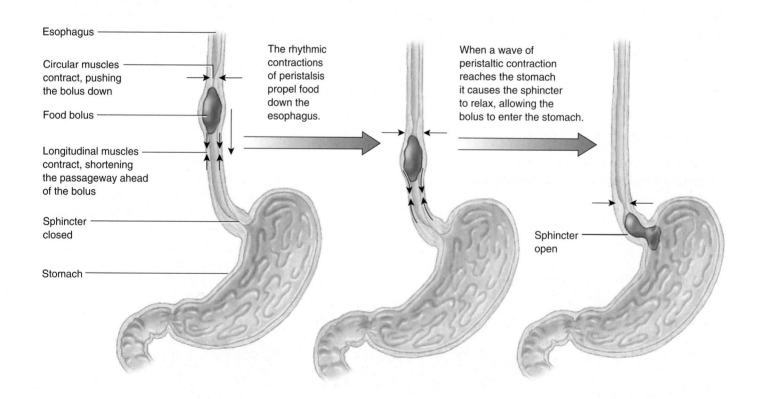

Esophagus

Circular muscles contract, pushing the bolus down

Food bolus

Longitudinal muscles contract, shortening the passageway ahead of the bolus

Sphincter closed

Stomach

The rhythmic contractions of peristalsis propel food down the esophagus.

When a wave of peristaltic contraction reaches the stomach it causes the sphincter to relax, allowing the bolus to enter the stomach.

Sphincter open

A Most of the gastrointestinal tract is surrounded by two layers of smooth muscle, one running longitudinally and one running horizontally, but the stomach contains a third smooth muscle layer running diagonally. The presence of this diagonal layer allows for the powerful contractions that churn and mix the stomach contents. The sphincter at the bottom of the stomach controls the flow of chyme into the small intestine.

B The lining of the stomach is covered with gastric pits. Inside these pits are the gastric glands, made up of different types of cells that produce the mucus, hydrochloric acid (parietal cells), and the inactive form of pepsin (chief cells) contained in gastric juice.

THE STOMACH

The stomach is an expanded portion of the gastrointestinal tract that serves as a temporary storage place for food. Here the bolus is mashed and mixed with highly acidic stomach secretions to form a semiliquid food mass called **chyme**. The mixing of food in the stomach is aided by an extra layer of smooth muscle in the stomach wall (FIGURE 3.7A). Some digestion takes place in the stomach, but, with the exception of some water, alcohol, and a few drugs, such as aspirin and acetaminophen (Tylenol), very little absorption occurs here.

Gastric juice Chemical digestion in the stomach is caused by **gastric juice** produced by gastric glands in pits that dot the stomach lining (FIGURE 3.7B). Gastric juice is a mixture of water, mucus, hydrochloric acid, and an inactive form of the protein-digesting enzyme **pepsin**. This enzyme is secreted in an inactive form so that it will not damage the gastric glands that produce it. The hydrochloric acid in gastric juice kills most of the bacteria present in food. It also stops the activity of the carbohydrate-digesting enzyme salivary amylase and helps begin the digestion of protein by activating pepsin and unfolding proteins. A thick layer of mucus protects the protein that makes up the stomach wall from the hydrochloric acid and pepsin in gastric juice.

The regulation of stomach motility and secretion FIGURE 3.8

 View in your WileyPLUS course

Process Diagram

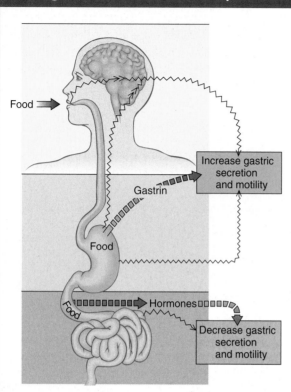

Stomach activity is affected by food that has not yet reached the stomach, by food that is in the stomach, and by food that has left the stomach.

1 Before food enters the stomach, the thought, smell, sight, or taste of food causes the brain to send nerve signals (zig-zag lines) that stimulate gastric secretions and increase the rate of stomach churning or motility, thereby preparing the stomach to receive food.

2 Food entering the stomach increases the rate of gastric secretion and motility by stimulating local nerves, sending signals to the brain, and stimulating the secretion of **gastrin**, a hormone that triggers an increase in the release of gastric juice.

3 Food leaving the stomach and entering the small intestine distends (stretches) the intestine, triggering hormonal and nervous signals that decrease stomach motility and slow the secretion of gastric juice. This ensures that the amount of chyme entering the small intestine does not exceed the intestine's ability to process it.

Regulation of stomach activity How much your stomach churns, how much gastric juice is released, and how fast material empties out of the stomach are regulated by signals from both nerves and hormones. These signals originate from three sites—the brain, the stomach, and the small intestine (**FIGURE 3.8**).

As chyme moves out of the stomach, signals sent by the small intestine help regulate the rate at which the stomach empties. The small intestine stretches as it fills with chyme; this distension inhibits the stomach from emptying. Chyme normally empties from the stomach within two to six hours, but this rate varies with the size and composition of the meal that has been consumed. A large meal takes longer to leave the stomach than does a small meal. Liquids empty quickly; solids, however, linger until they are well mixed with gastric juice and liquefied; hence, solids leave the stomach more slowly than liquids.

The nutritional composition of a meal also affects how long it stays in the stomach. A meal that consists primarily of carbohydrate from starch and sugar leaves quickly, but a meal that is high in fiber or protein takes

longer to leave the stomach. A high-fat meal stays in the stomach the longest. Because the nutrient composition of a meal affects how quickly it leaves your stomach, it affects how soon after eating you will feel hungry again (**FIGURE 3.9**).

Hunger and meal composition FIGURE 3.9

What you choose for breakfast can affect how soon you become hungry for lunch. A small, carbohydrate-rich meal of toast and coffee will leave your stomach far more quickly than a larger meal containing more protein, fiber, and fat, such as a vegetable-and-cheese omelet with whole-wheat toast and butter.

THE SMALL INTESTINE

The small intestine, a narrow tube about 20 feet long, is the main site for the chemical digestion of food, completing the process that the mouth and stomach have started. It is also the primary site for the absorption of water, vitamins, minerals, and the products of carbohydrate, fat, and protein digestion.

The small intestine has a number of unique structural features that contribute to its digestive function and enhance the amount of surface area available for absorption (FIGURE 3.10). Together these features pro-

vide a surface area that is about the size of a tennis court (250 m², or about 2,700 ft²).

Secretions that aid digestion

In the small intestine, secretions from the pancreas, the gallbladder, and the small intestine itself aid digestion. The pancreas secretes **pancreatic juice**, which contains **bicarbonate**, and digestive enzymes. Bicarbonate, which is a base, neutralizes the acid in the chyme, making the environment in the small intestine neutral or slightly basic rather than acidic, as in the stomach. This neutrality allows enzymes from the pancreas and small intestine to function.

Visualizing

The structure of the small intestine FIGURE 3.10

A The wall of the small intestine is arranged in large circular folds, which increase the surface area in contact with nutrients. ▼

SMALL INTESTINE

Large circular folds

Lumen
Microvilli
Mucosal cell
Lacteal
Capillary
Artery
Vein
Lymph vessel

Villi

Microvilli

C Each villus is covered with tiny projections of the mucosal cell membrane called **microvilli**, often referred to as the **brush border**. Some of the digestive enzymes produced by the small intestine are located in the membrane, and some are located inside the mucosal cells.

B The entire inner surface of the ▶ small intestine is covered with fingerlike projections called **villi** (the singular is *villus*). Each villus contains a **capillary** (small blood vessel) and a **lacteal** (small lymph vessel). Nutrients must cross only the single-cell layer of the mucosa to reach the blood or lymph for delivery to the tissues of the body.

Digestion and Absorption of Nutrients   67

Pancreatic amylase is an enzyme that continues the job of breaking down starches into sugars, which was started in the mouth by salivary amylase. Pancreatic **proteases** (protein-digesting enzymes), such as trypsin and chymotrypsin, break protein into shorter and shorter chains of amino acids, and fat-digesting enzymes called **lipases** break down fats into fatty acids. The pancreatic proteases, like the pepsin produced by the stomach, are released in an inactive form so that they will not digest the glands that produce them. Intestinal digestive enzymes, found in the cell membranes or inside the cells lining the small intestine, aid the digestion of double sugars (those containing two sugar units) into single sugar units and the digestion of short amino acid chains into single amino acids. The sugars from carbohydrate digestion and the amino acids from protein digestion pass into the blood and are delivered to the liver (FIGURE 3.11).

Process Diagram

Digestion in the small intestine FIGURE 3.11

Most digestion occurs in the small intestine.

HOW IT WORKS
View in your WileyPLUS course

1 The digestion of starch to double sugars and short glucose chains is completed by the enzyme pancreatic amylase.

2 Fiber, which cannot be digested by human enzymes, passes to the large intestine.

3 Enzymes in the brush border digest double sugars into single sugars, which are absorbed into the blood for transport to the liver.

4 The digestion of proteins into amino acids and short amino acid chains is completed by pancreatic protein-digesting enzymes (proteases).

5 Enzymes in the brush border break short amino acid chains into single amino acids and into chains containing only two or three amino acids. These are absorbed into the mucosal cells where they are digested into single amino acids. The amino acids pass into the blood.

6 Bile helps divide large fat globules. Pancreatic lipases digest the fat molecules into fatty acids and other breakdown products that combine with bile to form small droplets.

7 Small lipid droplets aid the absorption of fatty acids and other fat-soluble substances into the mucosal cell.

8 Absorbed fats are incorporated into transport particles that pass into the lymph.

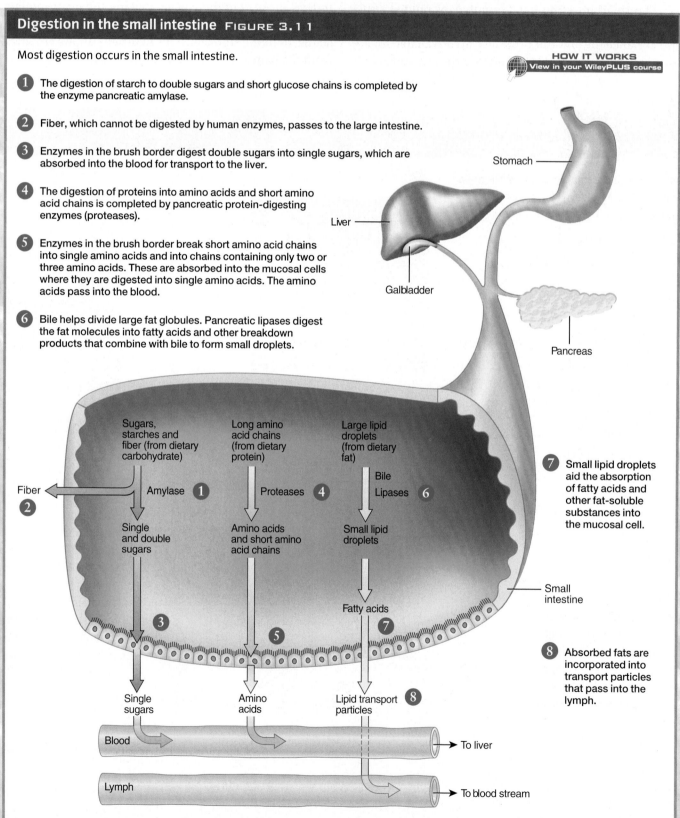

Absorption mechanisms FIGURE 3.12

A In **simple diffusion**, substances pass freely across a cell membrane from an area of higher concentration to an area of lower concentration, and no energy is required. Here the purple balls represent molecules that move by means of simple diffusion. Vitamin E and fatty acids are absorbed by simple diffusion.

B **Osmosis** is the passage of water molecules (purple arrow) from an area with a lower concentration of dissolved substances (blue dots) to an area with a higher concentration of dissolved substances. Water can move both into and out of the lumen of the GI tract by osmosis.

C **Facilitated diffusion** is a type of passive diffusion that requires a carrier molecule. Here the yellow cubes represent molecules that move from an area of higher concentration to an area of lower concentration, with the help of a carrier molecule. The sugar fructose found in fruit is absorbed by facilitated diffusion.

D **Active transport** requires energy and a carrier molecule. The red pyramids represent molecules that are transported from an area of lower concentration to an area of higher concentration. Active transport allows glucose and amino acids to be absorbed even when they are present in higher concentrations in the mucosal cell than in the lumen.

> **bile** A digestive fluid made in the liver and stored in the gallbladder that is released into the small intestine, where it aids in fat digestion and absorption.

The gallbladder stores and secretes **bile**, a substance that is produced in the liver and is necessary for the digestion and absorption of fat. Bile that is secreted into the small intestine mixes with fat and divides it into small globules, allowing lipases to access and digest the fat molecules more efficiently. The bile and digested fats then form small droplets that facilitate the absorption of fat into the mucosal cells. Once inside the mucosal cells, the products of fat digestion are incorporated into transport particles. These are absorbed into the lymph before passing into the blood (Figure 3.11).

Absorption
The small intestine is the main site for the absorption of nutrients. To be absorbed, nutrients must pass from the lumen of the GI tract into the mucosal cells lining the tract and then into either the blood or the lymph. Several different mechanisms are involved (**FIGURE 3.12**). Some rely on **diffusion**, which is the net movement of substances from an area of higher concentration to an area of lower concentration. **Simple diffusion**, in which material moves freely across the cell membrane; **osmosis**, which is the diffusion of water; and **facilitated diffusion**, in which a carrier molecule is needed for the substance to cross the membrane, depend on diffusion and are passive, requiring no energy. **Active transport** requires energy and a carrier molecule. This process can transport material from an area of lower concentration to one of higher concentration.

THE LARGE INTESTINE

Materials not absorbed in the small intestine pass through a sphincter between the small intestine and the large intestine. This sphincter prevents material from the large intestine from reentering the small intestine.

> **simple diffusion** The unassisted diffusion of a substance across the cell membrane.

> **osmosis** The unassisted diffusion of water across the cell membrane.

> **facilitated diffusion** Assisted diffusion of a substance across the cell membrane.

> **active transport** The transport of substances across a cell membrane with the aid of a carrier molecule and the expenditure of energy.

Bacteria on the Menu

The human gut is home to 300 to 500 species of bacteria. The right mix of bacteria is important for immune function, proper growth and development of colon cells, and optimal intestinal motility and transit time.[1] A healthy microflora can inhibit the growth of harmful bacteria and has been shown to prevent the diarrhea associated with antibiotic use and to reduce the duration of diarrhea resulting from intestinal infections and other causes.[2,3] There is also evidence that a healthy microflora may relieve constipation, reduce allergy symptoms, modify the risk of colon cancer, and affect body weight.[4,5,6] Consuming these beneficial bacteria, called **probiotics**, is one way of promoting a healthy microflora. Another way is to consume **prebiotics**, substances that serve as a food supply for beneficial bacteria. Why might consuming a prebiotic increase the numbers of healthy bacteria in the gut?

A Ads claim that eating yogurt will help regulate the digestive system. Consumers see these products as a tasty way to provide nutrients and help regulate digestion.

B Scientists recognize that yogurt contains beneficial bacteria, including *Lactobacillus* and *Bifidobacterium*. When these living microorganisms are consumed in adequate amounts, they live temporarily in the colon where they inhibit the growth of harmful bacteria and confer other health benefits on the host. However, the bacteria must be consumed frequently because they are flushed out in the feces.

● Beneficial bacteria ● Harmful bacteria

Colon mucosa

Without probiotics   With probiotics

The large intestine is about 5 feet long and is divided into the colon, which makes up the majority of the large intestine, and the rectum, the last 8 inches. The large intestine opens to the exterior of the body at the anus. Although most nutrient absorption occurs in the small intestine, water and some vitamins and minerals are also absorbed in the colon.

Peristalsis occurs more slowly in the large intestine than in the small intestine. Water, nutrients, and fecal matter may spend 24 hours in the large intestine, in contrast to the 3 to 5 hours it takes these materials to move through the small intestine. This slow movement favors the growth of bacteria. These bacteria, called the **intestinal microflora**, are permanent, beneficial residents of this part of the gastrointestinal tract (see *What a Scientist Sees*). They break down unabsorbed portions of food, such as fiber, producing nutrients that can be used by the microflora or, in some cases, absorbed into the body. For example, the microflora synthesize small amounts of certain B vitamins and vitamin K, some of which can be absorbed. As the microflora break down material in the colon, they produce gas, which causes flatulence. In a

healthy adult, between 200 and 2000 ml of gas is produced in the intestine each day.

Material that is not absorbed in the colon passes into the rectum, where it is stored temporarily and then evacuated through the anus as feces. The feces are a mixture of undigested, unabsorbed matter, dead cells, secretions from the GI tract, water, and bacteria. The amount of bacteria varies but can make up more than half the weight of the feces. The amount of water in the feces is affected by fiber and fluid intake. Because fiber retains water, when adequate fiber and fluids are consumed, feces have a higher water content and are more easily passed.

CONCEPT CHECK **STOP**

How does food move through the GI tract?

How do the villi and microvilli aid absorption?

What are the functions of the stomach?

Why is active transport needed for the complete absorption of some nutrients?

Digestion in Health and Disease

LEARNING OBJECTIVES

Explain how the gastro-intestinal tract protects us from infection.

Describe the causes of food allergies.

Discuss the causes and consequences of ulcers, heartburn, and GERD.

Explain how dental problems and gallstones might affect food intake.

The health of the GI tract is essential to our overall health. The gut acts as a defense against invasion by disease-causing organisms and other contaminants and allows us to obtain nutrients efficiently. Food allergies, which can be life threatening, have their origins in the GI tract, but most common gastrointestinal problems are minor and do not affect long-term health.

THE DIGESTIVE SYSTEM AND DISEASE PREVENTION

Food almost always contains bacteria and other contaminants, but it rarely makes us sick. This is because the mucosa of the GI tract contains tissue that is part of the immune system (**FIGURE 3.13A**). This tissue prevents disease-causing bacteria and toxins from taking over the GI tract and invading the body.

If an invading substance, or **antigen**, enters the lumen or is absorbed into the mucosa, the immune system can use a number of weapons to destroy it. These include various types of white blood cells, which circulate in the blood and reside in the mucosa of the gastrointestinal tract, where they can quickly destroy most antigens that enter the body through the mucosa.

When an antigen is present, **phagocytes** are the first type of white blood cell to come to the body's defense (**FIGURE 3.13B**). If the invader is not eliminated by the phagocytes, more specific white blood cells called **lymphocytes** join the battle. Some lymphocytes destroy specific antigens by binding to them. This type of lymphocyte helps eliminate cancer cells, foreign tissue, and cells that have been infected by viruses and bacteria. Other lymphocytes produce and secrete protein molecules called **antibodies**. Antibodies bind to antigens and help destroy them. Each antibody is designed to fight off only one type of antigen. Once antibodies to a specific antigen have been made, the immune system remembers and is ready to fight that antigen any time it enters the body again.

If harmful organisms infect the GI tract, the body may help out the immune system by using diarrhea or vomiting to flush them out.

> **antigen** A foreign substance that, when introduced into the body, stimulates an immune response.

> **antibodies** Proteins, released by a type of lymphocyte, that interact with and deactivate specific antigens.

Immune function in the small intestine FIGURE 3.13

HOW IT WORKS
View in your WileyPLUS course

A This immune system tissue embedded throughout the mucosa of the small intestine is called a Peyer's patch. It contains cells that participate in the immune system's efforts to prevent harmful organisms or materials present in the GI tract from making us ill.

B The large cells shown here in yellow are phagocytes, which can engulf and destroy invading substances. The smaller cells shown in blue, are lymphocytes, which are specific with regard to which invaders they can attack. Some lymphocytes directly kill invaders, while others secrete antibodies, which help destroy antigens.

Peyer's patch

Phagocyte

Red blood cell

Lymphocyte

Foods that commonly cause allergic reactions
FIGURE 3.14

Food allergies affect about 2% of adults and 4 to 8% of children and are responsible for 150 deaths in the U.S. each year.[7] To protect consumers, food manufacturers are required to clearly state on the label whether a product contains any of the eight major ingredients that are most likely to cause allergic reactions: peanuts, tree nuts, milk, eggs, fish, shellfish, soy, and wheat.

Our immune system protects us from many invaders without our being aware of it. Unfortunately, the response of the immune system to a foreign substance is also to blame for allergic reactions. An allergic reaction occurs when the immune system produces antibodies to a substance, called an **allergen**, that is present in our diet or environment. **Food allergies** occur when the body sees proteins present in food as foreign substances and therefore initiates an immune response. The immune response causes symptoms that range from hives to life-threatening reactions such as breathing difficulties or a drop in blood pressure.

> **allergen** A substance that causes an allergic reaction.

The first time a food is consumed, it does not trigger an allergic reaction, but in a susceptible person, this first exposure begins the process. As the food is digested, tiny fragments of undigested protein trigger the production of antibodies. When the food protein is eaten again, it binds to the antibodies, signaling the release of chemicals that cause redness, swelling, and other allergy symptoms. When the protein enters the mouth, the allergic person may experience an itching or tingling sensation on the tongue or lips. As the protein travels down to the stomach and intestines, the allergic response may lead to vomiting and cramps. After the protein fragments are absorbed and travel through the blood, they may cause a drop in blood pressure, hives, and breathing difficulties.

The best way to avoid allergy symptoms is to avoid foods to which you are allergic (FIGURE 3.14).

DIGESTIVE SYSTEM PROBLEMS AND DISCOMFORTS

Almost everyone experiences digestive system problems from time to time. These problems often cause discomfort and frequently limit the types of foods the person can consume (FIGURE 3.15A). They also can interfere with nutrient digestion and absorption. Problems may occur anywhere in the digestive tract, from the mouth to the anus, and can affect the accessory organs that provide the secretions that are essential for proper GI function.

Heartburn and GERD

Heartburn occurs when the acidic contents of the stomach leak back into the esophagus (FIGURE 3.15B). The medical term for the leakage of stomach contents into the esophagus is *gastroesophageal reflux*. Occasional heartburn is common, but if it occurs more than twice a week, it may indicate a condition called **gastroesophageal reflux disease (GERD)**. If left untreated, GERD can eventually lead to more serious health problems, such as bleeding, ulcers, and cancer.

> **heartburn**
> A burning sensation in the chest or throat caused when acidic stomach contents leak back into the esophagus.

> **gastroesophageal reflux disease (GERD)** A chronic condition in which acidic stomach contents leak into the esophagus, causing pain and damaging the esophagus.

The discomforts of heartburn and GERD can be avoided by limiting the amounts and types of foods consumed. Eating small meals and consuming beverages between rather than with meals prevents heartburn by reducing the volume of material in the stomach. Avoiding fatty and fried foods, chocolate, peppermint, and caffeinated beverages, which increase stomach acidity or slow stomach emptying, can help minimize symptoms. Remaining upright after eating, wearing loose clothing, avoiding smoking and alcohol, and losing weight may also help prevent heartburn. For many people, medications that neutralize acid or reduce acid secretion are needed to manage symptoms.

A Tooth loss and dental pain can make chewing difficult. This may limit the intake of certain foods and reduce nutrient absorption because poorly chewed food may not be completely digested. Tooth decay and gum disease are more likely when saliva production is reduced. Reduced saliva production is a side effect of many medications and can cause changes in taste and difficulty in swallowing.

Esophagus

Stomach wall

Sphincter

Acidic stomach contents

B Heartburn and GERD occur when stomach acid leaks back through the sphincter and irritates the lining of the esophagus. Stomach contents also pass through this sphincter during vomiting. Vomiting may be caused by an illness, a food allergy, medication, an eating disorder, or pregnancy.

C Peptic ulcers occur when the mucosa is destroyed, exposing underlying tissues to gastric juices. Damage that reaches the nerve layer causes pain, and bleeding can occur if the small blood vessels of the mucosa are damaged. If the stomach or esophagus wall is perforated because of an ulcer, a serious abdominal infection can occur.

Gallstones

Gallbladder

D Gallstones, visible in this image of the abdomen, are deposits of cholesterol, bile pigments, and calcium that can be in the gallbladder or the bile duct. They can block bile from entering the small intestine, causing pain when the gallbladder contracts and reducing fat digestion and absorption.

E Constipation, in which the feces are hard and dry, is often due to a diet that is too low in fiber and fluids. It increases pressure in the colon and can lead to outpouches in the colon wall, shown here, called diverticula (discussed further in Chapter 4). ▼

Colon wall

Diverticula

Peptic ulcers

Peptic ulcers occur when the mucus barrier protecting the stomach, esophagus, or upper small intestine is penetrated and the acid and pepsin in digestive secretions damage the gastrointestinal lining (**FIGURE 3.15C**). Mild ulcers cause abdominal pain; more severe ulcers can cause life-threatening bleeding.

Peptic ulcers can result from GERD or from misuse of medications such as aspirin or nonsteroidal anti-inflammatory drugs (Motrin, Advil) but are more often caused by infection with the bacterium *Helicobacter pylori* (*H. pylori*). These bacteria burrow into the mucus and destroy the protective mucosal layer.[8] Over half of the world's population is infected with *H. pylori*, but not everyone who is infected develops ulcers.[9] *H. pylori* can be treated using antibiotics.

peptic ulcers
Open sores in the lining of the stomach, esophagus, or upper small intestine.

Gallstones

Clumps of solid material that accumulate in either the gallbladder or the bile duct are referred to as **gallstones** (**FIGURE 3.15D**). They can cause pain when the gallbladder contracts in response to fat in the intestine. Gallstones can interfere with bile secretion and reduce fat absorption. They are usually treated by removing the gallbladder. After the gallbladder has been removed, bile, which is produced in the liver, drips directly into the intestine as it is produced rather than being stored and squeezed out in larger amounts when fat enters the intestine.

Diarrhea and constipation

Diarrhea and constipation are common discomforts that are related to problems in the intestines. **Diarrhea** refers to frequent, watery stools. It occurs when material moves through the colon too quickly for sufficient water to be absorbed or when water is drawn into the lumen from cells lining the intestinal tract.

Diarrhea can be caused by bacterial or viral infections, irritants that inflame the lining of the GI tract, the passage of undigested food into the large intestine, medications, and chronic intestinal diseases. Diarrhea causes loss of fluids and minerals. Severe diarrhea lasting more than a day or two can be life threatening.

Constipation refers to hard, dry stools that are difficult to pass; it occurs when the water content of the stool is too low. Constipation can be caused by a diet that contains insufficient fluid or fiber, lack of exercise, a weakening of the muscles of the large intestine, and a variety of medications (**FIGURE 3.15E**). It can be prevented by drinking plenty of fluids, consuming a high-fiber diet, and getting enough exercise (see *What Should I Eat?* and the *Case Study*).

WHAT SHOULD I EAT?   **For Digestive Health**

Use iProfile to find the fiber content of your favorite fruits and vegetables.

Reduce your risk of adverse reactions
- Read food labels to avoid foods that you are allergic to.
- Chew each bite thoroughly to maximize digestion and avoid choking.
- Don't talk with food in your mouth.
- Learn the Heimlich maneuver: You could save a life.

Reduce the chances of heartburn
- Eat enough to satisfy your hunger but not so much that you are stuffed.
- Wait 10 minutes between your first and second courses to see how full you feel.
- Stay upright after you eat—don't flop on the couch in front of the television.

Avoid constipation by consuming enough fiber and fluid
- Choose whole-grain cereals such as oatmeal or raisin bran.
- Double your servings of vegetables at dinner.
- Eat two pieces of fruit with your lunch.
- Choose whole-grain bread.
- Have one or two beverages with or before each meal.

HOW DO CHANGES IN THE GI TRACT AFFECT HEALTH?

Mary is a registered dietitian. Often patients come to her with gastrointestinal problems. For each patient described here, think about how digestion and absorption are affected and the consequences for the patient's nutritional health.

A 50-year-old man is taking medication that reduces the amount of saliva he produces.

What effect might this have on his nutrition and health?

Your answer:

An 80-year-old woman wearing dentures that don't fit well likes raw carrots but can't chew them thoroughly.

How might this affect the digestion and absorption of nutrients contained in the carrots?

Your answer:

A 47-year-old woman undergoes treatment for colon cancer, which requires that most of her large intestine be surgically removed.

How does this change affect the amount of fluid she needs to consume?

Your answer:

A 56-year-old man has gallstones, which cause pain when his gallbladder contracts.

What type of foods should he avoid and why?

Your answer:

A 40-year-old woman weighing 350 pounds has undergone a surgical procedure called gastric bypass. The diagram shows how her stomach and small intestine were altered.

Why can't she eat as much food as before or absorb all the nutrients from the food she eats?

Your answer:

Food
Esophagus
Staple line
Unused portion of stomach
New stomach pouch
Outlet to intestines
Unused portion of small intestine
Small intestine

Gastric bypass surgery involves stapling off the top portion of the stomach and attaching it directly to the small intestine.

(Check your answers in Appendix K.)

CONCEPT CHECK **STOP**

Why is the immune function of the GI tract so important?

How can food allergy symptoms be prevented?

What foods should be avoided by people with heartburn? by people with gallstones?

When can ulcers be treated with antibiotics?

Delivering Nutrients and Eliminating Wastes

LEARNING OBJECTIVES

Trace the path of blood circulation.

Discuss how blood flow is affected by eating and activity.

Explain the functions of the lymphatic system.

List four ways in which waste products are eliminated from the body.

A fter food has been digested and the nutrients absorbed, they must be delivered to the cells. This delivery is handled by the **cardiovascular system**, which consists of the heart and blood vessels. Amino acids from protein, single sugars from carbohydrate, and the water-soluble products of fat digestion are absorbed into **capillaries** in the villi of the small intestine and transported via the blood to the liver (see Figure 3.10B). The products of digestion that are not water soluble, such as cholesterol and large fatty acids, are absorbed into **lacteals,** which are part of the **lymphatic system,** before entering the blood.

capillaries Small, thin-walled blood vessels through which blood and the body's cells exchange gases and nutrients.

lacteals Lymph vessels in the villi of the small intestine that pick up particles containing the products of fat digestion.

Process Diagram

Blood circulation FIGURE 3.16

Blood pumped to the lungs picks up oxygen and delivers nutrients. Blood pumped to the rest of the body delivers oxygen and nutrients.

1. Oxygen-poor blood that reaches the heart from the rest of the body is pumped through the arteries to the capillaries of the lungs.

2. In the capillaries of the lungs, oxygen from inhaled air is picked up by the blood, and carbon dioxide is released into the lungs and exhaled.

3. Oxygen-rich blood returns to the heart from the lungs via veins.

4. Oxygen-rich blood is pumped out of the heart into the arteries that lead to the rest of the body.

5. In the capillaries of the body, nutrients and oxygen move from the blood to the body's tissues, and carbon dioxide and other waste products move from the tissues to the blood, to be carried away.

6. Oxygen-poor blood returns to the heart via veins.

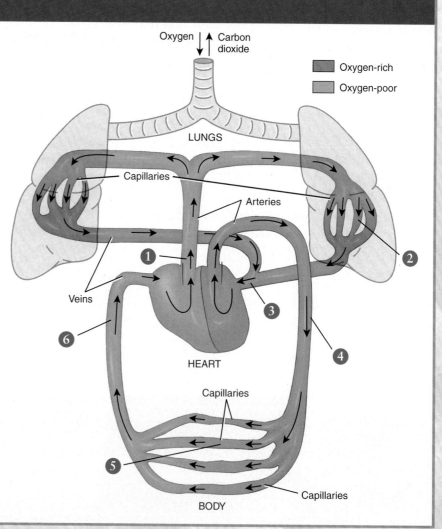

A At rest between meals, the amount of blood directed to the abdomen, which includes the organs, muscles, and glands of the digestive system, is similar to the amount that goes to the skeletal muscles.[10]

B During exercise, the demands of the muscles take priority, and only a small proportion of the blood is directed to the abdomen.[10] This is why you may get cramps if you exercise right after eating a big meal: Your body cannot direct enough blood to the intestines and the muscles at the same time. The muscles win out, and food remains in your intestines, often causing cramps.

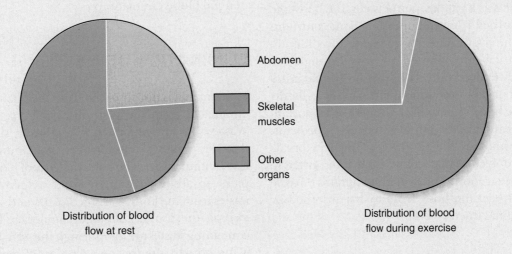

Abdomen

Skeletal muscles

Other organs

Distribution of blood flow at rest

Distribution of blood flow during exercise

THE CARDIOVASCULAR SYSTEM

The cardiovascular system circulates blood throughout the body. Blood carries nutrients and oxygen to the cells of all the organs and tissues of the body and removes carbon dioxide and other waste products from these cells. Blood also carries other substances, such as hormones, from one part of the body to another.

The heart and blood vessels The heart is the workhorse of the cardiovascular system. It is a muscular pump with two circulatory loops—one that carries blood to and from the lungs and one that carries blood to and from the rest of the body (Figure 3.16).

The blood vessels that transport blood and dissolved substances toward the heart are called **veins**, and those that transport blood and dissolved substances away from the heart are called **arteries**. As arteries carry blood away from the heart, they branch many times to form smaller and smaller blood vessels. The smallest arteries are called **arterioles**. Arterioles branch to form capillaries. Blood from capillaries then flows into the smallest veins, the **venules**, which converge to form larger and larger veins for returning blood to the heart.

The exchange of nutrients and gases occurs across the thin walls of the capillaries. In most body tissues, oxygen and nutrients carried by the blood pass from the capillaries into the cells, and carbon dioxide and other waste products pass from the cells into the capillaries. In the capillaries of the lungs, blood releases carbon dioxide to be exhaled and picks up oxygen to be delivered to the cells. In the capillaries of the GI tract, blood delivers oxygen and picks up water-soluble nutrients absorbed from the diet.

The amount of blood, and hence the amounts of nutrients and oxygen, delivered to a specific organ or tissue depends on the need. When you are resting, about 25% of your blood goes to your digestive system, about 20% to your skeletal muscles, and the rest to the heart, kidneys, brain, skin, and other organs.[10] This distribution changes when you eat or exercise. When you have eaten a large meal, a greater proportion of your blood goes to your digestive system to provide the oxygen and nutrients needed by the GI muscles and glands for digestion of the meal and absorption of nutrients. When you are exercising strenuously, about 70% of your blood is directed to your skeletal muscles to deliver nutrients and oxygen and remove carbon dioxide and other waste products (Figure 3.17).

DELIVERING NUTRIENTS TO THE LIVER

Water-soluble molecules in the small intestine, including amino acids, sugars, water-soluble vitamins, and the water-soluble products of fat digestion, cross the mucosal cells of the villi and enter the capillaries (see Figure 3.10). Once in the capillaries, these molecules are carried to the liver via the **hepatic portal vein** (FIGURE 3.18).

The liver acts as a gatekeeper between the body and substances absorbed from the intestine. Some nutrients are stored in the liver, some are changed into different forms, and others are allowed to pass through unchanged. The liver determines whether individual nutrients are stored or delivered immediately to the cells, depending on the body's needs. The liver is also important in the synthesis and breakdown of amino acids, proteins, and lipids. It modifies the products of protein breakdown to form molecules that can be safely transported to the kidney for excretion. The liver also contains enzyme systems that protect the body from toxins absorbed by the gastrointestinal tract.

THE LYMPHATIC SYSTEM

The lymphatic system consists of a network of tubules (lymph vessels) and lymph organs that contain infection-fighting cells. Fluid that collects in tissues and between cells drains into the lymphatic system. This prevents the fluid from accumulating and causing swelling.

The lymphatic system is an important part of the immune system. Fluid collected in the lymph vessels is filtered past a collection of infection-fighting cells before being returned to the blood. If the fluid contains antigen, an immune response is triggered. White blood cells and antibodies produced by this response enter the blood and help destroy the foreign substance.

In the small intestine, the lymph vessels aid in the absorption and transport of fat-soluble substances such as cholesterol, fatty acids, and fat-soluble vitamins. These pass from the intestinal mucosa into the lacteals located in the villi (see Figure 3.10B). The lacteals drain into larger lymph vessels. Lymph vessels from the intestine and most other organs drain into the thoracic duct, which empties into the blood near the neck. Therefore, substances absorbed into the lymphatic system do not pass through the liver before entering the general blood circulation.

ELIMINATION OF WASTES

Material that is not absorbed from the gut into the body is eliminated from the gastrointestinal tract in the feces. Wastes that are generated in the body, such as carbon dioxide, minerals, and nitrogen-containing wastes, must also be eliminated. The same highway of blood vessels that picks up absorbed nutrients and oxygen helps remove wastes from the body. Carbon dioxide and some water are lost via the lungs, and water, minerals, and nitrogen-containing wastes are lost through the skin, but the kidney is the primary site for the excretion of metabolic wastes. Water, minerals, and the nitrogen-containing by-products of protein breakdown are filtered out of the blood by the kidneys and excreted in urine. FIGURE 3.19 illustrates how the circulatory system is involved in both the delivery of nutrients and oxygen and the elimination of wastes.

Hepatic portal circulation FIGURE 3.18

The hepatic portal circulation delivers nutrients to the liver. Water-soluble substances absorbed into the capillaries of the villi move into venules, which merge to form larger veins that eventually form the hepatic portal vein.

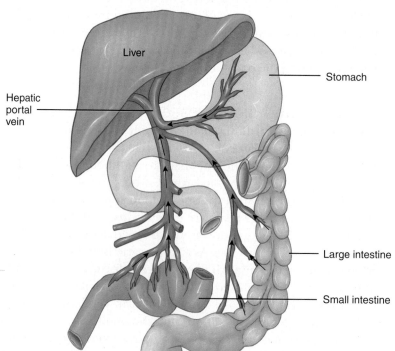

Liver

Stomach

Hepatic portal vein

Large intestine

Small intestine

Organ systems involved in elimination of wastes FIGURE 3.19

The nutrients taken in by the digestive system and the oxygen taken in by the respiratory system are both distributed to all the cells in the body by the circulatory system. Unabsorbed materials are eliminated in the feces. Metabolic wastes are transferred to the outside environment by the skin and the urinary and respiratory systems.

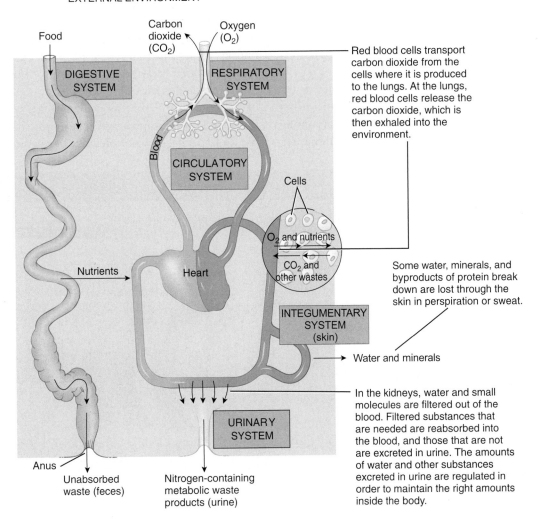

EXTERNAL ENVIRONMENT

Food

Carbon dioxide (CO₂)

Oxygen (O₂)

DIGESTIVE SYSTEM

RESPIRATORY SYSTEM

Blood

CIRCULATORY SYSTEM

Cells

Red blood cells transport carbon dioxide from the cells where it is produced to the lungs. At the lungs, red blood cells release the carbon dioxide, which is then exhaled into the environment.

Nutrients

Heart

O₂ and nutrients

CO₂ and other wastes

INTEGUMENTARY SYSTEM (skin)

Some water, minerals, and byproducts of protein break down are lost through the skin in perspiration or sweat.

Water and minerals

URINARY SYSTEM

Anus

Unabsorbed waste (feces)

Nitrogen-containing metabolic waste products (urine)

In the kidneys, water and small molecules are filtered out of the blood. Filtered substances that are needed are reabsorbed into the blood, and those that are not are excreted in urine. The amounts of water and other substances excreted in urine are regulated in order to maintain the right amounts inside the body.

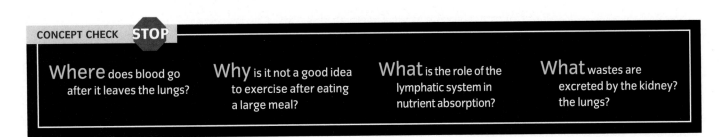

CONCEPT CHECK STOP

Where does blood go after it leaves the lungs?

Why is it not a good idea to exercise after eating a large meal?

What is the role of the lymphatic system in nutrient absorption?

What wastes are excreted by the kidney? the lungs?

An Overview of Metabolism

 nce they are inside the body's cells, nutrients are used either for energy or to synthesize all the structural and regulatory molecules needed for growth and maintenance.

Together, the chemical reactions that break down molecules to provide energy and those that synthesize larger molecules are referred to as **metabolism**. Many of the reactions of metabolism occur in series known as **metabolic pathways**. Molecules that enter these pathways are modified at each step with the help of enzymes. Some of the pathways use energy to build body structures, whereas others break large molecules into smaller ones, releasing energy. Reactions that synthesize molecules occur in different cellular compartments from those that break down molecules for energy. For example, ribosomes are cellular structures that specialize in the synthesis of proteins, and **mitochondria** are cell organs that are responsible for breaking down molecules to release energy.

Process Diagram

Producing ATP FIGURE 3.20

Cellular respiration uses oxygen to convert glucose, fatty acids, and amino acids into carbon dioxide, water, and energy, in the form of ATP.

HOW IT WORKS
View in your WileyPLUS course

① In the presence of oxygen, glucose, fatty acids, and amino acids can be metabolized to produce a two-carbon molecule (acetyl-CoA).

② Each acetyl-CoA molecule enters a circular pathway that produces two molecules of carbon dioxide (CO_2).

③ In the final step of this metabolic pathway, most of the energy released from the glucose, fatty acid, or amino acid molecules is used to produce ATP, and oxygen combines with hydrogen to form water.

RELEASING ENERGY

In the mitochondria, the glucose, fatty acids, and amino acids derived from carbohydrates, fats, and proteins, respectively, are broken down in the presence of oxygen to produce carbon dioxide and water and release energy. This process, called **cellular respiration**, is like cell breathing: Oxygen goes into the cell, and carbon dioxide comes out. The energy released by cellular respiration is used to make a molecule called **ATP (adenosine triphosphate)** (FIGURE 3.20). ATP can be thought of as the cell's energy currency. The chemical bonds of ATP are very high in energy, and when they break, the energy is released and can be used either to power body processes, such as muscle contraction or the transport of molecules across membranes, or to synthesize new molecules needed to maintain and repair body tissues.

> ■ **ATP (adenosine triphosphate)**
> A high-energy molecule that the body uses to power activities that require energy.

SYNTHESIZING NEW MOLECULES

Glucose, fatty acids, and amino acids that are not broken down for energy are used, with the input of energy from ATP, to synthesize structural, regulatory, or storage molecules. Glucose molecules are used to synthesize the glucose-storage molecule glycogen and, in some cases, fatty acids. Fatty acids are used to make body fat, cell membranes, and regulatory molecules, and amino acids are used to synthesize the various proteins that the body needs and, when necessary, to make glucose. Excess amino acids can also be converted into fatty acids and stored as body fat.

CONCEPT CHECK STOP

How are nutrients used to produce ATP?

Why can cellular respiration be thought of as cell breathing?

What types of molecules can be made from amino acids?

SUMMARY

1 The Organization of Life

1. Our bodies and the foods we eat are all made from the same building blocks—**atoms**. Atoms are linked together by chemical bonds to form **molecules**. Molecules can form **cells**. Cells with similar structures and functions are organized into **tissues**, and tissues are organized into the **organs** and **organ systems** that make up an organism. The 11 body organ systems work together; the passage of food through the digestive system and the secretion of digestive substances are regulated by the nervous and endocrine systems.

2 The Digestive System

1. The digestive system has two major functions: **digestion** and **absorption**. Digestion breaks down food and nutrients into units that are small enough to be absorbed. Absorption transports nutrients into the body. The main component of the digestive system is the **gastrointestinal tract**, which consists of a hollow tube that begins at the mouth and continues through the pharynx, esophagus, stomach, small intestine, and large intestine, ending at the anus.

2. The digestion of food and absorption of nutrients are aided by the secretion of **mucus** and **enzymes**.

3 Digestion and Absorption of Nutrients

1. The processes involved in digestion begin in response to the smell or sight of food and continue as food enters the digestive tract at the mouth, where it is broken down into smaller pieces by the teeth and mixed with **saliva** to form a **bolus**. Carbohydrate digestion is begun in the mouth by **salivary amylase**. From the mouth, the **bolus** passes through the **pharynx** and into the esophagus. The rhythmic contractions of **peristalsis** propel it down the esophagus to the stomach.

2. The stomach is a temporary storage site for food. The muscles of the stomach mix the food into a semiliquid mass called **chyme**, and **gastric juice**, which contains hydrochloric acid and **pepsin**,

begins the digestion of protein. The rate at which the stomach empties varies with the amount and composition of food consumed and is regulated by nervous and hormonal signals.

3. The small intestine is the primary site for nutrient digestion and absorption. The structural features of the small intestine ensure a large absorptive surface area. In the small intestine, bicarbonate from the pancreas neutralizes stomach acid, and pancreatic and intestinal enzymes digest carbohydrate, fat, and protein. The digestion and absorption of fat in the small intestine are aided by **bile** from the gallbladder.

4. The absorption of food across the intestinal **mucosa** occurs by means of several different transport mechanisms. **Simple diffusion**, **osmosis**, and

Microvilli

facilitated diffusion do not require energy, but **active transport** does.

5. Components of **chyme** that are not absorbed in the small intestine pass on to the large intestine, where some water and nutrients are absorbed. The large intestine is populated by **intestinal microflora** that digest some of the unabsorbed materials, such as fiber, producing small amounts of nutrients and gas. The remaining unabsorbed materials are eliminated in the **feces**.

---

4 Digestion in Health and Disease

1. Immune system cells and tissues located in the gastrointestinal tract help prevent disease-causing organisms or chemicals from entering the body. An **antigen** entering the digestive tract is attacked first by **phagocytes**. If it is not eliminated by the phagocytes, **lymphocytes** respond specifically to the antigen by

producing **antibodies**. The immune system protects us from disease but can also cause **food allergies**.

2. Diseases or discomforts at any point in the digestive system can interfere with food intake, digestion, or nutrient absorption. Common problems include dental problems, reduced saliva production, **heartburn**, **GERD**, **peptic ulcers**, **gallstones**, vomiting, **diarrhea**, and **constipation**.

---

5 Delivering Nutrients and Eliminating Wastes

1. Absorbed nutrients are delivered to the cells by the **cardiovascular system**. The heart pumps blood to the lungs to pick up oxygen and release carbon dioxide. From the lungs, blood returns to the heart and is then pumped to the rest of the body to deliver oxygen and nutrients and remove carbon dioxide and other wastes before returning to the heart. Exchange of nutrients and gases occurs at the **capillaries**.

2. The products of carbohydrate and protein digestion and the water-soluble products of fat digestion enter capillaries in the intestinal **villi** and are transported to the liver via the **hepatic portal vein**. The liver removes the absorbed substances for storage, converts them into other forms, or allows them to pass unaltered. The liver also protects the body from toxic substances that may have been absorbed.

3. The fat-soluble products of digestion enter **lacteals** in the intestinal villi.

Lacteals join larger lymph vessels. The nutrients absorbed via the **lymphatic system** enter the blood without first passing through the liver.

4. Unabsorbed materials are eliminated in the feces. The waste products of metabolism are excreted by the lungs, skin, and kidneys.

Cells

O_2 and nutrients

CO_2 and other wastes

6 An Overview of Metabolism

1. In the cells, glucose, **fatty acids**, and amino acids absorbed from the diet can be broken down by means of **cellular respiration** to provide energy in the form of **ATP**.

2. In the presence of ATP, glucose, fatty acids, and amino acids can be used either to synthesize structural or regulatory molecules or to synthesize energy-storage molecules.

ATP

KEY TERMS

- atoms p. 56
- molecules p. 56
- cells p. 56
- tissues p. 56
- organs p. 57
- organ systems p. 57
- hormones p. 57
- digestion p. 60
- absorption p. 60
- fatty acids p. 60
- feces p. 60
- gastrointestinal tract p. 60
- lumen p. 60
- mucosal cells p. 60
- mucosa p. 60
- transit time p. 60
- mucus p. 60
- enzymes p. 62
- saliva p. 63

- salivary amylase p. 63
- pharynx p. 63
- bolus p. 63
- epiglottis p. 63
- peristalsis p. 64
- sphincter p. 64
- chyme p. 65
- gastric juice p. 65
- pepsin p. 65
- gastrin p. 66
- pancreatic juice p. 67
- bicarbonate p. 67
- villi p. 67
- capillary p. 67
- lacteal p. 67
- microvilli p. 67
- brush border p. 67
- pancreatic amylase p. 68
- proteases p. 68

- lipases p. 68
- bile p. 69
- diffusion p. 69
- simple diffusion p. 69
- osmosis p. 69
- facilitated diffusion p. 69
- active transport p. 69
- probiotics p. 70
- prebiotics p. 70
- intestinal microflora p. 70
- antigen p. 71
- phagocytes p. 71
- lymphocytes p. 71
- antibodies p. 71
- allergen p. 72
- food allergies p. 72
- heartburn p. 72
- gastroesophageal reflux disease (GERD) p. 72

- peptic ulcers p. 74
- gallstones p. 74
- diarrhea p. 74
- constipation p. 74
- cardiovascular system p. 76
- capillaries p. 76
- lacteals p. 76
- lymphatic system p. 76
- veins p. 77
- arteries p. 77
- arterioles p. 77
- venules p. 77
- hepatic portal vein p. 78
- metabolism p. 80
- metabolic pathways p. 80
- mitochondria p. 80
- cellular respiration p. 81
- ATP (adenosine triphosphate) p. 81

CRITICAL AND CREATIVE THINKING QUESTIONS

1. For lunch, a college student has a smoothie made with blended fruit and juice. His friend has a burger, fries, and a milkshake. Which person's stomach will empty faster? Why?

2. After reading about the benefits of a high-fiber diet, a 23-year-old man decides to double his fiber intake by taking a fiber supplement that provides 15 grams of fiber. How might this dramatic increase affect the feces? How might it affect the amount of intestinal gas produced?

3. Your grandmother's favorite snack is a crisp fresh apple, but she has difficulty chewing because of tooth loss and dental pain. How might you modify her snack to make it easier for her to eat?

4. Starting in the esophagus, trace the path of food through the digestive system. At each organ, indicate anatomical adaptations of the general GI tract tube structure that enable the functions of that organ. For example, how does the structure of the small intestine aid absorption?

5. Water is absorbed from the small intestine and colon by osmosis. What might happen to the body's water balance if a large number of small, unabsorbed molecules ended up in the colon?

6. What path does an amino acid follow from absorption to delivery to a cell? Compare this path with the path followed by a large fatty acid.

(See *What is happening in this picture?* on page 84)

This man's digestive tract is not working, so nutrients are being infused into his blood through a process called total parenteral nutrition (TPN).

Would the TPN solution delivered meet his needs if it contained intact starches and proteins? Why or why not?

What would happen to him if an essential nutrient were missing from the TPN solution?

How would waste products from the TPN be excreted?

SELF-TEST

(Check your answers in Appendix L.)

1. Which of the following is the smallest unit of life?

   a. atom   d. tissue
   b. molecule   e. organism
   c. cell

2. Which of the following statements about saliva is false?

   a. It lubricates the mouth.
   b. It helps protect the teeth from decay.
   c. It moistens food so that it can be tasted and swallowed.
   d. It contains the enzyme salivary amylase.
   e. It contains the protein-digesting enzyme pepsin.

Use the diagram to answer questions 3 and 4.

3. Which letter in this illustration points to the organ in which carbohydrate digestion begins?

   a. A   c. C   e. E
   b. B   d. D

4. Which letter in this illustration points to the organ in which bile is stored?

   a. A   c. E   e. G
   b. C   d. F

5. The tissue layer labeled C _____.

a. secretes mucus
b. contains nerves and blood vessels
c. mixes and propels food through the GI tract
d. provides external support to the gut

6. The _____ prevents food from entering the passageway to the lungs during swallowing.

a. gallbladder
b. pancreas
c. epiglottis
d. tongue

7. The secretion of digestive juices does not begin until food enters the mouth.

a. True   b. False

8. The rhythmic contractions that propel food through the GI tract are called _____.

a. peristalsis
b. enzymatic digestion
c. swallowing
d. gastroesophageal reflux
e. chewing

9. Which of the following is most likely to inhibit stomach secretions and stomach motility?

a. the release of gastrin
b. the smell of freshly baked cookies
c. the entry of food into the small intestine
d. the entry of food into the stomach

10. The diffusion of water across a membrane is called _____.

a. simple diffusion
b. osmosis
c. facilitated diffusion
d. active transport

11. Which of the following is not true of the microvilli?

a. They help increase the surface area available for absorption.
b. They contain digestive enzymes.
c. Each contains a capillary and a lacteal.
d. They are referred to as the brush border.

12. This diagram could represent all the following except _____.

a. heartburn
b. diarrhea
c. GERD
d. vomiting

13. Which of the numbers on this illustration label blood that is rich in oxygen?

a. 1 and 2
b. 2 and 5
c. 3 and 4
d. 5 and 6

14. Most digestion and absorption occur in the _____.

a. small intestine
b. stomach
c. mouth
d. large intestine

15. All absorbed nutrients go directly to the liver.

a. True   b. False

Carbohydrates: Sugars, Starches, and Fibers

4

A fragrant loaf of bread fresh from the oven, a plate of *al dente* pasta, a steaming bowl of sticky rice, piping-hot noodles. What quality do these tantalizing foods share? All are important dietary basics produced from high-carbohydrate grains. Grains are so fundamental to the world's food supply that every culture relies on them as a readily available, inexpensive source of calories. Grains have long been cultural symbols: Bread is the "staff of life," and "breaking bread together" is a universal sign of friendship. The Chinese word for rice also means *food*, and the Japanese word for cooked rice means *meal*.

Grains such as rice, oats, corn, and wheat are an important carbohydrate source. They can be transformed into noodles, tortillas, couscous, and breakfast cereals or baked into breads, cakes, crackers, and chips. We smother them with sauces; we wrap and hold them around fillings, both savory and sweet. Carbohydrates also come from fruits, milk, and starchy vegetables like potatoes, peas, and beans. All told, carbohydrate-rich foods provide more than half the calories in the U.S. diet.

Many of us in Western societies have a love–hate relationship with carbohydrates. We're told to "carbo-load" before serious, sustained exercise, such as a marathon, yet we're admonished by health and fitness authorities to moderate our intake of carbohydrate-rich foods. Many people have come to fear carbohydrates as a cause of unwanted weight gain and other health problems. Can such a fundamental dietary staple contribute to today's chronic diseases? Can't humans and carbohydrates just learn to get along?

Carbohydrates in Our Food

LEARNING OBJECTIVES

Distinguish refined carbohydrates from unrefined carbohydrates.

Define enrichment.

Explain how added refined sugars and naturally occurring sugars differ from each other.

Our hunter-gatherer ancestors ate very differently from the way we eat. Their diet consisted almost entirely of **unrefined foods**—foods eaten either just as they are found in nature or with only minimal processing, such as cooking. Today we still consume some unrefined sources of carbohydrate, but many of the foods we consume are made with **refined** grains and contain added refined sugar (FIGURE 4.1).

The increased consumption of refined carbohydrates that has occurred around the world over the past few decades has been implicated as one of the causes of the current obesity epidemic and the rising incidence of chronic diseases. Recommendations for a healthy diet suggest that we select more unrefined sources of carbohydrates, including whole grains, vegetables, and fruits, and that we limit foods high in refined carbohydrates, such as candies, cookies, and sweetened beverages.

refined Refers to foods that have undergone processing to remove the coarse parts of the original food.

WHAT IS A WHOLE GRAIN?

When you eat a bowl of oatmeal or a slice of whole-wheat toast, you are consuming a **whole-grain product**. Whole-grain products include the entire kernel of the grain; the **germ**, the **bran**, and the **endosperm** (FIGURE 4.2). Refined grain products, such as white bread, include just the endosperm. The bran and germ are discarded during refining, and along with them the fiber and some vitamins and minerals are lost. To make up some of these losses, refined grains sold in the United States are enriched. **Enrichment**, which is a type of **fortification**, adds back some, but not all, of the nutrients lost in processing. For example, thiamin and iron are lost when grains are milled, and they are later added back to even higher levels through enrichment. Vitamin E and vitamin B_6 are also removed by milling, but they are not added back. Therefore, foods made with refined grains contain more of some nutrients and less of others than foods made from whole grains.

enrichment The addition of specific amounts of thiamin, riboflavin, niacin, and iron to refined grains. Since 1998 folic acid has also been added to enriched grains.

fortification The addition of nutrients to foods.

Unrefined and refined foods FIGURE 4.1

Corn is an unrefined source of carbohydrate, but it can be refined by washing, cooking, extruding, and drying to eventually end up as cornflakes in your cereal bowl. The sugar you sprinkle on cornflakes is also a refined carbohydrate; it has been refined from sugar cane or sugar beets.

Unrefined

Refined

Unrefined

Refined

Whole grains FIGURE 4.2

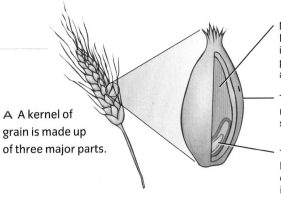

A A kernel of grain is made up of three major parts.

Most of the kernel is endosperm. It is made up of primarily starch, but it also contains most of the kernel's protein, along with some vitamins and minerals.

The outermost bran layers contain most of the fiber and are a good source of many vitamins and minerals.

The germ, located at the base of the kernel, is the embryo where spouting occurs. It is a source of oil and is rich in vitamin E.

WHOLE GRAIN
8g or more per serving
WholeGrainsCouncil.org

EAT 48g OR MORE OF WHOLE GRAINS DAILY

The product may contain some refined grain.

100% WHOLE GRAIN
16g or more per serving
WholeGrainsCouncil.org

EAT 48g OR MORE OF WHOLE GRAINS DAILY

All grain ingredients are whole grains.

B These whole-grain stamps were developed by the Whole Grains Council to help consumers identify products that provide either a half serving (8g) or a whole serving (16g) of whole grain.

WHAT IS ADDED REFINED SUGAR?

Refined sugars added to food during processing or at the table account for about 16% of the calories consumed in the typical American diet. Refined sugars are nutritionally and chemically identical to sugars that occur naturally in foods. When separated from their plant sources, however, refined sugars no longer come with the fiber, vitamins, minerals, and other substances found in the original plant. Therefore, added refined sugars contribute **empty calories** to the diet. Foods that naturally contain sugars, such as fruits and milk, provide vitamins, minerals, and phytochemicals along with the calories from the sugar, making them higher in nutrient density (**FIGURE 4.3**).

empty calories
Energy with few additional nutrients.

CONCEPT CHECK STOP

What is the difference between a whole-grain product and a product made with a refined grain?

Why are foods high in added refined sugars said to contribute empty calories?

How do enriched grains differ from whole grains?

Empty calories FIGURE 4.3

A 12-ounce soda contains about 140 Calories from sugar but almost no other nutrients. Three medium kiwis also provide about 140 Calories along with plenty of other nutrients including vitamin C, folate, and calcium, making the kiwis more nutrient dense than the soda.

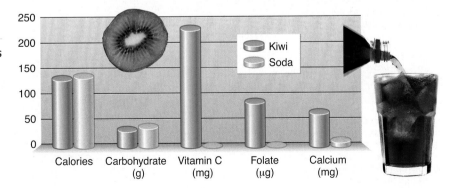

Types of Carbohydrates

Chemically, carbohydrates are a group of compounds made up of one or more **sugar units** that contain carbon (*carbo*) as well as hydrogen and oxygen in the same two-to-one proportion found in water (*hydrate*, H_2O). Carbohydrates made up of only one sugar unit are called **monosaccharides**, those made up of two sugar units are called **disaccharides**, and those made up of more than two sugar units are called **polysaccharides**.

sugar unit A sugar molecule that cannot be broken down to yield other sugars.

monosaccharide A carbohydrate made up of a single sugar unit.

disaccharide A carbohydrate made up of two sugar units.

polysaccharide A carbohydrate made up of many sugar units linked together.

Visualizing

Carbohydrates FIGURE 4.4

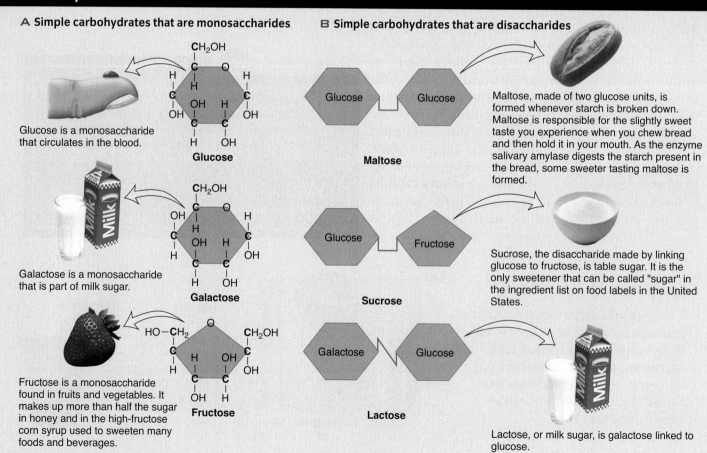

A Simple carbohydrates that are monosaccharides

Glucose is a monosaccharide that circulates in the blood.

Glucose

Galactose is a monosaccharide that is part of milk sugar.

Galactose

Fructose is a monosaccharide found in fruits and vegetables. It makes up more than half the sugar in honey and in the high-fructose corn syrup used to sweeten many foods and beverages.

Fructose

B Simple carbohydrates that are disaccharides

Glucose — Glucose

Maltose

Maltose, made of two glucose units, is formed whenever starch is broken down. Maltose is responsible for the slightly sweet taste you experience when you chew bread and then hold it in your mouth. As the enzyme salivary amylase digests the starch present in the bread, some sweeter tasting maltose is formed.

Glucose — Fructose

Sucrose

Sucrose, the disaccharide made by linking glucose to fructose, is table sugar. It is the only sweetener that can be called "sugar" in the ingredient list on food labels in the United States.

Galactose — Glucose

Lactose

Lactose, or milk sugar, is galactose linked to glucose.

SIMPLE CARBOHYDRATES

glucose A 6-carbon monosaccharide that is the primary form of carbohydrate used to provide energy in the body.

glycogen The storage form of carbohydrate in animals, made up of many glucose molecules linked together in a highly branched structure.

Monosaccharides and disaccharides are classified as **simple carbohydrates**. The three most common monosaccharides in the diet are **glucose**, **fructose**, and **galactose**. Each contains 6 carbon, 12 hydrogen, and 6 oxygen atoms ($C_6H_{12}O_6$), but these three sugars differ in the arrangement of these atoms (FIGURE 4.4A). Glucose, often called *blood sugar*, is the most important carbohydrate fuel for the human body.

The most common disaccharides in our diet are **maltose**, **sucrose**, and **lactose** (FIGURE 4.4B).

COMPLEX CARBOHYDRATES

Complex carbohydrates are polysaccharides; they are generally not sweet-tasting the way simple carbohydrates are. They include **glycogen** in animals and starches and fibers in plants (FIGURE 4.4C). Glycogen is the storage form of glucose in humans and other animals. It is found in the liver and muscles, but we don't consume it in our diet because the glycogen in animal muscles is broken down soon after the animal is slaughtered.

Starch is made up of glucose molecules linked together in either straight or branched chains (Figure 4.4C). It is the storage form of carbohydrate in plants and provides energy for plant growth and reproduction. When we eat

starch A carbohydrate found in plants, made up of many glucose molecules linked in straight or branched chains.

C **Complex carbohydrates**

Glycogen

The polysaccharide glycogen is made of highly branched chains of glucose. This branched structure allows glycogen to be broken down quickly when the body needs glucose.

Starches

Different types of starch consist of either straight chains or branched chains of glucose. We consume a mixture of starches in grains, legumes, and other starchy vegetables.

Fiber (cellulose)

Most fiber is made of either straight or branched chains of monosaccharides, but the bonds that link the sugar units cannot be broken by human digestive enzymes. For example, **cellulose** is a fiber made up of straight chains of glucose molecules.

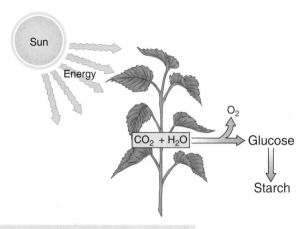

Photosynthesis FIGURE 4.5

Glucose is produced in plants through the process of **photosynthesis**, which uses energy from the sun to convert carbon dioxide and water to glucose. Plants most often convert glucose to starch. When a human eats plants, digestion converts the starch back to glucose.

plants, we consume the energy stored in the starch (FIGURE 4.5).

Fiber is a type of complex carbohydrate that cannot be digested by human digestive enzymes. Thus fiber cannot be absorbed in the human small intestine, and it passes into the large intestine. Fiber includes several chemical substances, some of which are soluble in water. **Soluble fiber**, found around and inside plant cells, dissolves in water to form viscous solutions. Although human enzymes can't digest soluble fiber, it is broken down by bacteria in the large intestine. Foods containing soluble fiber include oats, apples, beans, and seaweed (FIGURE 4.6).

Fiber that does not dissolve in water is called **insoluble fiber**. Insoluble fiber comes primarily from structural parts of plants, such as cell walls. This type of fiber adds bulk to fecal matter because it passes, unchanged, through the gastrointestinal tract. Food sources of insoluble fiber include wheat and rye bran, broccoli, and celery.

soluble fiber
Fiber that dissolves in water or absorbs water and can be broken down by intestinal microflora. It includes pectins, gums, and some hemicelluloses.

insoluble fiber
Fiber that, for the most part, does not dissolve in water and cannot be broken down by bacteria in the large intestine. It includes cellulose, some hemicelluloses, and lignin.

Soluble fiber FIGURE 4.6

A Jams and jellies are thickened with pectin, which is a soluble fiber found in fruits and vegetables. Foods are also thickened with gums because they combine with water to keep solutions from separating. Gums you might see in an ingredient list include gum arabic, gum karaya, guar gum, locust bean gum, xanthan gum, and gum tragacanth, which are extracted from shrubs, trees, and seedpods, and agar, carrageenan, and alginates, which are gums derived from seaweed.

B Beans contain soluble fiber and small polysaccharides that cannot be broken down by human digestive enzymes. Both of these pass into the large intestine, where their digestion by bacteria creates gas. Over-the-counter enzyme tablets and solutions (such as Beano®) can be taken to digest the small polysaccharides and thus reduce the amount of gas produced.

CONCEPT CHECK **STOP**

Which monosaccharide circulates in the blood?

What is glycogen?

How do the bonds that link the sugar units in starch differ from the bonds that link the units in fiber?

Which type of fiber is plentiful in beans?

Carbohydrate Digestion and Absorption

Disaccharides and complex carbohydrates must be digested to monosaccharides before they can be absorbed into the body. Carbohydrates that cannot be completely digested cannot be absorbed but still have an impact on the gastrointestinal tract and overall health. Once absorbed, carbohydrates travel in the blood to the liver.

CARBOHYDRATE DIGESTION

Carbohydrate digestion begins in the mouth, but most digestion occurs in the small intestine (**FIGURE 4.7**). Carbohydrate that cannot be digested passes into the colon. Some of this is broken down by bacteria. Material that cannot be absorbed is excreted in the feces.

Carbohydrate digestion FIGURE 4.7

During digestion, enzymes break starches and sugars into monosaccharides, which are absorbed. Most of the fiber and other indigestible carbohydrates are excreted in the feces.

HOW IT WORKS
View in your WileyPLUS course

1. In the mouth, the enzyme salivary amylase starts breaking starch into shorter polysaccharides.

2. In the stomach, salivary amylase is inactivated by acid so no carbohydrate digestion occurs.

3. In the small intestine, most starch digestion and breakdown of disaccharides occur. Here pancreatic amylase completes the job of breaking down starch into disaccharides, and short chains of sugar units called oligosaccharides.

4. Enzymes attached to the brush border of the small intestinal villi complete the digestion of carbohydrates. Here, disaccharides and oligosaccharides are broken down into monosaccharides.

5. In the large intestine, fiber and other indigestible carbohydrates are partially broken down by bacteria to form short chain fatty acids and gas. Some fiber is excreted in the feces.

Salivary glands

Liver

Stomach

Pancreas

Small intestine

Large intestine

Oligosaccharide

Disaccharide

Monosaccharides

Intestinal villi

Capillaries

Vein

Artery

To liver

Process Diagram

Lactose intolerance FIGURE 4.8

This map illustrates the dramatic variation in the incidence of lactose intolerance around the world. In the United States, between 30 and 50 million people are lactose intolerant, but certain ethnic and racial populations are more affected than others. Up to 80% of African Americans, 80 to 100% of Native Americans, and 90 to 100% of Asian Americans are lactose intolerant, but only about 15% of Caucasian Americans are.[1]

Lactose Intolerance
71–100%
51–70%
31–50%
11–30%
0–10%
No Data

Lactose intolerance

The disaccharide lactose is broken down by the enzyme lactase in the small intestine. We are all born with adequate levels of lactase, but in many people levels decline so much with age that lactose cannot be completely digested, a condition called **lactose intolerance**. When these individuals consume dairy products, the lactose passes into the large intestine, where it draws in water and is metabolized by bacteria, producing gas and causing abdominal distension, cramping, and diarrhea. The incidence of lactose intolerance varies among populations (FIGURE 4.8).

Because milk is the primary source of calcium in the U.S. diet, lactose-intolerant individuals may have difficulty meeting calcium needs. Those who can tolerate small amounts of lactose can meet their calcium needs by consuming smaller portions of milk throughout the day. Cheese and yogurt may also be tolerated because some of the lactose originally present in the milk is either digested by bacteria or lost in processing. Those who cannot tolerate any lactose can choose tofu and fish consumed with bones to supply calcium. Calcium-fortified foods and supplements and lactase-treated milk are also available. Another option is to take lactase tablets with or before consuming milk products to digest the lactose before it passes into the large intestine.

> **lactose intolerance**
> The inability to digest lactose due to a reduction in the levels of the enzyme lactase.

Indigestible carbohydrates

Fiber and some **oligosaccharides** are not digested because they cannot be broken down by human enzymes. **Resistant starch** is not digested either because the natural structure of the grain protects the starch molecules or because cooking and processing alter their digestibility. Legumes, unripe bananas, and cold cooked potatoes, rice, and pasta are high in resistant starch.

As indigestible carbohydrates pass through the gastrointestinal tract, they slow the rate at which nutrients are absorbed (FIGURE 4.9A). Fiber can also bind to certain minerals, preventing their absorption. For instance, wheat bran fiber binds zinc, calcium, magnesium, and iron. Indigestible carbohydrates also speed transit through the intestine by increasing the amount of fluid and the volume of material in the intestine. This stimulates peristalsis, causing the muscles of the large intestine to work more, and function better (FIGURE 4.9B).

Some carbohydrates that are not digested by human enzymes are digested by intestinal bacteria when they reach the large intestine, producing fatty acids and gas. The fatty acids can be used as a fuel source for cells in the colon and other body tissues; they may play a role in regulating cellular processes (FIGURE 4.9C).

> **oligosaccharides**
> Short carbohydrate chains containing 3 to 10 sugar units.

> **resistant starch**
> Starch that escapes digestion in the small intestine of healthy people.

A The bulk and volume of a fiber-rich meal dilutes the gastrointestinal contents. This dilution slows the digestion of food and absorption of nutrients (green dots), causing a delay and a blunting of the rise in blood glucose that occurs after a meal. With a low-fiber meal, nutrients are more concentrated; digestion and absorption occur more rapidly, causing a quicker, sharper rise in blood glucose. ▼

▲

B Stool weights are greater and transit times shorter for Ugandan villagers, who consume a diet high in fiber, than for British subjects, who consume a more refined, low-fiber diet. (Source: Adapted from Burkitt, D.P., Walker, A.R.P., and Painter, N.S. Dietary fiber and disease. JAMA 229:1068–1074, 1974.)

▲

C Indigestible carbohydrates are a food source for the bacteria in the colon. When bacteria break down these carbohydrates, fatty acids are formed. The acidic conditions inhibit the growth of undesirable bacteria and favor the growth of healthy ones, such as the *Bifidobacteria* shown here.[2] In addition to inhibiting the growth of disease-causing bacteria, these fatty acids may help prevent and treat inflammation in the bowel, which causes diarrhea, and protect against colon cancer.[3,4]

Glycemic Index

Potatoes are a source of unrefined carbohydrate, but scientists know that the effect potatoes have on blood glucose is very different from the effect beans have. Beans are also a source of unrefined carbohydrate but they are much higher in fiber and protein, both of which slow digestion and absorption and therefore reduce the glycemic response.

The glycemic response of beans versus potatoes is shown here graphically, but it can also be expressed using the **glycemic index**, which is a ranking of how a food affects blood glucose relative to the effect of an equivalent amount of carbohydrate from a reference food, such as white bread or pure glucose. For example, on a glycemic index scale on which white bread is 100, potatoes are 90, and kidney beans are about 25.

A shortcoming of the glycemic index is that it is measured using a portion of food that contains a set amount of carbohydrate (usually 50 grams), not a typical food portion. To overcome this shortcoming, **glycemic load** can be used to rank the effect of a food on blood sugar. This method considers the glycemic response of a typical portion of food.

A shortcoming of both the glycemic index and glycemic load is that they are determined for individual foods rather than for meals, which contain mixtures of foods. What do you think the glycemic response graph would look like for a stew containing potatoes, beef, carrots, and onions?

CARBOHYDRATE ABSORPTION

After a meal, the monosaccharides from carbohydrate digestion enter the portal circulation and travel to the liver. The liver uses fructose and galactose for energy. Glucose can be used for energy, stored as liver glycogen, or delivered via the general blood circulation to other body tissues, causing blood glucose levels to rise. **Glycemic response** is a measure of how quickly and how high blood glucose levels rise after carbohydrate is consumed. Glycemic response is affected by how long it takes a food to leave the stomach and by how fast it is digested and the glucose absorbed.

glycemic response The rate, magnitude, and duration of the rise in blood glucose that occurs after food is consumed.

Refined sugars and starches generally cause a greater glycemic response than unrefined carbohydrates because sugars and starches consumed alone leave the stomach quickly and are rapidly digested and absorbed. For example, when you drink a bottle of sugary soda, your blood glucose increases within minutes. Because fiber takes longer to leave the stomach and slows absorption in the small intestine, fiber-containing foods cause a lower glycemic response (see *What a Scientist Sees*). When carbohydrate, fat, and protein are consumed together, stomach emptying is slowed, delaying both digestion and absorption of carbohydrate, so blood glucose rises more slowly than when carbohydrate is consumed alone. For instance, after a meal of chicken, brown rice, and green beans, which contains carbohydrate, fat, protein, and fiber, blood glucose doesn't begin to rise for 30 to 60 minutes.

CONCEPT CHECK STOP

What steps are involved in starch digestion?

What foods are good sources of calcium for someone with lactose intolerance?

Why are carbohydrates that cannot be digested important for health?

How does fiber affect glycemic response?

Carbohydrate Functions

LEARNING OBJECTIVES

Name the main function of carbohydrate in the body.

Explain how insulin and glucagon help regulate blood glucose levels.

Compare anaerobic and aerobic metabolism.

Discuss what happens to protein and fat metabolism when dietary carbohydrate is insufficient.

The main function of carbohydrates is to provide energy, but carbohydrates also play other roles in the body. The sugar galactose, for example, is needed by nerve tissue, and in breast-feeding women, galactose combines with glucose to produce the milk sugar lactose. The monosaccharides ribose and deoxyribose play nonenergy roles as components of RNA and DNA, respectively, the two molecules that contain the cell's genetic information. Ribose is also a component of the B vitamin riboflavin. Oligosaccharides are associated with cell membranes, where they help signal information about cells, and large polysaccharides found in connective tissue provide cushioning and lubrication.

insulin A hormone made in the pancreas that allows glucose to enter cells and stimulates the synthesis of protein, fat, and liver and muscle glycogen.

GETTING ENOUGH GLUCOSE TO CELLS

Glucose is an important fuel for body cells. Many body cells can use energy sources other than glucose, but brain cells, red blood cells, and a few others must have glucose to stay alive. In order to provide a steady supply of glucose, the concentration of glucose in the blood is regulated by the liver and by hormones secreted by the pancreas. The rise in blood glucose levels after eating stimulates the pancreas to secrete the hormone **insulin**, which allows glucose to be taken into body cells, causing blood glucose levels to drop. Once inside cells, glucose can be used immediately for energy or converted into energy-storage molecules for future use. In both muscle cells and liver cells,

Blood glucose regulation FIGURE 4.10

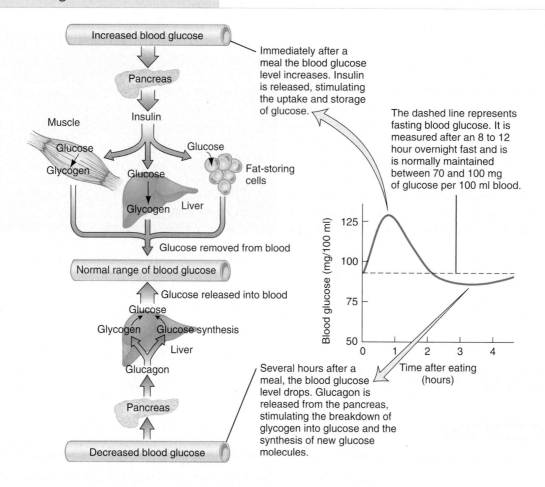

Immediately after a meal the blood glucose level increases. Insulin is released, stimulating the uptake and storage of glucose.

The dashed line represents fasting blood glucose. It is measured after an 8 to 12 hour overnight fast and is is normally maintained between 70 and 100 mg of glucose per 100 ml blood.

Several hours after a meal, the blood glucose level drops. Glucagon is released from the pancreas, stimulating the breakdown of glycogen into glucose and the synthesis of new glucose molecules.

insulin promotes the conversion of glucose into glycogen for storage. In the liver and in fat-storing cells, it promotes the conversion of glucose to fat for storage (FIGURE 4.10).

A few hours after eating, blood glucose levels—and consequently the amount of glucose available to the cells—begin to decrease. This triggers the pancreas to secrete the hormone **glucagon** (Figure 4.10). Glucagon raises blood glucose by signaling liver cells to break down glycogen into glucose, which is released into the blood. At the same time, glucagon signals the liver to synthesize new glucose molecules, which are also released into the blood, bringing blood glucose levels back to normal.

glucagon
A hormone made in the pancreas that raises blood glucose levels by stimulating the breakdown of liver glycogen and the synthesis of glucose.

GLUCOSE AS A SOURCE OF ENERGY

Cells use glucose to provide energy via cellular respiration (see Chapter 3). Cellular respiration, uses oxygen to convert glucose to carbon dioxide and water and provide energy in the form of ATP (FIGURE 4.11).

The first step in cellular respiration is **glycolysis**.

glycolysis An anaerobic metabolic pathway that splits glucose into two three-carbon pyruvate molecules; the energy released from one glucose molecule is used to make two molecules of ATP.

Because oxygen isn't needed for this reaction, glycolysis is sometimes called anaerobic glycolysis, or **anaerobic metabolism**. Glycolysis can rapidly produce two molecules of ATP from each glucose molecule. When oxygen is limited, no further metabolism of glucose and production of ATP occurs. When oxygen is available, the complete breakdown of glucose can proceed. This **aerobic metabolism** produces about 36 molecules of ATP for each glucose molecule, 18 times more ATP than is generated by anaerobic glycolysis.

Cellular respiration FIGURE 4.11

The reactions of cellular respiration split the bonds between carbon atoms in glucose, releasing energy that is used to synthesize ATP. ATP is used to power the energy-requiring processes in the body.

1 Glycolysis splits glucose, a six-carbon molecule, into two molecules of pyruvate, a three-carbon molecule. This step produces high-energy electrons (dashed lines) and a small amount of ATP. Each pyruvate is then either broken down to produce more ATP or used to make glucose.

2 When oxygen is available, pyruvate can be used to produce more ATP. One carbon is removed from each pyruvate, producing carbon dioxide. High-energy electrons are released and the remaining two carbons form a molecule called acetyl-CoA, which continues through aerobic metabolism.

3 A circular pathway breaks each acetyl-CoA molecule into two molecules of carbon dioxide and produces high-energy electrons.

HOW IT WORKS
View in your WileyPLUS course

4 In the final step of aerobic metabolism, the energy in the high-energy electrons released in previous steps is transferred to ATP, and the electrons are combined with oxygen and hydrogen to form water.

Process Diagram

Ketone formation FIGURE 4.12

Fatty acids are broken down into two-carbon units that form acetyl-CoA. To proceed through aerobic metabolism, acetyl-CoA must combine with a molecule derived primarily from carbohydrate. When carbohydrate is in short supply, molecules of acetyl-CoA react with each other to form ketones. The presence of carbohydrate allows fatty acids to be completely broken down to yield ATP.

Fatty acids

C—C
Acetyl-CoA

Carbohydrate unavailable

Carbohydrate available

Ketones

Used for energy

Excreted in urine

Accumulate in blood

CO_2

CO_2

O_2

H_2O

ATP

Carbohydrate and protein breakdown

Glucose is an essential fuel for brain cells and red blood cells. If adequate amounts are not available, glucose can be synthesized from three-carbon molecules (see Figure 4.11, step 1). Fatty acids cannot be used to make glucose because the reactions that break them down produce two-carbon, rather than three-carbon, molecules. Amino acids from protein breakdown can supply the three-carbon molecules. However, because protein is not stored in the body, this use of amino acids takes away functioning body proteins. Body proteins that are broken down to make glucose are no longer available to do their job, whether that job is to speed up a chemical reaction or contract a muscle. Sufficient dietary carbohydrate ensures that protein is not utilized in this way; carbohydrate is therefore said to *spare* protein.

Carbohydrate and fat breakdown

Most of the energy stored in the body is stored as fat. In order to fully access the energy from fatty acids, carbohydrate is required. If carbohydrate is not available, molecules called either **ketones** or **ketone bodies** are formed (**FIGURE 4.12**). Small amounts of ketones can be used for energy by the heart, muscle, and kidney. Even the brain, which requires some glucose, can obtain a portion of its energy from ketones.

ketones or **ketone bodies** Acidic molecules formed when there is not sufficient carbohydrate to completely metabolize the acetyl-CoA produced from fatty acid breakdown.

Ketones not used for energy can be excreted in the urine. However, when high levels of ketones build up in the blood, a condition known as **ketosis**, they can increase the blood's acidity so much that normal body processes are disrupted. Mild ketosis can occur during starvation or when consuming a low-carbohydrate weight-loss diet and can cause symptoms such as reduced appetite, headaches, dry mouth, and odd-smelling breath. Severe ketosis can occur with untreated diabetes and can cause coma and even death.

ketosis High levels of ketones in the blood.

CONCEPT CHECK STOP

Why is it important to keep blood glucose levels in the normal range?

How do insulin and glucagon affect blood glucose levels?

What process breaks down glucose in the presence of oxygen to yield ATP?

Why is carbohydrate said to spare protein?

Carbohydrates in Health and Disease

re carbohydrates good for you or bad for you? On the one hand, they have been blamed for everything from diabetes to obesity. On the other hand, U.S. guidelines for a healthy diet recommend that people base their diet on carbohydrate-rich foods in order to reduce disease risk. This incongruity relates to the health effects of different types of dietary carbohydrates: Diets high in whole grains, fruits, and vegetables are associated with a lower incidence of a variety of chronic diseases, whereas diets high in refined carbohydrates, such as refined grains and foods high in added sugars, may contribute to chronic disease risk.

DIABETES

Diabetes mellitus, commonly referred to simply as diabetes, is a disease characterized by high blood glucose levels (FIGURE 4.13). Uncontrolled diabetes damages the heart, blood vessels, kidneys, eyes, and nerves. It is the leading cause of adult blindness and accounts for 40% of new cases of kidney failure

diabetes mellitus
A disease characterized by elevated blood glucose due to either insufficient production of insulin or decreased sensitivity of cells to insulin.

Blood glucose levels in diabetes FIGURE 4.13

Normal blood glucose is less than 100 mg/100 ml blood after an eight-hour fast; a fasting blood level between 100 and 125 mg/100 ml is defined as prediabetes; a fasting level of 126 mg /100 ml or above is defined as diabetes. Two hours after consuming 75 g of glucose, normal blood levels are less than 140 mg/100 ml; prediabetes levels are between 140 and 199 mg/100 ml; diabetes levels are 200 mg/100 ml or greater.

Incidence of diabetes FIGURE 4.14

The incidence of diabetes in the United States is rising, and certain racial and ethnic groups are affected disproportionately.[5] This graph compares the age-adjusted prevalence of type 2 diabetes in adults of different groups. Reducing diabetes in minority groups will require culturally sensitive strategies to modify diet and lifestyle.

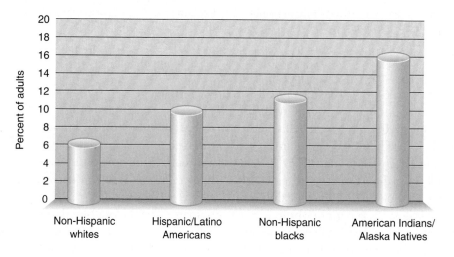

and more than 60% of nontraumatic lower-limb amputations. Nearly 24 million people in the United States have been diagnosed with diabetes, and another 6 million of them have undiagnosed diabetes. The incidence of diabetes is greater in minority populations (**FIGURE 4.14**).[5]

Types of diabetes Type 1 diabetes
is an **autoimmune disease** in which the insulin-secreting pancreatic cells are destroyed by the body's immune system. This form of diabetes accounts for only 5 to 10% of diagnosed cases and is usually diagnosed before age 30. Because no insulin is produced, people with type 1 diabetes must inject insulin in order to keep blood glucose levels in the normal range.

The more common form of diabetes is **type 2 diabetes**, which accounts for 90 to 95% of all cases. It occurs either when the body does not produce enough insulin or when body cells lose their sensitivity to it, a condition called **insulin resistance**. Therefore, the amount of insulin released is insufficient to allow enough glucose to enter the cells and blood glucose levels remain high. Type 2 diabetes is believed to be due to both

type 1 diabetes
The form of diabetes caused by auto-immune destruction of insulin-producing cells in the pancreas, usually leading to absolute insulin deficiency.

autoimmune disease A disease that results from immune reactions that destroy normal body cells.

type 2 diabetes
The form of diabetes characterized by insulin resistance and relative (rather than absolute) insulin deficiency.

genetic and lifestyle factors. A progressive disease, it usually begins with **prediabetes**, a condition in which glucose levels are above normal but not high enough to be diagnosed as diabetes (see Figure 4.13). In many cases, adjustments in diet and lifestyle can keep prediabetes from progressing to type 2 diabetes.

Gestational diabetes is an elevation of blood sugar that is first recognized during pregnancy.[6] The high levels of glucose in the mother's blood are passed to the fetus, frequently resulting in a baby who is large for gestational age and at increased risk of complications. Gestational diabetes usually resolves after the pregnancy, but women with gestational diabetes are at increased risk of developing type 2 diabetes later in life.

Symptoms and complications of diabetes The symptoms and complications of all types of diabetes result from the inability to use glucose normally and from high glucose levels in the blood. Cells that require insulin in order to take up glucose are starved for glucose, and cells that can use glucose without insulin are exposed to damaging high levels.

The early symptoms of diabetes include frequent urination, excessive thirst, blurred vision, and weight loss. Frequent urination and excessive thirst occur because, as blood glucose levels rise, the kidneys excrete the extra glucose and as a result must also excrete extra water, increasing the volume of urine. The additional loss of water from the body makes the individual thirsty. Blurred vision occurs when excess glucose enters the lens of the eye, drawing in water and causing the lens to swell. Weight loss occurs because cells are unable to use glucose for energy and so the body must break down fat to obtain the energy it needs.

The long-term complications of diabetes include damage to the heart, blood vessels, kidneys, eyes, and nerves. Damage to the large blood vessels leads to an increased risk of heart attack and stroke. Changes in small blood vessels, cells, and nerves can lead to blindness, kidney failure, and nerve dysfunction. For example, accumulation of glucose in the eye damages small blood vessels in the retina, leading to blindness. In addition to these problems, infections are more common in people with diabetes because high blood glucose levels favor microbial growth. Infections may lead to amputations of the toes, feet, and legs.

Managing blood glucose
The goal in treating diabetes is to maintain blood glucose levels within the normal range. This requires a program of diet, exercise, and, in many cases, medication, along with frequent monitoring of blood glucose levels.[7] Carbohydrate intake must be coordinated with exercise and medication schedules so that glucose and insulin are available in the right proportions.

Dietary management involves limiting the amount of carbohydrate consumed to prevent a rapid or prolonged rise in blood glucose.[7] A diet providing unrefined carbohydrates is recommended because these carbohydrate sources cause a slower rise in blood glucose than refined carbohydrates. Diets for individuals with diabetes should also be limited in saturated fat, *trans* fat, and cholesterol in order to reduce the risk for cardiovascular disease. Weight management is an important component of diabetes care because excess body fat increases the resistance of body cells to insulin. Exercise is important not only because it helps to achieve and maintain a healthy body weight but also because it increases the sensitivity of body cells to insulin.[8]

Individuals with type 1 diabetes require insulin injections because they no longer make insulin. Insulin must be given by injection because it is a protein that would be digested in the gastrointestinal tract if taken orally. Individuals with type 2 and gestational diabetes are often able to manage blood glucose levels with diet and exercise but may also require oral medications and/or insulin injections.

Carbohydrate intake and the risk of diabetes
Evidence is accumulating that carbohydrate consumption may play a role in the development of type 2 diabetes in susceptible individuals.[9,10] In populations where the diet is high in whole grains, there is a lower risk of developing type 2 diabetes than in populations where the diet is high in refined starches and added sugars.[11,12] The reason for this is not fully understood. However, it has been proposed that because insulin needs are increased when the diet is high in refined carbohydrates, the insulin-producing cells in the pancreas may wear out over time.[12]

HYPOGLYCEMIA

Another condition that involves blood glucose is **hypoglycemia**. Symptoms of hypoglycemia include low blood sugar (below 70 mg glucose/ 100 ml blood), irritability, sweating, shakiness, anxiety, rapid heartbeat, headache, hunger, weakness, and sometimes seizures and coma. Hypoglycemia occurs most frequently in people with diabetes as a result of overmedication. It can also be caused by abnormalities in insulin production or by abnormalities in the way the body responds to insulin or to other hormones.

> **hypoglycemia**
> Abnormally low blood glucose levels.

Fasting hypoglycemia, which occurs when an individual has not eaten, is often related to some underlying condition, such as excess alcohol consumption, hormonal deficiencies, or tumors. Treatment involves identifying and treating the underlying disease. **Reactive hypoglycemia** occurs in response to the consumption of high-carbohydrate foods. The rise in blood glucose from the carbohydrate meal stimulates insulin release. However, too much insulin is secreted, resulting in a rapid fall in blood glucose to abnormally low levels. To prevent the rapid changes in blood glucose that occur with reactive hypoglycemia, the diet should consist of small, frequent meals that are low in carbohydrate and high in protein and fiber.

Tooth decay FIGURE 4.15

The regions on these teeth that are stained brown indicate the presence of dental plaque. The main component of dental plaque is bacterial colonies. If the plaque is not brushed, flossed, or scraped off, the bacteria metabolize the carbohydrates in food, producing acid. This acid can dissolve tooth enamel and the underlying tooth structure, forming dental caries.

DENTAL CARIES

Dental caries, or cavities, are the best-documented health problem associated with carbohydrate intake. Eighty-five percent of people 18 years and older have had caries. They occur when bacteria on the teeth metabolize carbohydrates, producing tooth-damaging acids (FIGURE 4.15). Simple carbohydrates, especially sucrose, are easiest for the bacteria to metabolize into acids, but starchy foods also promote tooth decay. The longer teeth are exposed to carbohydrates—for example, through frequent snacking, consuming foods that stick to the teeth, sucking hard candy, and slowly sipping soda—the greater the risk of caries. Limiting intake of sweet or sticky foods and proper dental hygiene can help prevent dental caries.

WEIGHT MANAGEMENT

As low-carbohydrate diets have gained in popularity, carbohydrates have gotten a reputation for being fattening. In reality, carbohydrates are no more fattening than other nutrients. Weight gain is caused by excess intake of calories, no matter whether the excess is from carbohydrate, fat, or protein. Carbohydrates provide only 4 Calories per gram, less than half the 9 Calories per gram provided by fat (FIGURE 4.16).

Carbohydrates and calorie intake FIGURE 4.16

A It is the fat we add to high-carbohydrate foods that increases their calorie count. A medium-sized baked potato provides about 160 Calories. Adding 2 tablespoons of sour cream brings the total to over 200 Calories, and adding 2 tablespoons of butter more than doubles the number of calories.

B A diet high in sugar-sweetened beverages may increase caloric intake because beverages do not induce satiety to the same extent as solid forms of carbohydrate.[13] A diet high in unrefined carbohydrates may help reduce total food intake because the fiber in these foods increases the sense of fullness by adding bulk and slowing digestion.

Consumers often recognize their favorite nonnutritive sweetener by the color of the packet.

Sucralose, the sweetener in Splenda, is 600 times sweeter than sucrose. The ADI is 5 mg/kg of body weight/day, and one packet contains about 12 mg of sucralose. A 154-lb (70-kg) person could consume 29 packets without exceeding the ADI.

Saccharin, the sweetener in Sweet'n Low, is 300 times sweeter than sucrose. The ADI is 5 mg/kg of body weight/day, and one packet contains 36 mg of saccharin. A 154-lb (70-kg) person would exceed the ADI by consuming 10 packets or about three 12-oz saccharin-sweetened beverages.

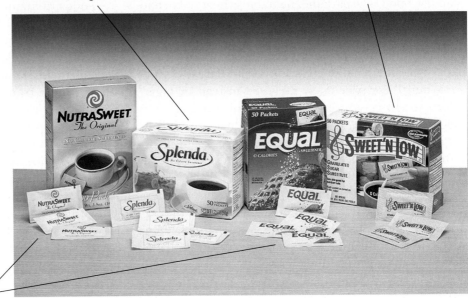

Aspartame, the sweetener in NutraSweet and Equal, is 200 times sweeter than sucrose. The ADI is 50 mg/kg of body weight/day, and one packet contains 37 mg of aspartame. To exceed the ADI, a 154-lb (70-kg) person would have to consume 95 packets or sixteen 12-oz aspartame-sweetened beverages.

Carbohydrates and weight loss

The type of carbohydrates you consume can affect how hungry you feel and whether you lose or gain weight. A diet high in unrefined carbohydrates is high in fiber, which is filling, allowing you to feel satisfied with less food. This can help promote weight loss. However, diets high in fiber may be problematic for children, who have a small stomach capacity, because they may become satiated before meeting their nutrient requirements.

Foods high in refined carbohydrates cause a rapid rise in blood glucose and therefore stimulate release of insulin. The more insulin you produce, the more fat you store, so a diet high in refined carbohydrate may shift metabolism toward fat storage. In contrast, a low-carbohydrate diet causes less insulin release and hence does not promote fat storage. Low-carbohydrate diets lead to weight loss because they reduce insulin levels and raise blood ketone levels, both of which supress appetite. In addition, these diets limit food choices to such an extent that the monotony results in a spontaneous reduction in calorie intake.[14]

The weight loss achieved with these diets, as with any other weight-loss diet, is therefore caused by consuming less energy than the body expends.

Nonnutritive sweeteners

One way to reduce the amount of refined sugar in the diet is to replace sugar with a **nonnutritive sweetener** (also called **artificial sweetener**), which provides no calories. The FDA has approved saccharin, aspartame, sucralose, acesulfame K, neotame, and rebiana as nonnutritive sweeteners and defined **acceptable daily intakes (ADIs)**—levels that should not be exceeded when using these products.[15]

Saccharin, aspartame, and sucralose are the products typically available to sweeten coffee (**FIGURE 4.17**). Saccharin, the oldest of the nonnutritive sweeteners, was once considered a carcinogen but was taken off the government's list of cancer-causing substances in 2000. Aspartame is made of two amino acids. Because it breaks down when heated, it is typically used in cold products or added after cooking. Sucralose is sucrose that has been modified so that it cannot be digested or absorbed. It is heat stable, so it can be used in cooking. Acesulfame K, the sweetener in Sunette and Sweet One, is also heat stable. It is 200 times sweeter than sucrose and is often used in combination with other sweeteners. Neotame, like aspartame, is made from two amino acids, but because the bond between them is harder to break than the bond in aspartame, neotame is heat stable and can be used in baking. The newest sweetener on the market is rebiana, which is a natural sweetener made from the leaf of the stevia plant.[16] It is about 300 times sweeter than sugar and is marketed as Truvia and PureVia.

When these sweeteners are used instead of sugar, calorie intake is reduced. Over time, this can help with weight loss. However, because foods that are high in added sugar tend to be nutrient poor, replacing them with artificially sweetened alternatives does not increase the nutrient density or overall quality of the diet.

Although the usefulness of nonnutritive sweeteners for weight loss depends on whether the calories they replace are added back from other food sources, these sweeteners can help reduce the incidence of dental caries and manage blood sugar levels.

HEART DISEASE

The impact of carbohydrates on heart disease risk depends on the type of carbohydrate. There is evidence that a diet high in sugar can raise blood lipid levels and thereby increase the risk of heart disease,[17] whereas diets high in fiber have been found to reduce the risk of heart disease.[18]

Foods containing soluble fiber, such as legumes, oats, flaxseed, and brown rice, may reduce the risk of heart disease by lowering blood cholesterol levels. In the digestive tract, soluble fiber binds dietary cholesterol and bile acids, which are made from cholesterol, preventing them from being absorbed (FIGURE 4.18). Soluble fiber may also help lower blood cholesterol because the by-products of the bacterial breakdown of the fiber may inhibit cholesterol synthesis in the liver or increase its removal from the blood.[19]

Insoluble fibers, such as wheat bran and cellulose, do not lower blood cholesterol, but a diet high in any type of fiber may help lower blood pressure, normalize blood glucose levels, prevent obesity, and affect a number of other parameters that help reduce the risk of heart disease.[20]

Cholesterol and soluble fiber FIGURE 4.18

A When the diet is low in soluble fiber, dietary cholesterol and bile, which contains cholesterol and bile acids made from cholesterol, are absorbed into the blood and transported to the liver, where they are reused.

B When soluble fiber is present in the digestive tract, the fiber binds cholesterol and bile acids so that they are excreted rather than absorbed. This helps reduce the amount of cholesterol in the body.

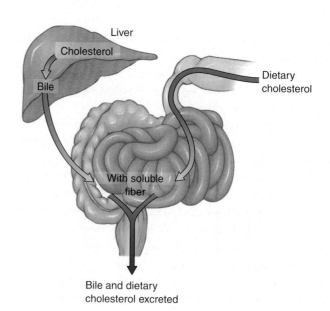

Diverticula FIGURE 4.19

Diverticula (the singular is *diverticulum*) are outpouches in the wall of the colon that form at weak points due to pressure exerted when the colon contracts. Fecal matter can accumulate in these pouches, causing irritation, pain, and inflammation—a condition known as **diverticulitis**.

Diverticulitis may lead to infection. Treatment usually includes antibiotics to eliminate the infection and a low-fiber diet to prevent irritation of inflamed tissues. Once the inflammation is resolved, a high-fiber diet is recommended to ease stool elimination and reduce future attacks of diverticulitis.

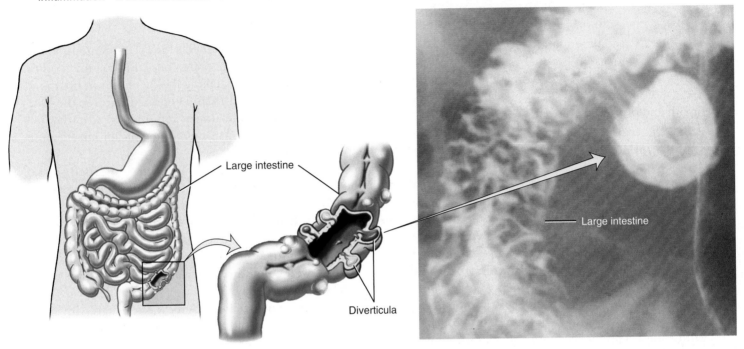

Large intestine

Diverticula

Large intestine

BOWEL HEALTH

Fiber and other indigestible carbohydrates add bulk and absorb water in the gastrointestinal tract, making the feces larger and softer and reducing the pressure needed for defecation. This helps reduce the incidence of constipation and **hemorrhoids**: the swelling of veins in the rectal or anal area. It also reduces the risk of developing **diverticulosis** (FIGURE 4.19).

> **diverticulosis**
> A condition in which outpouches (or sacs) form in the wall of the large intestine.

Although fiber speeds movement of the intestinal contents, when the diet is low in fluid, fiber can contribute to constipation. The more fiber in the diet, the more water is needed to keep the stool soft. When too little fluid is consumed, the stool becomes hard and difficult to eliminate. In severe cases of excessive fiber intake and low fluid intake, intestinal blockage can occur.

A diet high in fiber, particularly from whole grains, may reduce the risk of colon cancer, although not all studies support this finding.[21-24] Fiber reduces contact between the cells lining the colon and potentially cancer-causing substances in the feces. Fiber in the colon also affects the intestinal microflora and their by-products. These by-products may directly affect colon cells or may change the environment of the colon in a way that can affect the development of colon cancer. Some of the protective effect may also be due to antioxidant vitamins and phytochemicals present in fiber-rich whole grains.

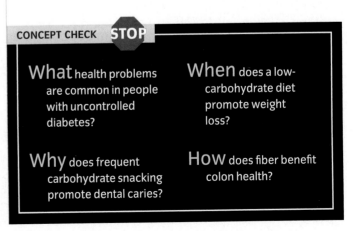

CONCEPT CHECK STOP

What health problems are common in people with uncontrolled diabetes?

When does a low-carbohydrate diet promote weight loss?

Why does frequent carbohydrate snacking promote dental caries?

How does fiber benefit colon health?

Meeting Carbohydrate Needs

LEARNING OBJECTIVES

Discuss how Americans' carbohydrate intake compares with recommendations.

Calculate the percentage of calories from carbohydrate in a food or in a diet.

Use food labels to identify foods high in fiber and low in added sugar.

Recommendations for carbohydrate intake focus on two main points: getting enough carbohydrate to meet the need for glucose and choosing the types that promote health and prevent disease.

CARBOHYDRATE RECOMMENDATIONS

The RDA for carbohydrate is 130 g/day, based on the average minimum amount of glucose used by the brain.[25] In a diet that meets energy needs, this amount provides adequate glucose and prevents ketosis. Additional carbohydrate provides an important source of energy in the diet and carbohydrate-containing foods can add vitamins, minerals, fiber, and phytochemicals. Therefore, the Acceptable Macronutrient Distribution Range for carbohydrate is 45 to 65% of total calorie intake. A diet within this range meets energy needs without excessive amounts of protein or fat (**FIGURE 4.20**).

The typical U.S. diet meets the recommendation for the amount of carbohydrate, but most of this comes from refined sources, making the diet lower in fiber and higher in added sugar than recommended (see the *Case Study*). The Adequate Intake for fiber is 38 g/day for men and 25 g/day for women; the typical intake is only about 15 g/day.

There is no RDA or Daily Value for added sugar, but the Dietary Guidelines and MyPyramid consider added sugar a component of discretionary calories. A 2000-Calorie diet allows only 267 discretionary Calories per day. If half of these discretionary calories came from added sugar, it would be equivalent to about 8 teaspoons, well below an American's average added sugar intake of 32 tsp a day.[26]

Because no specific toxicity is associated with high intake of any type of carbohydrate, no UL has been established for total carbohydrate intake, for fiber intake, or for added sugar intake.

How much carbohydrate do you eat? FIGURE 4.20

To calculate the percentage of calories from carbohydrate in a diet, first determine the number of grams of carbohydrate and multiply this value by 4 Calories per gram. For example, this vegetarian diet provides about 300 grams of carbohydrate:

300 g × 4 Calories/g = 1200 Calories from carbohydrate

Next divide the number of Calories from carbohydrate by the total number of Calories in the diet and multiply by 100 to convert it to a percentage. In this example, the diet contains 2000 total Calories, and so it provides:

(1200 Calories from carbohydrate/2000 Calories total) × 100 = 60% of Calories from carbohydrate

BECOMING LESS REFINED

Guadalupe thinks a good diet is important. She is concerned that she eats too much added refined sugar and not enough fiber. To see if this is a problem, she records what she eats for a day and uses iProfile to determine her energy and nutrient intake. Guadalupe finds that her daily diet provides 2340 Calories, 67 grams of protein, 80 grams of fat, 350 grams of carbohydrate, and 12 grams of fiber.

How does her intake compare with the recommended amounts of carbohydrate and fiber?
▼

By calculating the percentage of calories from carbohydrate (350 grams carbohydrate × 4 Calories/gram ÷ 2340 Calories × 100 = 60%), Guadalupe finds that she is within the recommended range of 45 to 65%. Her fiber intake is low, however. She eats 12 grams of fiber, 13 grams less than the 25 grams recommended for women her age.

Guadalupe is 23 years old and exercises 30 to 60 minutes per day. She eats about 6 ounces of grains, 1.5 cups of vegetables, and 1 cup of fruit per day.

How does her intake of grains, fruits, and vegetables compare with MyPyramid recommendations?
▼

Your answer:

To increase her fiber intake Guadalupe looks at the grains, fruits, and vegetables in her diet. She decides to switch to whole-grain bread and cereal but is not sure which fruits and vegetables are the best sources of fiber. She therefore looks up the fiber content of some of her favorites.

Choose a combination of fruits and vegetables from this list that will add at least 13 grams of fiber to Guadalupe's diet.

Food	Fiber (grams)	Food	Fiber (grams)
Black beans, 1/2 cup	7.5	Canned pears, 1/2 cup	3
Green beans, 1/2 cup	2	Kiwi, 2 small	5
Iceberg lettuce, 1 cup	0.8	Broccoli, 1/2 cup	2.4
Apple, 1 medium	3.7	Banana, 1 medium	2.8
Asparagus, 1/2 cup	1.4	Raw spinach, 1 cup	0.8
Orange, 1 medium	3	Watermelon, 1 cup	0.8

Your answer:

Guadalupe sees that much of the added sugar in her diet comes from soda and candy. She decides she can reduce her intake of added sugar and boost her fiber intake by drinking water and eating dried fruit and granola bars as snacks.

What are the carbohydrate pluses and minuses of these two choices?
▼

Your answer:

Nutrition Facts
Serving Size 1/4 Cup (40g)
Servings Per Container about 28

Amount Per Serving

Calories 110	**Calories from Fat** 0
	% Daily Value
Total Fat 0g	**0%**
Saturated Fat 0g	**0%**
Trans Fat 0g	
Cholesterol 0mg	**0%**
Sodium <5mg	**0%**
Total Carbohydrate 26g	**9%**
Dietary Fiber 2g	**8%**
Sugars 15g	
Protein 1g	

Vitamin A 15%	●	Vitamin C 2%
Calcium 2%	●	Iron 4%

Ingredients: Dried apricots, naturals flavors, sulfur dioxide added as a preservative.

Nutrition Facts
Serving Size 1 Bar Cup (42g)
Servings Per Container 6

Amount Per Serving

Calories 180	**Calories from Fat** 50
	% Daily Value
Total Fat 6g	**9%**
Saturated Fat 0.5g	**3%**
Trans Fat 0g	
Cholesterol 0mg	**0%**
Sodium 167mg	**7%**
Total Carbohydrate 29g	**10%**
Dietary Fiber 2g	**8%**
Sugars 11g	
Protein 4g	

Iron	**6%**

Not a significant source of vitamin A, vitamin C, and calcium

Ingredients: Whole grain rolled oats, sugar, canola oil, crisp rice with soy protein (rice flour, soy protein concentrate, sugar malt, salt), honey, brown sugar syrup, soy lecithin, baking soda, natural flavor, peanut flour, almond flour, pecan flour.

(Check your answers in Appendix K.)

EAT LESS →←

| Baked goods high in added sugar; refined grain products, such as white bread, white rice, and pasta | Sweetened vegetable dishes such as candied yams carrot cake, and zucchini bread | Fruit with added sugar, such as fruit pies and tarts; and fruit juices because fiber has been removed or sugar added | Sweetened dairy products such as sweetened yogurt, flavored milk, and ice cream | Few foods in this group contain added sugar or have fiber removed in processing |

GRAINS   VEGETABLES   FRUITS   MILK   MEAT & BEANS

| Whole grains | Fresh leafy and starchy vegetables | Fresh and dried fruit | Low-fat milk and unsweetened yogurt | Dried peas and beans |

← **EAT MORE** →

Healthy MyPyramid carbohydrate choices FIGURE 4.21

The healthiest carbohydrate choices are carbohydrate-containing foods at the base of each MyPyramid food group, such as whole grains, legumes, and fresh fruits and vegetables, which are low in added sugar and often good sources of fiber. Carbohydrate-containing foods at the tip of each group should be limited because they may contain added sugar or may have had fiber removed in processing.

CHOOSING CARBOHYDRATES WISELY

To promote a healthy, balanced diet, the Dietary Guidelines and MyPyramid recommend increasing consumption of whole grains, vegetables, and fruits and limiting bakery products, candy, soft drinks, and other foods high in added sugars.

Using MyPyramid to make healthy choices

For a 2000-Calorie diet, MyPyramid recommends 6 ounces of grains (half of which should be whole grains), 2 cups of fruit, and 2½ cups of vegetables. As FIGURE 4.21 suggests, refined carbohydrates can be replaced with unrefined ones to make the diet health-ier. For example, an apple provides about 80 Calories and 3.7 grams of fiber, making it a better choice than a cup of apple juice, which has the same amount of energy but almost no fiber (0.2 gram).

Interpreting food labels

Food labels can help in choosing the right mix of carbohydrates (FIGURE 4.22). The Nutrition Facts panel helps find foods that are good sources of fiber. The ingredient list helps identify whole-grain products and sources of added sugar. Nutrient content claims such as "high in fiber" or "no sugar added" and health claims identify foods that help meet the recommendations for fiber and added sugar intake (see *What Should I Eat?* on page 112) (see Appendix F).

A

Whole Wheat Bread

Nutrition Facts

Serving Size 1 Slice (27g)
Servings Per Container 17
Calories 70
Calories from Fat 10

Amount/Serving	%DV*	Amount/Serving	%DV*
Total Fat 1g	2%	**Total Carb.** 12g	4%
Sat. Fat 0g	0%	Dietary Fiber 2g	8%
Trans Fat 0g	0%	Sugars 2g	
Cholesterol 0mg	0%	**Protein** 2g	
Sodium 10mg	0%		

Vitamin A 0% • Vitamin C 0% • Calcium 4% • Iron 4%
Thiamin 4% • Riboflavin 2% • Niacin 4%

*Percent Daily Values (DV) are based on a 2,000-calorie diet. Your daily values may be higher or lower depending on your calorie needs:

	Calories:	2,000	2,500
Total Fat	Less than	65g	80g
Sat Fat	Less than	20g	25g
Cholesterol	Less than	300mg	300mg
Sodium	Less than	2,400mg	2,400mg
Total Carbohydrate		300g	375g
Dietary Fiber		25g	30g

NOT A SODIUM FREE FOOD

INGREDIENTS: WHOLE WHEAT FLOUR, WATER, SWEETENERS (HIGH FRUCTOSE CORN SYRUP MOLASSES), WHEAT GLUTEN, SOYBEAN, CONTAINS 2% OR LESS OF THE FOLLOWING: YEAST, DOUGH CONDITIONERS (MONO DIGLYCERIDES, ETHOXYLATED MONO & GLYCERIDES, CALCIUM STEAROYL-2-LACTYLATE), YEAST NUTRIENTS (CALCIUM SULFATE, MONO- CALCIUM PHOSPHA, CALCIUM PROPIONATE (A PRESERVATIVE).

The Nutrition Facts panel of a food label lists the number of grams of total carbohydrate, fiber, and sugars. The total carbohydrate and fiber values are also given as a percentage of the Daily Value.

The Daily Value for total carbohydrate is 60% of the diet's energy content, or 300 g for a 2000-Calorie diet. The Daily Value for fiber in a 2000-Calorie diet is 25 g.

To identify products made mostly from whole grains, look for the word whole before the name of the grain. If this is the first ingredient listed, the product is made from mostly whole grains.

Foods labeled "good source of fiber" contain between 10% and 19% of the Daily Value per serving.

Foods labeled "high fiber" or "excellent source of fiber" contain 20% or more of the Daily Value per serving.

B

The ingredient list helps identify added sugars. Many products have more than one added sweetener. The closer the name of each sweetener appears to the beginning of the list, the more of it has been added.

INGREDIENTS: CULTURED PASTEURIZED GRADE A REDUCED FAT MILK, SUGAR, NONFAT MILK, HIGH FRUCTOSE CORN SYRUP, STRAWBERRY PUREE, MODIFIED CORN STARCH, KOSHER GELATIN, TRICALCIUM PHOSPHATE, NATURAL FLAVOR, COLORED WITH CARMINE, VITAMIN A ACETATE, VITAMIN D3

On the ingredient list, all these mean added sugar: Brown sugar, corn sweetener, corn syrup, dextrose, fructose, fruit juice, glucose, high fructose corn syrup, honey, invert sugar, lactose, maltose, malt syrup, molasses, raw sugar, sucrose, and sugar syrup concentrates.

Thick & Creamy Lowfat Yogurt STRAWBERRY

Products labeled "reduced sugar" contain 25% less sugar than the regular, or reference, product.

Nutrition Facts

Serving Size 1 Container

Amount Per Serving	
Calories 190	**Calories from Fat** 30

Amount/Serving	% DV*
Total Fat 3.5g	5%
Saturated Fat 2g	10%
Trans Fat 0g	
Cholesterol 15mg	4%
Sodium 100mg	4%
Potassium 310g	9%
Total Carbohydrate 32g	11%
Sugars 28g	
Protein 7g	14%

Vitamin A 15% ● Calcium 30%

*Percent Daily Values (DV) are based on a 2,000 calorie diet.

Foods labeled "sugar free" contain less than 0.5 g of sugar per serving.

The number of grams of sugars listed under Nutrition Facts tells you the total amount of monosaccharides plus disaccharides in a food, but this number does not distinguish between added sugar and the sugar occurring naturally in the food.

Use iProfile to look up the fiber content of some of your favorite foods.

Choose more unrefined carbohydrates

- Pass on the white bread and have your sandwich on whole wheat, oat bran, rye, or pumpernickel.
- Add extra vegetables to your stir fry and serve over brown rice.
- Fill your cereal bowl with oatmeal.
- Satisfy your sweet tooth with a fresh fruit salad.

Increase your fiber

- Don't forget beans—kidney beans, chickpeas, black beans, and others have more fiber and resistant starch than any other vegetables.
- Add berries, bananas, and oats to cereal and desserts.
- Pop some corn.

Limit added sugars

- Switch to a 12-ounce can instead of a 20-ounce bottle when you grab a soft drink or, better yet, have a glass of low-fat milk.
- Use one-quarter less sugar in your recipe next time you bake.
- Snack on a piece of fruit instead of a candy bar.
- Switch to an unsweetened breakfast cereal.

CONCEPT CHECK **STOP**

How does the U.S. diet compare with recommendations for fiber and added sugar?

What types of carbohydrate are recommended by MyPyramid?

Where on a food label can you find information about added sugars?

SUMMARY

1 Carbohydrates in Our Food

1. Unrefined whole grains, fruits, and vegetables are good sources of fiber and micronutrients. When these foods are **refined**, nutrients and fiber are lost. Whole grains contain the **bran**, **germ**, and **endosperm**; refined grains include only the endosperm. **Enrichment**, one type of **fortification**, adds back some but not all of the nutrients lost in refining.

2. Refined sugars contain calories but few nutrients; for this reason, foods high in added refined sugar are low in nutrient density.

2 Types of Carbohydrates

1. Carbohydrates contain carbon as well as hydrogen and oxygen, in the same proportion as water. **Simple carbohydrates** include **monosaccharides** and **disaccharides** and are found in foods such as table sugar, honey, milk, and fruit. **Complex carbohydrates** are **polysaccharides**; they include **glycogen** in animals and **starch** and **fiber** in plants.

2. Fiber cannot be digested in the stomach or small intestine and therefore is not absorbed into the body. **Soluble fiber** dissolves in water to form a viscous solution and is digested by bacteria in the colon; **insoluble fiber** is not digested by bacteria and adds bulk to fecal matter.

3 Carbohydrate Digestion and Absorption

1. Disaccharides and starches must be digested to monosaccharides before they can be absorbed. In individuals with **lactose intolerance**, low levels of the enzyme lactase allow lactose to pass into the colon undigested, causing cramps, gas, and diarrhea. Indigestible complex carbohydrates, including fiber, some **oligosaccharides**, and **resistant starch**, can increase intestinal gas, but they benefit health by increasing bulk in the stool, promoting growth of healthy microflora, and slowing nutrient absorption.

2. After a meal, blood **glucose** levels rise. The rate and duration of this rise are referred to as the **glycemic response**. Glycemic response is affected by the amount and type of carbohydrate consumed and by other nutrients ingested with the carbohydrate.

4 Carbohydrate Functions

1. Carbohydrate, primarily as glucose, provides energy to the body. Blood glucose levels are maintained by the hormones **insulin** and **glucagon**. When blood glucose levels rise, insulin from the pancreas allows cells to take up glucose from the blood and promotes the synthesis of glycogen, fat, and protein. When blood glucose levels fall, glucagon increases them by causing glycogen breakdown and glucose synthesis.

2. Glucose is metabolized through cellular respiration. It begins with **glycolysis**, which breaks each six-carbon glucose molecule into two three-carbon pyruvate molecules, producing ATP even when oxygen is unavailable. The complete breakdown of glucose through **aerobic metabolism** requires oxygen and produces carbon dioxide, water, and more ATP than glycolysis.

3. When carbohydrate intake is limited, amino acids from the breakdown of body proteins can be used to synthesize glucose. Therefore, an adequate carbohydrate intake is said to spare protein. Limited carbohydrate intake also results in the formation of **ketones (ketone bodies)** by the liver. These can be used as an energy source by other tissues. Ketones that accumulate in the blood can cause symptoms that range from headache and lack of appetite to coma and even death if levels are extremely high.

Blood glucose (mg/100 ml)

- Diabetes
- Prediabetes
- Normal

Fasting
- ≥126
- 100–125
- <100

2 hrs.
- ≥200
- 140–199
- <140

5 Carbohydrates in Health and Disease

1. **Diabetes** is characterized by high blood glucose levels that occur either because insufficient insulin is produced or because of a decrease in the body's sensitivity to insulin. Over time, high blood glucose levels damage tissues and contribute to the development of heart disease, kidney failure, blindness, and infections that may lead to amputations. Treatment includes diet, exercise, and medication to keep glucose levels in the normal range.

2. **Hypoglycemia**, or low blood glucose, causes symptoms such as sweating, headaches, and rapid heartbeat.

3. Diets high in carbohydrate, particularly refined sugars, increase the risk of dental caries. The carbohydrate provides a food supply for bacteria that form plaque on the teeth.

4. Gram for gram, carbohydrates provide less energy than fat. High-fiber diets can prevent weight gain by making you feel full longer so that you eat less. Low-carbohydrate diets promote weight loss by causing a spontaneous reduction in food intake. **Nonnutritive sweeteners** aid weight loss if the sugar calories they replace are not added back from other food sources.

5. Diets high in unrefined carbohydrates from whole grains, vegetables, fruits, and legumes may reduce the risk of heart disease, bowel disorders, and colon cancer. Soluble fiber helps prevent heart disease because it can lower blood cholesterol.

6 Meeting Carbohydrate Needs

1. Guidelines for a healthy diet recommend 45 to 65% of energy from carbohydrates. Most of this should come from whole grains, legumes, fruits, and vegetables. Foods high in added sugar should be consumed in moderation.

2. The recommendations of MyPyramid and the information on food labels can be used to select healthy amounts and sources of carbohydrate.

KEY TERMS

CRITICAL AND CREATIVE THINKING QUESTIONS

1. Adam is 14 and plays basketball. Recently, he has been thirsty all the time, and he needs to get up several times a night to urinate. He has lost 10 pounds and is so tired that he has been missing basketball practice. What type of diabetes is most likely affecting Adam? How does it need to be managed? Why is it important to keep blood sugar levels within the normal range in both type 1 and type 2 diabetes?

2. Are carbohydrates good for you? Explain why or why not.

3. Imagine that you have gained 20 pounds over the past 5 years, and you decide to use a low-carbohydrate diet to return to a healthy weight. You are happy with your initial weight loss but begin to have headaches and bad breath. What is causing these symptoms and why?

4. Your breakfast cereal provides 20% of the Daily Value for fiber and lists whole oats as the first ingredient and brown sugar as the second ingredient. What does this tell you about whether it is a whole-grain product? What does this tell you about the amount of added sugar it contains? Would you recommend this product to a friend? Why or why not?

5. Record everything you eat for three days. Next to each high-carbohydrate food, record whether the food is unrefined, minimally processed, or highly processed. Suggest some changes that would increase your intake of less-refined carbohydrates. List some foods in your diet that are high in added sugars. Suggest some changes that would reduce your intake of these sugars. How could you increase your fiber intake?

What is happening in this picture ?

You don't usually think of sugar when you see a field of corn, but all these products contain high-fructose corn syrup (HFCS), an inexpensive sweetener produced by modifying cornstarch to produce a syrup that is approximately 55% fructose and 45% glucose.

- How do you think America's intake of HFCS compares with sucrose intake?

- Are the monosaccharides in HFCS any different from those in sucrose?

- What could you do to reduce the amount of HFCS in your diet?

SELF-TEST

(Check your answers in Appendix L.)

1. Which of the following is a source of unrefined carbohydrate?

   a. white bread
   b. white rice
   c. corn on the cob
   d. donut

2. Which of these molecules is a disaccharide?

   a. A
   b. B
   c. C
   d. D

3. Which of the following is most likely to occur soon after you eat a large carbohydrate-rich meal?

   a. You break down body fat stores.
   b. Your pancreas releases insulin.
   c. Your pancreas releases glucagon.
   d. Your liver breaks down glycogen.
   e. You produce ketones.

4. If curve B on the graph shows the glycemic response after eating kidney beans, which of the following foods is most likely to cause a glycemic response similar to that shown by curve A?

   a. saltine crackers
   b. pat of butter
   c. egg
   d. bowl of bran cereal

5. A diet that provides about half of its calories from carbohydrate .

   a. contains too much carbohydrate to be healthy
   b. is bad for your heart
   c. increases the risk of diabetes
   d. contains the recommended percentage of carbohydrate

6. Which part of a whole grain contains most of the grain's fiber as well as many vitamins?

   a. A
   b. B
   c. C

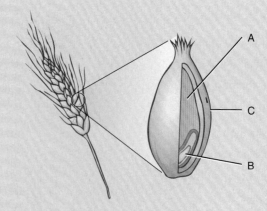

7. Foods high in added sugar provide _____.

  a. many vitamins in each calorie

  b. empty calories

  c. soluble fiber

  d. insoluble fiber

8. Which statement about simple carbohydrates is false?

  a. Fructose is found in fruit.

  b. Lactose is milk sugar.

  c. Glucose is blood sugar.

  d. Maltose is table sugar.

9. The digestive enzymes that break disaccharides into monosaccharides are located in the _____.

  a. stomach

  b. saliva

  c. brush border

  d. colon

10. When blood glucose levels drop, all except which of the following may occur?

  a. Glucagon is released.

  b. Glycogen is broken down.

  c. Fatty acids are used to make glucose.

  d. Amino acids from protein are used to make glucose.

11. Which one of the following statements about soluble fiber is false?

  a. It holds water in the gastrointestinal tract.

  b. It is not digested by bacteria in the colon.

  c. It dissolves in water and forms a viscous solution.

  d. It slows the absorption of nutrients.

12. People who are lactose intolerant do not produce enough of the enzyme _____.

  a. lactase

  b. lactose

  c. galactose

  d. amylase

13. This graph shows an individual's glycemic response after consuming a sugar-sweetened beverage. Which of the following individuals does this graph represent?

  a. a person who has a normal glycemic response

  b. a person who has hypoglycemia

  c. a person who has prediabetes

  d. a person who has diabetes

14. Which steps in the diagram proceed in the absence of oxygen?

  a. only step 1

  b. steps 1, 2, and 3

  c. only step 4

  d. steps 1 and 2

15. A high-fiber diet may help protect against which of the following?

  a. heart disease

  b. diverticulosis

  c. large swings in blood glucose

  d. all of the above

Lipids: Fats, Phospholipids, and Sterols

5

"**S**ausages taste good. Pork chops taste good," wrote filmmaker Quentin Tarantino in the original screenplay of *Pulp Fiction*. Fat makes foods taste good, smell good, and feel good to our palate. Tarantino understands the appeal of fat. As for its function, we have to rely on study, not entertainment.

The word *fat* has come to be associated with unhealthiness, unfitness, and obesity. Fitness gurus and enthusiastic celebrities declare that "fat is bad," whether you are considering which fast-food meal to choose or trying to remove it from your waist. Their 30-second commercial or half-hour program for a new diet regimen or exercise contraption—or both—gives little consideration to the vital role that fats play in healthy nutrition. There is, in reality, nothing intrinsically "bad" about dietary fats. The body uses fats as building blocks for other molecules, as a source of energy, and for energy storage. Fats are as important to a well-balanced diet as carbohydrates, proteins, and vitamins, and without them the body cannot function. Unfortunately, the amount of dietary fat we require and the amount we desire are often two very different things. In the case of the body's requirements for these substances, moderation is key. Whatever our bodies don't use remains in stored reserves. Depending on our lifestyle choices, these abundant unused reserves may become not only unnecessary but unhealthy.

Fats in Our Food

LEARNING OBJECTIVES

Describe the qualities that fat adds to foods.

Identify sources of hidden fat in the diet.

Discuss how fat intake in the United States has changed since the 1970s.

The fats in our foods contribute to their texture, flavor, and aroma. It is the fat that gives ice cream its smooth texture and rich taste. Olive oil imparts a unique flavor to salads and many traditional Italian and Greek dishes. Sesame oil gives egg rolls and other Chinese foods their distinctive aroma. But while the fats in our foods contribute to their appeal, they also add to their caloric content and can affect our health.

SOURCES OF FAT IN OUR FOOD

Sometimes the fat in our food is obvious. You can see the stripes of fat in a slice of bacon sizzling in a frying pan, for example, or the layer of fat around the outside of your steak. Other visible sources of fat in our diets are the fats we add to foods at the table—the pat of butter melting on your steaming baked potato and the dressing you pour over your salad.

Some other sources of fat are less obvious. Cheese, ice cream, and whole milk are high in fat, and foods such as crackers, doughnuts, cookies, and muffins, which we think of as sources of carbohydrate, may also be quite high in fat (FIGURE 5.1). We also add invisible fat when we fry foods: French fries start as potatoes, which are low in fat, but when they are immersed in hot oil for frying, they soak up fat.

AMERICA'S CHANGING FAT INTAKE

Eating patterns in the United States have changed significantly over the past 40 years, even though total fat intake hasn't changed much. Beginning in the 1950s Americans were told that too much fat made them fat, increased their risk of heart disease, and maybe even increased their risk of cancer. In response to these messages, many Americans switched from whole milk to low-fat, chose chicken in place of beef, consumed fewer eggs, and used less butter and high-fat salad dressing. But in addition to these changes, we consumed more hidden fats from foods such as pizza, pasta dishes, snack foods, and fried potatoes.[1] Thus, even though the sources of fat in our diet have changed between 1970 and the present, the types of fat and the number of grams of fat we consume daily have changed little.

What has changed in the past 40 years is our energy intake: It has increased. While the number of calories we eat has increased, the number of grams of fat we eat has remained constant, causing the percentage of calories from fat to drop from about 37% to 33% (FIGURE 5.2).[2]

Visible and hidden fats FIGURE 5.1

The amount of fat in a food is not always obvious. The two strips of bacon in this breakfast provide a total of 8 grams of fat, and the muffin provides 16 grams.

U.S. food intake in the 1970s and today FIGURE 5.2

◀ A In the 1970s, a typical dinner included high-fat meat, bread with butter, and mashed potatoes with lots of gravy, and it was usually served with a glass of whole milk.

B Today we drink low-fat milk and eat leaner meats, but we eat more fat from takeout Chinese and Mexican foods and fast-food pizza, French fries, hamburgers, and cheeseburgers than we did in the 1970s.[1] ▼

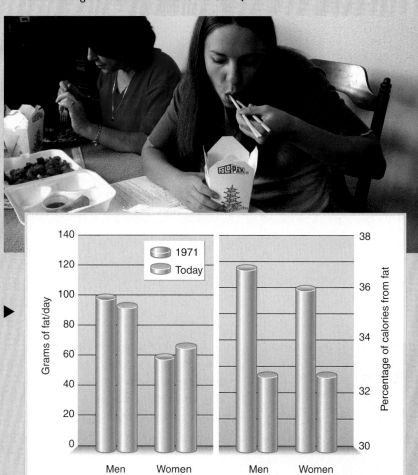

C In 1971, U.S. men consumed an average of 2450 Calories/day and women 1540 Calories/day. Today men consume over 2600 Calories/day and women almost 1900 Calories/day.[2] Because of this increase in energy intake, the percentage of calories from fat decreased, but we don't consume any less fat today than we did in the 1970s.

Efforts to reduce chronic disease risk by cutting fat from our diets have failed not just because we haven't really cut our fat intake but because fat does not deserve its bad reputation. Changing the kinds of foods we choose without paying attention to calories hasn't promoted weight loss. Limiting visible fats without considering hidden fats, the types of fats, and our intake of other dietary components, such as whole grains, fruits, and vegetables, doesn't reduce the incidence of heart disease or cancer. A healthy diet requires eating the right kinds of fats and making healthy choices from all the food groups.

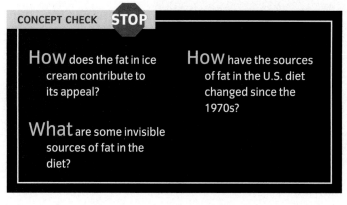

CONCEPT CHECK STOP

HOW does the fat in ice cream contribute to its appeal?

What are some invisible sources of fat in the diet?

HOW have the sources of fat in the U.S. diet changed since the 1970s?

Types of Lipids

L ipids are substances that do not dissolve in water. We tend to use the term *fat* to refer to lipids, but we are usually referring to types of lipids called **triglycerides**. Triglycerides make up most of the lipids in our food and in our bodies. The structure of triglycerides includes lipid

lipids
A group of organic molecules, most of which do not dissolve in water. They include fatty acids, triglycerides, phospholipids, and sterols.

Visualizing

Triglycerides and fatty acids FIGURE 5.3

A A triglyceride contains glycerol and three fatty acids. The carbon chains of the fatty acids vary in length from short-chain fatty acids (4 to 7 carbons) to medium-chain (8 to 12 carbons) and long-chain fatty acids (more than 12 carbons). The types of fatty acids in triglycerides determine their texture, taste, and physical characteristics.

The amounts and types of fatty acids in the triglycerides of chocolate allow it to remain brittle at room temperature, snap when bitten into, and then melt quickly and smoothly in your mouth.

Triglyceride

Oils are fats that are liquid at room temperature. The properties of the fatty acids in vegetable oil allow it to remain a liquid.

triglycerides
The major form of lipid in food and the body; consist of three fatty acids attached to a glycerol molecule.

fatty acids
Molecules made up of a chain of carbons linked to hydrogens, with an acid group at one end of the chain.

phospholipids
Types of lipids whose structure includes a phosphorus atom.

sterols Types of lipids with a structure composed of multiple chemical rings.

molecules called **fatty acids**. Two other types of lipids that are important in nutrition but are present in the body in smaller amounts are **phospholipids** and **sterols**.

TRIGLYCERIDES AND FATTY ACIDS

A triglyceride consists of the three-carbon molecule glycerol with three fatty acids attached to it (FIGURE 5.3A).

A fatty acid is a chain of carbon atoms with an acid group at one end of the chain (FIGURE 5.3B). Fatty acids vary in the length of their carbon chains and the types and locations of carbon–carbon bonds within the chain. Fatty acids are what we are really talking about when we refer to *trans* fat or saturated fat—these terms really mean *trans* **fatty acids** and saturated fatty acids. Triglycerides may contain any combination of fatty acids. The fatty acids in a triglyceride determine its function in the body and the properties it gives to food.

B Most fatty acids in plants and animals contain between 14 and 22 carbons. Each carbon atom in the carbon chain is attached to up to four other atoms. At the methyl or omega end of the carbon chain, three hydrogen atoms are attached to the carbon (CH_3). At the other end of the chain, an acid group (COOH) is attached to the carbon. Each of the carbon atoms in between is attached to two carbon atoms and up to two hydrogen atoms. If there is only one hydrogen atom attached to adjacent carbon atoms, a double bond forms between them.

A fatty acid is saturated when each carbon atom is attached to as many hydrogen atoms as possible so that no double bonds form. The fat on the outside of a steak is solid at room temperature because it is high in saturated fatty acids.

A **monounsaturated fatty acid** contains one carbon–carbon double bond. Canola, olive, and peanut oils, as well as nuts and avocados, are high in monounsaturated fatty acids.

A **polyunsaturated fatty acid** contains more than one carbon–carbon double bond. When the first double bond occurs between the sixth and seventh carbon atoms (from the omega end), the fatty acid is called an **omega-6 (ω-6) fatty acid**. Corn oil, safflower oil, soybean oil, and nuts are sources of omega-6 polyunsaturated fatty acids.

If the first double bond in a polyunsaturated fatty acid occurs between the third and fourth carbon atoms (from the omega end), the fatty acid is an **omega-3 (ω-3) fatty acid**. Fish oils, flaxseed, soybean and canola oils, nuts, and leafy green vegetables are sources of omega-3 polyunsaturated fatty acids.

Saturated fatty acid: palmitic acid

Monounsaturated fatty acid: oleic acid (omega-9)

Polyunsaturated fatty acid: linoleic acid (omega-6)

Polyunsaturated fatty acid: alpha-linolenic acid (omega-3)

Fatty acid composition of foods FIGURE 5.4

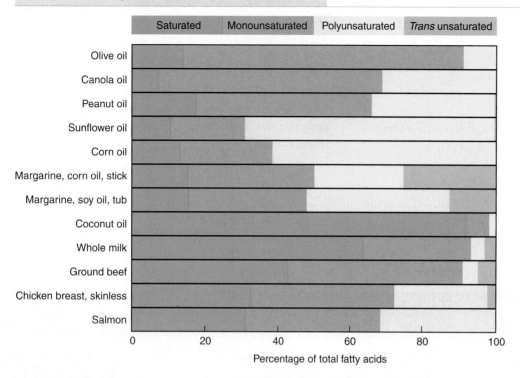

The fats and oils in our diets contain combinations of saturated, monounsaturated, and polyunsaturated fatty acids. Vegetable oils are good sources of mono- and polyunsaturated fatty acids. Animal fats, as well as coconut oil and other tropical oils, are high in saturated fatty acids, while margarines, especially solid margarines, contain more *trans* fatty acids.

Types of fatty acids

Fatty acids are classified as **saturated fatty acids** or **unsaturated fatty acids**, depending on whether they contain carbon–carbon double bonds (see Figure 5.3B). The number and location of these double bonds affect the characteristics that fatty acids give to food and the health effects they have on the body. Triglycerides that are high in saturated fatty acids, such as those found in butter and lard, tend to be solid at room temperature, whereas triglycerides that are higher in unsaturated fatty acids, such as those found in corn, safflower, and sunflower oils, are liquid at room temperature.

Saturated fatty acids are more plentiful in animal foods, such as meat and dairy products, than in plant foods. Plant oils are generally low in saturated fatty acids (FIGURE 5.4). Exceptions include palm oil, palm kernel oil, and coconut oil, which are saturated plant oils. These are often called **tropical oils** because they are found in plants that are common in tropical climates. Saturated plant oils are useful in food processing because they are less susceptible to spoilage than are more unsaturated oils. Spoilage of fats and oils, referred to as *rancidity*, occurs when the unsaturated bonds in fatty acids are damaged by oxygen. When fats go rancid, they give food an "off" flavor.

Food manufacturers can increase the shelf life of oils by using a process called **hydrogenation**, which makes unsaturated oils more saturated. This improves the storage properties of the oils and makes them more solid at room temperature. Products such as hard margarine and shortening have undergone hydrogenation. A disadvantage of this process is that in addition to converting some double bonds into saturated bonds, it transforms some double bonds from the *cis* to the *trans* configuration (FIGURE 5.5). As discussed later, consumption of *trans* fats increases the risk of developing heart disease.

saturated fatty acid A fatty acid in which the carbon atoms are bonded to as many hydrogen atoms as possible; it therefore contains no carbon–carbon double bonds.

unsaturated fatty acid A fatty acid that contains one or more carbon–carbon double bonds; may be either monounsaturated or polyunsaturated.

hydrogenation A process whereby hydrogen atoms are added to the carbon–carbon double bonds of unsaturated fatty acids, making them more saturated.

Cis and trans fatty acids FIGURE 5.5

The orientation of hydrogen atoms around the double bond distinguishes *cis* fatty acids from **trans fatty acids**. Most unsaturated fatty acids found in nature have double bonds in the *cis* configuration.

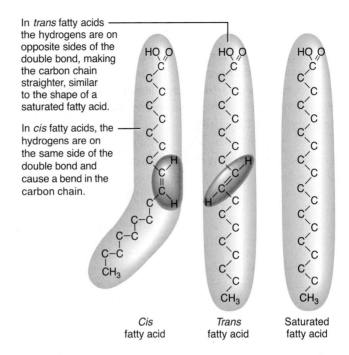

In *trans* fatty acids the hydrogens are on opposite sides of the double bond, making the carbon chain straighter, similar to the shape of a saturated fatty acid.

In *cis* fatty acids, the hydrogens are on the same side of the double bond and cause a bend in the carbon chain.

Cis fatty acid

Trans fatty acid

Saturated fatty acid

Essential fatty acids The body is capable of synthesizing most of the fatty acids it needs from glucose or other sources of carbon, hydrogen, and oxygen. However, humans are not able to synthesize fatty acids that have double bonds in the omega-6 and omega-3 positions. Therefore, the fatty acids **linoleic acid** (omega-6) and **alpha-linolenic acid (α-linolenic acid)** (omega-3)

essential fatty acids Fatty acids that must be consumed in the diet because they cannot be made by the body or cannot be made in sufficient quantities to meet needs.

are considered **essential fatty acids**. They must be consumed in the diet if they are to be available to carry out their essential functions and make other omega-6 and omega-3 fatty acids needed by the body (**FIGURE 5.6**). If the diet is low in linoleic acid and/or α-linolenic acid, any fatty acids that the body would normally synthesize from them become dietary essentials as well.

Essential fatty acids FIGURE 5.6

Linoleic acid is an omega-6 fatty acid that is found in vegetable oils, such as corn and safflower oils. **Arachidonic acid** is an omega-6 fatty acid that is found in both animal and vegetable fats. It is essential only when the diet does not provide enough linoleic acid for the body to synthesize adequate

amounts of it. α-linolenic acid is an omega-3 fatty acid that is found in flaxseed, canola oil, and nuts. **Eicosapentaenoic acid (EPA)** and **docosahexaenoic acid (DHA)** are omega-3 fatty acids that are synthesized from α-linolenic acid; in our diet they are found in fatty fish.

Omega-6

Linoleic acid

↓

Arachidonic acid

Omega-3

α-linolenic acid

Eicosapentaenoic acid (EPA)   Docosahexaenoic acid (DHA)

Phospholipids FIGURE 5.7

A Like a triglyceride, a phospholipid, such as the lecithin molecule shown here, has a backbone of glycerol, but it contains two fatty acids rather than three. Instead of the third fatty acid, a phospholipid has a chemical group containing phosphorus, called a **phosphate group**. The fatty acids at one end of a phospholipid molecule are soluble in fat, while the phosphate-containing region at the other end is soluble in water.

B Phospholipids act as emulsifiers because they can surround droplets of oil, allowing them to remain suspended in a watery environment. The salad dressing shown here does not contain an emulsifier, so it separates into a layer of oil and vinegar and must be shaken before it is poured on your salad. Ranch salad dressings are emulsified so that they do not separate when left standing.

C Phospholipids are an important component of cell membranes. They form a double-layered sheet called the **lipid bilayer** by orienting the water-soluble, phosphate-containing "heads" toward the aqueous (water) environments inside and outside the cell and the fatty acid "tails" toward each other to form the lipid center of the membrane.

PHOSPHOLIPIDS

Phospholipids, though present in small amounts, are important in food and in the body because they allow water and fat to mix. They can do this because one side of the molecule dissolves in water, and the other side dissolves in fat (**FIGURE 5.7A**). In foods, substances that allow fat and water to mix are referred to as **emulsifiers**. For example, the phospholipids in egg yolks allow the oil and water in cake batter to mix; phospholipids in salad dressings prevent the oil and vinegar in the dressing from separating.

One of the best-known phospholipids is **lecithin**. Eggs and soybeans are natural sources of lecithin. The food industry uses lecithin as an emulsifier in margarine,

Cholesterol FIGURE 5.8

Cholesterol

▲ A The cholesterol structure shown here illustrates the four interconnected rings of carbon atoms that form the backbone structure that is common to all sterols.

B Egg yolks and organ meats such as liver and ▶ kidney are high in cholesterol. Lean red meats and skinless chicken are low in total fat but still contain some cholesterol. Cholesterol is not found in plant cell membranes, so even high-fat plant foods, such as nuts, peanut butter, and vegetable oils, do not contain cholesterol.

salad dressings, chocolate, frozen desserts, and baked goods to prevent oil from separating from the other ingredients (FIGURE 5.7B). In the body, lecithin is a major constituent of cell membranes (FIGURE 5.7C). It is also used to synthesize the neurotransmitter acetylcholine, which activates muscles and plays an important role in memory.

STEROLS

The best-known sterol is **cholesterol** (FIGURE 5.8). It is needed in the body, but because the liver manufactures it, it is not essential in the diet. More than 90% of the cholesterol in the body is found in cell membranes (see Figure 5.7C). It is also part of myelin, the insulating coating on many nerve cells. Cholesterol is needed to synthesize other sterols, including vitamin D; bile acids, which are emulsifiers in bile; cortisol, which is a hormone that regulates our physiological response to stress; and testosterone and estrogen, which are hormones necessary for reproduction.

In the diet, cholesterol is found only in foods from animal sources. Plant foods do not contain cholesterol unless it has been added in the course of cooking or processing. Plants do contain other sterols, however, and these **plant sterols** have a role similar to that of cholesterol in animals: They help form plant cell membranes. Plant sterols are found in small quantities in most plant foods; when consumed in the diet, they can help reduce cholesterol levels in the body.

cholesterol
A sterol, produced by the liver and consumed in the diet, which is needed to build cell membranes and make hormones and other essential molecules.

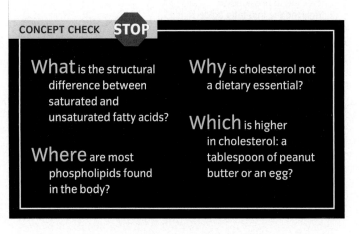

CONCEPT CHECK **STOP**

What is the structural difference between saturated and unsaturated fatty acids?

Where are most phospholipids found in the body?

Why is cholesterol not a dietary essential?

Which is higher in cholesterol: a tablespoon of peanut butter or an egg?

Absorbing and Transporting Lipids

LEARNING OBJECTIVES

Discuss the steps involved in the digestion and absorption of lipids.

Describe how lipids are transported in the blood and delivered to cells.

Compare the functions of LDLs and HDLs.

The fact that oil and water do not mix poses a problem for the digestion of lipids in the watery environment of the small intestine and their transport in the blood, which is mostly water. Therefore, the body has special mechanisms that allow it to digest and transport lipids.

DIGESTION AND ABSORPTION OF FAT

In healthy adults, most fat digestion and absorption occurs in the small intestine (FIGURE 5.9). Here, bile acts as an emulsifier, breaking down large lipid droplets into small globules. The triglycerides in the globules

Process Diagram

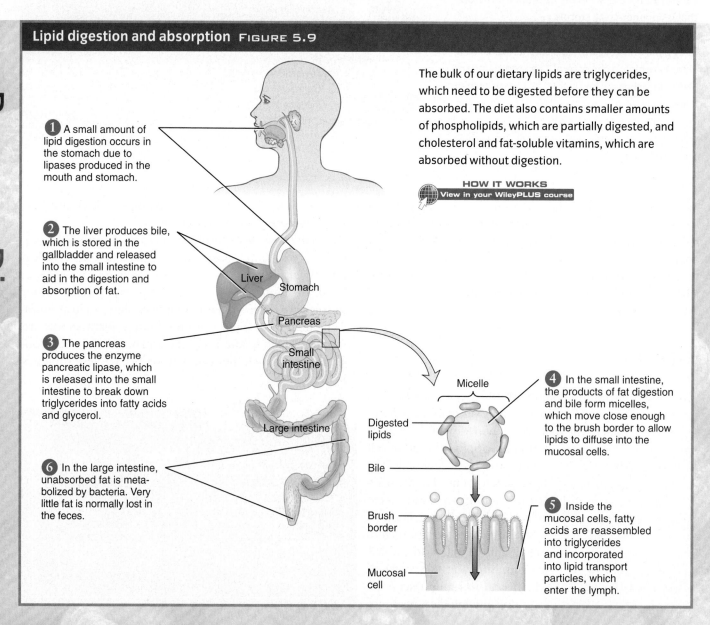

Lipid digestion and absorption FIGURE 5.9

The bulk of our dietary lipids are triglycerides, which need to be digested before they can be absorbed. The diet also contains smaller amounts of phospholipids, which are partially digested, and cholesterol and fat-soluble vitamins, which are absorbed without digestion.

HOW IT WORKS
View in your WileyPLUS course

1 A small amount of lipid digestion occurs in the stomach due to lipases produced in the mouth and stomach.

2 The liver produces bile, which is stored in the gallbladder and released into the small intestine to aid in the digestion and absorption of fat.

3 The pancreas produces the enzyme pancreatic lipase, which is released into the small intestine to break down triglycerides into fatty acids and glycerol.

6 In the large intestine, unabsorbed fat is metabolized by bacteria. Very little fat is normally lost in the feces.

Liver
Stomach
Pancreas
Small intestine
Large intestine

Micelle

Digested lipids

Bile

4 In the small intestine, the products of fat digestion and bile form micelles, which move close enough to the brush border to allow lipids to diffuse into the mucosal cells.

Brush border

Mucosal cell

5 Inside the mucosal cells, fatty acids are reassembled into triglycerides and incorporated into lipid transport particles, which enter the lymph.

Lipoproteins consist of a core of triglycerides and cholesterol surrounded by a shell of protein, phospholipids, and cholesterol. Phospholipids orient with their fat-soluble "tails" toward the interior and their water-soluble "heads" toward the outside.

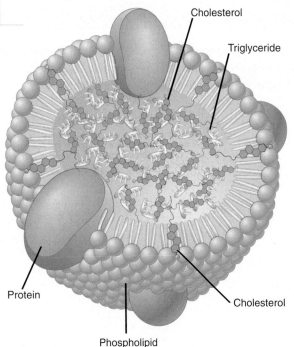

Cholesterol

Triglyceride

Cholesterol

Phospholipid

Protein

micelles Particles that are formed in the small intestine when the products of fat digestion are surrounded by bile. They facilitate the absorption of lipids.

can then be digested by enzymes from the pancreas. The resulting mixture of fatty acids, partially digested triglycerides, cholesterol, and bile forms smaller droplets called **micelles**, which facilitate absorption (see Figure 5.9). The bile in the micelles is also absorbed and returned to the liver to be reused. Once inside the mucosal cells of the intestine, the fatty acids, cholesterol, and other fat-soluble substances must be processed further before they can be transported in the blood.

The fat-soluble vitamins (A, D, E, and K) are absorbed through the same process as other lipids. These vitamins are not digested but must be incorporated into micelles to be absorbed. The amounts absorbed can be reduced if dietary fat is very low or if disease, medications, or other dietary components interfere with fat absorption.

TRANSPORTING LIPIDS IN THE BLOOD

Lipids that are consumed in the diet are absorbed into the intestinal mucosal cells. From here, small fatty acids, which are soluble in water, are absorbed into the blood

and travel to the liver for further processing. Long-chain fatty acids, cholesterol, and fat-soluble vitamins, which are not soluble in water, are not absorbed directly into the blood and must be packaged for transport. They are covered with a water-soluble envelope of protein, phospholipids, and cholesterol to form particles called **lipoproteins** (FIGURE 5.10). Different types of lipoproteins transport dietary lipids from the small intestine to body cells, from the liver to body cells, and from body cells back to the liver for disposal.

lipoproteins Particles that transport lipids in the blood.

Transport from the small intestine After long-chain fatty acids (from the digestion of triglycerides) have been absorbed into the mucosal cells, they are reassembled into triglycerides. These triglycerides, along with cholesterol and fat-soluble vitamins, are packaged with phospholipids, cholesterol, and protein to form lipoproteins called **chylomicrons**. Chylomicrons are too large to enter the capillaries in the small intestine, so they pass from the intestinal mucosa into the lymph, which then delivers them to the

chylomicrons Lipoproteins that transport lipids from the mucosal cells of the small intestine and deliver triglycerides to other body cells.

Lipid transport and delivery FIGURE 5.11

Chylomicrons and very-low-density lipoproteins transport triglycerides and deliver them to body cells. Low-density lipoproteins transport and deliver cholesterol, while high-density lipoproteins help return cholesterol to the liver for reuse or elimination.

HOW IT WORKS
View in your WileyPLUS course

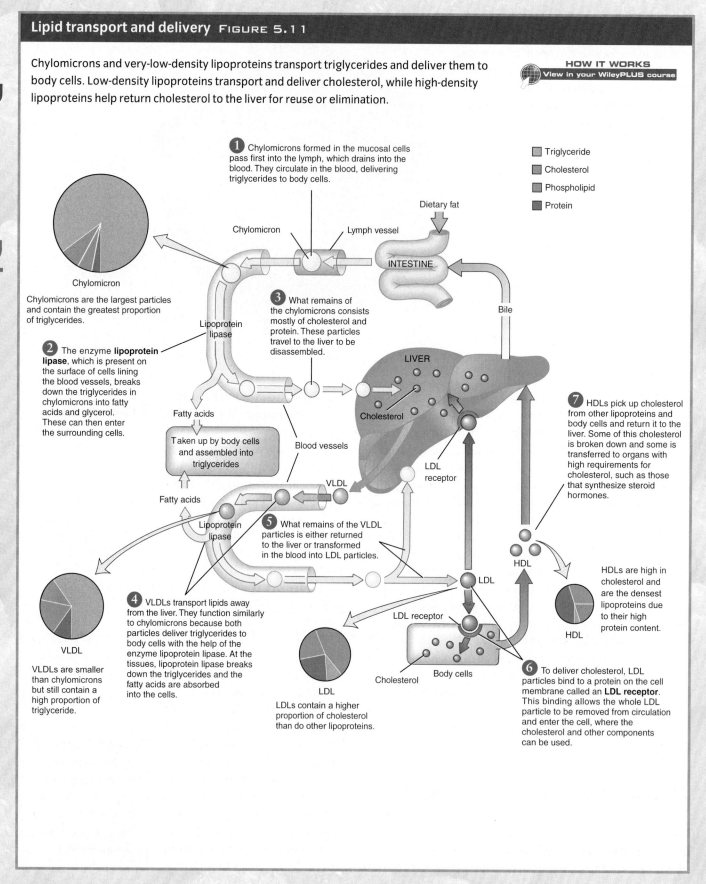

① Chylomicrons formed in the mucosal cells pass first into the lymph, which drains into the blood. They circulate in the blood, delivering triglycerides to body cells.

☐ Triglyceride
☐ Cholesterol
☐ Phospholipid
☐ Protein

Chylomicron

Dietary fat

Chylomicron   Lymph vessel

INTESTINE

Chylomicrons are the largest particles and contain the greatest proportion of triglycerides.

③ What remains of the chylomicrons consists mostly of cholesterol and protein. These particles travel to the liver to be disassembled.

Bile

Lipoprotein lipase

② The enzyme **lipoprotein lipase**, which is present on the surface of cells lining the blood vessels, breaks down the triglycerides in chylomicrons into fatty acids and glycerol. These can then enter the surrounding cells.

LIVER

Fatty acids

Taken up by body cells and assembled into triglycerides

Blood vessels

Cholesterol

⑦ HDLs pick up cholesterol from other lipoproteins and body cells and return it to the liver. Some of this cholesterol is broken down and some is transferred to organs with high requirements for cholesterol, such as those that synthesize steroid hormones.

LDL receptor

VLDL

Fatty acids

Lipoprotein lipase

⑤ What remains of the VLDL particles is either returned to the liver or transformed in the blood into LDL particles.

HDL

HDLs are high in cholesterol and are the densest lipoproteins due to their high protein content.

HDL

VLDL

VLDLs are smaller than chylomicrons but still contain a high proportion of triglyceride.

④ VLDLs transport lipids away from the liver. They function similarly to chylomicrons because both particles deliver triglycerides to body cells with the help of the enzyme lipoprotein lipase. At the tissues, lipoprotein lipase breaks down the triglycerides and the fatty acids are absorbed into the cells.

LDL

LDL receptor

Body cells

Cholesterol

LDL

LDLs contain a higher proportion of cholesterol than do other lipoproteins.

⑥ To deliver cholesterol, LDL particles bind to a protein on the cell membrane called an **LDL receptor**. This binding allows the whole LDL particle to be removed from circulation and enter the cell, where the cholesterol and other components can be used.

blood (FIGURE 5.11). They circulate in the blood, delivering triglycerides to body cells. To enter the cells, the triglycerides must first be broken down into fatty acids and glycerol, which can diffuse across the cell membrane. Once inside the cells, fatty acids can either be used to provide energy or reassembled into triglycerides for storage.

Transport from the liver

The liver can synthesize lipids. Lipids are transported from the liver in **very-low-density lipoproteins (VLDLs)**. Like chylomicrons, VLDLs are lipoproteins that circulate in the blood, delivering triglycerides to body cells. When the triglycerides have been removed from the VLDLs, a denser, smaller particle remains. About two-thirds of these particles are returned to the liver, and the rest are transformed in the blood into **low-density lipoproteins (LDLs)**. LDLs are the primary cholesterol delivery system for cells. They contain a higher proportion of cholesterol than do chylomicrons or VLDLs (see Figure 5.11). High levels of LDLs in the blood have been associated with an increased risk for heart disease. For this reason, they are sometimes referred to as "bad cholesterol."

■ **low-density lipoproteins (LDLs)** Lipoproteins that transport cholesterol to cells.

Eliminating cholesterol

Because most body cells have no system for breaking down cholesterol, it must be returned to the liver to be eliminated from the body. This reverse cholesterol transport is accomplished by **high-density lipoproteins (HDLs)**. HDL cholesterol is often called "good cholesterol" because high levels of HDL in the blood are associated with a reduction in the risk of heart disease.

■ **high-density lipoproteins (HDL)** Lipoproteins that pick up cholesterol from cells and transport it to the liver so that it can be eliminated from the body.

CONCEPT CHECK STOP

How does bile help in the digestion and absorption of lipids?

Why are lipoproteins needed to transport lipids?

What is the primary function of LDL cholesterol?

Lipid Functions

Fat is necessary to maintain health. In our diet, fat is needed to absorb fat-soluble vitamins and is a source of essential fatty acids and energy. In our bodies, lipids form structural and regulatory molecules and are broken down to provide ATP. As discussed earlier, cholesterol plays both regulatory and structural roles: It is used to make steroid hormones, and it is an important component of cell membranes and the myelin coating that is necessary for brain and nerve function.

Most lipids in the body are triglycerides stored in **adipose tissue**, which is body fat that lies under the skin and around internal organs (FIGURE 5.12). The triglycerides in our adipose tissue provide a lightweight energy storage molecule, help cushion our internal organs, and insulate us from changes in temperature. Triglycerides are also found in oils that lubricate body surfaces, keeping the skin soft and supple.

Adipose tissue FIGURE 5.12

A The amount and location of adipose tissue affect our body size and shape. Adipose tissue is an important source of stored energy, insulates the body from changes in temperature, and provides a cushion to protect against shock.

B Adipose tissue cells contain large droplets of triglyceride that push the other cell components to the perimeter of the cell. As weight is gained, the triglyceride droplets enlarge.

THE ROLE OF ESSENTIAL FATTY ACIDS

Essential fatty acids are important for the formation of the phospholipids that give cell membranes their structure and functional properties. As such, they are important for growth, skin integrity, fertility, and maintaining red blood cell structure. They are particularly important in cell membranes in the retina of the eye and in the central nervous system. Arachidonic acid and DHA are necessary for normal brain development in infants and young children. Essential fatty acids also serve as regulators of fatty acid and glucose metabolism through their role in gene expression.

eicosanoids
Regulatory molecules that can be synthesized from omega-3 and omega-6 fatty acids.

Longer-chain omega-6 and omega-3 polyunsaturated fatty acids made from linoleic and α-linolenic acid are used to make hormonelike molecules called **eicosanoids**. Eicosanoids help regulate blood clotting, blood pressure, immune function, and other body processes. The effect of an eicosanoid on these functions depends on the fatty acid from which it is made. For example, when the omega-6 fatty acid arachidonic acid is the starting material, the eicosanoid synthesized increases blood clotting; when the eicosanoid is made from the omega-3 fatty acid EPA, it decreases blood clotting. The ratio of dietary omega-6 to omega-3 fatty acids affects the balance of the omega-6 and omega-3 fatty acids in the body and, therefore, the balance of the omega-6 and omega-3 eicosanoids produced.

The U.S. diet contains a higher ratio of omega-6 to omega-3 fatty acids than is optimal for health.[3] Increasing consumption of foods that are rich in omega-3 fatty acids increases the proportion of omega-3 eicosanoids. This reduces the risk of heart disease by decreasing inflammation, lowering blood pressure, and reducing blood clotting. The American Heart Association recommends eating two or more servings per week of fish, which is a good source of EPA and DHA, along with plant sources of omega-3 fatty acids, such as walnuts, canola oil, and flaxseed.[4]

Process Diagram

Metabolism of fat FIGURE 5.13

HOW IT WORKS
View in your WileyPLUS course

Digestion of dietary triglycerides yields fatty acids and a small amount of glycerol. Fatty acids provide most of the energy stored in a triglyceride molecule. Inside the mitochondria, the fatty acid chains are broken down to form acetyl-CoA, which can be further metabolized to generate carbon dioxide, water, and ATP. The glycerol molecules, which contain three carbon atoms, can also be used to produce ATP or small amounts of glucose.

1. Beta-oxidation splits fatty acids into two-carbon units that form acetyl-CoA and produces high-energy electrons (dashed lines).

2. If oxygen and enough carbohydrate are available, acetyl-CoA enters a circular pathway, releasing two molecules of carbon dioxide and more high-energy electrons.

3. In the final step of aerobic metabolism, the energy in the high-energy electrons released in beta-oxidation and the circular pathway is trapped and used to produce ATP and water.

When we eat too much, excess energy is stored in the form of triglycerides. When we don't eat enough, triglycerides in adipose tissue are broken down, releasing fatty acids, which can be used to provide energy.

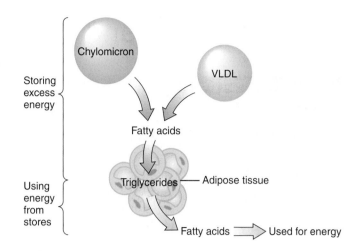

FAT AS A SOURCE OF ENERGY

Fat is an important source of energy in the body (**FIGURE 5.13**). Because each gram of fat provides 9 Calories, compared with only 4 Calories per gram from carbohydrate or protein, a large amount of energy can be stored in the body as fat without a great increase in body size or weight. Even a lean man stores over 50,000 Calories of energy in the form of triglycerides.

Triglycerides that are consumed in the diet can be either used immediately to fuel the body or stored in adipose tissue. Throughout the day, triglycerides are continuously stored and then retrieved from storage to be broken down, depending on the body's immediate energy needs. For example, after a meal, some triglycerides will be stored; then, between meals, some of the stored triglycerides will be broken down to provide energy. When the energy consumed in the diet equals the body's energy requirements, the net amount of body fat does not change.

Storing triglycerides

Excess calories that are consumed in the diet as fat can be transported directly from the intestines to the adipose tissue in chylomicrons. This is demonstrated by the fact that the fatty acid composition of your adipose tissue varies, depending on the types of fatty acids in the food you eat. Excess calories that are consumed as carbohydrate or protein must first go to the liver, where they can be used to synthesize fatty acids, which are then assembled into triglycerides and transported in VLDLs to adipose tissue (**FIGURE 5.14**).

The ability of the body to store excess triglycerides is theoretically limitless. Cells in your adipose tissue can increase in weight by about 50 times, and new fat cells can be made when existing cells reach their maximum size.

Retrieving energy from fat stores

When you eat fewer calories than you use, your body takes energy from its fat stores. In this situation, an enzyme inside the fat cells receives a signal to break down stored triglycerides. The fatty acids and glycerol that result are released directly into the blood and circulate throughout the body. They are taken up by cells and used to produce ATP (see Figure 5.14).

If there is not enough carbohydrate to allow the acetyl-CoA produced by fatty acid breakdown to enter aerobic metabolism, it will be used to make *ketones* (see Chapter 4). Muscle and adipose tissue can use ketones as an energy source. During prolonged starvation or fasting, the brain can adapt itself to use ketones to meet about half of its energy needs. For the other half, it continues to require glucose. Fatty acids cannot be used to make glucose, and only a small amount of glucose can be made from the glycerol released from triglyceride breakdown.

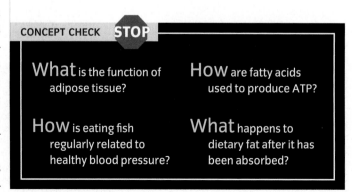

CONCEPT CHECK **STOP**

What is the function of adipose tissue?

How are fatty acids used to produce ATP?

How is eating fish regularly related to healthy blood pressure?

What happens to dietary fat after it has been absorbed?

Lipids in Health and Disease

LEARNING OBJECTIVES

Define essential fatty acid deficiency.

Describe the events that lead to the development of atherosclerosis.

Evaluate your risk of heart disease.

Discuss the role of dietary fat in promoting weight gain.

The amount and types of fat you eat can affect your health. A diet that is too low in fat can reduce the absorption of fat-soluble vitamins, slow growth, and impair the functioning of the skin, eyes, liver, and other body organs. Eating the wrong types of fat can contribute to chronic diseases such as heart disease and cancer. Consuming too much fat can increase calorie intake and contribute to extra body fat storage and therefore weight gain. Excess body fat, in turn, is associated with an increased risk of diabetes, cardiovascular disease, and high blood pressure.

ESSENTIAL FATTY ACID DEFICIENCY

If adequate amounts of linoleic and α-linolenic acid are not consumed, an **essential fatty acid deficiency** will result. Symptoms include scaly, dry skin, liver abnormalities, poor healing of wounds, impaired vision and hearing, and growth failure in infants. Because the require-

essential fatty acid deficiency A condition characterized by dry, scaly skin and poor growth that results when the diet does not supply sufficient amounts of linoleic acid and α-linolenic acid.

Process Diagram

Development of atherosclerosis FIGURE 5.15

The inflammation that occurs in response to an injury to the artery wall precipitates the development of atherosclerotic plaque. The presence of plaque can eventually lead to a heart attack or stroke.

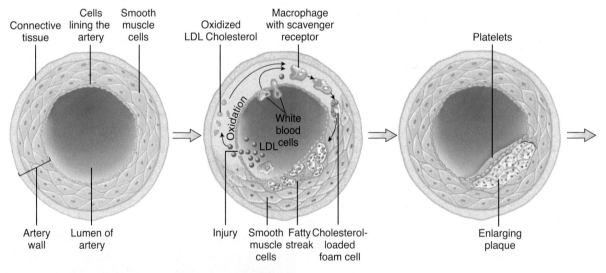

Normal artery

① The wall of a normal, healthy artery consists of a layer of epithelial cells surrounded by smooth muscle.

Fatty streak formation

② Plaque formation begins when the lining of the artery is damaged. An injury makes the lining more permeable to LDL particles, which migrate into and are retained in the artery wall. Here they are modified to form **oxidized LDL cholesterol**, which promotes inflammation.

③ Oxidized LDL cholesterol causes white blood cells to stick to and migrate into the artery wall, where they mature into large cells called **macrophages. Scavenger receptors** on the surface of macrophages transport oxidized LDL cholesterol into the cell. As macrophages fill with oxidized LDL cholesterol, they become **foam cells.** These cholesterol-filled cells accumulate in the artery wall and then burst, forming a fatty streak.[7,8]

Plaque accumulation

④ Macrophages and foam cells in the artery wall secrete chemicals that continue the inflammatory process and promote growth of the plaque. Smooth muscle cells migrate into the fatty streak and secrete fibrous proteins. **Platelets,** cell fragments involved in blood clotting, clump together around the plaque. As plaque builds up, it causes the artery to narrow and lose its elasticity.

ment for essential fatty acids is well below the typical intake in the United States, essential fatty acid deficiencies are rare in this country. However, deficiencies have occurred in infants and young children consuming low-fat diets and in individuals who are unable to absorb lipids.

HEART DISEASE

More than 80 million people in the United States suffer from some form of **cardiovascular disease**, which is any disease that affects the heart and blood vessels. It is the number-one cause of death for both men and women in the United States.[5] **Atherosclerosis** is a type of cardiovascular disease in which cholesterol is deposited in the artery walls, reducing their elasticity and eventually blocking the flow of blood. The development of atherosclerosis

> ■ **atherosclerosis**
> A type of cardio-vascular disease that involves the buildup of fatty material in the artery walls.

has been linked to diets that are high in cholesterol, saturated fat, and *trans* fat.[6]

How atherosclerosis develops

Inflammation, the process whereby the body responds to injury, is what drives the formation of **atherosclerotic plaque**. For example, cutting yourself triggers an inflammatory response. White blood cells, which are part of the immune system, rush to the injured area, blood clots form, and soon new tissue grows to heal the wound. Similar inflammatory responses occur when an artery is injured, but instead of resulting in healing, they lead to the development of atherosclerotic plaque (**FIGURE 5.15**). Therefore, the atherosclerotic process begins with an injury and the response to this injury causes changes in the lining of the artery wall.

> ■ **atherosclerotic plaque** Cholesterol-rich material that is deposited in the arteries of individuals with atherosclerosis. It consists of cholesterol, smooth muscle cells, fibrous tissue, and eventually calcium.

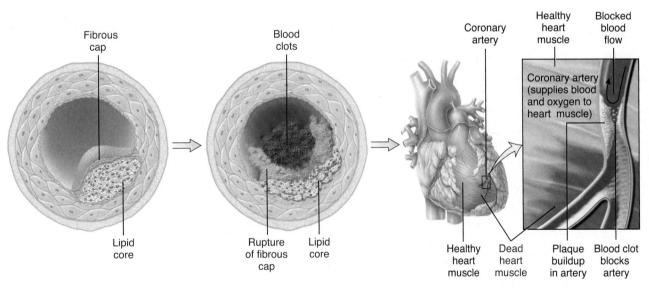

Fibrous cap formation

⑤ As the process progresses, a cap of smooth muscle cells and fibrous proteins forms over the plaque, walling it off from the lumen of the artery. If the inflammation continues, substances secreted by immune system cells can cause the cap to degrade.[7,8]

Fibrous cap rupture

⑥ If the cap ruptures or erodes, exposing the inner core, blood clots can rapidly form around it. The blood clots can completely block the artery at that spot or break loose and block an artery elsewhere.

Heart attack

⑦ If blood flow in a coronary artery is blocked, a heart attack results. Heart muscle cells that are cut off from their blood supply die, causing pain and reducing the heart's ability to pump blood. If the blood flow to the brain is interrupted, a stroke results. Brain cells are cut off from their blood supply and die.

The exact cause of the injuries that initiate the development of atherosclerosis is not known but may be related to elevated blood levels of LDL cholesterol, glucose, or the amino acid homocysteine or to high blood pressure, smoking, diabetes, genetic alterations, or infection.[8] The specific cause may be different in different people.

Risk factors for heart disease
Diabetes, high blood pressure, obesity, and high blood cholesterol levels are considered primary risk factors for heart disease because they directly increase risk. Other factors that affect risk include age, gender, genetics, and lifestyle factors such as smoking, exercise, and diet (TABLE 5.1).

Diet and heart disease risk
Individual nutrients, such as saturated fat and cholesterol; particular whole foods, such as nuts and fish; and dietary patterns, such as diets that are high in plant foods, affect heart disease risk. For example, diets that are high in fiber, **antioxidants**, and B vitamins can reduce the risk of developing heart disease. On the other hand, too much salt or saturated fat can increase heart disease risk. Intake of fish, nuts, and whole grains may decrease risk, while diets that are high in red meat may increase risk. More important than any individ-

antioxidant
A substance that is able to neutralize reactive oxygen molecules and thereby prevent cell damage.

ual dietary factor, though, are overall dietary and lifestyle patterns. The importance of these patterns is exemplified by the fact that the incidence of heart disease is lower in Asian and Mediterranean countries than in the United States (FIGURE 5.16). The heart-protective effect that these traditional diets seem to have has prompted nutrition experts to promote a Mediterranean dietary pattern to reduce the risk of heart disease in the United States.

Frequently, diet affects heart disease risk because it alters blood cholesterol levels. High intakes of saturated fat and cholesterol from high-fat meats and dairy products can cause an increase in blood levels of total and LDL cholesterol. High intakes of *trans* fat from products such as shortening that contain hydrogenated vegetable oils increase blood levels of LDL cholesterol and the risk of heart attack. Replacing these unhealthy fats with monounsaturated and polyunsaturated fats from nuts and vegetable oils lowers total and LDL cholesterol.[13] Consuming plant sterols reduces cholesterol absorption in the small intestine, lowering total and LDL cholesterol levels.[13] Small quantities of plant sterols are present in many fruits, vegetables, nuts, seeds, cereals, legumes, and vegetable oils. Larger amounts have been added to products such as margarines, salad dressings, and orange juice.

What's your risk of heart disease? TABLE 5.1

Risk Factor	How It Affects Your Risk
Obesity	Obesity increases blood pressure, blood cholesterol levels, and the risk of developing diabetes. It also increases the amount of work the heart must do to pump blood throughout the body.
Diabetes	High blood glucose damages blood vessel walls, initiating atherosclerosis.
High blood pressure	High blood pressure can damage blood vessel walls, initiating atherosclerosis. It forces the heart to work harder, causing it to enlarge and weaken over time.
Gender	Men and women are both at risk for heart disease, but men are generally affected a decade earlier than are women. This difference is due in part to the protective effect of the hormone estrogen in women. As women age, the effects of menopause—including a decline in estrogen level and a gain in weight—increase heart disease risk.
Age	Risk is increased in men age 45 and older and in women age 55 and older.
Family history	Individuals with a male family member who exhibited heart disease before age 55 or a female family member who exhibited heart disease before age 65 are considered to be at increased risk. African Americans have a higher risk of heart disease than the general population, in part due to the high incidence of high blood pressure among African Americans.[9]
Blood lipid level	Blood levels of total cholesterol, LDL cholesterol, HDL cholesterol, and triglycerides are all used to assess risk.[10]

	Low risk/Optimal	Near optimal	Borderline high	High risk
Cholesterol (mg/100 ml)	<200		200–239	≥240
LDL cholesterol (mg/100ml)	<100	100–129	130–159	≥160
HDL cholesterol (mg/100 ml)	≥60			<40
Triglycerides (mg/100 ml)	<150			

Risk Factor	How It Affects Your Risk
Lifestyle	Smoking increases risk. Regular exercise decreases risk by reducing blood pressure, increasing healthy HDL cholesterol levels, reducing the risk of diabetes, and promoting a healthy weight. Diet, including the types of lipids and the amounts of fiber, antioxidants, B vitamins, salt, sugar, and alcohol included in the diet, can affect the risk of heart disease.

Mediterranean Diet Pyramid
A contemporary approach to delicious, healthy eating

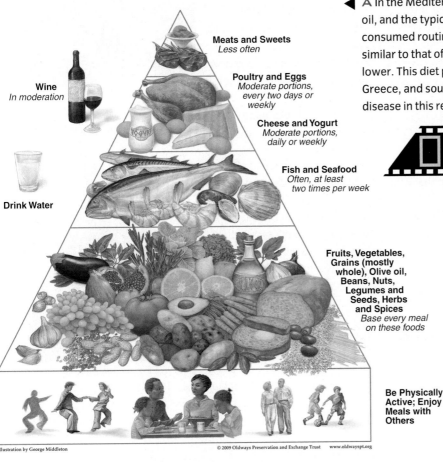

Meats and Sweets
Less often

Wine
In moderation

Poultry and Eggs
*Moderate portions,
every two days or
weekly*

Cheese and Yogurt
*Moderate portions,
daily or weekly*

Drink Water

Fish and Seafood
*Often, at least
two times per week*

Fruits, Vegetables,
Grains (mostly
whole), Olive oil,
Beans, Nuts,
Legumes and
Seeds, Herbs
and Spices
*Base every meal
on these foods*

Be Physically
Active; Enjoy
Meals with
Others

Illustration by George Middleton   © 2009 Oldways Preservation and Exchange Trust   www.oldwayspt.org

Traditional dietary patterns and heart disease
FIGURE 5.16

◀ **A** In the Mediterranean region, the main source of dietary fat is olive oil, and the typical diet is high in nuts, vegetables, and fruits. Fish is consumed routinely and red meat rarely. Despite a fat intake that is similar to that of the U.S. diet, the incidence of heart disease is much lower. This diet pyramid is based on the dietary patterns of Crete, Greece, and southern Italy around 1960, when the rates of chronic disease in this region were among the lowest in the world.

B In Asian countries, plant foods that are rich in fiber and antioxidants form the base of the diet, and animal products are more peripheral. Traditional Asian diets include more fish and seafood than red meat. Combined with small amounts of vegetable oil, this pattern produces a balance of omega-3 to omega-6 fatty acids that helps prevent heart disease.[11] Routine consumption of green tea, which is high in antioxidants, may also contribute to the low rate of chronic disease, in the region.[12] This diet pyramid was inspired by the traditional cuisines of southern and eastern Asia. ▶

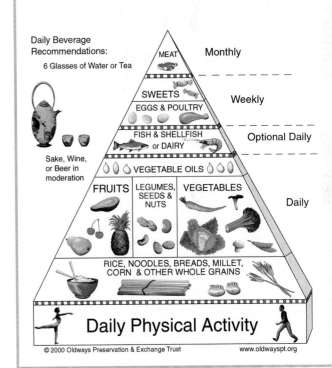

The Traditional Healthy Asian Diet Pyramid

Daily Beverage
Recommendations:
6 Glasses of Water or Tea

MEAT — Monthly

SWEETS
EGGS & POULTRY — Weekly

FISH & SHELLFISH
or DAIRY — Optional Daily

Sake, Wine,
or Beer in
moderation

VEGETABLE OILS

FRUITS | LEGUMES, SEEDS & NUTS | VEGETABLES — Daily

RICE, NOODLES, BREADS, MILLET,
CORN & OTHER WHOLE GRAINS

Daily Physical Activity

© 2000 Oldways Preservation & Exchange Trust   www.oldwayspt.org

◀ **C** Traditional Asian and Mediterranean diets often protect against heart disease, but as younger generations abandon these long-established dietary patterns for more modern ones, the incidence of high blood pressure, elevated blood lipids, diabetes, and obesity is likely to rise.

Lipids in Health and Disease   137

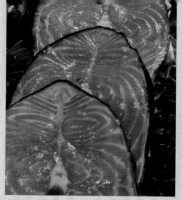

A Omega-3 fatty acids found in fish, flaxseed, and vegetable oils reduce the risk of heart disease and decrease mortality from heart attacks. In addition to lowering triglyceride levels, they protect against heart disease by decreasing the stickiness of platelets, lowering blood pressure, improving the function of the cells lining blood vessels, reducing inflammation, and modulating heartbeats.[14]

B Nuts, olives, and avocados are all good sources of monounsaturated fat, which lowers LDL cholesterol and makes it less susceptible to oxidation. Nuts are also high in omega-3 fatty acids, fiber, vegetable protein, antioxidants, and plant sterols. Diets containing nuts may lower heart disease risk by decreasing total and LDL cholesterol, increasing HDL, and improving the functioning of cells lining the artery wall.[15,16]

C Diets that are high in fruits, vegetables, and whole grains reduce the risk of heart disease.[17] Fruits and vegetables add fiber, antioxidants, and phytochemicals. Whole grains provide fiber, omega-3 fatty acids, B vitamins, and antioxidants, as well as other phytochemicals that may protect against heart disease.

D Moderate alcohol consumption—that is, one drink a day for women and two a day for men (one drink is equivalent to 5 ounces wine, 12 ounces beer, or 1.5 ounces distilled spirits)—reduces blood clotting and increases HDL cholesterol but also raises blood triglyceride levels. Higher alcohol intake increases the risk of heart disease and causes other health and societal problems.

Eating to reduce the risk of heart disease FIGURE 5.17

Diet can also affect heart disease risk through mechanisms unrelated to blood cholesterol level. Much of the heart-protective effect of omega-3 fatty acids, such as those found in fish, is due to the eicosanoids made from them, which prevent the growth of atherosclerotic plaque, reduce blood clotting and blood pressure, and decrease inflammation (FIGURE 5.17).[14] Diets that are high in soluble fiber may reduce heart disease risk by lowering cholesterol or by helping to lower triglyceride levels, blood pressure, and body weight.[13]

Diets that are high in plant foods are good sources of fiber as well as vitamins, minerals, and phytochemicals, some of which protect against heart disease because they perform antioxidant functions. Antioxidants decrease the oxidation of LDL cholesterol and, therefore, the development of plaque in artery walls.[18] Adequate intakes of vitamin B_6, vitamin B_{12}, and folic acid also help protect against heart disease because they help maintain low blood levels of the amino acid homocysteine (discussed further in chapter 7). Elevated homocysteine levels are associated with a higher incidence of heart disease.[19]

CANCER

Cancer is the second leading cause of death in the U.S. As with heart disease, there is evidence that the risk of cancer can be reduced with changes in diet and activity patterns.[20] Populations consuming diets that are high in fruits and vegetables tend to have a lower risk of cancer than populations with lower intakes. These foods are rich in antioxidants such as vitamin C, vitamin E, and β-carotene. In contrast, in populations that consume diets that are high in fat, particularly animal fats, the incidence of cancer is higher.

The good news is that the same type of diet that protects you from cardiovascular disease may also reduce the risk of certain forms of cancer. For example, the incidence of breast cancer in Mediterranean women whose diet is high in monounsaturated fat, is low despite a total fat intake similar to that in the United States.[21] *Trans* fatty acids, on the other hand, not only raise LDL cholesterol levels but are also believed to increase the risk of breast cancer.[22] Diets that are high in omega-3 fats from fish are associated with a lower incidence of colon cancer.[23]

OBESITY

Excess dietary fat consumption contributes to weight gain and obesity. One reason is that fat contains 9 Calories per gram, more than twice the calorie content of carbohydrate or protein. Therefore, a high-fat meal contains more calories in the same volume than does a lower-fat meal. Because people have a tendency to eat a certain weight or volume of food, consuming meals that are high in fat causes more calories to be consumed.[24,25] Dietary fat may also contribute to weight gain because it is stored very efficiently as body fat.

Despite the fact that fat is fattening, the fat content of the U.S. diet is unlikely to be the sole reason for the high rate of obesity in the United States.[26] Weight gain occurs when energy intake exceeds energy expenditure, regardless of whether the extra energy comes from fat, carbohydrate, or protein. The increasing prevalence of overweight and obesity in the United States and worldwide is likely due to a general increase in calorie intake combined with a decrease in energy expenditure.[27]

CONCEPT CHECK STOP

Why does a deficiency of essential fatty acids cause health problems?

What are three dietary factors that increase the risk of heart disease?

How is oxidized LDL cholesterol involved in the formation of atherosclerotic plaque?

Why might eating a high-fat diet increase the number of calories you consume?

Meeting Lipid Needs

LEARNING OBJECTIVES

Discuss the recommendations for fat and cholesterol intake.

Classify fats as either healthy or unhealthy.

Name a food that is high in cholesterol, saturated fat, or *trans* fat.

Use food labels to choose healthy fats.

The amount of fat the body requires from the diet is small, but a diet that provides only the minimum amount would be very high in carbohydrate, not be very palatable, and not necessarily be any healthier than diets with more fat. Therefore, the recommendations for fat intake focus on getting enough to meet the need for essential fatty acids and choosing the amounts and types of fat that will promote health and prevent disease.

FAT AND CHOLESTEROL RECOMMENDATIONS

The DRIs recommend a total fat intake of 20% to 35% of calories for adults. Of this, a small proportion needs to come from the essential fatty acids. The AI for linoleic acid is 12 grams per day for women and 17 grams per day for men. You can meet your requirement by consuming a half-cup of walnuts or 2 tablespoons of safflower oil. For α-linolenic acid, the AI is 1.1 grams per day for women and 1.6 grams per day for men. Your requirement can be met by eating a quarter-cup of walnuts or 1 tablespoon of ground flaxseeds. Consuming these amounts provides the recommended ratio of linoleic to α-linolenic acid of between 5:1 and 10:1.[6]

The DRIs recommend that cholesterol, saturated fat, and *trans* fat intake be kept to a minimum because the risk of heart disease increases with higher intakes (see the *Case Study* on the next page). The Daily Values used on food labels give more specific recommendations.

Children need more fat to allow for growth and development, so their acceptable ranges of fat intake are higher: 30% to 40% of calories for ages 1 to 3 and 25% to 35% of calories for ages 3 to 18. Like adults, adolescents and children over age 2 should consume a diet that is low in saturated fat, cholesterol, and *trans* fat.[28]

CHOOSING FATS WISELY

The typical American diet falls within the recommended 20% to 35% of calories from fat, and meets cholesterol guidelines. Our *trans* fat intake is declining because food manufacturers have reduced the *trans* fat content of fats and oils used in processing. However, our intake of saturated fat exceeds recommendations, and most people don't get enough omega-3 fatty acids.[29]

IMPROVING HEART HEALTH

Rafael is a financial advisor who spends much of his day sitting at his computer. When he is home with his family, he enjoys watching his children play soccer and basketball but rarely finds time to exercise himself. Rafael's doctor recently told him that his blood cholesterol levels are elevated. His blood lipids and other information about his medical history are given below:

Sex	Male
Age	35
Family history	Mother had heart attack at age 60.
Height/weight	68 inches/160 lb
Blood pressure	145/80 (optimal is < 120/80)
Smoker	Yes
Activity level	Sedentary
Blood values	
Total cholesterol	210 mg/100 ml
LDL cholesterol	160 mg/100 ml
HDL cholesterol	34 mg/100 ml
Triglycerides	120 mg/100 ml

Which of the factors listed here increase Rafael's risk of developing cardiovascular disease?

▼

Your answer:

Rafael meets with a dietitian. A diet recall reveals that his breakfast typically consists of a bagel with cream cheese and coffee with cream and sugar. For lunch, he goes out with his colleagues for fast food. Dinner at home with his family consists of beef or chicken, a green or orange vegetable, and rice or potatoes.

An analysis of his diet indicates that his total fat intake is within the recommended range of 20% to 35% of calories, but he consumes more saturated fat than is recommended, and his intake of omega-3 and monounsaturated fatty acids is low.

To reduce Rafael's intake of saturated fat, the dietitian suggests that he switch to cereal with low-fat milk for breakfast and make better fast-food choices at lunchtime. For lunch, he frequents a burger fast-food restaurant, a taco shop, or a pizza restaurant.

What could he choose at his favorite fast-food restaurants to reduce his intake of saturated fat?

▼

Your answer:

At home, to increase intake of omega-3 and monounsaturated fatty acids, the family switches to canola oil and olive oil for cooking and has fish or seafood twice a week. Because these changes have reduced the calories in Rafael's diet and he did not need to lose weight, he starts bringing fruit and other snacks to work with him.

Which of the following snack choices is the most heart healthy? Give two reasons.

▼

Your answer:　　　(Check your answers in Appendix K.)

Cheese Sandwich Crackers

Nutrition Facts

Serving Size 1 Package (43g)
Servings Per Container 12

Amount/Serving	
Calories 230 Calories from Fat 120	
	% Daily Value*
Total Fat 14g	**22%**
Saturated Fat 3.5g	**18%**
Trans Fat 4g	
Polyunsaturated Fat 5.5g	
Monounsaturated Fat 1g	
Cholesterol 5mg	**2%**
Sodium 410mg	**17%**
Total Carbohydrate 23g	**8%**
Dietary Fiber less than 1g	**2%**
Sugars 6g	
Protein 3g	

Vitamin A 0%	•	Vitamin C 0%
Calcium 6%	•	Iron 6%

*Percent Daily Values are based on a 2,000 calorie diet. Your daily values may be higher or lower depending on your calorie needs:

		Calories:	2,000	2,500
Total Fat	Less than		65g	80g
Sat Fat	Less than		20g	25g
Cholesterol	Less than		300mg	300mg
Sodium	Less than		2,400mg	2,400mg
Total Carbohydrate			300g	375g
Dietary Fiber			25g	30g

Dried Fruit and Nut Mix

Nutrition Facts

Serving Size 1/4 cup (28g)
Servings Per Container 9

Amount/Serving	
Calories 170 Calories from Fat 50	
	% Daily Value*
Total Fat 6g	**9%**
Saturated Fat 1g	**5%**
Trans Fat 0g	
Polyunsaturated Fat 1.5g	
Monounsaturated Fat 3.5g	
Cholesterol 0mg	**0%**
Sodium 0mg	**0%**
Total Carbohydrate 15g	**5%**
Dietary Fiber 2g	**8%**
Sugars 11g	
Protein 3g	

Vitamin A 0%	•	Vitamin C 0%
Calcium 0%	•	Iron 4%

*Percent Daily Values are based on a 2,000 calorie diet. Your daily values may be higher or lower depending on your calorie needs:

		Calories:	2,000	2,500
Total Fat	Less than		65g	80g
Sat Fat	Less than		20g	25g
Cholesterol	Less than		300mg	300mg
Sodium	Less than		2,400mg	2,400mg
Total Carbohydrate			300g	375g
Dietary Fiber			25g	30g

Processed grains such as frozen pizzas, macaroni and cheese, flavored rice dishes, crackers, and baked goods, which can be hidden sources of total fat, saturated fat, and *trans* fat.	French fries and breaded fried vegetables, such as onion rings, zucchini, and mushrooms, which are high in fat and energy and can be a source of saturated fat or *trans* fat.	Fruit pies and tarts, which are high in refined sugar and can add total fat, saturated fat, and *trans* fat as well as refined sugar to the diet.	Solid fats such as lard, butter, stick margarine, and shortening. These are high in saturated fat, cholesterol, or *trans* fat and are considered discretionary calories.	Whole-fat milk products like whole milk, ice cream, cheese, and cream are high in total and saturated fat as well as cholesterol.	Fatty and fried meats. Trimming the fat from meat, choosing lean cuts, and removing the skin from poultry can reduce the amount of total fat, saturated fat, and cholesterol in the diet.

GRAINS **VEGETABLES** **FRUITS** **OILS** **MILK** **MEAT & BEANS**

Whole grains	Fresh leafy, green, and orange vegetables. These have little or no fat unless it is added in cooking or processing.	Fresh and dried fruit most of which is low in fat. Avocados are high-fat fruit that provides heart healthy monounsaturated fats.	Liquid vegetable oils such as olive, canola, soybean, and corn oil, which are good sources of mono and polyunsaturated fat.	Nonfat or low-fat milk and milk products.	Legumes, which are low in fat, nuts and seeds, which add omega-3 and monounsaturated fat and fish which provides long-chain omega-3 fatty acids.

EAT MORE

Healthy MyPyramid choices FIGURE 5.18

Foods at the base of each MyPyramid food group are low in solid fats and may be low in total fat or may be good sources of healthy liquid oils. Those at the tip of each group may contain solid fat and added sugar.

Shifting the sources of dietary fat can improve the proportion of healthy fats in your diet. Limiting solid fats such as those in red meat and cheese will reduce your intake of saturated fat and cholesterol. Avoiding hydrogenated fats from foods such as hard margarines and baked goods will limit your intake of *trans* fat. Eating more nuts and avocados and cooking with canola and olive oils will boost your intake of monounsaturated fat, and eating more fish will boost your omega-3 intake.

Making wise MyPyramid choices Your choices from each food group can have a significant impact on the amounts and types of fats in your diet (FIGURE 5.18). Generally, grains, fruits, and vegetables are low in total fat and saturated fat and they contain no cholesterol. However, choices from these groups need to be made with care to avoid fats that are added in processing or preparation. Smart choices from the meat and beans and milk groups can

Looking for Lean Meat

Fresh meats are not required to carry Nutrition Facts labels, but they often provide information about the fat content of the meat. The terms *lean* and *extra lean* are used to describe the fat content of packaged meats, such as hot dogs and lunch meat, and fresh meats, such as pork chops and steaks. "Lean" means that the meat contains less than 10% fat by weight, and "extra lean" means that it contains less than 5% fat by weight (see Appendix F). So a package of ground beef like this one that is 85% lean looks like a good choice.

Ground beef that is 85% lean looks like a healthy, low-fat choice.

☐ % Fat ☐ % Protein ☐ % Water

Weight   Calories

The chart on the left shows what percentage of the weight of the ground beef consists of fat, protein, and water. The graph on the right shows the percentage of calories contributed by fat, protein, and water. Because each gram of fat contributes 9 Calories, compared to only 4 Calories/g for protein and none for water, the fat in this meat contributes almost two-thirds of its calories.

What a scientist sees is that "percent lean" and "lean" are not the same thing. "Percent lean" refers to the weight of the meat that is lean, not the percentage of calories provided by lean meat. So when the label says it is 85% lean, it means that 15% of the weight of the meat is fat, or that there are 15 grams of fat in 100 grams (3.5 ounces) of raw hamburger. This is a relatively small percentage by weight, but because fat contains 9 Calories per gram, the fat contributes 63% of the calories in the meat. If you want to purchase ground beef that fits the definition of a "lean" meat, what "percent lean" should you look for on the label?

reduce your intake of unhealthy fats (see *What a Scientist Sees*).

Oils, butter, margarine, fatty sauces, and salad dressings used in cooking or added at the table are the most concentrated sources of fat in the diet. Limiting these can reduce your total fat and calorie intake, and choosing liquid oils rather than solid fat can increase the proportion of unsaturated fats in your diet. Because solid fats such as butter, shortening, beef fat, and lard are high in saturated or *trans* fats, the Dietary Guidelines and MyPyramid consider these discretionary calories—calories that are left over after you have met your nutrient needs by choosing the right amounts of nutrient-dense foods from each of the food groups. If you consume a 2000-Calorie diet you can include only about 270 discretionary Calories. Spreading 1 tablespoon of butter on your morning toast uses up 100 Calories, over one third of your discretionary calories.

Refer to food labels
Food labels are an accessible source of information about the fat content of packaged foods. The Nutrition Facts panel shows the amounts of total fat, saturated fat, and *trans* fat, and the ingredient list indicates the source of the fat—for example, whether a food contains corn oil, soybean oil, coconut oil, or partially hydrogenated vegetable oil. Nutrient content claims such as "low fat," "fat free," and "low cholesterol" on food labels can also be used to identify foods that help you meet the recommendations for fat intake. Health claims can help you choose foods that will meet your nutritional goals. For example, foods that are low in saturated fat and cholesterol may state that they help reduce the risk of heart disease (**FIGURE 5.19** and Appendix F).

Lipids on food labels FIGURE 5.19

A Understanding how to use food labels can help you make more informed choices about the foods you include in your diet. By noting the grams of fat and the total number of Calories, you can determine the percentage of calories from fat in a product as follows:

1. Multiply the grams of fat by 9 Calories/gram. For example, this product provides about 11 grams of fat:

   11 grams × 9 Calories/gram =
   99 Calories from fat

2. Divide Calories from fat by total Calories and multiply by 100 to obtain the percentage.

   For example, this food contains 100 Calories/serving and 99 Calories from fat:

   99 Calories ÷ 100 Calories × 100 =
   99% Calories from fat

A % Daily Value is listed for total fat, saturated fat, and cholesterol. This allows consumers to tell how a food fits the recommendations. Generally, <5% of the Daily Value is low; >20% is high. There are no Daily Values for *trans*, polyunsaturated, and monounsaturated fat.

The Nutrition Facts panel lists Calories from fat; grams of total fat, saturated fat, and *trans* fat; and milligrams of cholesterol in a serving. The amount of monounsaturated and polyunsaturated fat is voluntarily included on the labels of some products, such as this one.

The Daily Values recommend consuming less than 30% of energy as fat, no more than 300 mg of cholesterol/day, and no more than 10% of energy as saturated fat. It is recommended that *trans* fat intake not increase above the current average level of 2.6% of calorie intake.[30]

The sources of fat in a product are listed in the ingredient list with the other ingredients in order of prominence by weight.

Mayonnaise

Nutrition Facts
Serving Size 1Tbsp (13g)
Servings Per Container 30

Amount/Serving	
Calories 100	Calories from Fat 99

	% Daily Value*
Total Fat 11g	**17%**
Saturated Fat 1.5g	**8%**
Trans Fat 0g	
Polyunsat Fat 6.5g	
Monounsat Fat 3g	
Cholesterol 5mg	**2%**
Sodium 70mg	**3%**
Total Carbohydrate 0g	**0%**
Dietary Fiber 0g	**0%**
Sugars 0g	
Protein 0g	

Vitamin A 0%	•	Vitamin C 0%
Calcium 0%	•	Iron 0%

*Percent Daily Values are based on a 2,000 calorie diet. Your daily values may be higher or lower depending on your calorie needs:

		Calories:	2,000	2,500
Total Fat	Less than		65g	80g
Sat Fat	Less than		20g	25g
Cholesterol	Less than		300mg	300mg
Sodium	Less than		2,400mg	2,400mg
Total Carbohydrate			300g	375g
Dietary Fiber			25g	30g

INGREDIENTS: SOYBEAN OIL, WHOLE EGG YOLKS, DISTILLED VINEGAR, WATER, SUGAR, SALT, CIDER VINEGAR AND SPICES.

Fat free: Contains <0.5 g fat per serving

Reduced fat: Contains at least 25% less fat per serving than the regular or reference product

Low fat: Contains ≤3 g fat per serving

B Food labeling regulations have developed standard definitions for descriptors such as "low fat" and "low cholesterol," and such terms can be used only in ways that will not confuse the consumer. For example, because saturated fat in the diet raises blood cholesterol, to be labeled "low cholesterol" a food must contain ≤20 mg cholesterol per serving and ≤2g saturated fat per serving. So crackers containing coconut oil, which are low in cholesterol but are high in saturated fat cannot be labeled "low cholesterol."

THE ROLE OF FAT REPLACERS

People often choose low-fat and reduced-fat products in order to reduce the total amount of fat in their diets. Some of these foods, such as low-fat and nonfat milk and yogurt, are made by simply removing the fat, but in other products, the fat is replaced with ingredients that mimic the taste and texture of the fat. A number of these fat replacers are carbohydrate based, a few are protein based, and others are made from fats that are modified to reduce or prevent absorption (FIGURE 5.20).[31] A prob-lem with nonabsorbable fats is that they reduce the absorption of the fat-soluble substance in the diet, including the fat-soluble vitamins, A, D, E, and K. To avoid depleting these vitamins, products made with Olestra, which is a nonabsorbable fat substitute, have been fortified with them. However, these products are not fortified with β-carotene and other fat-soluble substances that may be important for health. Another potential problem with Olestra is that it can cause abdominal cramping and loose stools in some individuals because it passes into the colon without being digested.

Fat replacers FIGURE 5.20

Both carbohydrate- and protein-based fat replacers add calories to foods because they are made from energy-yielding nutrients. Some fat replacers are made from fats that have been modified to reduce how well they can be digested and absorbed. The calories they provide depend on how much is absorbed.

The artificial fat Olestra (sucrose polyester) is made from sucrose with fatty acids attached. Olestra cannot be digested by either human enzymes or bacterial enzymes in the gastro-intestinal tract. Therefore, it is excreted in the feces without being absorbed.

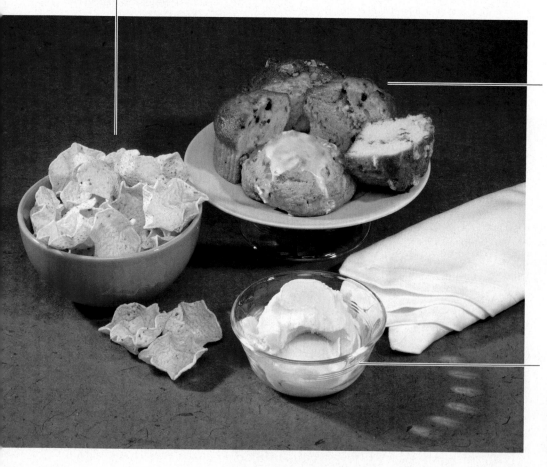

Polysaccharides such as pectins and gums are often used in baked goods, as well as salad dressings, sauces, and ice cream, to mimic the texture that fat provides. They reduce the amount of fat in a product and at the same time add soluble fiber.

Protein-based fat replacers are made from milk and egg proteins processed to form millions of microscopic balls that slide over each other, mimicking the creamy texture of fat.[31] They are used in frozen desserts, cheese foods, and other products, but cannot be used for frying because they break down at high temperatures.

Use iProfile to find the varieties of nuts and fish that are highest in omega-3 fatty acids.

Limit your intake of cholesterol, *trans* fat, and saturated fat
- Use low-fat dairy products.
- Trim the fat from your meat and serve chicken and fish but don't eat the skin.
- Cut in half your usual amount of butter and use soft rather than stick margarine.
- Use beans instead of meat in your chili, soups, and casseroles.

Increase the proportion of polyunsaturated and monounsaturated fats
- Use olive, peanut, or canola oil for cooking and salad dressing.
- Use corn, sunflower, or safflower oil for baking.
- Snack on nuts and seeds.
- Add olives and avocados to your salads.

Up your omega-3 intake
- Bake flaxseeds into breads and sprinkle them on your cereal or yogurt.
- Add another serving of fatty fish, such as mackerel, lake trout, herring, sardines, tuna, or salmon, to your weekly menu.
- Have a leafy green vegetable with dinner.
- Add walnuts to your salad or cereal.

Will using low-fat and reduced-fat products improve your diet? Some low-fat foods make an important contribution to a healthy diet. Low-fat dairy products are recommended because they provide all the essential nutrients contained in the full-fat versions but have fewer calories and less saturated fat and cholesterol. Using these products increases the nutrient density of the diet as a whole. However, not all reduced-fat foods are nutrient dense. Some are just lower-fat versions of nutrient-poor choices such as baked goods and chips. If these reduced-fat desserts and snack foods replace whole grains, fruits, and vegetables, the resulting diet could be low in fat but also low in fiber, vitamins, minerals, and phytochemicals (see *What Should I Eat?*).

Using low-fat foods does not necessarily transform a poor diet into a healthy one or improve overall diet quality, but if used appropriately, fat-modified foods can be part of a healthy diet.[31] For example, if a low-fat salad dressing replaces a full-fat version, it allows you to enhance the appeal of a nutrient-rich salad without as much added fat and calories from the dressing. Low-fat

products can also be used in conjunction with weight-loss diets because they are often lower in calories. But check the label. Although they are lower in calories, they are by no means calorie free and cannot be consumed liberally without adding calories to the diet and possibly contributing to weight gain.

CONCEPT CHECK　STOP

How much fat is recommended in a healthy diet?

Why is fatty fish a healthier choice than fatty beef?

Which food groups contribute the most foods that are high in saturated fat and cholesterol?

How can labels help you identify foods that are low in cholesterol and saturated fat?

SUMMARY

1 Fats in Our Food

1. Fat adds calories, texture, and flavor to foods. Some of the fats we eat are visible, but others are hidden.

2. Over the past 40 years, Americans have changed the sources of fat in their diets, but the number of grams of fat consumed daily has changed little, and the incidence of obesity and other chronic diseases has continued to rise.

2 Types of Lipids

1. **Lipids** are a diverse group of organic compounds, most of which do not dissolve in water. **Triglycerides**, commonly referred to as fat, are the type of lipid that is most abundant in our food and in our **adipose tissue**. A triglyceride

contains three **fatty acids** attached to a molecule of glycerol.

2. The structure of fatty acids affects their chemical properties and functions in the body. Each carbon atom in the carbon chain of a **saturated fatty acid** is attached to as many hydrogen atoms as possible, so no carbon–carbon double bonds form. Saturated fatty acids are found primarily in animal products. Exceptions include saturated plant oils often called **tropical oils**. A **monounsaturated fatty acid** contains one carbon–carbon double bond. A **polyunsaturated fatty acid** contains more than one carbon–carbon double bond. The location of the first double bond determines whether it is an **omega-3 (ω-3)** or an **omega-6 (ω-6) fatty acid**. The orientation of hydrogen atoms around a carbon–carbon double

bond distinguishes *cis* fatty acids from *trans* fatty acids. **Hydrogenation** transforms some carbon–carbon double bonds to the *trans* configuration.

3. A **phospholipid** contains a **phosphate group** and two fatty acids attached to a backbone of glycerol. One end of the molecule is water soluble, and one end is lipid soluble. Phospholipids therefore make good **emulsifiers**. In the human body, they are an important structural component of cell membranes and **lipoproteins**.

4. **Sterols**, of which **cholesterol** is the best known, are made up of multiple chemical rings. Cholesterol is made by the body and consumed in animal foods in the diet. In the body, it is a component of cell membranes and is used to synthesize vitamin D, bile acids, and some hormones.

3 Absorbing and Transporting Lipids

1. In the small intestine, muscular churning mixes chyme with bile from the gallbladder to break fat into small globules. This allows pancreatic lipase to access these fats for digestion. The products of triglyceride digestion, cholesterol, phospholipids, and other fat-soluble substance combine with bile to form **micelles**, which facilitate the absorption of these materials.

2. Lipids absorbed from the intestine are packaged with protein to form **chylomicrons**. The triglycerides in

chylomicrons are broken down by **lipoprotein lipase** on the surface of cells lining the blood vessels. The fatty acids released are taken up by surrounding cells, and what remains is taken up by to the liver.

3. **Very-low-density lipoproteins (VLDLs)** are synthesized by the liver. With the help of lipoprotein lipase, they deliver triglycerides to body cells. **Low-density lipoproteins (LDLs)** deliver cholesterol to tissues by binding to **LDL receptors** on the cell surface. **High-density lipoproteins (HDLs)** help remove cholesterol from cells and transport it to the liver for disposal.

Micelle

Digested lipids

Bile

Brush border

Mucosal cell

4 Lipid Functions

1. Dietary fat is needed for the absorption of fat-soluble vitamins and to provide essential fatty acids. In the body, triglycerides in adipose tissue provide a concentrated source of energy and insulate the body against shock and temperature changes. **Essential fatty acids** are needed for normal structure and function of cell membranes, particularly those in the retina and central nervous system. Long-chain omega-6 and omega-3 polyunsaturated fatty acids are used to synthesize **eicosanoids**, which help regulate blood clotting, blood pressure, immune function, and other body processes. The ratio of dietary omega-6 to omega-3 fatty acids affects the balance of omega-6 and omega-3 eicosanoids made and hence their overall physiological effects.

2. Throughout the day, triglycerides are continuously stored in adipose tissue and then broken down to release fatty acids, depending on the immediate energy needs of the body. To generate ATP from fatty acids, the carbon chain is broken into two carbon units that form acetyl-CoA, which can then be metabolized by aerobic pathways.

5 Lipids in Health and Disease

1. **Essential fatty acid deficiency** causes symptoms such as scaly, dry skin, liver abnormalities, poor healing of wounds, impaired vision and hearing, and growth failure.

2. **Atherosclerosis** is a disease characterized by the formation of **atherosclerotic plaque** in the artery wall. It is begun by an injury to the artery wall that triggers **inflammation**, leading to plaque formation. A key event in the process is the oxidation of LDL cholesterol in the artery wall. **Oxidized LDL cholesterol** promotes inflammation and attracts white blood cells, which fill with cholesterol, forming **foam cells** that deposit in the artery wall. High blood levels of total and LDL cholesterol are risk factors for heart disease. High blood HDL cholesterol protects against heart disease. The risk of atherosclerosis is also increased by diabetes, high blood pressure, and obesity.

3. Diets high in saturated fat, *trans* fat, and cholesterol increase the risk of heart disease. Diets high in omega-6 and omega-3 polyunsaturated fatty acids, monounsaturated fatty acids, certain B vitamins, and plant foods containing fiber, antioxidants, and phytochemicals reduce the risk of heart disease. The total dietary and lifestyle pattern is more important than any individual dietary factor in reducing heart disease risk.

4. Diets high in fat correlate with an increased incidence of certain types of cancer. In general, the same types of lipids and other dietary components that protect you from heart disease will also protect you from certain forms of cancer.

5. Fat contains 9 Calories per gram. A high-fat diet may therefore increase energy intake and promote weight gain, but it is not the primary cause of obesity. Consuming more energy than expended leads to weight gain, regardless of whether the energy is from fat, carbohydrate, or protein.

Blood clots

Rupture of fibrous cap

Lipid core

6 Meeting Lipid Needs

1. The DRIs recommend that adults consume a diet that provides 20% to 35% of energy from fat and is low in cholesterol, saturated fat, and *trans* fat.

2. The U.S. diet is not too high in fat, but it often does not contain the healthiest types of fats. To reduce saturated fat and cholesterol intake, limit solid fats and choose liquid oils, fish, and nuts and seeds often. Use food labels to avoid processed foods that are high in saturated and *trans* fat. A diet based on whole grains, fruits, vegetables, and lean meats and low-fat dairy products will meet the recommendations for fat intake.

3. Fat replacers are used to create reduced-fat products with taste and texture similar to the original. Some low-fat products are made by using mixtures of carbohydrates or proteins to simulate the properties of fat, and some use lipids that are modified to reduce their digestion and absorption. Products containing fat replacers can help reduce fat and energy intake when used in moderation as part of a balanced diet.

KEY TERMS

CRITICAL AND CREATIVE THINKING QUESTIONS

1. The percentage of calories from fat in the typical American diet has decreased since the 1970s. Nevertheless, there has been an increase in the incidence of obesity in the United States over this same period. Discuss how is it possible that people are cutting down on the percentage fat in their diet and still gaining weight.

2. Record everything you eat for three days or refer to a previous food record. List the dairy products in your diet and indicate whether they are full fat or reduced fat. List the grain products you typically consume. How many of them are baked goods with added fats? How many of them are eaten with an added high-fat spread or sauce? Suggest changes you could make to reduce the fats added to your carbohydrates. List the vegetables in your diet. Underline those that are cooked or prepared in a way that increases their fat intake. For example, are they fried or topped with butter or margarine? List the high-protein foods in your diet. Use iProfile to determine the types and amounts of lipids they provide. Substitute some high-protein foods that would increase your intake of monounsaturated and omega-3 fatty acids.

3. Ka Ming is 54 years old and has lived in the United States since 1964. A physical exam reveals that his total blood cholesterol is 280 mg/100 ml and his HDL cholesterol is 25 mg/100 ml. He is at a healthy weight and does not smoke. He gets little exercise and consumes a diet that is a mixture of American foods and traditional Chinese foods. A medical history reveals that none of Ka Ming's relatives in China have had cardiovascular disease. Why might the lack of cardiovascular disease in his family history not be a true indication of Ka Ming's risk?

4. Compare and contrast the structure and functions of chylomicrons and VLDLs.

5. What are the similarities and differences in how the body responds to a cut on the finger and to an injury to the inside of an artery wall?

6. Why might taking fish oil supplements reduce the rate at which your blood clots?

7. How could a person who is a vegan and therefore consumes no dietary cholesterol still have elevated blood cholesterol?

What is happening in this picture ?

This individual has familial hypercholesterolemia, a rare genetic disease in which there are no LDL receptors on cells. It causes cholesterol levels so high that the cholesterol deposits in body tissues, seen here as raised lumps.

■ Why would this condition cause elevated blood cholesterol?

■ How would this condition affect the risk of developing heart disease?

SELF-TEST

(Check your answers in Appendix L.)

1. What type of fatty acid is labeled C in the illustration?

  a. saturated

  b. monounsaturated

  c. omega-3 polyunsaturated

  d. omega-6 polyunsaturated

2. Which one of the following is unlikely to occur after you eat a fatty meal?

  a. Fatty acids stored in adipose tissue are released into the blood and taken up by body cells as an energy source.

  b. The gallbladder releases bile into the small intestine.

  c. Micelles are formed in the small intestine.

  d. Pancreatic lipase releases fatty acids from triglycerides.

  e. The concentration of chylomicrons in the blood increases.

3. Omega-3 fatty acids have a beneficial effect on blood lipid levels but also reduce the risk of cardiovascular diseases because they _____.

  a. inhibit the absorption of cholesterol from the diet

  b. increase the formation of oxidized LDL cholesterol

  c. cause mutations in cellular DNA

  d. break down *trans* fatty acids

  e. are converted into eicosanoids

4. Which of the following statements about cholesterol is false?

  a. It is used to synthesize vitamin D.

  b. It is needed to make bile.

  c. It is an essential component of animal cell membranes.

  d. It is found in peanut butter, leafy green vegetables, and avocados.

  e. It is needed to make the hormones estrogen and testosterone.

5. Which two fatty acids are considered essential?

  a. saturated and unsaturated

  b. linoleic and α-linolenic

  c. stearic and palmitic

  d. EPA and DHA

  e. short and medium chain

Use the diagram to answer questions 6 and 7.

6. Which of the following statements about dietary sources of fat is false.

  a. Canola oil is high in monounsaturated fat.

  b. Coconut oil is high in polyunsaturated fat.

  c. Salmon is high in unsaturated fatty acids.

  d. Whole milk is high in saturated fat.

  e. Stick margarine is a source of *trans* fatty acids.

7. Which of the following is the best source of monounsaturated fatty acids and is also low in saturated and *trans* fatty acids.

  a. corn oil

  b. whole milk

  c. olive oil

  d. stick margarine

  e. ground beef

8. Which one of the following is associated with an increased risk of developing heart disease?

   a. a high concentration of HDL in the blood
   b. daily exercise
   c. a high-fiber, low-fat diet
   d. a diet made up mostly of plant foods
   e. a high concentration of LDL in the blood

9. Which of the following contribute to the lower heart disease risk associated with eating nuts?

   a. They are high in monounsaturated fat and omega-3 fatty acids.
   b. They are a good source of fiber and vegetable protein.
   c. They provide antioxidants.
   d. They contain plant sterols.
   e. All of the above are correct.

10. The transport of cholesterol to the liver for elimination is accomplished by _____.

    a. chylomicrons
    b. VLDLs
    c. HDLs
    d. LDLs

11. Which of the following statements about *trans* fatty acids is false?

    a. They have carbon–carbon double bonds, with the hydrogen atoms on the same side of the bond.
    b. They have straighter carbon chains than a corresponding *cis* fatty acid.
    c. They are formed during the hydrogenation of vegetable oils.
    d. High levels in the diet increase the risk of heart disease.

12. What is the approximate percentage of calories from saturated fat in this product?

    a. 99%
    b. 18%
    c. 14%
    d. 17%
    e. 24%

Cheese Sandwich Crackers

Nutrition Facts

Serving Size 1 Package (43g)
Servings Per Container 12

Amount/Serving	
Calories 230	Calories from Fat 120

	% Daily Value*
Total Fat 14g	**22%**
Saturated Fat 3.5g	**18%**
Trans Fat 4g	
Polyunsat. Fat 5.5g	
Monounsat. Fat 1g	
Cholesterol 5mg	**2%**

13. Which one of the following statements about micelles is true?

    a. They help facilitate the absorption of lipids in the small intestine.
    b. They help transport lipids in the bloodstream.
    c. They are essential in the diet.
    d. They break the bonds that hold fatty acids to glycerol.
    e. They are transformed into chylomicrons in the blood.

14. Which of the following statements about fat replacers is false?

    a. Some fat replacers are made from carbohydrate.
    b. Some fat replacers are made from protein.
    c. Some fat replacers stimulate metabolism so the body burns off the extra calories.
    d. Some fat replacers are made from fats that cannot be absorbed.

15. Identify the molecule in the animal cell membrane labeled A.

    a. cholesterol
    b. protein
    c. starch
    d. phospholipid

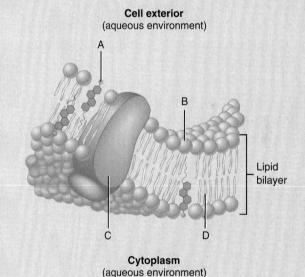

Cell exterior
(aqueous environment)

Cytoplasm
(aqueous environment)

Proteins and Amino Acids

The word *protein* comes from the Greek *proteios*, meaning "of primary importance." This is an apt name because proteins are essential to every process that takes place in our cells. They catalyze chemical reactions, are fundamental components of muscular and skeletal tissue, and are vital in the body's immune response. Because of this primary importance, the generation, development, processing, and renewal of protein resources are major human activities.

Although protein is found in both plants and animals, in Western culture, people fulfill most of their protein needs from animal products. As affluence has increased in non-Western societies, they have adopted many Western habits, including increasing the amount of beef in their diets, a trend that places greater demands on agriculture to provide grain to feed to cattle, which will then convert it to the preferred beef protein.

Now agricultural production is facing a challenge from another front: biofuels. In the United States today, more and more grain crops are being grown not as food (for either humans or farm animals) but to be converted into biofuel. One may argue that it is inefficient to feed grain protein to cattle in order to consume the beef protein the cattle will produce, but at least this process is a nutrition cycle. Corn that is converted into ethanol to fuel an automobile feeds neither cattle nor humans. The challenge of obtaining enough protein and maintaining an adequate balance of plant and animal protein for the world's population, like protein itself, is clearly of primary importance.

NATIONAL GEOGRAPHIC

Proteins in Our Food

LEARNING OBJECTIVES

Describe which types of foods provide the most concentrated sources of protein.

Compare the nutrients in plant sources of protein with those in animal sources of protein.

When we think of protein, we usually think of a steak, a plate of scrambled eggs, or a glass of milk. These animal foods provide the most concentrated sources of protein in our diet, but plant foods such as grains, nuts, and **legumes** are also important sources of dietary protein. The proteins found in plants are made up of different combinations of **amino acids** than proteins found in animals. Because of this difference, most plant proteins are not used as efficiently as animal proteins to build proteins in the human body. Nevertheless, a diet that includes a variety of plant proteins can easily meet most people's protein needs.

legumes
The starchy seeds of plants that produce bean pods; include peas, peanuts, beans, soybeans, and lentils.

amino acids
The building blocks of proteins. Each contains an amino group, an acid group, and a unique side chain.

The sources of protein in your diet have an impact not only on the amount of protein and variety of amino acids available to your body but also on what other nutrients are consumed in the diet (**FIGURE 6.1**). Animal products provide B vitamins and readily absorbable sources of minerals such as iron, zinc, and calcium. They are low in fiber, however, and are often high in saturated fat and cholesterol—a nutrient mix that increases the risk of heart disease.

Plant sources of protein provide most, but not all, B vitamins and also supply iron, zinc, and calcium, but in less absorbable forms. Plant foods are generally excellent sources of fiber, phytochemicals, and unsaturated fats—nutrients that should be increased in our diets to promote health. Recommendations for a healthy diet, including the Dietary Guidelines and MyPyramid, suggest that our diets be based on whole-grain products, vegetables, and fruits and include smaller amounts of meats and dairy products. Following these guidelines will provide plenty of protein from a mixture of plant and animal sources.

CONCEPT CHECK STOP

Which is higher in protein, an egg or a cup of rice?

What nutrients are plentiful in meat and milk? in grains and legumes?

Animal versus plant proteins FIGURE 6.1

A Animal products are high in protein, iron, zinc, and calcium but also add saturated fat and cholesterol to the diet.

One cup milk: 8 grams protein

One egg: 7 grams protein

3 ounces meat: over 20 grams protein

B Plant sources of protein are rich in fiber, phytochemicals, and monounsaturated and polyunsaturated fats.

1 slice bread: about 2 grams protein

½ cup legumes: 6–10 grams protein

½ cup rice, pasta, or cereal: 2–3 grams protein

¼ cup nuts or seeds: 5–10 grams protein

The Structure of Amino Acids and Proteins

What do the proteins in a lamb chop, a kidney bean, and your thigh muscle have in common? They are all constructed of amino acids linked together to form one or more folded, chainlike strands. Twenty amino acids are commonly found in proteins. Each kind of protein contains a different number, combination, and sequence of these amino acids. These differences give specific proteins their unique functions in living organisms and their unique characteristics in foods.

AMINO ACID STRUCTURE

Each amino acid consists of a carbon atom that is bound to a hydrogen atom; an amino group, which contains nitrogen; an acid group; and a side chain (FIGURE 6.2A on the next page). The nitrogen in amino acids distinguishes protein from carbohydrates and lipids; all three contain carbon, hydrogen, and oxygen, but only protein contains nitrogen. The side chains of amino acids vary in size and structure; they are what give different amino acids their unique properties.

Nine of the amino acids needed by the adult human body must be consumed in the diet because they cannot be made in the body (FIGURE 6.2B). If the diet is deficient in one or more of these **essential amino acids** (also called **indispensable amino acids**), the body cannot make new proteins without breaking down existing proteins to provide the needed amino acids. The other 11 amino acids that are commonly found in protein are **nonessential**, or **dispensable**, **amino acids** because they can be made in the body.

essential amino acids (also called **indispensable amino acids**) Amino acids that cannot be synthesized by the body in sufficient amounts to meet its needs and therefore must be included in the diet.

Under certain conditions, some of the nonessential amino acids cannot be synthesized in sufficient amounts to meet the body's needs. These are therefore referred to as **conditionally essential amino acids**. For example, the amino acid tyrosine can be made in the body from the essential amino acid phenylalanine. In individuals who have the inherited disease **phenylketonuria (PKU)**, phenylalanine cannot be converted into tyrosine, so tyrosine is an essential amino acid for these individuals (see *What a Scientist Sees* on page 157).

phenylketonuria (PKU) A genetic disease in which the amino acid phenylalanine cannot be metabolized normally, causing it to build up in the blood. If untreated, the condition results in brain damage.

PROTEIN STRUCTURE

To form proteins, amino acids are linked together by **peptide bonds**, which join the acid group of one amino acid to the amino group of another amino acid (FIGURE 6.2C). Many amino acids bonded together constitute a **polypeptide**. A protein is made up of one or more polypeptide chains that are folded into three-dimensional shapes. The order and chemical properties of the amino acids in a polypeptide determine its final shape because the folding of the chain occurs in response to forces that attract or repel amino acids from one another or from water (FIGURE 6.2D). The folded polypeptide chain may constitute the final protein, or it may join with several other folded polypeptide chains to form the final structure of the protein (FIGURE 6.2E).

polypeptide A chain of amino acids linked by peptide bonds that is part of the structure of a protein.

Visualizing

Amino acid and protein structure FIGURE 6.2

A The general structure ▶ of an amino acid.

H Hydrogen

Amino group H₂N — C — C $=$ O / OH Acid group

Side chain, which is unique to each amino acid

B Twenty amino acids are commonly found in proteins. The table shown here lists them based on whether they are essential or nonessential and indicates those that are conditionally essential. ▼

Essential Amino Acids	Nonessential Amino Acids
Histidine	Alanine
Isoleucine	Arginine*
Leucine	Asparagine
Lysine	Aspartic acid
Methionine	Cysteine*
Phenylalanine	Glutamic acid
Threonine	Glutamine*
Tryptophan	Glycine*
Valine	Proline*
	Serine
	Tyrosine*

*Considered conditionally essential by the Institute of Medicine, Food and Nutrition Board

Amino acids bond to form polypeptides

Peptide bond

◀ C Amino acids linked by peptide bonds are called **peptides**. When two amino acids are linked, they form a **dipeptide**; three form a **tripeptide**. Many amino acids bonded together constitute a polypeptide. Polypeptide chains may contain hundreds of amino acids.

Polypeptide chains fold to form 3-dimensional shapes

D The order and ▶ chemical properties of the amino acids in a polypeptide chain determine how the polypeptide folds and, hence, the three-dimensional shape of the protein.

E The final ▶ structure of a protein molecule may consist of several folded polypeptide chains.

NATIONAL GEOGRAPHIC

Phenylketonuria

This warning on a can of diet soda probably doesn't mean much unless you have the genetic disease phenylketonuria (PKU). Individuals with PKU must limit their intake of the amino acid phenylalanine. Usually this means limiting their consumption of high-protein foods. When a scientist looks at this label, she recognizes that the artificial sweetener aspartame in this soda is the source of the phenylalanine. The breakdown of aspartame in the digestive tract releases phenylalanine, which cannot be properly metabolized by individuals with PKU. If they consume large amounts of this amino acid, compounds called phenylketones build up in their blood. In infants and young children, phenylketones interfere with brain development, and in pregnant women they cause birth defects in the baby. To prevent this, these individuals must consume a diet that provides just enough phenylalanine to meet the body's needs but not so much that phenylketones build up in their blood. Why do you think this warning appears on diet soda labels but not on high-protein foods such as meat and milk?

Phenylketonurics: Contains phenylalanine

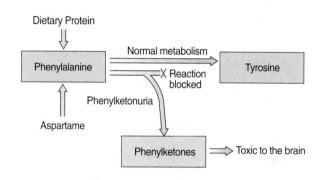

The shape of a protein is essential to its function. For example, the elongated shape of the proteins collagen and alpha-keratin, found in connective tissue, helps them give strength to tendons and ligaments. The spherical shape of the protein hemoglobin contributes to the proper functioning of red blood cells, and the long shape of muscle proteins allows them to overlap and shorten muscles during contraction.

Protein denaturation FIGURE 6.3

When an egg is cooked, the heat denatures the protein. The protein in a raw egg white forms a clear, viscous liquid, but when cooking denatures it, the egg white becomes white and firm and cannot be restored to its original form. Other factors that denature the proteins in food include mechanical agitation, such as when cream is whipped to make whipped cream, and the addition of acid, such as when milk is curdled by the addition of an acid such as lemon juice.

When the shape of a protein is altered, the protein no longer functions normally. For example, when salivary amylase, which is an enzyme protein, enters the stomach, the acid causes the structure of the protein to change, and it no longer functions in the digestion of starch. This change in structure is called **denaturation**, referring to a change from the natural. Proteins in food are often denatured during processing and cooking (**FIGURE 6.3**).

denaturation
Alteration of a protein's three-dimensional structure.

CONCEPT CHECK STOP

Which chemical element is found in protein but not in carbohydrate or lipid?

What determines the shape of a protein?

Why must only some of the 20 amino acids that the body needs to make proteins be consumed in the diet?

How does denaturation affect the function of proteins?

Protein digestion and absorption FIGURE 6.4

Protein must be broken down into small peptides and amino acids to be absorbed into the mucosal cells.

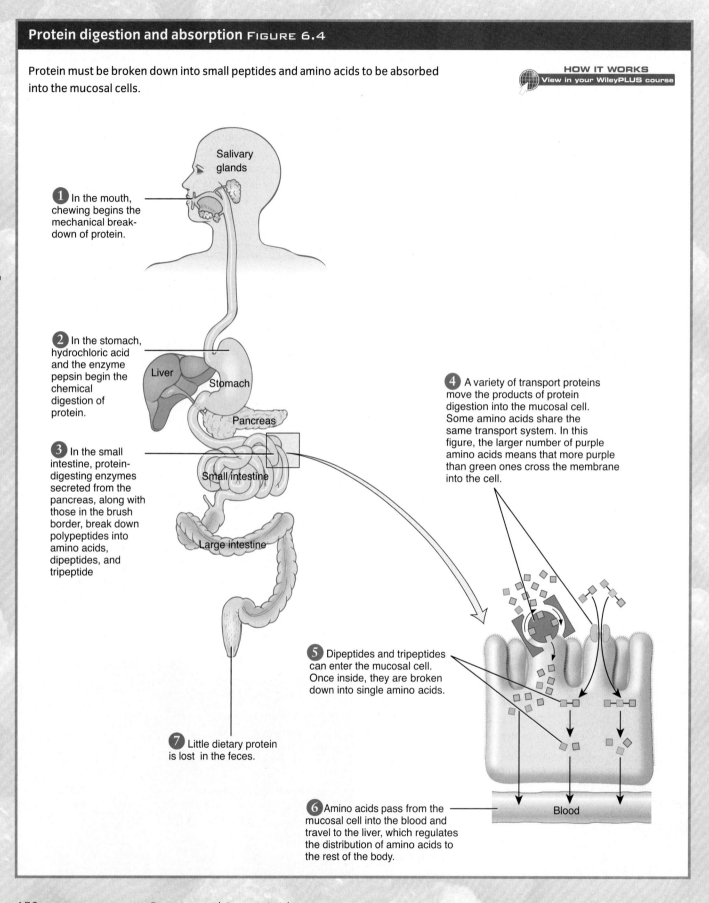

Salivary glands

1 In the mouth, chewing begins the mechanical break-down of protein.

2 In the stomach, hydrochloric acid and the enzyme pepsin begin the chemical digestion of protein.

Liver

Stomach

Pancreas

3 In the small intestine, protein-digesting enzymes secreted from the pancreas, along with those in the brush border, break down polypeptides into amino acids, dipeptides, and tripeptide

Small intestine

Large intestine

4 A variety of transport proteins move the products of protein digestion into the mucosal cell. Some amino acids share the same transport system. In this figure, the larger number of purple amino acids means that more purple than green ones cross the membrane into the cell.

5 Dipeptides and tripeptides can enter the mucosal cell. Once inside, they are broken down into single amino acids.

7 Little dietary protein is lost in the feces.

6 Amino acids pass from the mucosal cell into the blood and travel to the liver, which regulates the distribution of amino acids to the rest of the body.

Blood

Protein Digestion and Absorption

Proteins must be digested before their amino acids can be absorbed into the body (**FIGURE 6.4**). The chemical digestion of protein begins in the acid environment of the stomach. Here, hydrochloric acid denatures proteins, opening up their folded structure to make the polypeptide chains more accessible for breakdown by enzymes. Stomach acid also activates the protein-digesting enzyme *pepsin*, which breaks some of the peptide bonds in the polypeptide chains, leaving shorter polypeptides. Most protein digestion occurs in the small intestine, where polypeptides are broken into even smaller peptides and amino acids by protein-digesting enzymes produced in the pancreas and small intestine. Single amino acids, dipeptides, and tripeptides are absorbed into the mucosal cells of the small intestine.

Amino acids enter your body by crossing from the lumen of the small intestine into the mucosal cells and then into the blood. This process involves one of several energy-requiring amino acid transport systems. Amino acids with similar structures use the same transport system (see Figure 6.4). As a result, amino acids may compete with one another for absorption. If there is an ex-cess of any one of the amino acids sharing a transport system, more of it will be absorbed, slowing the absorption of competing amino acids. This competition for absorption is usually not a problem because foods contain a variety of amino acids, none of which are present in excessive amounts. However, when people consume amino acid supplements, the supplemented amino acid may clog the transport system, reducing the absorption of other amino acids that share the same transport system. For example, weight lifters often take supplements of the amino acid arginine. Because arginine shares a transport system with lysine, large doses of arginine can inhibit the absorption of lysine, upsetting the balance of amino acids in the body.

CONCEPT CHECK **STOP**

Where does the chemical digestion of protein begin?

Why might supplementing one amino acid reduce the absorption of other amino acids?

Protein Synthesis and Functions

LEARNING OBJECTIVES

Explain what is meant by the term limiting amino acid.

Discuss the steps involved in synthesizing proteins.

Name four functions of body proteins.

Describe the conditions under which the body uses protein to produce energy.

As discussed earlier, proteins are made from amino acids. Amino acids are also used to make other nitrogen-containing molecules, including neurotransmitters; the units that make up DNA and RNA; the skin pigment melanin; the vitamin niacin; creatine, which is used to fuel muscle contrac-tion; and histamine, which causes blood vessels to dilate. In some situations, amino acids from proteins are also used to provide energy or synthesize glucose or fatty acids.

The amino acids available for these functions come from the proteins consumed in the diet and from the break-down of body proteins. These amino acids are referred to

amino acid pool All the amino acids in body tissues and fluids that are available for use by the body.

collectively as the **amino acid pool** (FIGURE 6.5). There is not actually a "pool" in the body containing a collection of amino acids, but these molecules are available in body fluids and cells to provide the raw materials needed to synthesize proteins and other molecules.

SYNTHESIZING PROTEINS

The instructions for making proteins are contained in the

gene A length of DNA that contains the information needed to synthesize a polypeptide chain.

nucleus of the cell in stretches of DNA called **genes**. When a protein is needed, the process of protein synthesis is turned on, and the information contained in the gene is used to make the necessary protein (FIGURE 6.6).

Regulating protein synthesis The types of proteins made and when they are made are carefully regulated by the turning on and off of the genes that code for each protein. When a gene is turned on, the protein is made, and the gene is said to be *expressed*. Not all genes are ex-

pressed in all cells or at all times; only the proteins that are needed are made at any given time. This allows the body to save energy and resources. For example, when your diet is high in iron, the gene that codes for the protein ferritin, which stores iron, is turned on. This causes ferritin to be made and allows the body to hold on to the iron by storing it in this protein. When the diet is low in iron, the production of ferritin is turned off so that we don't waste amino acids and energy making a protein that we don't need.

Limiting amino acids During the synthesis of a protein, a shortage of one amino acid can stop the process. Just as on an assembly line, if one part is missing, the line stops—a different part cannot be substituted. If the missing amino acid is a nonessential amino acid, it can be made in the body, and protein synthesis can continue. Most nonessential amino acids are made through a process called **transamination**, which involves transferring the amino group from one amino acid to a carbon-containing molecule to form the needed amino acid (see FIGURE 6.6A). If the missing amino acid is an essential amino acid, the body can break down its own protein to obtain it. If an amino acid cannot be supplied, protein synthesis will stop.

transamination The process by which an amino group from one amino acid is transferred to a carbon compound to form a new amino acid.

Amino acid pool FIGURE 6.5

Amino acids enter the available pool from the diet and from the breakdown of body proteins. Of the approximately 300 grams of protein synthesized by the body each day, only about 100 grams are made from amino acids consumed in the diet. The other 200 grams are produced by the recycling of amino acids from protein broken down in the body. Amino acids in the pool can be used to synthesize body proteins and other nitrogen-containing molecules, to provide energy, or to synthesize glucose or fatty acids.

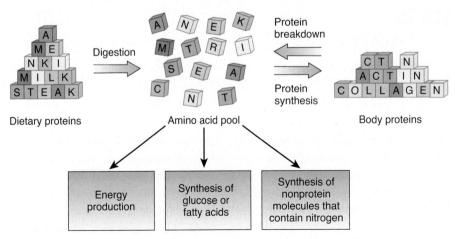

A Amino acids can be thought of as building blocks. Protein consumed in the diet and body proteins that are broken down supply these building blocks to the amino acid pool. Most nonessential amino acids can be made from carbon compounds by adding an amino group through transamination.

Dietary proteins

Digestion

Amino acid pool

Protein breakdown

Protein synthesis

Body proteins

Transamination

Carbon compound

NH₂

Carbon compound

Amino acid

B Essential and nonessential amino acids are used to synthesize body proteins.

1. The first step in protein synthesis occurs inside the nucleus. It involves transferring, or transcribing, the blueprint or code for the protein from the DNA gene into a molecule of messenger RNA (mRNA). This process is called **transcription**.

Cell

Transcription

Translation

Growing chain of amino acids

transfer RNA

mRNA

Nucleus

mRNA

Ribosome

DNA

Cytoplasm

2. The mRNA takes the genetic information from the nucleus of the cell to structures called ribosomes in the cytoplasm of the cell, where proteins are made.

3. Transfer RNA reads the genetic code and delivers the needed amino acids to the ribosome to form a polypeptide chain. This process is called **translation**.

C The amino acids needed for protein synthesis come from the amino acid pool. If the protein to be made requires more of a particular amino acid than is available, that amino acid limits protein synthesis and is referred to as the *limiting amino acid*.

Amino acid pool

A shortage of the amino acid represented by the orange blocks limits the ability to synthesize a protein that is high in this amino acid.

Protein

The essential amino acid that is present in shortest supply relative to the body's need for it is called the **limiting amino acid** because lack of this amino acid limits the ability to synthesize protein (**FIGURE 6.6C**). Different food sources of protein provide different combinations of amino acids. The limiting amino acid in a food is the one supplied in the lowest amount relative to the body's need. For example, the limiting amino acid in wheat is lysine, whereas the limiting amino acid in peanut butter is methionine. When the diet provides adequate amounts of all the essential amino acids needed to synthesize a specific protein,

synthesis of the polypeptide chains that make up the protein can be completed.

PROTEINS PROVIDE STRUCTURE AND REGULATION

When you think of the protein in your body, you probably think of muscle, but muscle contains only a few of the many types of proteins found in your body. There are more than 500,000 proteins in the human body, each with a unique function. Some perform important structural roles, and others help regulate specific body processes.

Structural proteins are found in skin, hair, ligaments, and tendons (**FIGURE 6.7A**). Proteins also provide

Visualizing

Protein functions FIGURE 6.7

A Collagen, which is the most abundant protein in the body, plays important structural roles. It is the major protein in ligaments, which hold our bones together, and in tendons, which attach muscles to bones, and it forms the protein framework of bones and teeth. ▼

B Enzymes, such as this one that speeds up the breakdown of starch, are protein molecules. All chemical reactions occurring within the body require the help of enzymes. The structure or shape of each enzyme allows it to interact with the molecules in the reaction it accelerates. Without enzymes, metabolic reactions would occur too slowly to support life. Each of the reactions of metabolism requires a unique enzyme. ▼

Enzyme → Enzyme

Femur

Tendon

Knee cap

Ligaments

Lower leg bones

C Proteins help transport materials throughout the body and into and out of cells. The protein hemoglobin, which gives these red blood cells their color, shuttles oxygen to body cells and carries away carbon dioxide.

structure to individual cells, where they are an integral part of the cell membrane, cytoplasm, and organelles. Proteins such as enzymes, which speed up biochemical reactions (FIGURE 6.7B) and transport proteins that travel in the blood or help materials cross membranes, regulate processes throughout the body (FIGURE 6.7C).

Proteins are an important part of the body's defense mechanisms. Skin, which is made up primarily of protein, is the first barrier against infection and injury. Foreign particles such as dirt or bacteria that are on the skin cannot enter the body and can be washed away. If the skin is broken and blood vessels are injured, blood-clotting proteins help prevent too much blood from being lost. If a foreign material does get into the body, *antibodies*, which are immune system proteins, help destroy it (FIGURE 6.7D).

Some proteins have contractile properties, which allow muscles to move various parts of the body (FIGURE 6.7E). Others are hormones, which regulate biological processes. The hormones insulin, growth hormone, and glucagon are made from amino acids. These protein hormones act rapidly because they affect the activity of proteins that are already present in the cell.

Proteins also help regulate fluid balance (FIGURE 6.7F) and prevent the level of acidity in body fluids from deviating from the normal range. The chemical reactions of metabolism require a specific level of acidity, or pH, to function properly. Inside the body, pH must be maintained at a relatively neutral level in order to allow metabolic reactions to proceed normally. If the pH changes, these reactions slow or stop. Proteins both within cells and in the blood help prevent large changes in acidity.

E Proteins help us move. The proteins actin and myosin in the arm and leg muscles of this rock climber are able to slide past each other to contract the muscles. A similar process causes contraction in the heart muscle and in the muscles of the digestive tract, blood vessels, and body glands. ▼

D Proteins help protect us ▲ from disease. This child is being immunized against measles. The vaccine contains a small amount of dead or inactivated measles virus. It does not make the child sick, but it does stimulate his immune system to make proteins called *antibodies*, which specifically attack the measles virus and prevent the child from contracting the disease.

F Proteins help regulate fluid balance ▲ through their effect on *osmosis*. Blood proteins contribute to the number of dissolved particles in the blood. If protein levels in the blood fall too low, osmosis causes fluid to leak out of the blood vessels and accumulate in the tissues, causing swelling known as **edema**, shown here. Proteins also regulate fluid balance because some are membrane transporters, which pump dissolved substances from one side of a membrane to the other.

Producing ATP from amino acids FIGURE 6.8

The compounds remaining after the amino group (NH₂) has been removed through a process called **deamination** are composed of carbon, hydrogen, and oxygen and can be broken down to produce ATP or used to make glucose or fatty acids.

Dietary proteins   Amino acid pool   Body proteins

Digestion

Protein synthesis

Protein breakdown

Glucose synthesis   **Aerobic Metabolism**

The amino group is removed by deamination and converted into the waste product **urea**: urea is removed from the blood by the kidneys and excreted in the urine.

Glucose

Amino acids

Deamination

NH₂ → Urea

CO₂

CO₂

O₂

H₂O

C—C—C
3 carbons
(pyruvate)

Acetyl-CoA
C—C

Fatty acids

ATP

2 Deamination of some amino acids results in three-carbon molecules that can be used to synthesize glucose.

3 Deamination of some amino acids results in acetyl-CoA that enters the circular pathway to yield two molecules of carbon dioxide. Deamination of other amino acids forms molecules that enter the circular pathway directly.

4 When excess calories are consumed, the acetyl-CoA derived from the breakdown of amino acids can be used to synthesize fatty acids.

5 In the final step of aerobic metabolism, the energy from the amino acid molecules is trapped and used to produce ATP and water.

Process Diagram

PROTEIN AS A SOURCE OF ENERGY

In addition to all the essential functions performed by body proteins, under some circumstances, proteins can be broken down and their amino acids used to provide energy or synthesize glucose or fatty acids (**FIGURE 6.8**). When the diet does not provide enough energy to meet the body's needs, such as during starvation or when consuming a weight-loss diet, body protein is used to provide energy. Because our bodies do not store protein, functional body proteins, such as enzymes and muscle proteins, must be broken down to yield amino acids, which can then be used as fuel or to make glucose. This ensures that cells have a constant energy supply but also robs the body of the functions performed by these proteins.

Amino acids are also used for energy when the amount of protein consumed in the diet is greater than that needed to make body proteins and other molecules. This occurs in most Americans every day because our typical diet contains more protein than we need. The body first uses amino acids from the diet to make body proteins and other nitrogen-containing molecules. Then, because extra amino acids can't be stored, they are metabolized to provide energy. When your diet includes more calories than you need, amino acids can be converted into fatty acids, which are stored as triglycerides, thus contributing to weight gain.

CONCEPT CHECK **STOP**

Why does protein synthesis stop when the supply of an amino acid is limited?

How does the body know in what order to assemble the amino acids when making a protein?

How do proteins help regulate body functions?

When is protein used as an energy source?

Protein in Health and Disease

LEARNING OBJECTIVES

Distinguish kwashiorkor from marasmus.

Explain why protein-energy malnutrition is more common in children than in adults.

Discuss the potential risks associated with high-protein diets.

Explain how a dietary protein can trigger a food allergy.

We need to eat protein to stay healthy. If we don't eat enough of it, less-essential body proteins are broken down, and their amino acids are used to synthesize proteins that are critical for survival. For example, when the diet is deficient in protein, muscle protein is broken down to provide amino acids to make hormones and enzymes for which there is an immediate need. If protein deficiency continues, eventually so much body protein is lost that all life-sustaining functions cannot be supported. In some cases too much protein or the wrong proteins can also contribute to health problems.

protein-energy malnutrition (PEM) A condition characterized by loss of muscle and fat mass and an increased susceptibility to infection that results from the long-term consumption of insufficient amounts of energy and/or protein to meet the body's needs.

PROTEIN DEFICIENCY

Protein deficiency is a great concern in the developing world but generally not a problem in economically developed societies, where plant and animal sources of protein are abundant. Usually, protein deficiency occurs along with a general lack of food and other nutrients. The term **protein-energy malnutrition (PEM)** is used to refer to a continuum of conditions ranging from pure protein deficiency, called **kwashiorkor**, to an overall energy deficiency, called **marasmus** (FIGURE 6.9).

A pure protein deficiency occurs when the diet is ex-

tremely limited or when protein needs are high, as they are in young children. Hence, kwashiorkor is typically a disease found in children (FIGURE 6.9A). The word *kwashiorkor* comes from the Ga tribe of the African Gold Coast. It means

Protein-energy malnutrition FIGURE 6.9

NATIONAL GEOGRAPHIC

A Kwashiorkor is characterized by a swollen belly, which results from fluid accumulating in the abdomen and fat accumulating in the liver. Growth is impaired, but because energy intake is not necessarily low, the child may not appear extremely thin. The lack of protein also causes poor immune function and an increase in infections, changes in hair color, and impaired nutrient absorption.

B Marasmus is characterized by depletion of fat stores and wasting of muscle. It has devastating effects on infants because most brain growth takes place in the first year of life; malnutrition in the first year causes decreases in intelligence and learning ability that persist throughout the individual's life.

C Protein-energy malnutrition is uncommon in the United States and other developed nations, but in developing countries it is a serious public health problem, resulting in high infant and child mortality. The highest prevalence is in sub-Saharan Africa and south Asia.

More than 20 percent of population are undernourished, and 75 or more of every 1,000 children die before age 5.

More than 20 percent of population are undernourished, and under-5 mortality rate is less than 75 per 1,000 children.

Less than 20 percent of population are undernourished, and 75 or more of every 1,000 children die before age 5.

"the disease that the first child gets when a second child is born."[1] When the new baby is born, the older child is no longer breast-fed. Rather than receiving protein-rich breast milk, the young child is fed a watered-down version of the diet eaten by the rest of the family. This diet is low in protein and often high in fiber and difficult to digest. The child, even if he or she is able to obtain adequate calories from their diet, may not be able to eat a large enough quantity to get adequate protein. Because children are growing, their protein needs per unit of body weight are higher than those of adults, and a deficiency occurs more quickly.

At the other end of the continuum of protein-energy malnutrition is marasmus, meaning "to waste away" (FIGURE 6.9B). Marasmus is caused by starvation; the diet doesn't supply enough calories or nutrients to meet the body's needs. Marasmus may have some of the same symptoms as kwashiorkor, but there are differences. In kwashiorkor, some fat stores are retained because energy intake is adequate. In marasmus, individuals appear emaciated because their stores of body fat have been depleted to provide energy. Although they are most common in children, both marasmus and kwashiorkor can occur in individuals of all ages.

HIGH-PROTEIN DIETS AND HEALTH

The recent popularity of high-protein, low-carbohydrate diets has raised questions about whether consuming too much protein can be harmful. As protein intake increases, so does the production of protein-breakdown products, such as urea, which must be eliminated from the body by the kidneys. To excrete more waste, more water must be lost in the urine. High-protein diets therefore increase water loss. Although not a concern for most people, this can be a problem if the kidneys are not able to concentrate urine, as is the case for infants. Feeding a newborn an infant formula that is too high in protein increases the amount of fluid lost in the urine and can lead to dehydration. High protein intake may also be detrimental for people with kidney disease; the increased wastes produced with a high-protein diet may speed the progression of renal failure.[2] However, there is little evidence that a high-protein diet will precipitate kidney disease in a healthy person.[3]

It has also been suggested that the amount and source of protein in the diet affect calcium status and bone health.[4] For healthy bone, intakes of both calcium and protein must be adequate. There is general agreement that diets that are moderate in protein (1.0 to 1.5 g/kg/day) are associated with normal calcium metabolism and do not alter bone metabolism.[4,5] However, a high protein intake may increase the amount of calcium lost in the urine. Some studies suggest that the amount of calcium lost in the urine is greater when protein comes from animal rather than vegetable sources.[6] These findings have contributed to a widely held belief that high-protein diets (especially diets that are high in animal protein) result in bone loss. However, clinical studies do not support the idea that animal protein has a detrimental effect on bone health or that vegetable-based proteins are better for bone health.[5] In fact, when calcium intake is adequate, high-protein diets are associated with greater bone mass and fewer fractures.[4] This is likely the case because in healthy adults, a high protein intake increases intestinal calcium absorption as well as urinary excretion, so the increase in the amount of calcium lost in the urine does not cause an overall loss of body calcium.

The increase in urinary calcium excretion associated with high-protein diets has led to speculation that a high protein intake may increase the risk of kidney stones. Kidney stones are deposits of calcium and other substances in the kidneys and urinary tract. Higher concentrations of calcium and acid in the urine increase the likelihood that the calcium will be deposited, forming these stones. Epidemiological studies suggest that diets that are rich in animal protein and low in fluid contribute to the formation of kidney stones.[7]

The best-documented concern with high-protein diets is related more to the rest of the diet than to the amount of protein consumed. Typically, high-protein diets are also high in animal products; this dietary pattern is high in saturated fat and cholesterol and low in fiber, and it therefore increases the risk of heart disease. These diets are also typically low in grains, vegetables, and fruits, a pattern associated with an increased risk of cancer.[8] Such diets are also usually high in energy and total fat, which may promote excess weight gain.

PROTEINS AND FOOD ALLERGIES AND INTOLERANCES

When a protein from the diet is absorbed without being completely digested, it can trigger a **food allergy**. The proteins from milk, eggs, peanuts, tree nuts, wheat, soy,

food allergy
An adverse immune response to a specific food protein.

Food allergy labeling FIGURE 6.10

Food labels provide life-saving information for individuals with food allergies. A label must indicate whether the product contains any of the eight major food allergens: milk, eggs, peanuts, tree nuts, fish, shellfish, soy, and wheat. Sometimes these are just included in the ingredient list, but often, as on this label, they are also highlighted at the end of the list in a statement such as "Contains soy ingredients." Warnings such as "manufactured in a facility that processes peanuts" are included on products that may be cross-contaminated with these allergens.

The ingredient list includes sources of protein in food as well as sources of **hydrolyzed protein** or **protein hydrolysates**. These are proteins that have been treated with acid or enzymes to break them down into amino acids and small peptides. They are added as flavorings, flavor enhancers, stabilizers, and thickening agents.

INGREDIENTS: CHICKEN BROTH, CARROTS, COOKED WHITE CHICKEN MEAT (WHITE CHICKEN MEAT, WATER, SALT, SODIUM PHOSPHATE, ISOLATED SOY PROTEIN, MODIFIED CORN STARCH, CORN STARCH, CARRAGEENAN), TOMATOES, WILD RICE, RICE, CELERY. LESS THAN 2% OF: SALT, MONOSODIUM GLUTAMATE, HYDROLYZED CORN PROTEIN, CHICKEN FAT, ONION POWDER, AUTOLYZED YEAST EXTRACT, PARSLEY FLAKES, NATURAL FLAVOR. **CONTAINS SOY INGREDIENTS.**

Nutrition Facts

Serving Size 1 cup (239g)
Servings Per Container about 2

Amount Per Serving	
Calories 100	Calories from Fat 30

	% Daily Value*
Total Fat 1.5g	2%
Saturated Fat 2g	10%
Trans Fat 0g	
Cholesterol 15mg	5%
Sodium 850mg	35%
Total Carbohydrate 15g	5%
Dietary Fiber 1g	4%
Sugars 1g	
Protein 7g	

Vitamin A 25%	•	Vitamin C 0%	
Calcium 0%	•	Iron 2%	

*Percent Daily Values (DV) are based on a 2,000 calorie diet.

There is little emphasis on protein in the Nutrition Facts panel, where the grams of protein are given without any % Daily Value. A % Daily Value for protein is required only on products that make a claim about the product's protein content.

fish, and shellfish are common causes of food allergies (FIGURE 6.10). The first time the protein is consumed and a piece of it is absorbed intact, it stimulates the immune system. When the same protein is consumed again, the immune system sees it as a foreign substance and mounts an attack, causing an allergic reaction (see Chapter 3). Allergic reactions cause symptoms throughout the body and can be life threatening.

Not all adverse reactions to proteins and amino acids are due to allergies; some are due to **food intolerances**, also called **food sensitivities**. These reactions do not involve the immune system. The symptoms of a food intolerance can range from minor discomfort, such as the abdominal distress some people feel after eating raw onions, to more severe reactions. For example, some people report having a reaction after consuming **monosodium glutamate (MSG)**. MSG is a flavor enhancer made up of the amino acid glutamic acid bound to sodium. It is used in meat tenderizers and commonly added to Chinese food. In sensitive individuals, it causes a collection of symptoms such as flushed face, tingling or burning sensations, headache, rapid heartbeat, chest pain, and general weakness that are collectively referred to as **MSG symptom complex**, commonly called **Chinese restaurant syndrome**.[9] Sensitive individuals should ask for food to be prepared without added MSG and should check in-

food intolerance, or food sensitivity
An adverse reaction to a food that does not involve the production of antibodies by the immune system.

gredient lists for monosodium glutamate or potassium glutamate before consuming packaged foods.

Gluten intolerance, also called **celiac disease**, celiac sprue, or gluten-sensitive enteropathy, is another form of food intolerance. Individuals with celiac disease cannot tolerate gluten, a protein found in wheat, rye, and barley. Celiac disease is an autoimmune disease in which gluten causes the body to attack the villi in the small intestine, causing symptoms such as diarrhea, abdominal bloating and cramps, weight loss, and anemia. Once thought to be a rare childhood disease, it is now known to affect more than 2 million people in the United States.[10] The only treatment is to avoid gluten by eliminating from the diet all products containing wheat, rye, or barley or proteins isolated from these foods.

celiac disease
A disorder that causes damage to the intestines when the protein gluten is eaten.

CONCEPT CHECK STOP

Why do children with marasmus appear more emaciated than those with kwashiorkor?

Who should be concerned about excessive protein intake?

Why is protein-energy malnutrition more common in children than in adults?

How can allergic reactions to food be avoided?

Meeting Protein Needs

I n order to stay healthy, you have to eat enough protein to replace the amount you lose every day. Most Americans get plenty of protein, and healthy diets can contain a wide range of intakes from both plant and animal sources. An individual's protein needs may be increased by growth, injury, and illness, as well as by some types of physical activity.

BALANCING PROTEIN INTAKE AND LOSSES

Current protein intake recommendations are based on **nitrogen balance** studies. These studies compare the amount of nitrogen consumed with the amount excreted. Studying nitrogen balance allows researchers to evaluate protein balance because protein is the only macronutrient that contains nitrogen. Most of the nitrogen we consume comes from dietary protein. Most of the nitrogen we lose is excreted in urine. Smaller amounts are lost in feces, skin, sweat, menstrual fluids, hair, and nails. When your body is in nitrogen balance, your nitrogen intake equals your nitrogen losses; in other words, you are consuming enough protein to replace losses. You are not gaining or losing body protein; you are maintaining it at a constant level. Nitrogen balance is negative if you're losing body protein and positive if the amount of body protein is increasing (**FIGURE 6.11**).

nitrogen balance The amount of nitrogen consumed in the diet compared with the amount excreted over a given period.

Nitrogen balance FIGURE 6.11

Nitrogen intake

Nitrogen output

A Nitrogen balance: Nitrogen intake = nitrogen output. This indicates that the amount of protein being synthesized is equal to the amount being broken down, so the total amount of protein in the body is not changing. Healthy adults who consume adequate amounts of protein and are maintaining a constant body weight are in nitrogen balance.

Nitrogen intake

Nitrogen output

B Negative nitrogen balance: Nitrogen intake < nitrogen output. This indicates that more protein is being broken down than is being synthesized so body protein is decreasing. Negative nitrogen balance occurs due to injury or illness as well as when the diet is too low in protein or calories.

Nitrogen intake

Nitrogen output

C Positive nitrogen balance: Nitrogen intake > nitrogen output. This indicates that there is more protein synthesis than degradation so the body is gaining protein. This occurs when the body is growing, during pregnancy, and in individuals who are increasing their muscle mass by lifting weights.

Protein requirements TABLE 6.1	
Age (years)	RDA (g/kg/day)
0–0.5	1.52
0.5–1	1.50
1–3	1.10
4–8	0.95
9–13	0.95
14–18	0.85
≥19	0.80

RECOMMENDED PROTEIN INTAKE

Most of us eat more protein than we need: The typical young adult in the United States consumes about 90 grams of protein/day.[11] The RDA for protein for adults is 0.8 g/kilogram of body weight. For a person weighing 70 kg (154 lbs), the RDA is 56 g of protein/day. This recommendation is expressed per unit of body weight because protein is needed to maintain and repair the body. The more a person weighs, the more protein he or she needs for these purposes. Because children are small, they need less total protein than adults do, but because new protein must be synthesized for growth to occur, protein requirements per unit of body weight are much greater for infants and children than for adults. During the first year of life, growth is rapid, so a large amount of protein is required. As growth rate slows, requirements per unit of body weight decrease but continue to be greater than adult require-

ments until age 19 (TABLE 6.1). To calculate protein needs per day, multiply weight in kilograms (which equals weight in pounds × 0.45 kg/lb) by the recommended amount for the individual's age.

Protein needs are also increased during pregnancy and lactation. Additional protein is needed during pregnancy to support the expansion of maternal blood volume, the growth of the uterus and breasts, the formation of the placenta, and the growth and development of the fetus. The RDA for pregnant women is 25 g of protein/day higher than the recommendation for non-pregnant women. An extra 25 g/day is also needed during lactation to provide protein for the production of breast milk.

Extreme stresses on the body, such as infections, fevers, burns, or surgery, increase the amount of protein that is broken down. For the body to heal and rebuild, the amount of protein lost must be replaced. The extra amount needed for healing depends on the injury. A severe infection may increase the body's protein needs by about 30%, whereas a serious burn can increase protein requirements by 200 to 400%.

Although most athletes can meet their protein needs by consuming the RDA of 0.8 g/kg of body weight, endurance athletes and strength athletes benefit from higher protein intakes (FIGURE 6.12).[12] Athletes often think they need supplements to meet their higher protein needs. However, because they typically also consume more calories, which increases the amount of dietary protein they consume, they can easily meet their protein needs through diet alone.

Protein needs of athletes FIGURE 6.12

A Endurance athletes need more protein than others because some protein is used for energy and to maintain blood glucose during endurance events, such as triathlons. Endurance athletes may benefit from the daily consumption of 1.2 to 1.4 g of protein/kilogram of body weight.

B Strength athletes, such as weight lifters and body builders, need extra protein because it provides the raw materials needed for muscle growth; 1.2 to 1.7 g/kilogram/day is recommended.

Protein and amino acid supplements FIGURE 6.13

Supplements are marketed to boost total protein intake, to add individual amino acids, and to provide enzyme activity.

Protein supplements are marketed to promote proper immune function, make hair healthy, and stimulate muscle growth, but increasing protein intake above the level required for good health does not protect you from disease, make your hair shine, or give you larger biceps.

Many promises are made about amino acid supplements, from aiding sleep to enhancing athletic performance. There is weak evidence to support some of these, but consuming large amounts of one amino acid may interfere with the absorption of others. Due to insufficient research, no ULs have been set for amino acids.

Supplements of enzymes that function inside body tissues provide no benefits because the enzyme is broken down into amino acids during digestion. Supplements of enzymes that function in the gut, such as lactase for lactose intolerance, retain enzyme activity long enough to breakdown the lactose but are also eventually digested.

RDAs have also been developed for each of the essential amino acids;[3] these are not a concern in typical diet planning but are important when developing solutions for intravenous feeding. Protein and amino acid supplements are rarely needed to meet individuals' protein needs (FIGURE 6.13).

In addition to the RDA, the DRIs include a recommendation for protein intake as a percentage of calories: The Acceptable Macronutrient Distribution Range for protein is 10% to 35% of calories.[3] This range allows for different food preferences and eating patterns. A protein intake in this range will meet protein needs and allow sufficient intakes of other nutrients to promote health. A diet that provides 10% of calories from protein will meet the RDA but is a relatively low-protein diet compared with typical eating patterns in the United States. The upper end of this healthy range—35% of calories—is a relatively high-protein diet, about twice as much protein as the average American eats. This amount of protein is not harmful, but if the diet is this high in protein, it is probably high in animal products, which tend to be high in saturated fat and cholesterol. Therefore, unless protein sources are chosen carefully, a diet that contains 35% protein would tend to include more saturated fat and cholesterol than would a diet with the same number of calories that contains only 10% protein.

CHOOSING PROTEIN WISELY

To evaluate protein intake, it is important to consider both the amount and the quality of protein in the diet. **Protein quality** is a measure of how good the protein in a food is at providing the essential amino acids the body needs to synthesize proteins. Because we are animals, it makes sense that animal proteins generally contain mixtures of amino acids more similar to those we need than do those found in plant proteins. This is why animal proteins are generally of higher quality than proteins from plant sources. Animal proteins also tend to be digested more easily than plant proteins; only protein that is digested can contribute amino acids to meet the body's requirements.[13] Because they are easily digested and supply essential amino acids in the proper proportions for human use, foods of animal origin are sources of **high-quality protein**, or **complete dietary protein**. When your diet contains high-quality protein, you don't have to eat as much total protein to meet your needs. This is because high-quality protein provides more of the essential amino acids in the proportions needed by the body than the same amount of low-quality protein would provide.

Compared to animal proteins, plant proteins are usually more difficult to digest and are lower in one or more of the essential amino acids. They are therefore referred to as **incomplete dietary protein**. An exception is soy protein, which is a high-quality plant protein—as high as egg or milk protein.

Complementary proteins

If you get your protein from a single source and that source is an incomplete protein, it will be difficult to meet your body's protein needs. However, combining proteins that are limited in different amino acids can supply a complete mixture of essential amino acids. For example, legumes are limited in methionine but high in lysine. When legumes are consumed with grains, which are high in methionine and low in lysine, the combination provides all the needed amino acids (**FIGURE 6.14**). Vegetarian

Protein complementation FIGURE 6.14

A The amino acids that are most often limited in plant proteins are lysine (lys), methionine (met), and cysteine (cys). As a general rule, legumes are deficient in methionine and cysteine but high in lysine. Grains, nuts, and seeds are deficient in lysine but high in methionine and cysteine. ▼

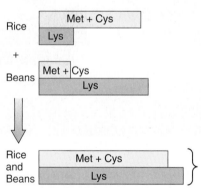

When rice, which is limited in lys but high in met and cys, is eaten with beans, which are high in lys but limited in met and cys, the combination provides all the amino acids needed by the body.

B Many traditional diets take advantage of complementary plant proteins, such as lentils and rice or chickpeas and rice in India, rice and beans in Mexico and South America, hummus (chickpeas and sesame seeds) in the Middle East, and bread and peanut butter (peanuts are a legume) in the United States. Complementary proteins do not have to be consumed in the same meal, so eating an assortment of plant foods throughout the day can provide enough of all the essential amino acids.[14]

Grains, Nuts, or Seeds + Legumes = Complete Protein

Choosing healthy protein sources FIGURE 6.15

The meat and beans group and the milk group provide the most concentrated sources of protein. Dry beans and peas are the most concentrated sources of plant protein. These may be included in the vegetables group or the meat and beans group. There is very little protein in fruits.

EAT LESS

Baked goods and refined grains, which supply small amounts of protein but add sugar and fat.	Fried vegetables and vegetables with cream sauces.	Whole milk and high-fat cheeses, which are high in saturated fat and cholesterol.	Fatty meats, which are high in saturated fat and cholesterol.

GRAINS   **VEGETABLES**   **MILK**   **MEAT & BEANS**

Whole grains, which supply small amounts of protein and add fiber, photochemicals, vitamins, and minerals.	Dry beans and peas such as kidney beans, pinto beans, lima beans, and lentils. These are excellent sources of plant protein and also provide fiber, iron, and zinc. Much of the fiber is soluble fiber, which helps lower blood cholesterol.	Nonfat or low-fat milk and milk products, which provide high-quality protein and calcium with little or no saturated fat or cholesterol.	Lean cuts of meat and skinless poultry, which add high-quality protein, iron, and zinc; fish, which provides heart-healthy omega-3 fatty acids; and nuts and seeds, which provide plant protein, heart-healthy mono-unsaturated fats, and fiber.

EAT MORE

protein complementation

The process of combining proteins from different sources so that they collectively provide the proportions of amino acids required to meet the body's needs.

diets rely on this technique, called **protein complementation**, to meet protein needs. By eating plant proteins that have complementary amino acid patterns, a person can meet his or her essential amino acid requirements without consuming any animal proteins.

MyPyramid recommendations

Choosing a diet that includes a variety of foods will provide enough protein and enough of each of the essential amino acids to meet the body's needs. If you follow the MyPyramid recommendations, your diet will include both animal and plant sources of protein (**FIGURE 6.15**). A cup of milk provides about 8 g of protein, and an ounce from the meat and beans group can add another 7 to 10 g. These two food groups contain the foods that are the highest in protein. Each serving from the grains group and the vegetables group provides 1 to 3 g, but because we eat a larger number of servings from these groups, they make an important contribution to our protein intake. However, just getting enough protein does not ensure a healthy diet. The

Use iProfile to look up the protein content of your favorite vegetarian entree.

Get protein without too much saturated fat
- Plan on poultry or fish.
- Choose lean cuts of red meat.
- Grill, roast, or broil so that the fat will end up in the pan or the fire.
- Choose low-fat or reduced-fat milk.

Eat both animal and plant proteins
- Have your beef or chicken in a stir-fry with lots of vegetables.
- Serve a small portion of meat over noodles.
- Add nuts and seeds to snacks and salads.
- Have a meatless meal at least once a week.

Go with beans
- Try hummus—made from ground chickpeas and sesame seeds.
- Add kidney beans or chickpeas to soups.
- Snack on soy beans.
- Enjoy tacos or burritos stuffed with pinto beans or black beans.

sources of your dietary proteins also affect the healthfulness of your diet, particularly how well it meets the recommendations for fat and fiber intake (see *What Should I Eat?*).

VEGETARIAN DIETS

vegetarian diets
Diets that include plant-based foods and eliminate some or all foods of animal origin.

In many parts of the world, diets based on plant proteins, called **vegetarian diets**, have evolved mostly out of necessity because animal sources of protein are limited, either physically or economically, in those areas. Animals require more land and resources to raise and are more expensive to purchase than are plants. The developing world relies on plant foods to meet protein needs. For example, in rural Mexico, most of the protein in the diet comes from beans, rice, and tortillas (corn), and in India protein comes from lentils and rice. As a population's economic prosperity rises, the proportion of animal foods in its diet typically increases, but in developed countries, vegetarian diets are followed for a variety of reasons other than economics, such as health, religion, personal ethics, or environmental awareness. **Vegan diets** eliminate all animal products, but there are other types of vegetarian diets that are less restrictive (TABLE 6.2).

vegan diets
Plant-based diets that eliminate all animal products.

Benefits of vegetarian diets A vegetarian diet can be a healthy, low-cost alternative to the traditional American meat-and-potatoes diet. Vegetarians have been shown to have lower body weight and a reduced incidence of obesity and of other chronic diseases, such as diabetes, cardiovascular disease, high blood pressure, and some types of cancer.[15,16] The lower body weight of vegetarians is a result of lower energy intake, primarily due to higher intake of

Types of vegetarian diets	TABLE 6.2
Diet	**What it excludes and includes**
Semivegetarian	Excludes red meat but may include fish and poultry, as well as dairy products and eggs.
Pescetarian	Excludes all animal flesh except fish.
Lacto-ovo vegetarian	Excludes all animal flesh but does include eggs and dairy products such as milk and cheese.
Lacto vegetarian	Excludes animal flesh and eggs but does include dairy products.
Vegan	Excludes all food of animal origin.

fiber, which makes the diet more filling. The reductions in the risk of other chronic diseases may be due to lower body weight and to the fact that these diets are lower in saturated fat and cholesterol, which increase disease risk. Or it could be that vegetarian diets are higher in grains, legumes, vegetables, and fruits, which add fiber, vitamins, minerals, antioxidants, and phytochemicals—substances that have been shown to lower disease risk. It is likely that the total dietary pattern, rather than a single factor alone, is responsible for the health-promoting effects of vegetarian diets.

In addition to reducing disease risks, diets that rely more heavily on plant protein than on animal protein are more economical. For example, a vegetarian stir-fry over rice costs about half as much as a meal of steak and potatoes. Yet both meals provide a significant portion of the day's protein requirement. A 6-ounce steak, a baked potato with sour cream, and a tossed salad provides about 50 grams of protein, whereas a dish of rice with tofu and vegetables provides about 30 g.

Risks of vegetarian diets
Despite the health and economic benefits of vegetarian diets, a poorly planned vegetarian diet can cause nutrient deficiencies. Protein deficiency is a risk when vegan diets that contain little high-quality protein are consumed by small children or by adults with increased protein needs, such as pregnant women and those recovering from illness or injury. Most people can easily meet their protein needs with lacto and lacto-ovo vegetarian diets. These diets contain high-quality animal proteins from eggs or milk, which complement the limiting amino acids in the plant proteins.

Vitamin and mineral deficiencies are a greater concern for vegetarians than is protein deficiency. Of primary concern to vegans is vitamin B_{12}. Because this B vitamin is found almost exclusively in animal products, vegans must take vitamin B_{12} supplements or consume foods fortified with vitamin B_{12} to meet their needs for this nutrient. Another nutrient of concern is calcium. Dairy products are the major source of calcium in the North American diet, so diets that eliminate these foods must rely on plant sources of calcium. Likewise, because most dietary vitamin D comes from fortified milk, this vitamin must be made in the body from exposure to sunlight or consumed in other sources. Iron and zinc may be deficient in vegetarian diets because red meat is an excellent source of these minerals, and they are poorly absorbed from plant sources. Because dairy products are low in iron and zinc, lacto-ovo and lacto vegetarians as well as vegans are at risk for deficiencies of these minerals. Omega-3 fatty acids, including EPA and DHA (see Chapter 5), are also a concern in vegan diets.[14] **TABLE 6.3** provides suggestions for how to meet the need for the nutrients just discussed.

Meeting nutrient needs with a vegan diet[14] TABLE 6.3

Nutrient at Risk	Sources in Vegan Diets
Protein	Soy-based products, legumes, seeds, nuts, grains, and vegetables
Vitamin B_{12}	Products fortified with vitamin B_{12}, such as soy beverages and breakfast cereals; nutritional yeast; dietary supplements
Calcium	Tofu processed with calcium; broccoli, kale, bok choy, and legumes; products fortified with calcium, such as soy beverages, grain products, and orange juice
Vitamin D	Sunshine; products fortified with vitamin D, such as soy beverages, breakfast cereals, and margarine
Iron	Legumes, tofu, dark green leafy vegetables, dried fruit, whole grains, iron-fortified grain products (absorption is improved when iron-containing foods are consumed with vitamin C found in citrus fruit, tomatoes, strawberries, and dark green vegetables)
Zinc	Whole grains, wheat germ, legumes, nuts, tofu, and fortified breakfast cereals
Omega-3 fatty acids	Canola oil, flaxseed and flaxseed oil, soybean oil, walnuts, sea vegetables (seaweed), and DHA-rich microalgae

Soy from products such as these provides high-quality protein that can help vegetarians meet their protein needs. Soy has also been suggested to protect against heart disease and cancer, diseases that are less common in Asian countries, where soy is a major source of protein. Recent studies have not supported soy's benefits in preventing or treating cancer and have shown that it causes only a slight decrease in LDL cholesterol, but soy may still protect the heart because it is high in polyunsaturated fat, fiber, vitamins, and minerals, and low in saturated fat.[17]

Soy milk can be substituted for cow's milk.

Soy flour can be incorporated into baked goods.

Texturized soy protein (TSP) also known as texturized vegetable protein (TVP) can be formed into chunks, woven or spun into fibers, or otherwise shaped and flavored to produce vegetarian versions of burgers, hot dogs, meatballs, and chicken.

Soy butter, which is similar to peanut butter, can be spread on crackers and sandwiches.

Tofu, also known as bean curd, can be enjoyed in soups, salads, and stir-fries.

Planning vegetarian diets

Well-planned vegetarian diets, including vegan diets, can meet nutrient needs at all stages of the life cycle, from infancy, childhood, and adolescence to early, middle, and late adulthood, and during pregnancy and lactation.[14] One way to plan a healthy vegetarian diet is to modify the selections from MyPyramid. The food choices and recommended amounts from the grains, vegetables, and fruits groups should stay the same for vegetarians. Including 1 cup of dark green leafy vegetables daily will help meet iron and calcium needs. The milk group and the meat and beans group include foods of animal origin. Vegetarians who consume eggs and milk can still choose these foods. Those who avoid all animal foods can choose dry beans, nuts, and seeds from the meat and beans group. Soy products provide high-quality plant protein (FIGURE 6.16). Fortified soymilk can be substituted for dairy foods. To obtain adequate vitamin B_{12}, vegans must take supplements or use products fortified with vitamin B_{12}. Obtaining plenty of omega-3 fatty acids from foods such as canola oil, nuts, and flaxseed ensures adequate synthesis of the long-chain omega-3 fatty acids DHA and EPA. (See the *Case Study*.)

CONCEPT CHECK **STOP**

What circumstances result in a positive nitrogen balance?

Why is the quality of animal protein considered to be higher than that of plant protein?

What protein source could you serve with pasta that would complement the wheat protein in the pasta?

Why are vegans at risk for vitamin B_{12} deficiency?

IS A VEGETARIAN DIET ALWAYS HEALTHY?

Simon is 26 years old and weighs 154 pounds. A year ago, he decided to stop eating meat for health reasons. Now that he is studying protein in his nutrition class, he has become concerned that his lacto vegetarian diet isn't meeting his needs.

What is the RDA for protein for someone of Simon's age and weight?

▼

Your answer:

Simon records his food intake for 1 day and then uses iProfile to assess his nutrient intake. He is pleased to discover that his diet provides 65.7 g of protein, which exceeds his RDA, but he is shocked to discover that his diet is high in saturated fat.

This is a photo of Simon's typical lunch. Why is it high in saturated fat?

▼

Your answer:

For breakfast Simon typically has cereal with milk, and for dinner he has cheese pizza or cheese lasagna. He snacks on chips and ice cream.

Is this diet providing all the health benefits of a vegetarian diet?

▼

Your answer:

When he sees his diet analysis, Simon decides to try a vegan diet.

What could be included in Simon's vegan diet to meet his needs for calcium and vitamin D?

▼

Your answer:

Suggest a sandwich Simon could have for lunch that makes use of complementary plant proteins.

▼

Your answer:

(Check your answers in Appendix K.)

SUMMARY

1 Proteins in Our Food

1. Dietary protein comes from both animal and plant sources. Animal sources of protein are generally good sources of iron, zinc, and calcium but are high in saturated fat and cholesterol. Plant sources of protein are higher in unsaturated fat, fiber, and phytochemicals.

2 The Structure of Amino Acids and Proteins

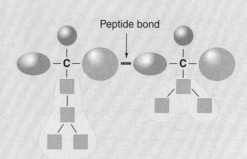

Peptide bond

1. **Amino acids** are the building blocks from which proteins are made. Each amino acid contains an amino group, an acid group, and a unique side chain. The amino acids that the body is unable to make in sufficient amounts are called **essential amino acids** and must be consumed in the diet.

2. Proteins are made of one or more chains of amino acid that fold to create unique three-dimensional structures. The shape of a protein determines its function.

3 Protein Digestion and Absorption

1. Digestion breaks dietary protein into small **peptides** and amino acids that can be absorbed. Because amino acids that share the same transport system compete for absorption, an excess of one can inhibit the absorption of another.

Blood

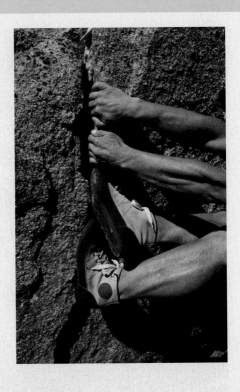

4 Protein Synthesis and Functions

1. Amino acids are used to synthesize proteins and other nitrogen-containing molecules. **Genes** located in the nucleus of the cell code for the order of amino acids in the **polypeptide** chains that make up proteins. Regulatory mechanisms ensure that proteins are made only when they are needed. For a protein to be synthesized, all the amino acids it contains must be available. The amino acid present in shortest supply relative to need is called the **limiting amino acid**.

2. In the body, protein molecules form structures, regulate body functions, transport molecules through the blood and in and out of cells, function in the immune system, and aid in muscle contraction, fluid balance, and acid balance.

3. When the diet is deficient in energy or when the diet contains more protein than needed, amino acids are used as an energy source and to synthesize glucose or fatty acids. Before amino acids can be used for these purposes, the amino group must be removed via **deamination**.

5 Protein in Health and Disease

1. **Protein-energy malnutrition (PEM)** is a health concern primarily in developing countries. **Kwashiorkor** occurs when the protein content of the diet is deficient but energy is adequate. It is most common in children. **Marasmus** occurs when total energy intake is deficient.

2. High-protein diets increase the production of urea and other waste products that must be excreted in the urine and therefore can increase water losses. High protein intakes increase urinary calcium losses, but when calcium intake is adequate, high-protein diets are associated with greater bone mass and fewer fractures. Diets high in animal proteins and low in fluid are associated with an increased risk of kidney stones. High-protein diets can be high in saturated fat and cholesterol.

3. If proteins are absorbed without being completely digested, they can trigger an immune system reaction, resulting in a **food allergy**. Some amino acids and proteins can also cause **food intolerances**.

6 Meeting Protein Needs

1. Protein requirements are determined by looking at **nitrogen balance**, the amount of nitrogen consumed as dietary protein compared with the amount excreted as protein waste products.

2. For healthy adults, the RDA for protein is 0.8 g/kilogram of body weight. Growth, pregnancy, lactation, illness, injury, and certain types of physical exercise increase requirements. Recommendations for a healthy diet are to ingest 10% to 35% of calories from protein.

3. Animal proteins are considered **high-quality proteins** because their amino acid composition matches that needed to synthesize body proteins. Most plant proteins are limited in one or more of the amino acids needed to make body protein; therefore, they are considered **incomplete proteins**. The **protein quality** of plant sources can be increased by **protein complementation**, which combines proteins with different limiting amino acids to supply enough of all the essential amino acids.

4. Compared with meat-based diets, **vegetarian diets** are lower in saturated fat and cholesterol and higher in fiber, certain vitamins and minerals, antioxidants, and phytochemicals. People consuming **vegan diets** must plan their diets carefully to meet their needs for vitamin B$_{12}$, calcium, vitamin D, iron, zinc, and omega-3 fatty acids.

KEY TERMS

1. Children with the genetic disease phenylketonuria must consume a low-phenylalanine diet to prevent the accumulation of damaging phenylketones. Why not just eliminate phenylalanine from the diet altogether?

2. Jack consumes about 120 grams of protein/day. Of this, about 30 grams is broken down and used to make ATP, and 30 grams is used to synthesize body fat. What does this tell you about Jack's protein and energy intake?

3. Syed is a body builder. He is concerned about his protein intake. If Syed weighs 200 pounds and consumes about 3600 Calories/day, 15% of which comes from protein, will his diet supply enough protein to meet the recommendation for strength athletes of 1.6 to 1.7 grams of protein/kilogram of body weight per day? How about if he consumed only 2500 Calories/day?

4. Fluid accumulates in the bellies of children with kwashiorkor. Use your understanding of how protein helps regulate fluid balance to explain why this occurs.

5. Suggest a breakfast, lunch, and dinner menu that supplies complementary sources of plant proteins.

6. At a recent physical, a blood test indicated that Taliah's blood urea concentration is elevated. What might be the cause of the elevation? What could she do to reduce the amount of urea produced?

7. Make a vegetarian meal plan for yourself for one day. Use iProfile to make sure it meets your calorie and protein needs. Then plan a day that includes meat. Go to the grocery store and calculate how much each day's meals will cost. Use this information to explain the economic benefits or pitfalls of these two eating plans.

What is happening in this picture ?

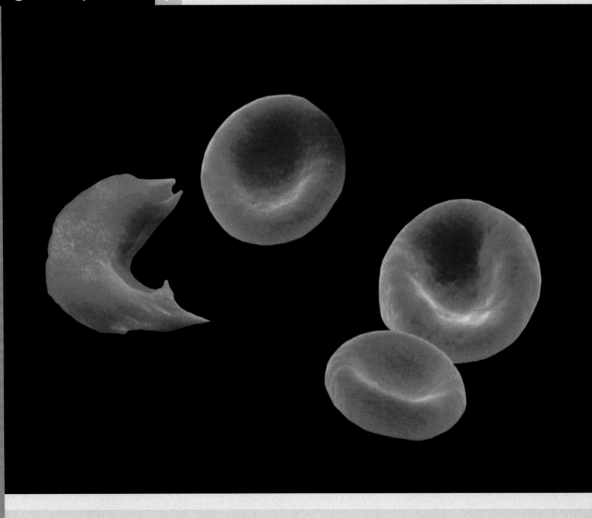

Sickle cell anemia is caused by an abnormality in the gene for the protein hemoglobin. It causes red blood cells to take on a sickle shape.

Sickle cell hemoglobin differs from normal hemoglobin by one amino acid. Why might this difference change the shape of the hemoglobin?

Do you think sickle-shaped red blood cells can travel easily through narrow capillaries?

How might this disorder affect the ability to get oxygen to the body's cells?

SELF-TEST

(Check your answers in Appendix L.)

1. Which part of this amino acid will differ, depending on the particular amino acid?

    a. A
    b. B
    c. C
    d. D

2. Amino acids that cannot be made by the adult human body in sufficient amounts are called _____.

    a. essential amino acids
    b. complete proteins
    c. incomplete amino acids
    d. hydrolyzed proteins
    e. nonessential amino acids

3. Based on the diagram, which letters label the parts of the digestive tract where chemical digestion of protein occurs?

    a. A and B
    b. A and C
    c. B and C
    d. B and D
    e. C and D

    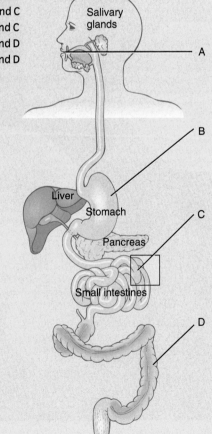

4. Which one of the following is made from amino acids?

    a. triglycerides
    b. glycogen
    c. lecithin
    d. cholesterol
    e. enzymes

5. Which of the following letters best labels transcription?

    a. A
    b. B
    c. C
    d. D

6. _____ is the process of transferring an amino group from an amino acid to another molecule to form a second amino acid.

    a. Deamination
    b. Transamination
    c. Denaturation
    d. Hydrogenation

7. Which color amino acid would be considered the most limiting for the synthesis of this specific protein?

   a. yellow
   b. green
   c. orange
   d. red
   e. blue

Amino acid pool → Protein

8. Which of the following groups requires the least protein per kilogram of body weight?

   a. adult men
   b. pregnant women
   c. infants
   d. young children

9. What element is found in proteins but not in carbohydrates and lipids?

   a. carbon
   b. nitrogen
   c. phosphorous
   d. oxygen
   e. hydrogen

10. Which of the following is least likely to be low in a vegan diet?

    a. calcium
    b. vitamin D
    c. iron
    d. fiber
    e. vitamin B$_{12}$

11. Which of the following values for nitrogen intake and output are most likely to belong to a healthy 9-year-old boy?

    a. nitrogen in = 14 g, nitrogen out = 16 g
    b. nitrogen in = 15 g, nitrogen out = 15 g
    c. nitrogen in = 14 g, nitrogen out = 10 g
    d. nitrogen in = 20 g, nitrogen out = 22 g

12. When amino acids are broken down to generate energy or synthesize glucose, the amino group must be removed. What waste product is generated from it?

    a. ketones
    b. urea
    c. free fatty acids
    d. carbon dioxide
    e. oxygen

13. Which of the following is *not* a good example of protein complementation?

    a. sunflower seeds and peanuts
    b. rice and beans
    c. chickpeas and sesame seeds
    d. corn and rice
    e. lentils and rice

14. When extra protein is consumed, it is stored in the muscle for later use.

    a. True
    b. False

15. Which one of the following statements about children with kwashiorkor is false?

    a. Their fat stores are completely depleted.
    b. They are more susceptible to infections than healthy children.
    c. They have swollen bellies.
    d. They have hair color changes.
    e. They do not grow well.

Vitamins

Britons have long been referred to as "Limeys." If you eat a lot of carrots, your night vision will improve. Mom says to go outside and get some sunshine.

These statements are related to an alphabet soup of essential compounds known as *vitamins*. British sailors on long voyages developed a debilitating disease called scurvy due to a lack of vitamin C. Consumption of adequate amounts of citrus fruits—such as limes—prevented them from developing this condition, and thus a nickname was born. Carrots are high in vitamin A, which is critical to the perception of light. And when exposed to sunlight, our bodies make the vitamin D we need; without vitamin D, we can't absorb enough calcium to build strong bones.

Populations enduring sunless Arctic winters have long acquired adequate amounts of vitamin D from a traditional diet of fish, bird eggs, seal, walrus, and whale blubber. But as their diet has changed over time—consumption of walrus and whale has been declining over the past 30 years—vitamin D deficiencies are increasing in these populations. If we who live in more temperate regions do not get enough sunlight, we must also obtain vitamin D from our diet, most often by consuming fortified milk.

As the British Royal Navy discovered—and diverse cultures, such as the Inuit, have appreciated for thousands of years—certain foods can counteract certain ailments. Only relatively recently have the agents in these foods been isolated and recognized for the significant role they play in preventing or alleviating illness and ensuring good health.

CHAPTER OUT

A Vitamin Primer

Vitamins are organic compounds that are essential in small amounts to promote and regulate body processes necessary for growth, reproduction, and the maintenance of health. When a vitamin is lacking in the diet, deficiency symptoms occur. When the vitamin is restored to the diet, the symptoms resolve.

Vitamins have traditionally been assigned to two groups, based on their solubility in water or fat. This chemical characteristic allows generalizations to be made about how the vitamins are absorbed, transported, excreted, and stored in the body. The **water-soluble vitamins** include the B vitamins and vitamin C. The **fat-soluble vitamins** include vitamins A, D, E, and K (**TABLE 7.1**). The vitamins were initially named alphabetically, in approximately the order in which they were identified. The B vitamins were first thought to be a single chemical substance but were later found to be many different substances. Vitamins B_6 and B_{12} are the only ones that are still routinely referred to by their numbers.

The vitamins TABLE 7.1	
Water-soluble vitamins	**Fat-soluble vitamins**
B vitamins	Vitamin A
• Thiamin (B_1)	Vitamin D
• Riboflavin (B_2)	Vitamin E
• Niacin (B_3)	Vitamin K
• Biotin	
• Pantothenic acid	
• Vitamin B_6 (pyridoxine)	
• Folate (folic acid)	
• Vitamin B_{12} (cobalamin)	
Vitamin C (ascorbic acid)	

VITAMINS IN OUR FOOD

Almost all foods contain some vitamins, and all the food groups contain foods that are good sources of a variety of vitamins (**FIGURE 7.1**). The amount of a vitamin in a

Vitamins in MyPyramid FIGURE 7.1

Vitamins are found in foods from all the food groups, as well as in oils, but some groups are lacking in specific vitamins. For example, grains, fruits, and vegetables lack vitamin B_{12}, and grains and meat and beans are low in vitamin C.

GRAINS	VEGETABLES	FRUITS	OILS	MILK	MEAT & BEANS
Thiamin	Riboflavin	Folate	Vitamin E	Riboflavin	Thiamin
Riboflavin	Niacin	Vitamin C		Vitamin A	Riboflavin
Niacin	Vitamin B_6	Vitamin A		Vitamin D	Niacin
Pantothenic acid	Folate			Vitamin B_{12}	Biotin
Vitamin B_6	Vitamin C				Pantothenic acid
Folate	Vitamin A				Folate
	Vitamin E				Vitamin B_{12}
	Vitamin K				Vitamin A
					Vitamin D
					Vitamin K

Fortification: Benefits and Risks

Fortified Breakfast Cereal

Nutrition Facts

Serving Size	1 Cup (50g/1.8 oz.)	
Servings per Container		About 10

Amount Per Serving	Cereal	Cereal with 1/2 Cup Vitamins A&D Fat Free Milk
Calories	180	220
Calories from Fat	5	5

	% Daily Value**	
Total Fat 0.5g*	1%	1%
Saturated Fat 0g	0%	0%
Trans Fat 0g		
Cholesterol 0mg	0%	0%
Sodium 280mg	12%	14%
Potassium 100mg	3%	9%
Total Carbohydrate 35g	12%	14%
Dietary Fiber 2g	9%	9%
Sugars 7g		
Other Carbohydrate 26g		
Protein 3g		
Vitamin A	15%	20%
Vitamin C	25%	25%
Calcium	0%	15%
Iron	100%	100%
Vitamin D	10%	25%
Vitamin E	100%	100%
Thiamin	100%	100%
Riboflavin	100%	110%
Niacin	100%	100%
Vitamin B_6	100%	100%
Folic Acid	100%	100%
Vitamin B_{12}	100%	110%
Pantothenate	100%	100%
Phosphorus	10%	20%
Magnesium	8%	10%
Zinc	100%	100%
Copper	4%	6%

The Nutrition Facts panel on a box of breakfast cereal shows an abundance of vitamins and minerals, many of which have been added through fortification. A consumer sees an easy way to meet nutrient needs. A scientist sees both the health benefits and the risks of fortification.

Fortification began as a way to address nutrient deficiencies. In the early 1900s, the niacin deficiency disease *pellagra* caused more than 3,000 deaths annually in the southern United States. In 1938, bakers voluntarily began enriching flour with B vitamins, a move that led to a decline in mortality from pellagra (see graph).[1] By 1943, enrichment of flour was becoming mandatory. Other government-supported fortification programs in the United States have helped to prevent vitamin A and D deficiencies.

Not all fortification is mandated by the government. Scientists recognize that indiscriminate fortification of many foods, such as breakfast cereals, can increase the risk of nutrient toxicities. Almost 20% of toddlers who take vitamin supplements have folate intakes that exceed the UL, and more than half of infants and children up to age 3 exceed the UL for zinc.[2,3] In view of these risks, should the government regulate all fortification of food?

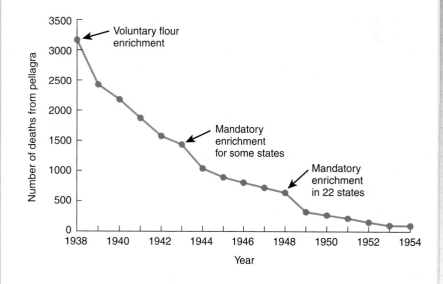

food depends on the amount that is naturally present in the food, what is added to it, and how the food is processed, cooked, and stored.

Fortification adds nutrients to foods. Sometimes nutrients are added to foods to comply with government fortification programs that mandate such additions in order to prevent vitamin or mineral deficiencies and promote health in the population (see *What a Scientist Sees*). For example, grains are *enriched* with B vitamins and iron to prevent deficiencies, and milk is fortified

Which choice is highest in vitamins? FIGURE 7.2

Because heat, light, air, and the passage of time all cause foods to lose nutrients, most of us try to purchase fresh produce, but is fresh always best?

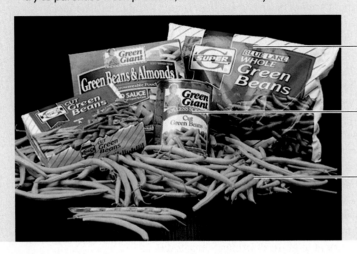

Frozen foods are often frozen in the field in order to minimize nutrient losses. Thus, frozen fruits and vegetables may supply more vitamins than "fresh" ones.

The high temperatures used in canning reduce nutrient content. However, because canned foods keep for a long time, do not require refrigeration, and are often less expensive than fresh or frozen foods, they provide an available, affordable source of nutrients that may be the best choice in some situations.

Sometimes "fresh" produce is lower in nutrients than you would expect because it has spent a week in a truck, traveling to the store, several days on the shelf, and maybe another week in your refrigerator.

with vitamin D to promote bone health. In other cases, manufacturers add nutrients with the goal of increasing product sales.

The vitamins in foods can be damaged by exposure to light or oxygen, washed away during preparation, or destroyed by cooking. Thus, processing steps used by food producers can cause nutrient losses, as can cooking and storage methods used at home (FIGURE 7.2). Vitamin losses can be minimized through food preparation methods that reduce exposure to heat and light, which destroy some vitamins, and to water, which washes away water-soluble vitamins (TABLE 7.2).

Tips for preserving the vitamins in your food
TABLE 7.2

- Store food away from heat and light and eat it soon after purchasing it.

- Cut fruits and vegetables as close as possible to the time when they will be cooked or served.

- Don't soak vegetables before you cook them.

- Cook vegetables with as little water as possible by microwaving, pressure-cooking, roasting, grilling, stir-frying, or baking rather than boiling them.

- If foods are cooked in water, use the cooking water to make soups and sauces so that you can retrieve some of the nutrients.

- Don't rinse rice before cooking, in order to avoid washing away water-soluble vitamins.

VITAMIN BIOAVAILABILITY

About 40 to 90% of the vitamins in food are absorbed, primarily from the small intestine (FIGURE 7.3). The composition of the diet and conditions in the digestive tract and the rest of the body influence vitamin **bioavailability**. For example, fat-soluble vitamins are absorbed along with dietary fat. If the diet is very low in fat, absorption of these vitamins is impaired.

> **bioavailability**
> The extent to which the body can absorb and use a nutrient.

Once they have been absorbed into the blood, vitamins must be transported to the cells. Most of the water-soluble vitamins are bound to blood proteins for transport. Fat-soluble vitamins are incorporated into chylomicrons for transport from the intestine. The bioavailability of a vitamin depends on the availability of these transport systems.

Some vitamins are absorbed in an inactive form called either a **provitamin** or a **vitamin precursor**. To perform vitamin functions, provitamins must be converted into active vitamin forms once they are inside the body. How much of each provitamin can be converted into the active vitamin and the rate at which this process occurs affect the amount of a vitamin available to function inside the body.

> **provitamin** or **vitamin precursor**
> A compound that can be converted into the active form of a vitamin in the body.

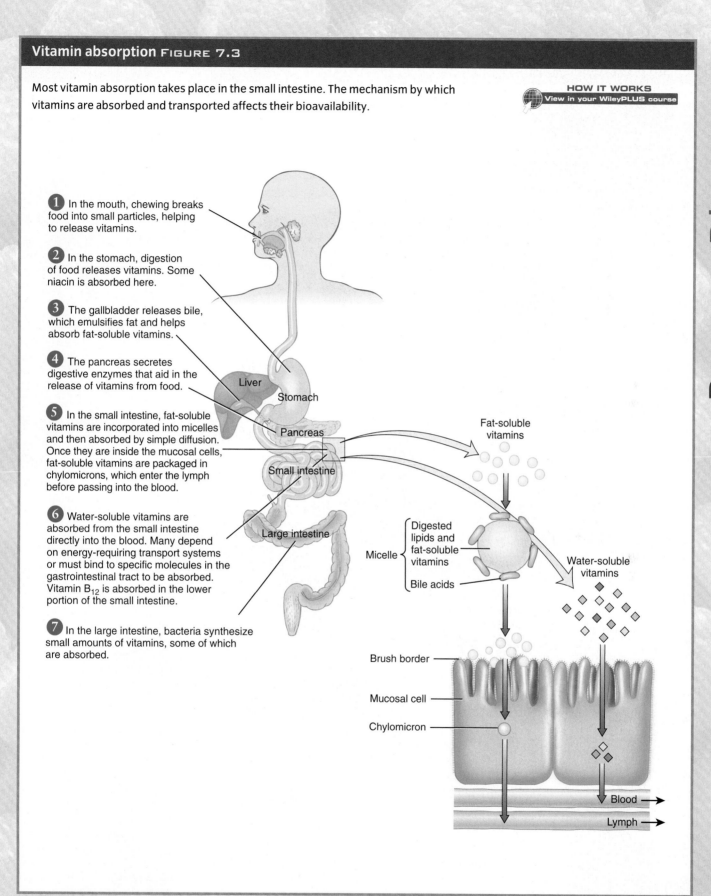

Vitamin absorption FIGURE 7.3

Most vitamin absorption takes place in the small intestine. The mechanism by which vitamins are absorbed and transported affects their bioavailability.

1 In the mouth, chewing breaks food into small particles, helping to release vitamins.

2 In the stomach, digestion of food releases vitamins. Some niacin is absorbed here.

3 The gallbladder releases bile, which emulsifies fat and helps absorb fat-soluble vitamins.

4 The pancreas secretes digestive enzymes that aid in the release of vitamins from food.

5 In the small intestine, fat-soluble vitamins are incorporated into micelles and then absorbed by simple diffusion. Once they are inside the mucosal cells, fat-soluble vitamins are packaged in chylomicrons, which enter the lymph before passing into the blood.

6 Water-soluble vitamins are absorbed from the small intestine directly into the blood. Many depend on energy-requiring transport systems or must bind to specific molecules in the gastrointestinal tract to be absorbed. Vitamin B_{12} is absorbed in the lower portion of the small intestine.

7 In the large intestine, bacteria synthesize small amounts of vitamins, some of which are absorbed.

Liver
Stomach
Pancreas
Small intestine
Large intestine

Fat-soluble vitamins

Micelle
Digested lipids and fat-soluble vitamins
Bile acids

Water-soluble vitamins

Brush border
Mucosal cell
Chylomicron
Blood →
Lymph →

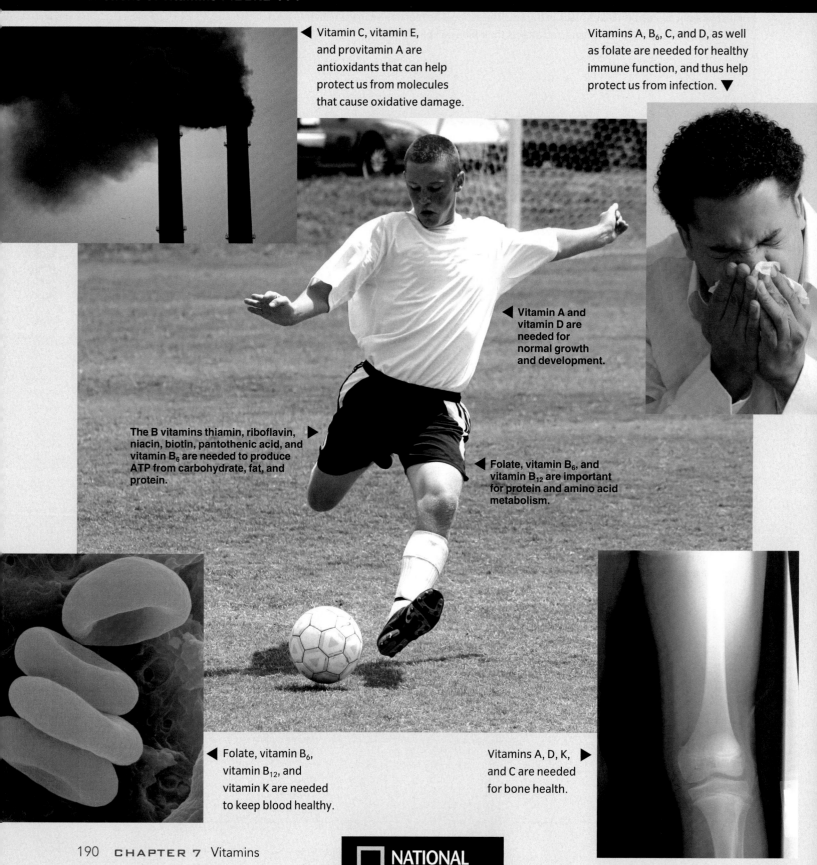

Vitamin C, vitamin E, and provitamin A are antioxidants that can help protect us from molecules that cause oxidative damage.

Vitamins A, B$_6$, C, and D, as well as folate are needed for healthy immune function, and thus help protect us from infection. ▼

Vitamin A and vitamin D are needed for normal growth and development.

The B vitamins thiamin, riboflavin, niacin, biotin, pantothenic acid, and vitamin B$_6$ are needed to produce ATP from carbohydrate, fat, and protein.

Folate, vitamin B$_6$, and vitamin B$_{12}$ are important for protein and amino acid metabolism.

Folate, vitamin B$_6$, vitamin B$_{12}$, and vitamin K are needed to keep blood healthy.

Vitamins A, D, K, and C are needed for bone health.

NATIONAL GEOGRAPHIC

VITAMIN FUNCTIONS

Vitamins promote and regulate the body's activities. Each vitamin has one or more important functions (**FIGURE 7.4**). For example, vitamin A is needed for vision as well as normal growth and development. Vitamin K is needed for blood clotting and bone health. Often more than one vitamin is needed to ensure the health of a particular organ or system. Some vitamins act in a similar manner to do their jobs. For example, all the B vitamins act as **coenzymes** (**FIGURE 7.5**).

A few vitamins function as **antioxidants**, substances that protect against **oxidative damage**. Oxidative damage is caused when reactive oxygen molecules steal electrons from other compounds, causing changes in their structure and function.

> **coenzymes**
> Organic nonprotein substances that bind to enzymes to promote their activity.

> **antioxidant**
> A substance that is able to neutralize reactive oxygen molecules and thereby prevent cell damage.

Coenzymes FIGURE 7.5

Coenzymes bind to enzymes to promote their activity. They act as carriers of electrons, atoms, or chemical groups that participate in the reaction. All the B vitamins are coenzymes, but there are also coenzymes that are not dietary essentials and therefore are not vitamins. Coenzymes are essential for the proper functioning of numerous enzymes involved in metabolism.

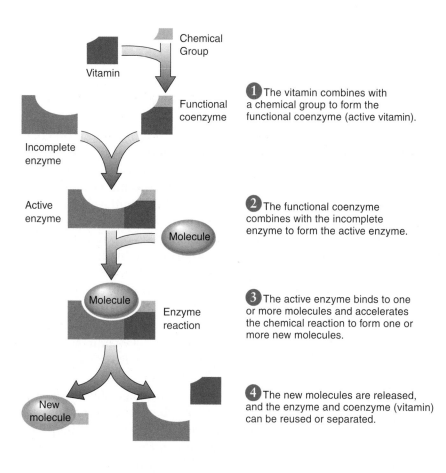

1 The vitamin combines with a chemical group to form the functional coenzyme (active vitamin).

2 The functional coenzyme combines with the incomplete enzyme to form the active enzyme.

3 The active enzyme binds to one or more molecules and accelerates the chemical reaction to form one or more new molecules.

4 The new molecules are released, and the enzyme and coenzyme (vitamin) can be reused or separated.

Process Diagram

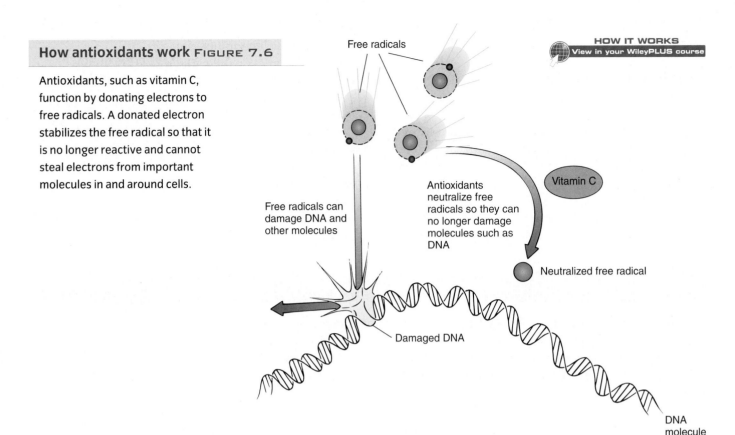

How antioxidants work FIGURE 7.6

Antioxidants, such as vitamin C, function by donating electrons to free radicals. A donated electron stabilizes the free radical so that it is no longer reactive and cannot steal electrons from important molecules in and around cells.

Free radicals

HOW IT WORKS
View in your WileyPLUS course

Antioxidants neutralize free radicals so they can no longer damage molecules such as DNA

Vitamin C

Free radicals can damage DNA and other molecules

Neutralized free radical

Damaged DNA

DNA molecule

---

free radicals
One type of highly reactive atom or molecule that causes oxidative damage.

Reactive oxygen molecules such as **free radicals** can be generated by normal oxygen-requiring reactions inside the body, such as cellular respiration, or can come from environmental sources such as air pollution or cigarette smoke. Free radicals cause damage by snatching electrons from DNA, proteins, carbohydrates, or unsaturated fatty acids. This loss of electrons results in changes in the structure and function of these molecules. Antioxidants act by destroying free radicals and other reactive oxygen molecules before they can do damage (**FIGURE 7.6**). Some antioxidants are produced in the body; others, such as vitamin C, vitamin E, and the mineral selenium, are consumed in the diet.[4]

MEETING VITAMIN NEEDS

The right amounts and combinations of vitamins and other nutrients are essential to health. Despite our knowledge of what vitamins do and how much of each we need, not everyone consumes the right amounts. In developing countries, vitamin deficiencies remain a major public health problem. In industrialized coun-

tries, thanks to the more varied food supply, along with fortification, vitamin-deficiency diseases have been almost eliminated. In these countries, concern now focuses on meeting the needs of high-risk groups, such as children and pregnant women; determining the consequences of marginal deficiencies, such as the effect of low B vitamin intake on heart disease risk; and evaluating the risk of consuming large amounts of certain vitamins.

The RDAs and AIs of the DRIs recommend amounts that provide enough of each of the vitamins to prevent a deficiency and promote health (see Chapter 2). Because more is not always better when it comes to nutrient intake, the DRIs have also established ULs as a guide to amounts that avoid the risk of toxicity (see Appendix A).

Food labels can help identify packaged foods that are good sources of vitamins. Labels are required to list the amounts of vitamin A and vitamin C in foods as a percentage of the Daily Values (**FIGURE 7.7**). Daily Values of other vitamins are often provided voluntarily. Fresh fruits, vegetables, fish, meat, and poultry, which are excellent sources of many vitamins, do not carry food labels. The FDA and USDA have therefore asked that grocery stores voluntarily provide nutrition information for the raw fruits, vegetables, fish, meat, and poultry that are most frequently purchased, and about 75% of stores comply.[5]

Vitamins on food labels FIGURE 7.7

As a general guideline, if the % Daily Value is 5% or less, the food is a poor source of that nutrient; if it is 10 to 19%, the food is a good source; and if the % Daily Value is 20% or more, the food is an excellent source.

To determine the exact amount of a vitamin in a food, look up the Daily Value (see Appendix F) and multiply it by the % Daily Value on the label.

Orange Juice

Nutrition Facts

Serving Size 8 fl oz (250 mL)
Servings Per Container 8

Amount Per Serving

Calories 110	Calories from Fat 0

	%Daily Value**
Total Fat 0g	2%
Sodium 0mg	0%
Potassium 450mg	13%
Total Carbohydrate 26g	9%
Sugars 7g	
Protein 2g	

Vitamin C 120%	•	Calcium	2%
Thiamin	10%	• Riboflavin	4%
Niacin	4%	• Vitamin B$_6$	6%
Folate	15%	• Magnesium	6%

Not a significant source or saturated fat, cholesterol, dietary fiber, vitamin A and iron.

*Percent Daily Values are based on a 2,000 calorie diet.

CONCEPT CHECK STOP

What food groups contain the greatest variety of vitamins?

Why might a low-fat diet affect the bioavailability of fat-soluble vitamins?

What is the principal function of coenzymes?

How do antioxidants protect our cells?

The Water-Soluble Vitamins

LEARNING OBJECTIVES

Discuss the role of thiamin, riboflavin, and niacin in producing ATP.

Explain why vitamin B$_6$ is so important for protein metabolism.

Compare the functions of folate and vitamin B$_{12}$.

Relate the role of vitamin C in the body to the symptoms of scurvy.

The water-soluble vitamins include the B vitamins and vitamin C. The B vitamins are directly involved in converting the energy in carbohydrate, fat, and protein into ATP, the form of energy that is used to run the body. Vitamin C is needed to synthesize connective tissue and to protect us from damage by oxidation.

Because water-soluble vitamins are not stored to any great extent, supplies of most of these vitamins are rapidly depleted. For this reason, water-soluble vitamins must be consumed regularly. Nevertheless, it takes more than a few days to develop deficiency symptoms, even when one of these vitamins is completely eliminated from the diet. For years, we thought that because most water-soluble vitamins are not stored in the body and are excreted in the urine, high doses were not harmful. However, we now recognize that high doses of some of these vitamins are toxic.

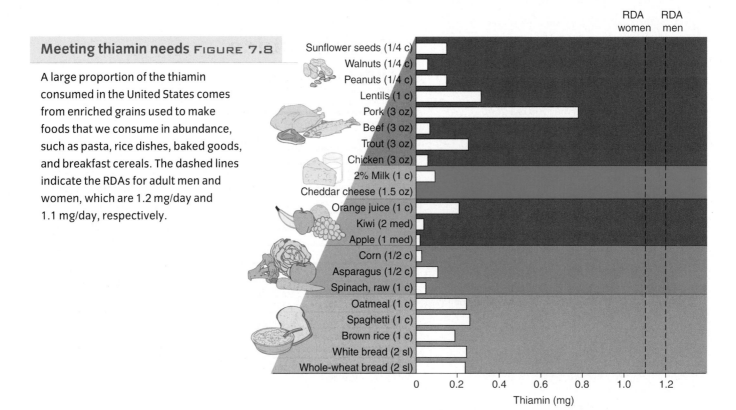

Meeting thiamin needs FIGURE 7.8

A large proportion of the thiamin consumed in the United States comes from enriched grains used to make foods that we consume in abundance, such as pasta, rice dishes, baked goods, and breakfast cereals. The dashed lines indicate the RDAs for adult men and women, which are 1.2 mg/day and 1.1 mg/day, respectively.

Thiamin (mg)

THIAMIN

Thiamin, the first of the B vitamins to be discovered, is sometimes called vitamin B_1. **Beriberi**, the disease that results from a deficiency of this vitamin, came to the attention of Western medicine in colonial Asia in the 19th century. It became such a problem that the Dutch East India Company sent a team of scientists to determine its cause. A young physician named Christian Eijkman worked on this problem for over 10 years. His success came as a result of a twist of fate. He ran out of food for his experimental chickens and, instead of the usual brown rice, fed them white rice. Shortly thereafter, the chickens displayed beriberi-like symptoms. When he fed them brown rice again, their health was restored. These results provided evidence that the cause of beriberi was not a poison or a microorganism as previously thought, but rather something that was missing from the diet.

Eijkman's studies enabled the prevention and cure of beriberi through feeding people a diet that was adequate in thiamin, but the vitamin itself was not isolated until 1926. We now know that polishing the bran layer off rice kernels to make white rice removes the thiamin-rich portion of the grain. Therefore, in populations where white rice was the staple of the diet, beriberi became a common health problem. The incidence of beriberi in eastern Asia increased dramatically in the late 1800s due to the rising popularity of polished rice.

Thiamin is a coenzyme that is needed for the breakdown of glucose to provide energy. It is particularly important for nerve function because glucose is the energy source for nerve cells. In addition to its role in energy production, thiamin is needed for the synthesis of **neurotransmitters**, the metabolism of other sugars and certain amino acids, and the synthesis of ribose, a sugar that is part of the structure of RNA (ribonucleic acid).

In addition to being found in the bran layer of brown rice and other whole grains, thiamin is added to enriched grains and is particularly abundant in pork, legumes, and seeds (FIGURE 7.8). When inadequate amounts of thiamin are consumed, the deficiency affects the nervous and cardiovascular systems. The neurological symptoms of beriberi can be related to the functions of thiamin (FIGURE 7.9). Beriberi can also

> **beriberi** A thiamin deficiency disease that causes weakness, nerve degeneration, and, in some cases, heart changes.

> **neurotransmitter** A chemical substance produced by a nerve cell that can stimulate or inhibit another cell.

How thiamin functions FIGURE 7.9

A The active thiamin coenzyme is needed to convert pyruvate, into acetyl-CoA. Acetyl-CoA can continue through cellular respiration to produce larger amounts of ATP. Acetyl-CoA is also needed to synthesize the neurotransmitter acetylcholine. Without thiamin, glucose, which is the primary fuel for the brain and nerve cells, cannot be used normally, and acetylcholine cannot be synthesized.

B For over 1000 years, beriberi flourished in East Asian countries. In Sri Lanka, the word *beriberi* means "I cannot," referring to the extreme weakness and depression that are the earliest symptoms of the disease. These symptoms may be caused by the inability of nerve cells to produce energy from glucose. Other neurological symptoms, such as poor coordination, tingling sensations, and paralysis, may be related to the body's inability to synthesize certain neurotransmitters when thiamin is deficient.

cause cardiovascular symptoms such as rapid heartbeat and enlargement of the heart, but it is not clear from the functions of thiamin why these cardiovascular symptoms occur.[6]

Beriberi is rare in North America today, but a form of thiamin deficiency called **Wernicke-Korsakoff syndrome** occurs in alcoholics. People with this condition experience mental confusion, psychosis, memory disturbances, and eventually coma. Alcoholics are particularly vulnerable because thiamin absorption is de-

creased due to the effect of alcohol on the gastrointestinal tract. In addition, their thiamin intake is low because alcohol contributes calories to the diet but brings with it almost no nutrients.

Although thiamin is needed to provide energy, unless the diet is deficient in thiamin, increasing thiamin intake does not increase the ability to produce ATP. There is no UL for thiamin because no toxicity has been reported when an excess of this vitamin is consumed from either food or supplements.[6]

RIBOFLAVIN

Riboflavin is a water-soluble vitamin that provides a visible indicator of excessive consumption; the excess is excreted in the urine, turning it a bright fluorescent yellow. The color may surprise you, but it is harmless. No adverse effects of high doses of riboflavin from either foods or supplements have been reported.

Riboflavin forms two active coenzymes that act as electron carriers. They function in the reactions needed to produce ATP from carbohydrate, fat, and protein. Riboflavin is also involved directly or indirectly in converting a number of other vitamins, including folate, niacin, vitamin B$_6$, and vitamin K, into their active forms.

One of the best sources of riboflavin in the diet is milk (**FIGURE 7.10**). When riboflavin is deficient, injuries heal poorly because new cells cannot grow to replace the damaged ones. The tissues that grow most rapidly, such as the skin and the linings of the eyes, mouth, and tongue, are the first to be affected. These tissues show symptoms such as cracking of the lips and at the corners of the mouth; increased sensitivity to light; burning, tearing, and itching of the eyes; and flaking of the skin around the nose, eyebrows, and earlobes.

Meeting riboflavin needs FIGURE 7.10

A Ever wonder why milk comes in opaque cardboard or cloudy plastic containers? The reason is that riboflavin is destroyed by light. If your milk was in a clear glass bottle and sat in a lighted grocery store display case for several days, much of the riboflavin would be destroyed. Translucent plastic containers block some of the light, but opaque containers are the most effective. Exposure to light can also cause an "off" flavor and losses of vitamins A and D.[7]

B Major dietary sources of riboflavin include dairy products, liver, red meat, poultry, fish, whole grains, and enriched breads and cereals. Vegetable sources include asparagus, broccoli, mushrooms, and leafy green vegetables such as spinach. The dashed lines indicate the RDAs for adult men and women, which are 1.3 mg/day and 1.1 mg/day, respectively.[6]

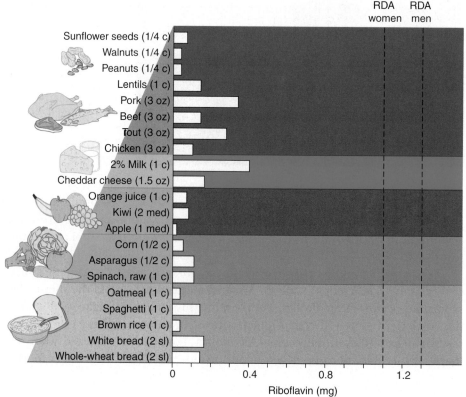

A deficiency of riboflavin usually occurs in conjunction with deficiencies of other B vitamins because the same foods are also sources of those vitamins and because riboflavin is needed to convert other vitamins into their active forms. Some of the symptoms seen in cases of riboflavin deficiency therefore reflect deficiencies of these other nutrients as well.

pellagra A disease resulting from niacin deficiency, which causes dermatitis, diarrhea, dementia, and, if not treated, death.

NIACIN

In the early 1900s, psychiatric hospitals in the southeastern United States were filled with patients with the niacin-deficiency disease **pellagra** (FIGURE 7.11). **Niacin** coenzymes are electron carriers that function in glucose metabolism and in reactions that synthesize fatty acids and cholesterol. The

Tracking down the cause of pellagra FIGURE 7.11

In 1914, Dr. Joseph Goldberger was appointed by the U.S. Public Health Service to investigate the pellagra epidemic in the South. He unraveled the mystery of its cause by using the scientific method. He observed that individuals in institutions such as hospitals, orphanages, and prisons suffered from pellagra, but the staff did not. If pellagra were an infectious disease, both populations would be equally affected. He therefore hypothesized that pellagra was due to a deficiency in the diet. He conducted a number of experiments, and the results supported his hypothesis. In 1937, the deficient dietary component was identified as the water-soluble B vitamin niacin.

Observation

Children in orphanages suffer from pellagra, but the staff does not

↓

Hypothesis

Pellagra is due to a deficiency of something in the diet

↓

Experiments

Experimental design: Nutritious foods including meat, milk, and vegetables are added to the diets of children in two orphanages.

Results: Those consuming the healthier diets recover from pellagra. Those without the disease who eat the new diet do not contract pellagra, supporting the hypothesis that it is caused by dietary deficiency.

Experimental design: Eleven volunteers are fed a diet believed to be lacking in the dietary substance that prevents pellagra.

Results: Six of the eleven develop symptoms of pellagra after 5 months of consuming the experimental diet, supporting the hypothesis that it is caused by a dietary deficiency.

Continued experiments: Various studies involving both animals and humans eventually reveal that nicotinic acid, better known as the B vitamin niacin, cures pellagra.

↓

Theory

Pellegra is caused by a deficiency of the B vitamin niacin.

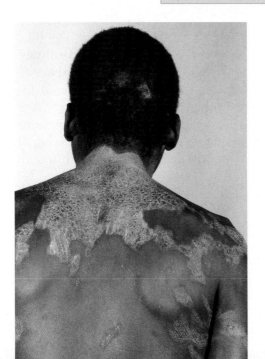

This photograph illustrates the cracked, inflamed skin that is characteristic of pellagra. The rash most commonly appears on areas of the skin that are exposed to sunlight or other stresses.

Meeting niacin needs FIGURE 7.12

Meat, fish, peanuts, and whole and enriched grains are the best sources of niacin. Other sources include legumes and wheat bran. Food composition tables and databases do not include the amount of niacin that could be made from the tryptophan in a food. The dashed lines indicate the RDAs for adult men and women, which are 16 mg NE/day and 14 mg NE/day, respectively.

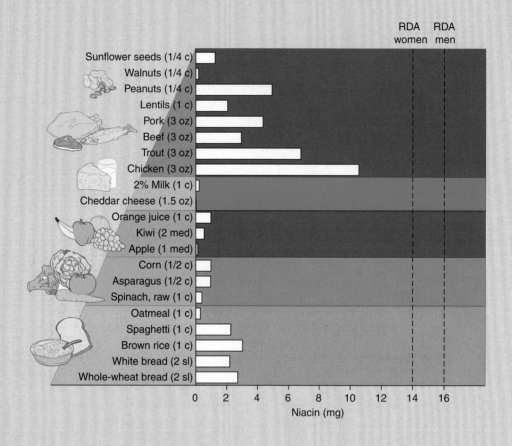

need for niacin is so widespread in metabolism that a deficiency causes major changes throughout the body. The early symptoms of pellagra include fatigue, decreased appetite, and indigestion. These are followed by symptoms that can be remembered as the three Ds: dermatitis, diarrhea, and dementia. If left untreated, niacin deficiency results in a fourth D—death.

Meats and grains are good sources of niacin (FIGURE 7.12). Niacin can also be synthesized in the body from the essential amino acid tryptophan. Tryptophan, however, is used to make niacin only if enough of it is available to first meet the needs of protein synthesis. When the diet is low in tryptophan, it is not used to synthesize niacin. Because some of the requirement for niacin can be met through the synthesis of niacin from tryptophan, the RDA is expressed as **niacin equivalents (NEs)**. One NE is equal to 1 mg of niacin or 60 mg of tryptophan, the amount needed to make 1 mg of niacin.[6]

The reason niacin deficiency was so prevalent in the South in the early 1900s is that the local diet among the poor was based on corn. Corn is low in tryptophan, and the niacin found naturally in corn is bound to other molecules and therefore not well absorbed. Today, as a result of the enrichment of grains with an available form of niacin, pellagra is rare in the United States, but it remains a problem in areas of Africa, where the diet is based on corn.[8] Despite the corn-based diet in Mexico and Central American countries, pellagra is uncommon in those countries, in part because the treatment of corn with limewater, as is done during the making of tortillas, enhances the availability of niacin. The diet in these regions also includes legumes, which provide both niacin and a source of tryptophan for the synthesis of niacin.

There is no evidence of any adverse effects due to the consumption of niacin that occurs naturally in foods, but niacin supplements can be toxic. Excess niacin supplementation can cause flushing of the skin, a tingling sensation in the hands and feet, a red skin rash, nausea, vomiting, diarrhea, high blood sugar levels, abnormalities in liver function, and blurred vision. The UL for adults is 35 mg. Doses of 50 mg or greater of one form of niacin are used as a drug to treat elevated blood cholesterol; this amount should be consumed only when prescribed by a physician.

BIOTIN

Biotin is a coenzyme that functions in energy production and glucose synthesis. It is also important in the metabolism of fatty acids and amino acids. Good sources of biotin in the diet include cooked eggs, liver, yogurt, and nuts. Fruit and meat are poor sources. Bacteria in the gastrointestinal tract synthesize biotin, and some of this is absorbed into the body and helps meet our biotin needs. An AI of 30 μg/day has been established for adults.[6]

Although biotin deficiency is uncommon, it has been observed in people with malabsorption or malnutrition and those taking certain medications for long periods.[6] Eating raw eggs can also cause biotin deficiency because raw egg whites contain a protein called avidin that tightly binds biotin and prevents its absorption. (Raw eggs should never be eaten anyway because they can contain harmful bacteria.) Thoroughly cooking eggs kills bacteria and denatures avidin so that it cannot bind biotin. Biotin deficiency in humans causes nausea, thinning hair, loss of hair color, a red skin rash, depression, lethargy, hallucinations, and tingling of the extremities. High doses of biotin have not resulted in toxicity symptoms; there is no UL for biotin.

PANTOTHENIC ACID

Pantothenic acid, which gets its name from the Greek word *pantothen* (meaning "from everywhere"), is widely distributed in foods. It is particularly abundant in meat, eggs, whole grains, and legumes, and it is found in lesser amounts in milk, vegetables, and fruits.

In addition to being "from everywhere" in the diet, pantothenic acid seems to be needed everywhere in the body. It is part of coenzyme A (CoA), which is needed for the breakdown of carbohydrates, fatty acids, and amino acids, as well as for the modification of proteins and the synthesis of neurotransmitters, steroid hormones, and hemoglobin. Pantothenic acid is also needed to form a molecule that is essential for the synthesis of cholesterol and fatty acids.

The wide distribution of pantothenic acid in foods makes deficiency rare in humans. The AI is 5 mg/day for adults. Pantothenic acid is relatively nontoxic, and there are insufficient data to establish a UL.[6]

VITAMIN B$_6$

Vitamin B$_6$ is particularly important for amino acid and protein metabolism. It is needed to synthesize nonessential amino acids, make neurotransmitters, synthesize hemoglobin, convert tryptophan into niacin, and break down glycogen to release glucose into the blood. There are three forms of vitamin B$_6$: pyridoxal, pyridoxine, and pyridoxamine. These can be converted into the active coenzyme **pyridoxal phosphate**, which is needed for the activity of more than 100 enzymes involved in the metabolism of carbohydrate, fat, and protein.

Vitamin B$_6$ deficiency leads to poor growth, skin lesions, decreased immune function, anemia, and neurological symptoms. Because vitamin B$_6$ is needed for amino acid metabolism, the onset of a deficiency can be hastened by a diet that is low in vitamin B$_6$ but high in protein. Many of the symptoms can be linked to the chemical reactions that depend on this vitamin coenzyme (**FIGURE 7.13** on the next page). For example, poor growth, skin lesions, and decreased antibody formation may occur with a diet that is low in vitamin B$_6$ because of the central role of vitamin B$_6$ in protein and energy metabolism.

A Vitamin B$_6$ is needed for *transamination* reactions, which synthesize nonessential amino acids by transferring an amino group to a carbon compound, and for *deamination* reactions, which remove the amino group from amino acids so that the remaining carbon compound can be used to provide energy or synthesize glucose. Vitamin B$_6$ is also needed to remove the acid group from amino acids so that the remaining molecule can be used to synthesize neurotransmitters.

B Vitamin B$_6$ is needed for the synthesis of lipids that are part of the **myelin** coating on nerves. Myelin is essential for nerve transmission. The role of vitamin B$_6$ in myelin formation and neurotransmitter synthesis may explain the neurological symptoms that occur with deficiency, such as numbness and tingling in the hands and feet, depression, headaches, confusion, and seizures.

◻ Vitamin B$_6$ is needed to synthesize hemoglobin, the oxygen-carrying protein in red blood cells. When vitamin B$_6$ is deficient, hemoglobin cannot be made; the result is a type of anemia characterized by small, pale red blood cells. Vitamin B$_6$ is also needed to form white blood cells, which are part of the immune system, so deficiency reduces immune function.

White blood cells   Red blood cells

◻ If vitamin B$_6$ status is low, homocysteine, which is formed from the amino acid methionine cannot be converted to cysteine so levels rise. Even a mild elevation in blood homocysteine levels has been shown to increase the risk of heart disease.[9]

Proteins

Amino acids

Methionine

Homocysteine

High levels in the blood increase cardiovascular disease risk

Vitamin B$_6$

Cysteine

Meat and fish are excellent sources of vitamin B$_6$, and whole grains and legumes are good plant sources (**Figure 7.14**). Refined grain products such as white rice and white bread are not good sources of vitamin B$_6$ because the vitamin is lost during refining but is not added back through enrichment. It is, however, added to many fortified breakfast cereals, which make an important contribution to vitamin B$_6$ intake.[10] Vitamin B$_6$ is destroyed by heat and light, so it can easily be lost during processing.

No adverse effects have been associated with high intake of vitamin B$_6$ from foods, but large doses found in supplements can cause severe nerve impairment. To prevent nerve damage, the UL for adults is set at 100 mg/day from food and supplements.[6] Despite the potential for toxicity, high-dose supplements of vitamin B$_6$ containing 100 mg/dose (5000% of the Daily Value) are available over the counter, making it easy to obtain a dose that exceeds the UL. People take vitamin B$_6$ supplements to reduce the symptoms of premenstrual syndrome (PMS), treat carpal tunnel syndrome, and strengthen immune function. There is little evidence that supplements consistently relieve the symptoms of carpal tunnel syndrome or provide significant benefit for women with PMS.[11,12] Vitamin B$_6$ supplements have been found to improve immune function in older adults.[6] However, because elderly people frequently have low intakes of vitamin B$_6$, it is unclear whether the beneficial effects of supplements are due to an improvement in vitamin B$_6$ status or to stimulation of the immune system.

FOLATE (FOLIC ACID)

Folate is a B vitamin that is important during embryonic development. Low folate intake during pregnancy increases the risk of birth defects called **neural tube defects** (**Figure 7.15**). The formation of the neural tube, which later develops into the brain and spinal cord, occurs very early during pregnancy. Therefore, to reduce the risk of neural tube defects, a woman's folate status must be adequate before she becomes pregnant and during the critical early days of pregnancy. To help ensure adequate folate intake in women of childbearing age, in 1998 the FDA mandated that the **folic acid** form of the vitamin be added to all enriched grains and cereal products. Since then, the incidence of neural tube defects in the United States has decreased by about 25%; a similar enrichment program in Canada has resulted in a decrease of almost 50%.[13,14]

neural tube defects Abnormalities in the brain or spinal cord that result from errors that occur during prenatal development.

folic acid An easily absorbed form of the vitamin folate that is used in dietary supplements and fortified foods.

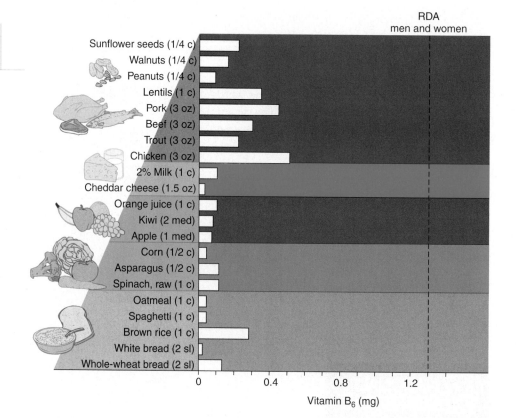

Meeting vitamin B$_6$ needs
Figure 7.14

Animal sources of vitamin B$_6$ include chicken, fish, pork, and organ meats. Good plant sources include whole-wheat products, brown rice, soybeans, sunflower seeds, and some fruits and vegetables, such as bananas, broccoli, and spinach. The dashed line indicates the RDA for adult men and women ages 19 to 50, which is 1.3 mg/day.[6]

RDA
men and women

Sunflower seeds (1/4 c)
Walnuts (1/4 c)
Peanuts (1/4 c)
Lentils (1 c)
Pork (3 oz)
Beef (3 oz)
Trout (3 oz)
Chicken (3 oz)
2% Milk (1 c)
Cheddar cheese (1.5 oz)
Orange juice (1 c)
Kiwi (2 med)
Apple (1 med)
Corn (1/2 c)
Asparagus (1/2 c)
Spinach, raw (1 c)
Oatmeal (1 c)
Spaghetti (1 c)
Brown rice (1 c)
White bread (2 sl)
Whole-wheat bread (2 sl)

0   0.4   0.8   1.2

Vitamin B$_6$ (mg)

Neural tube defects FIGURE 7.15

Day 19 — Neural tissue

Day 20 — Fold to form a groove

Day 22 — Sides almost touch to form a tube

Day 28 — Neural tube closure complete

◀ **A** During embryonic development, a groove forms in the plate of neural tissue; then the edges fold up to form the neural tube, which will become the brain and spinal cord. If this does not occur normally, the baby is born with a neural tube defect.

Normal spine — Vertebrae, Spinal cord

Spine with mild spina bifida — Vertebrae, Spinal cord

Spine with severe spina bifida — Vertebrae, Spinal cord

▲

B If a lower portion of the neural tube does not close normally, the result is **spina bifida**, a condition in which the spinal cord forms abnormally. Many babies with spina bifida have learning disabilities and nerve damage that causes varying degrees of paralysis of the lower limbs. If the head end of the neural tube does not close properly, the brain doesn't form completely; the result is anencephaly (partial or total absence of the brain). Babies with anencephaly are usually blind, deaf, and unconscious, and they die soon after birth.

Folate and *folacin* are general terms for compounds whose chemical structures and nutritional properties are similar to those of folic acid. The folic acid form, which is added to enriched grains and other fortified products and used in dietary supplements, is more easily absorbed, so its bioavailability is about twice that of folate found naturally in foods. The RDA for folate is expressed in **dietary folate equivalents (DFEs)**. This measure corrects for differences in the bioavailability of different forms of folate. One DFE is equal to 1 microgram (μg) of food folate, 0.6 μg of synthetic folic acid from fortified food or supplements con-

> **macrocytic anemia** or **megaloblastic anemia** A reduction in the blood's capacity to carry oxygen that is characterized by abnormally large immature and mature red blood cells.

sumed with food, or 0.5 μg of synthetic folic acid consumed on an empty stomach.

Folate coenzymes are needed for the synthesis of DNA and the metabolism of some amino acids. Cells must synthesize DNA in order to replicate, so folate is particularly important in tissues in which cells are dividing rapidly, such as the intestines, skin, embryonic and fetal tissues, and bone marrow, where red blood cells are made. When folate is deficient, cells cannot divide normally. One of the most notable symptoms of folate deficiency is a type of anemia called **macrocytic anemia**, or **megaloblastic anemia**

Folate deficiency and anemia FIGURE 7.16

Folate is needed for DNA replication. Without folate, developing red blood cells cannot divide. Instead, they just grow bigger. The abnormally large immature red blood cells, called megaloblasts, then mature into abnormally large red blood cells called macrocytes. Because fewer mature red cells are produced when folate is deficient, the blood's oxygen-carrying capacity is reduced.

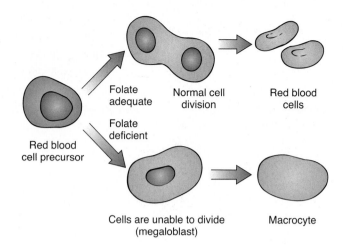

(FIGURE 7.16). Other symptoms of folate deficiency include poor growth, problems with nerve development and function, diarrhea, and inflammation of the tongue.

Low folate status may also increase the risk of developing heart disease and cancer of the ovary, pancreas, breast, and colon.[15–17] Folate's connection with heart disease has to do with the metabolism of homocysteine. Elevated levels of homocysteine have been associated with increased risk of heart disease. Folate and vitamin B_{12} are both needed to prevent homocysteine levels from rising (FIGURE 7.17).[9]

Population groups most at risk of folate deficiency include pregnant women and premature infants (because of their rapid rates of cell division and growth), the elderly (because of their limited intake of foods high in folate), alcoholics (because alcohol inhibits the absorption of folate), and tobacco smokers (because smoke inactivates folate in the cells lining the lungs).[6]

The relationship between folate and vitamin B_{12} FIGURE 7.17

Vitamin B_{12} deficiency prevents folate from being converted into one of its active forms. This interrelationship has raised concerns that our folate-fortified food supply will prevent folate-deficiency symptoms and allow B_{12} deficiencies to go unnoticed. The UL for adults, set at 1000 µg/day of folic acid from supplements and/or fortified foods, is based on an amount that will not mask the macrocytic anemia caused by vitamin B_{12} deficiency.

Supplemental folic acid can prevent macrocytic anemia, thus "hiding" vitamin B_{12} deficiency. Untreated vitamin B_{12} deficiency can cause irreversible nerve damage.

This form of folate, needed for the synthesis of DNA, cannot be made if vitamin B_{12} is deficient. The resulting folate deficiency causes macrocytic anemia.

Folate and vitamin B_{12} are both needed to convert homocysteine to methionine. When either is deficient, homocysteine levels rise.

High levels in the blood increase cardiovascular disease risk

Meeting folate needs FIGURE 7.18

Folate is named after the Latin word for *foliage* because leafy greens such as spinach are good sources of this vitamin. Fair sources include grains, corn, snap beans, mustard greens, and broccoli, as well as some nuts. Only small amounts of folate are found in meats, cheese, milk, fruits, and other vegetables. The dashed line indicates the RDA for adult men and women, which is 400 µg/day.

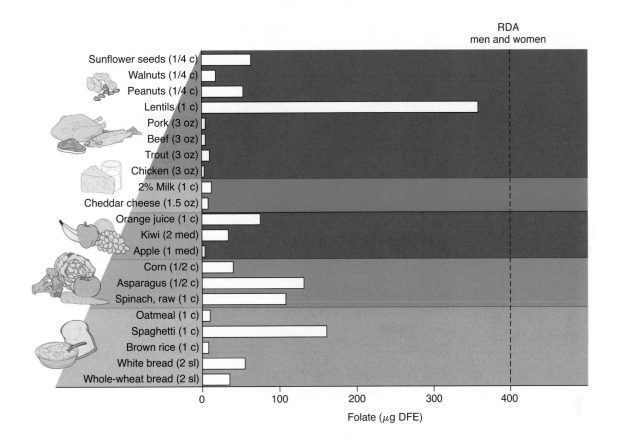

Asparagus, oranges, legumes, liver, and yeast are excellent food sources of folate (FIGURE 7.18). Whole grains are a fair source, and, as discussed earlier, folic acid is added to enriched grain products, including enriched breads, flours, corn meal, pasta, grits, and rice. Because supplementing folic acid early in pregnancy has been shown to reduce neural tube defects in the fetus, it is recommended that women who are capable of becoming pregnant consume 400 µg of synthetic folic acid from fortified foods and/or supplements in addition to the food folate consumed in a varied diet. To get 400 µg of folic acid, women of childbearing age would need to eat four to six servings of fortified grain products each day or take a supplement containing folic acid.

VITAMIN B₁₂

In the early 1900s, **pernicious anemia** amounted to a death sentence. There was no cure. In the 1920s, researchers George Minot and William Murphy pursued their belief that pernicious anemia could be cured by something in the diet. They discovered that they could restore patients' health by feeding them about 4 to 8 ounces of slightly cooked liver at every meal. Today we know that eating liver cured pernicious anemia

pernicious anemia
A macrocytic anemia resulting from vitamin B₁₂ deficiency that occurs when dietary vitamin B₁₂ cannot be absorbed due to a lack of intrinsic factor.

because liver is a concentrated source of **vitamin B$_{12}$**. Individuals with pernicious anemia lack a protein produced in the stomach called **intrinsic factor** that enhances vitamin B$_{12}$ absorption (**FIGURE 7.19**). Today, pernicious anemia is treated with injections of vitamin B$_{12}$ rather than with plates full of liver.

Vitamin B$_{12}$, also known as **cobalamin**, is necessary for the production of ATP from certain fatty acids, to convert homocysteine

to methionine (see Figure 7.17), and to maintain the myelin coating on nerves (see Figure 7.13B). When vitamin B$_{12}$ is deficient, homocysteine levels rise, and folate cannot be converted into its active form. The lack of folate causes macrocytic anemia. Lack of vitamin B$_{12}$ also leads to degeneration of the myelin that coats the nerves in the spinal cord and brain, resulting in symptoms such as numbness and tingling, abnormalities in gait, memory loss, and disorientation. If not

> ■ **intrinsic factor**
> A protein produced in the stomach that is needed for the absorption of adequate amounts of vitamin B$_{12}$.

Process Diagram

Vitamin B$_{12}$ digestion and absorption FIGURE 7.19

The body stores and reuses vitamin B$_{12}$ more efficiently than it does most other water-soluble vitamins, so deficiency is typically caused by poor absorption rather than by low intake alone. Absorption of adequate amounts of vitamin B$_{12}$ depends on the presence of stomach acid, protein-digesting enzymes, and intrinsic factor.

Stomach

Small intestine

Large intestine

1 Vitamin B$_{12}$ in food is bound to protein.

2 In the stomach, acid and pepsin help release vitamin B$_{12}$ from food proteins.

3 Cells in the stomach lining release intrinsic factor (IF).

4 In the upper portion of the small intestine (duodenum), intrinsic factor binds to vitamin B$_{12}$.

5 In the lower part of the small intestine (ileum), the vitamin B$_{12}$-intrinsic factor complex binds to receptors on cells, allowing absorption. A small amount of B$_{12}$ not bound to intrinsic factor can be absorbed through passive diffusion.

6 In the colon, vitamin B$_{12}$ is synthesized by microorganisms but cannot be absorbed.

treated, vitamin B_{12} deficiency eventually causes paralysis and death.

Vitamin B_{12} is found naturally only in animal products (**FIGURE 7.20**). Therefore, meeting vitamin B_{12} needs is a concern among vegans—those who consume no animal products. Vegans must consume supplements or foods fortified with vitamin B_{12} in order to meet their needs for this vitamin.[18] Vitamin B_{12} deficiency is also a concern in older adults because of a condition called **atrophic gastritis**, which reduces the secretion of stomach acid. Without sufficient stomach acid, the enzymes that release the vitamin B_{12} bound to proteins in food can-

atrophic gastritis
An inflammation of the stomach lining that results in reduced secretion of stomach acid, microbial overgrowth, and, in severe cases, a reduction in the production of intrinsic factor.

not function properly, so vitamin B_{12} remains bound to the food proteins and cannot be absorbed (see Figure 7.19). In addition, lack of stomach acid allows large numbers of microbes to grow in the gut and compete for available vitamin B_{12}, reducing absorption. Atrophic gastritis affects 10 to 30% of adults over age 50. To ensure adequate B_{12} absorption, it is recommended that individuals over age 50 meet their RDA by consuming foods fortified with vitamin B_{12} or taking vitamin B_{12} supplements.[6] The vitamin B_{12} in these products is not bound to proteins, so it is absorbed even when stomach acid levels are low.

Meeting vitamin B_{12} needs FIGURE 7.20

Animal foods provide vitamin B_{12}, but plant foods do not unless they have been fortified with it or contaminated by bacteria, soil, insects, or other sources of B_{12}. The dashed line indicates the RDA for adult men and women of all ages, which is 2.4 µg/day. No toxic effects have been reported for vitamin B_{12} intakes of up to 100 µg/day from food or supplements. Insufficient data are available to establish a UL for vitamin B_{12}.[6]

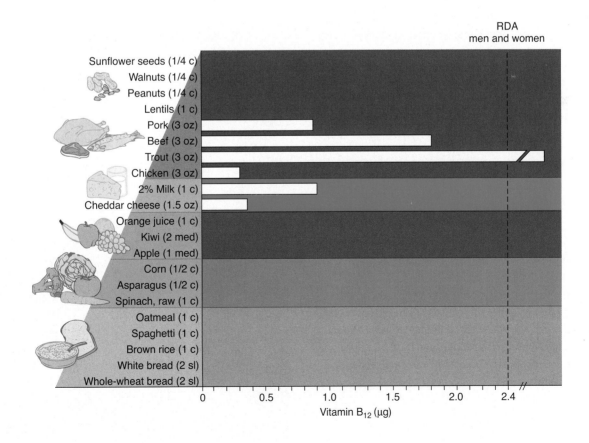

VITAMIN C

Vitamin C, also known as **ascorbic acid**, is best known for its role in the synthesis and maintenance of **collagen** (FIGURE 7.21). Collagen, the most abundant protein in the body, can be thought of as the glue that holds the body together. It forms the base of all connective tissue. It is the framework for bones and teeth; it is the main component of ligaments, tendons, and the scars that bind a wound together; and it gives structure to the walls of blood vessels. When vitamin C is lacking, collagen cannot be formed and maintained, and the symptoms of **scurvy** appear. In the 17th and 18th centuries, sailors were far more likely to die of scurvy than to be killed in shipwrecks or battles.

scurvy A vitamin C deficiency disease characterized by bleeding gums, tooth loss, joint pain, bleeding into the skin and mucous membranes, and fatigue.

In addition to its role in the synthesis and maintenance of collagen, vitamin C is needed in reactions that synthesize neurotransmitters, hormones, bile acids, and carnitine, which is needed for breakdown of fatty acids. It is also an antioxidant that acts in the blood and other body fluids. Because its antioxidant properties help maintain the immune system, the ability to fight infection is decreased when this vitamin is deficient. Vitamin C's antioxidant action also regenerates the active antioxidant form of vitamin E and enhances iron absorption in the small intestine by keeping iron in its more readily absorbed form.

Vitamin C, collagen synthesis, and scurvy FIGURE 7.21

A A reaction requiring vitamin C is essential for the formation of bonds that hold adjacent collagen strands together and give the protein strength. Like all other body proteins, collagen is continuously being broken down and reformed. Without vitamin C, the bonds holding adjacent collagen molecules together cannot be formed and maintained, so the collagen that is broken down cannot be replaced. The inability to form healthy collagen causes the symptoms of scurvy.

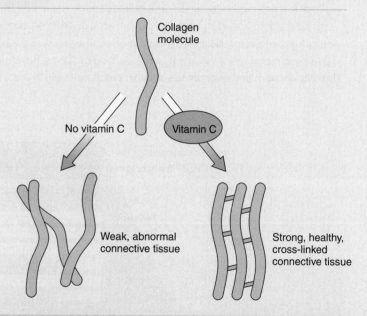

Collagen molecule

No vitamin C

Vitamin C

Weak, abnormal connective tissue

Strong, healthy, cross-linked connective tissue

B When vitamin C intake is below 10 mg/day, the symptoms of scurvy begin to appear. The gums become inflamed, swell, and bleed. The teeth loosen and eventually fall out. The capillary walls weaken and rupture, causing bleeding under the skin and into the joints. This causes raised red spots on the skin, joint pain and weakness, and easy bruising. Wounds do not heal, old wounds may reopen, and bones fracture. People with scurvy become tired and depressed, and they suffer from hysteria.

Citrus fruits are an excellent source of vitamin C. A large orange contains enough vitamin C to meet the RDA of 90 mg/day for men and 75 mg/day for women.[4] Other fruits and vegetables are also good sources of this vitamin (FIGURE 7.22).

Vitamin C is destroyed by oxygen, light, and heat, so it is readily lost in cooking. This loss is accelerated in low-acid foods and by the use of copper or iron cooking utensils. Although most Americans consume enough vitamin C to prevent severe deficiency, marginal vitamin C deficiency is a concern for individuals who consume few fruits and vegetables. Cigarette smoking increases the requirement for vitamin C because the vitamin is used to break down compounds in cigarette smoke. It is recommended that cigarette smokers consume an extra 35 mg of vitamin C daily—an amount that can easily be supplied by a half-cup of broccoli.[4]

One-third of the population of the United States takes vitamin C supplements—usually in the hope that they will prevent the common cold. Although vitamin C does not prevent colds, it may help reduce the duration and severity of cold symptoms.[19] It has also been suggested that vitamin C supplements reduce the risk of cardiovascular disease and cancer, but there is insufficient evidence to support this claim.[4]

Excessive vitamin C supplementation can cause diarrhea, nausea, and abdominal cramps, and it may increase the risk of kidney stone formation. In individuals who are unable to regulate iron absorption, excess vitamin C can increase absorption, allowing amounts of iron in the body to reach toxic levels. For those with sickle cell anemia, excess vitamin C can worsen symptoms. And doses greater than 3 g/day may interfere with drugs prescribed to slow blood clotting. In chewable form, large doses of vitamin C can dissolve tooth enamel. The UL for vitamin C has been set at 2000 mg/day from food and supplements.[4]

Meeting vitamin C needs FIGURE 7.22

Fruits that are high in vitamin C include citrus fruits, strawberries, kiwis, and cantaloupe. Vegetables in the cabbage family, such as broccoli, cauliflower, bok choy, and Brussels sprouts, as well as leafy green vegetables, green and red peppers, okra, tomatoes, and potatoes, are also good sources of vitamin C. Meat, fish, poultry, eggs, dairy products, and grains are poor sources.

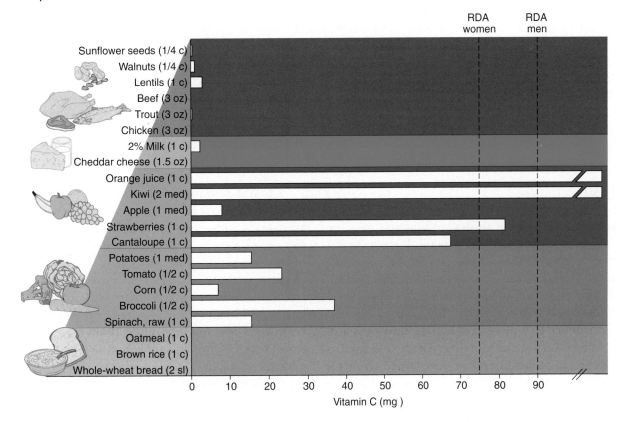

Vitamin	Sources	Recommended intake for adults	Major functions	Deficiency diseases and symptoms	Groups at risk of deficiency	Toxicity	UL
Thiamin (vitamin B$_1$, thiamin mononitrate)	Pork, whole and enriched grains, seeds, nuts, legumes	1.1–1.2 mg/day	Coenzyme in glucose and energy metabolism; needed for neurotransmitter synthesis and normal nerve function	Beriberi: weakness, apathy, irritability, nerve tingling, poor coordination, paralysis, heart changes	Alcoholics, those living in poverty	None reported	ND
Riboflavin (vitamin B$_2$)	Dairy products, whole and enriched grains, leafy green vegetables, meats	1.1–1.3 mg/day	Coenzyme in energy and lipid metabolism	Inflammation of the mouth and tongue, cracks at corners of the mouth	None	None reported	ND
Niacin (nicotinamide, nicotinic acid, vitamin B$_3$)	Beef, chicken, fish, peanuts, legumes, whole and enriched grains; can be made from tryptophan	14–16 mg NE/day	Coenzyme in energy metabolism and lipid synthesis and breakdown	Pellagra: diarrhea, dermatitis on areas exposed to sun, dementia	Those consuming a limited diet based on corn; alcoholics	Flushing, nausea, rash, tingling extremities	35 mg/day from fortified foods and supplements
Biotin	Liver, egg yolks; synthesized in the gut	30 µg/day	Coenzyme in glucose production and lipid synthesis	Dermatitis, nausea, depression, hallucinations	Those consuming large amounts of raw egg whites; alcoholics	None reported	ND
Pantothenic acid (calcium pantothenate)	Meat, legumes, whole grains; widespread in foods	5 mg/day	Coenzyme in energy metabolism and lipid synthesis and breakdown	Fatigue, rash	Alcoholics	None reported	ND
Vitamin B$_6$ (pyridoxine, pyridoxal phosphate, pyridoxamine)	Meat, fish, poultry, legumes, whole grains, nuts and seeds	1.3–1.7 mg/day	Coenzyme in protein and amino acid metabolism, neurotransmitter and hemoglobin synthesis, many other reactions	Headache, convulsions, other neurological symptoms, nausea, poor growth, anemia	Women, alcoholics	Numbness, nerve damage	100 mg/day

CHOLINE

Choline is a water-soluble substance that you may see included in supplements called "vitamin B complex." It is needed to synthesize a number of important molecules in the body, including the neurotransmitter acetylcholine, but because it can be synthesized to a limited extent by humans, it is not currently classified as a vitamin. There is evidence that it is essential in healthy men and women, but it is not yet clear whether it is also essential in the diets of infants and children.[6,20] The DRIs have set an AI for this compound: 550 mg/day for men, and 425 mg/day for women.[6]

Choline is found in many foods, with large amounts in egg yolks, broccoli, nuts, and wheat germ. Because the average daily choline intake in the United States exceeds the recommended intake, a deficiency is unlikely in healthy humans in this country.[6]

Excess choline intake can cause a fishy body odor, sweating, reduced growth rate, low blood pressure, and liver damage. The amounts needed to cause these symptoms are much higher than can be obtained from foods. The UL for choline for adults is 3.5 g/day.[6]

A summary of the water-soluble vitamins and choline is provided in TABLE 7.3.

TABLE 7.3 (CONTINUED)

Vitamin	Sources	Recommended intake for adults	Major functions	Deficiency diseases and symptoms	Groups at risk of deficiency	Toxicity	UL
Folate (folic acid, folacin, pteroylglutamic acid)	Leafy green vegetables, legumes, seeds, enriched grains, orange juice	400 µg DFE/day	Coenzyme in DNA synthesis and amino acid metabolism	Macrocytic anemia, inflammation of tongue, diarrhea, poor growth, neural tube defects	Pregnant women, alcoholics	Masks B_{12} deficiency	1000 µg/day from fortified food and supplements
Vitamin B_{12} (cobalamin, cyanocobalamin)	Animal products	2.4 µg/day	Coenzyme in folate metabolism; nerve function	Pernicious anemia, macrocytic anemia, nerve damage	Vegans, elderly, people with stomach or intestinal disease	None reported	ND
Vitamin C (ascorbic acid, ascorbate)	Citrus fruit, broccoli, strawberries, greens, peppers	75–90 mg/day	Coenzyme in collagen (connective tissue) synthesis; hormone and neurotransmitter synthesis; antioxidant	Scurvy: poor wound healing, bleeding gums, loose teeth, bone fragility, joint pain, pinpoint hemorrhages	Alcoholics, elderly men	GI distress, diarrhea	2000 mg/day
Choline*	Egg yolks, organ meats, leafy greens, nuts, synthesis in the body	425–550 mg/day	Synthesis of cell membranes and neurotransmitters	Liver dysfunction	None	Sweating, low blood pressure, liver damage	3500 mg/day

* Choline is technically not a vitamin, but recommendations have been made for its intake.

Note: UL, Tolerable Upper Intake Level; NE, niacin equivalent; DFE, dietary folate equivalent; ND, not determined due to insufficient data

CONCEPT CHECK STOP

Why do people think B vitamin supplements give them energy?

What is the role of vitamin B_6 in amino acid metabolism?

How can folate and vitamin B_{12} deficiency both cause macrocytic anemia?

What is the role of vitamin C in collagen formation?

The Fat-Soluble Vitamins

The fat-soluble vitamins—A, D, E, and K—are found along with fats in foods. They require special handling for absorption into and transport through the body. Because excesses of these vitamins can be stored in the liver and fatty tissues, intakes can vary without a risk of deficiency as long as average intake over a period of weeks or months meets the body's needs. Their solubility in fat, however, limits their routes of excretion and therefore increases the risk of toxicity.

VITAMIN A

Did you ever hear that eating carrots would help you see in the dark? It turns out to be true. Carrots are a good source of **beta-carotene (β-carotene)**, a provitamin that can be converted into vitamin A in your body. **Vitamin A** is needed for vision and healthy eyes.

Vitamin A in the diet Vitamin A is found both preformed and in provitamin form in our diet. Preformed vitamin A compounds are known as **retinoids**. Three retinoids are active in the body: retinal, retinol, and retinoic acid. **Carotenoids** are

retinoids The chemical forms of preformed vitamin A: retinol, retinal, and retinoic acid.

carotenoids Natural pigments synthesized by plants and many microorganisms. They give yellow and red-orange fruits and vegetables their color.

Meeting vitamin A needs FIGURE 7.23

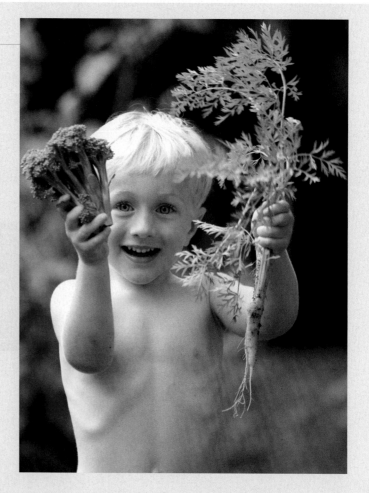

A Provitamin A is found in fruits and vegetables. Beta-carotene is plentiful in carrots, squash, apricots, and other orange and yellow vegetables and fruits. It is also found in leafy green vegetables such as spinach and broccoli, in which the yellow-orange pigment is masked by green chlorophyll. Other carotenoids that provide some provitamin A activity include α-carotene, found in leafy green vegetables, carrots, and squash, and β-cryptoxanthin, found in papaya, sweet red peppers, and winter squash.

yellow-orange pigments found in plants, some of which are vitamin A precursors; once inside the body, they can be converted into retinoids (**Figure 7.23A**). Beta-carotene is the most potent vitamin A precursor. **Alpha-carotene (α-carotene)** and **beta-cryptoxanthin (β-cryptoxanthin)** are also provitamin A carotenoids, but are not converted into retinoids as efficiently as β-carotene. Carotenoids that are not converted into retinoids may function as antioxidants and thus may play a role in protecting against cancer and heart disease.

You can meet your needs for vitamin A by eating animal products, such as eggs and dairy products, that are sources of retinoids, and by eating fruits and vegetables that are sources of provitamin A carotenoids (**Figure 7.23B**) (see the *Case Study* on page 214). Because carotenoids are not absorbed as well as retinoids and are not completely converted into vitamin A in the body, you get less functional vitamin A from this form. To account for this difference, a correction factor, referred to as **retinol activity equivalents (RAE)**, is used to express the amount of usable vitamin A in foods; 1 RAE is the amount of retinol, β-carotene, α-carotene,

or β-cryptoxanthin that provides vitamin A activity equal to 1 μg of retinol (see Appendix J).[21]

Because carotenoids and retinoids must combine with bile acids and other dietary fats in order to be absorbed, vitamin A absorption is impaired when dietary fat intake is very low (less than 10 g/day). This is rarely a problem in the United States and other industrialized countries, where typical fat intake is greater than 50 g/day. However, in developing countries, vitamin A deficiency may occur not only because the diet is low in vitamin A but also because the diet is too low in fat for the vitamin to be absorbed efficiently. Diseases that cause fat malabsorption can also interfere with vitamin A absorption and cause a deficiency.

Protein and zinc status are also important in preventing vitamin A deficiency. To move from liver stores to other body tissues, vitamin A must be bound to a protein called **retinol-binding protein**. When protein is deficient, inadequate amounts of retinol-binding protein are made, and vitamin A cannot be transported to the tissues where it is needed. Likewise, when zinc is deficient, a vitamin A deficiency may occur because zinc is needed to make proteins involved in vitamin A transport and metabolism.

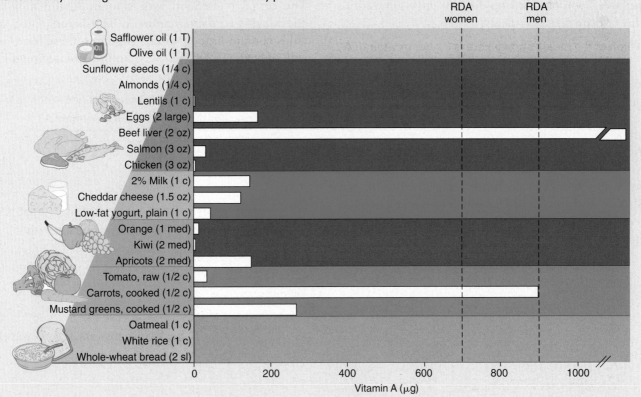

B Grains and meats are generally poor sources of vitamin A. The dashed lines indicate the RDA for adult men and women, which are 900 μg/day and 700 μg/day, respectively. No specific recommendations have been made for intakes of carotenoids; their intake is considered only with regard to the amount of retinol they provide.

HOW MUCH VITAMIN A IS IN YOUR FAST-FOOD MEAL?

John lives on his own, goes to school, and works part time. He eats breakfast at home and usually takes a sandwich for lunch; dinner is always fast food. He recently heard that fast food is low in some vitamins, particularly vitamin A. To check on his vitamin A intake, John uses iProfile to look up the nutrient compositions of his favorite fast-food meals.

Which of the meals shown here is higher in vitamin A? Which ingredients are sources of the vitamin?

▼

Your answer:

John doesn't want to give up his fast food, so he looks at his other meals to make sure they provide plenty of vitamin A. For breakfast he has Cheerios with milk, toast with jelly, and coffee, and for lunch he packs a ham-and-cheese sandwich on whole-wheat bread, potato chips, an apple, and a soda.

Which foods in John's breakfast and lunch are good sources of vitamin A?

▼

The cereal is fortified with vitamin A, the milk and cheese also contain vitamin A. The bread, meat, and chips contain little or none. Together, these foods provide only about 20% of the vitamin A John should consume on an average day.

What could John add to his breakfast and lunch to provide some good sources of vitamin A?

▼

Your answer:

John's meals are also low in vitamin C. What could he add to his breakfast and lunch to increase his intake of vitamin C?

▼

Your answer:

(Check your answers in Appendix K.)

Vitamin A functions and deficiency

Vitamin A is needed for vision and eye health because it is involved in the perception of light and because it is needed for normal **cell differentiation**, the process whereby immature cells change in structure and function to become specialized.

Vitamin A helps us see because retinal is part of **rhodopsin**, a visual pigment in the eye. When light strikes rhodopsin, it initiates a series of events that result in a nerve signal being sent to the brain, which allows us to see (**FIGURE 7.24**). After the light stimulus has passed, rhodopsin is re-formed. Because some retinal is lost in these reactions, it must be replaced by vitamin A from the blood. If blood levels of vitamin A are low, as they are in someone who is vitamin A deficient, there is a delay in the regeneration of rhodopsin. This delay causes difficulty seeing in dim light, a condition called **night blindness**. Night blindness is one of the first and most easily reversible symptoms of vitamin A deficiency. If the deficiency progresses, more serious and less reversible symptoms can occur.

Vitamin A affects cell differentiation through its role in **gene expression**: It can turn on or off certain genes. When a specific gene is turned on, it instructs the cell to make a particular protein. Proteins have structural and regulatory functions within cells and throughout the body. This turning on (or off) of specific genes increases (or decreases) the production of certain proteins and thereby affects various cellular and body functions. By affecting gene expression, vitamin A can determine what type of cell an immature cell will become.

> **gene expression**
> The events of protein synthesis in which the information coded in a gene is used to synthesize a protein.

The visual cycle FIGURE 7.24

Looking into the bright headlights of an approaching car at night is temporarily blinding for all of us, but for someone with vitamin A deficiency, the blindness lasts a lot longer. This occurs because of the role of vitamin A in the visual cycle.

1. Light strikes the visual pigment rhodopsin, which is formed by combining retinal with the protein opsin.

2. The retinal molecule changes from a bent to a straight configuration.

3. A nerve signal is sent to the brain, telling us that there is light, and retinal is released from opsin.

4. Some retinal is lost from the cycle.

5. Some retinal returns to its original configuration and binds opsin to begin the cycle again.

6. When vitamin A status is normal, vitamin A from the blood replaces any retinal lost from the cycle.

7. When vitamin A is deficient, not enough vitamin A is available in the blood, and the regeneration of rhodopsin is delayed. Until it is reformed, light cannot be perceived.

Light energy

Eye

Signal to brain

Light causes a change in retinal, which initiates a signal to the brain

Light energy

Rhodopsin

Opsin

Retinal

Opsin

Opsin

Retinal

Retinal

Low blood vitamin A

Vitamin A deficiency

Vitamin A from blood

Healthy vitamin A status

Process Diagram

Vitamin A is necessary for the maintenance of epithelial tissue, which makes up the skin, and the tissues that line the eyes, intestines, lungs, vagina, and bladder. When vitamin A is deficient, epithelial cells do not differentiate normally because vitamin A is not there to turn on or off the production of particular proteins. All epithelial tissues are affected by vitamin A deficiency, but the eye

■ **xerophthalmia**
A spectrum of eye conditions resulting from vitamin A deficiency that may lead to blindness.

is particularly susceptible (FIGURE 7.25). The eye disorders associated with vitamin A deficiency are collectively known as **xerophthalmia**. Night blindness is an early stage of xeropthalmia and can be treated by increasing vitamin A intake. If left untreated, xerophthalmia affects the epithelial lining of the eye and can result in permanent blindness.

Visualizing

Vitamin A deficiency FIGURE 7.25

The lining of the eye normally contains cells that secrete mucus, which lubricates the eye. When these cells die, immature cells differentiate to become new mucus-secreting cells that replace the dead ones. Without vitamin A, the immature cells can't differentiate normally, and instead of mucus-secreting cells, they become cells that produce a hard protein called keratin. ▶

Epithelial tissue

Normal vitamin A status

Mucus (moist and lubricating)

Keratin (hard and dry)

Vitamin A deficiency

New cells Differentiated cells

▲
When mucus-secreting cells are replaced by keratin-producing cells, the surface of the eye becomes dry and cloudy. As xerophthalmia progresses, the drying of the cornea results in ulceration and infection. If left untreated, the damage is irreversible and causes permanent blindness.

NATIONAL GEOGRAPHIC

Vitamin A deficiency is a threat to the health, sight, and lives of millions of children in the developing world. It is estimated that more than 250 million preschool children worldwide are vitamin A deficient and that 250,000 to 500,000 children go blind annually due to vitamin A deficiency. Children who are deficient in vitamin A have poor appetites, are anemic, are more susceptible to infections, and are more likely to die in childhood.[22]

Degree of public health importance of vitamin A deficiency

Clinical
Severe sub-clinical
Moderate sub-clinical
Mild sub-clinical
Under control
No data available

Vitamin A and carotenoid toxicity FIGURE 7.26

A Foods generally do not naturally contain large enough amounts of nutrients to be toxic. Polar bear liver is an exception. It contains about 100,000 µg of vitamin A in just 1 ounce and has caused vitamin A toxicity in Arctic explorers who consumed it. Although polar bear liver is not a common dish at most dinner tables, supplements of preformed vitamin A also have the potential to deliver a toxic dose.

B Because preformed vitamin A can be toxic, supplements typically contain β-carotene. Carotenoids are not toxic because when they are consumed in high doses, their absorption from the diet decreases, and their conversion to active vitamin A is limited. β-carotene supplements or regular consumption of large amounts of carrot juice, however, can cause hypercarotenemia. This harmless buildup of carotenoids in the adipose tissue makes the skin look yellow-orange, particularly on the palms of the hands and the soles of the feet.

The ability of vitamin A to regulate the growth and differentiation of cells makes it essential throughout life for normal reproduction, growth, and immune function. In reproduction, vitamin A is needed to direct cells to differentiate and to form the shapes and patterns needed for the development of a complete organism. In growing children, vitamin A affects the activity of cells that form and break down bone; a deficiency early in life can cause abnormal jawbone growth, resulting in crooked teeth and poor dental health. In the immune system, vitamin A is needed for the differentiation that produces the different types of immune cells. When vitamin A is deficient, the activity of specific immune cells cannot be stimulated; the result is increased susceptibility to infections.

Vitamin A toxicity

Preformed vitamin A is toxic in large doses, causing symptoms such as nausea, vomiting, headache, dizziness, blurred vision, and a lack of muscle coordination (**FIGURE 7.26A**). Excess vitamin A is a particular concern for pregnant women because it may contribute to birth defects. Derivatives of vitamin A that are used to treat acne (Retin A and Accutane) should never be used by pregnant women because they cause birth defects. High intakes of vitamin A have also been found to increase the incidence of bone fractures.[23] The UL is set at 2800 µg/day of preformed vitamin A for 14- to 18-year-olds and 3000 µg/day for adults.[20]

Although carotenoids are not considered toxic, large daily intakes can lead to a condition known as **hypercarotenemia** (**FIGURE 7.26B**). β-carotene supplements have also been associated with an increase in lung cancer in cigarette smokers.[24] Therefore, smokers are advised to avoid β-carotene supplements and rely on food sources to obtain carotenoids in their diet. There is no UL for carotenoids, and the small amounts found in standard-strength multivitamin supplements are not likely to be harmful for any group.

hypercarotenemia A condition caused by the accumulation of carotenoids in the adipose tissue, causing the skin to appear yellow-orange.

Vitamin D activation and function
FIGURE 7.27

We get vitamin D from the diet and from synthesis in the skin. In order to function, it must be chemically modified, first by the liver and then by the kidneys. Active vitamin D helps maintain blood levels of calcium and phosphorus that support bone mineralization (light blue arrow). In the intestine, active vitamin D increases the absorption of calcium and phosphorus from the diet. When blood calcium levels are low, vitamin D increases bone breakdown, and calcium and phosphorus are released into the blood.

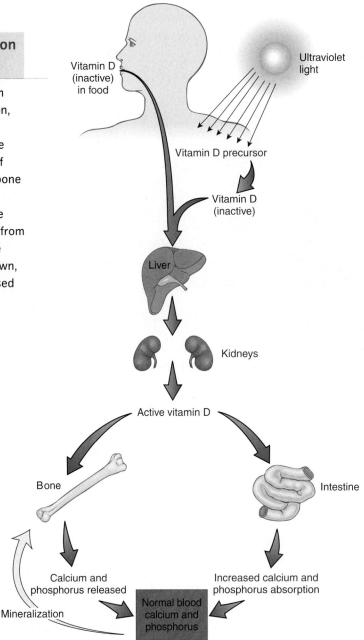

Vitamin D (inactive) in food

Ultraviolet light

Vitamin D precursor

Vitamin D (inactive)

Liver

Kidneys

Active vitamin D

Bone

Intestine

Calcium and phosphorus released

Increased calcium and phosphorus absorption

Mineralization

Normal blood calcium and phosphorus

VITAMIN D

Vitamin D is known as the sunshine vitamin because it can be made in the skin with exposure to ultraviolet (UV) light. Because vitamin D can be made in the body, it is essential in the diet only when exposure to sunlight is limited or the body's ability to synthesize it is reduced.

Vitamin D functions and deficiency

Vitamin D, whether from the diet or from synthesis in the skin, is inactive until it is modified by biochemical reactions in both the liver and the kidney (**FIGURE 7.27**). Active vitamin D is needed to maintain normal levels of the miner-

als calcium and phosphorus in the blood. Calcium is important for bone health, but it is also needed for proper functioning of nerves, muscles, glands, and other tissues. Blood levels of calcium are regulated so that a steady supply of the mineral is available when and where it is needed.

When calcium levels in the blood drop too low, the body responds immediately to correct the problem. The response starts with the release of **parathyroid hormone (PTH)**,

parathyroid hormone (PTH)
A hormone released by the parathyroid gland that acts to increase blood calcium levels.

which stimulates the activation of vitamin D by the kidney. Active vitamin D enters the blood and travels to its major target tissues—intestine and bone—where it acts to increase calcium and phosphorus levels in the blood (see Figure 7.27). Vitamin D, like vitamin A, acts through its role in gene expression. In the intestine, it turns on genes that make a protein that is needed for the absorption of calcium. In the bone, it turns on genes that are needed for the differentiation of cells that break down bone.

When vitamin D is deficient, only about 10 to 15% of the calcium in the diet can be absorbed. Without adequate calcium, bone structure becomes abnormal. In children, vitamin D deficiency is called **rickets**; it is characterized by narrow rib cages known as pigeon breasts and by bowed legs (**FIGURE 7.28**). In adults, vitamin D deficiency disease is called **osteomalacia**. It does not cause bone deformities because

rickets A vitamin D deficiency disease in children, characterized by poor bone development because of inadequate calcium absorption.

osteomalacia A vitamin D deficiency disease in adults, characterized by loss of minerals from bone, bone pain, muscle aches, and an increase in bone fractures.

adults are no longer growing, but bones are weakened because not enough calcium is available to form the mineral deposits needed to maintain healthy bone. Insufficient bone mineralization leads to fractures of the weight-bearing bones, such as those in the hips and spine. This lack of calcium in bones can precipitate or exacerbate **osteoporosis**, which is a loss of total bone mass, not just minerals (discussed further in Chapter 8). Osteomalacia is common in adults with kidney failure because the conversion of vitamin D to the active form is reduced in these patients.

Vitamin D also plays a role in preventing cells from being transformed into cancerous cells.[25] It has been recognized for many years that the risk of certain cancers is increased in people who live at higher latitudes, where less vitamin D can be synthesized in the skin. Studies now support the hypothesis that vitamin D deficiency increases the risk of developing and dying from colon, breast, ovarian, and prostate cancers.[26] There is also evidence that vitamin D may play a role in the increased risk of type 1 diabetes, multiple sclerosis, and high blood pressure in people who live at higher latitudes.[27]

Meeting vitamin D needs
Vitamin D is not very widespread in the diet. It is found naturally in liver, egg yolks, and oily fish such as salmon (**FIGURE 7.29A** on the next page). Foods fortified with vitamin D include milk, margarine, and some yogurts, cheeses, and breakfast cereals. The major source of vitamin D for most humans is exposure to sunlight.[28] Anything that interferes with the transmission of UV radiation to Earth's surface or its penetration into the skin will affect the synthesis of vitamin D. Therefore, individuals who live at higher latitudes, do not spend time outdoors, or cover their skin when they are outdoors are at risk of vitamin D deficiency (**FIGURE 7.29B–D**).

The recommended intake of vitamin D for young adult men and women is set at 5 μg/day—the amount contained in about 2 cups of vitamin D-fortified milk.[30] This is based on the assumption that no vitamin D is synthesized in the skin. The recommended intake is increased for older adults: 10 μg/day for those ages 50 to 70 and 15 μg/day for those over 70. However, our expanding understanding of the role of vitamin D in health and disease prevention has led many experts to agree that in the absence of adequate exposure to sunlight, 20 to 25 μg of vitamin D is needed per day for all adults and children.[27]

Vitamin D deficiency FIGURE 7.28

The vitamin D deficiency disease rickets causes short stature and bone deformities. The characteristic bowed legs occur because the bones are too weak to support the body. It is seen in children with poor diets and little exposure to sunlight, in those with disorders that affect fat absorption, and in some vegan children who do not receive adequate exposure to sunlight.

A Only a few foods are natural sources of vitamin D. Without adequate sun exposure, supplements, or fortified foods, it is difficult to meet the body's needs for this vitamin. The dashed line indicates the AI for adults ages 19 to 50, which is 5 µg/day. The requirement is expressed in µg, but the vitamin D content of foods and supplements may also be given as International Units (IUs); one IU is equal to 0.025 µg of vitamin D (40 IU = 1 µg of vitamin D; see Appendix J).

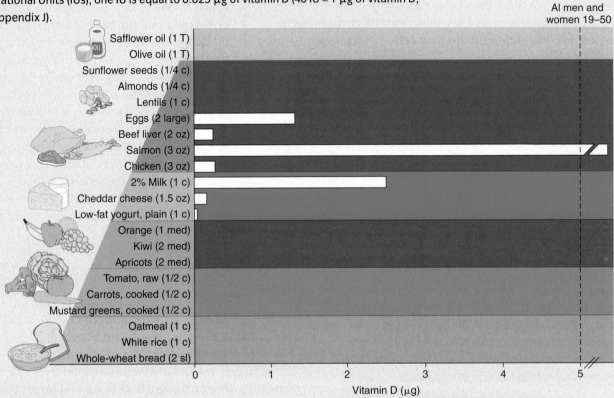

B The angle at which the sun strikes the earth affects the body's ability to synthesize vitamin D in the skin. During the winter at latitudes greater than about 40 degrees north or south, there is not enough UV radiation to synthesize adequate amounts. However, during the spring, summer, and fall at 42 degrees latitude, as little as 5 to 10 minutes of midday sun exposure three times weekly can provide a light-skinned individual with adequate vitamin D.[29]

C Sunscreen with an SPF of 15 will decrease vitamin D synthesis by 99%.[27] Sunscreen is important for reducing the risk of skin cancer, but some time in the sun without sunscreen may be needed to meet vitamin D needs. In the summer, children and active adults usually spend enough time outdoors without sunscreen to meet their vitamin D requirements. ▼

D Dark skin pigmentation prevents UV light rays from penetrating into the layers of the skin where vitamin D is formed and reduces the body's ability to make vitamin D in the skin by as much as 99%. Dark-skinned individuals living in temperate climates have a higher rate of vitamin D deficiency than do those living near the equator. ▼

◄ **E** Concealing clothing worn by certain cultural and religious groups prevents sunlight from striking the skin. This explains why vitamin D deficiency is common in women and children in some of the sunniest regions of the world. The elderly also typically cover their skin with clothing when they are outdoors. Risk of vitamin D deficiency in elderly people is further compounded because they consume a diet that is low in vitamin D, and the ability to synthesize vitamin D in the skin declines with age.

The antioxidant role of vitamin E FIGURE 7.30

By neutralizing free radicals, vitamin E guards not only cell membranes, as shown here, but also body proteins, DNA, and cholesterol, helping to prevent heart disease, cancer, macular degeneration, and other chronic diseases.

Membrane damage

Free radicals

Neutralized free radical

Vitamin E

Neutralized free radical

Vitamin E

Undamaged membrane

Vitamin E

minus e⁻

minus e⁻

Vitamin C

To neutralize reactive electron-scavenging molecules, such as free radicals, vitamin E donates one of its electrons.

The antioxidant function of vitamin E can be restored by another antioxidant vitamin—vitamin C, which gives an electron back to vitamin E.

Too much vitamin D in the body can cause high calcium concentrations in the blood and urine, deposition of calcium in soft tissues such as the blood vessels and kidneys, and cardiovascular damage. Synthesis of vitamin D from exposure to sunlight does not produce toxic amounts because the body regulates vitamin D formation. The UL for adults for vitamin D is currently 50 μg (2000 IU)/day. However, based on the fact that sunshine can provide an adult with vitamin D in an amount equivalent to daily oral consumption of 250 μg (10,000 IU)/day, it is now believed that intakes this high will not cause adverse reactions in the majority of healthy people.[31]

VITAMIN E

Vitamin E is an antioxidant that protects lipids throughout the body by neutralizing reactive oxygen compounds before they can cause damage (**FIGURE 7.30**). Vitamin E protects membranes in red blood cells, white blood cells, nerve cells, and lung cells, where it is particularly important because oxygen concentrations in lung cells are high.[32] Vitamin E can also defend cells against damage caused by heavy metals, such as lead and mercury, and toxins, such as carbon tetrachloride, benzene, and a variety of drugs.

Vitamin E deficiency Because vitamin E is needed to protect cell membranes, a deficiency causes those membranes to break down. Red blood cells and nerve tissue are particularly susceptible. With a vitamin E deficiency, red blood cell membranes may rupture, causing a type of anemia called **hemolytic anemia**. This is most common in premature infants. All newborn infants have low blood vitamin E levels because there is little transfer of this vitamin from mother to fetus until the last weeks of pregnancy. The levels are lower in premature infants because they are born before much vitamin E has been transferred from the mother. To prevent vitamin E deficiency in premature infants, special formulas for these infants contain higher amounts of vitamin E.

Vitamin E deficiency is rare in adults, occurring only when other health problems interfere with fat absorption, which reduces vitamin E absorption. In such cases, the vitamin E deficiency is usually characterized by symptoms associated with nerve degeneration, such as poor muscle coordination, weakness, and impaired vision.

The antioxidant role of vitamin E suggests that it may help reduce the risk of heart disease, cancer, Alzheimer's disease, macular degeneration, and a variety of other chronic diseases associated with oxidative damage. Particular attention has been paid to its potential benefits in guarding against heart disease. In addition to its antioxidant function, vitamin E has anti-inflammatory properties, and vitamin E supplements have been shown to decrease LDL oxidation and platelet stickiness.[33,34] Individuals with the highest vitamin E levels in their blood have been found to have the lowest risk of death,[35] yet studies examining the effects of vitamin E supplements have not found them to be beneficial in preventing heart disease or other chronic diseases, and some studies have shown an increase in the risk of death.[36,37] It seems that the best approach is to get plenty of dietary vitamin E. Unfortunately, most Americans do not consume enough vitamin E to meet the RDA (see *What Should I Eat?*).[38]

WHAT SHOULD I EAT?   Vitamins

Use iProfile to calculate your vitamin C intake for a day.

Focus on foliage for folate, vitamin A, and vitamin K
- Have a heaping helping of leafy greens.
- Snack on an orange—you'll get your folate.
- Eat beans—such as lentils and kidneys—in soups and stews.
- Utilize a hidden source of β-carotene by eating something dark green and leafy.

B (vitamin) sure
- Don't forget the whole grains to get vitamin B_6.
- Enrich your diet with some enriched grains.
- Have a bowl of fortified breakfast cereal for B_{12} insurance.

Get your antioxidants
- Go with nuts and seeds to increase your vitamin E.
- Think color when choosing your five fruits and veggies each day.
- Add carrot sticks to your lunch or snack to increase your vitamin A intake.
- Savor some strawberries and kiwis for dessert—they are loaded with vitamin C.

Soak up some D
- Get outside to stay fit and make some vitamin D.
- Have three servings of dairy per day to ensure that you get enough vitamin D.

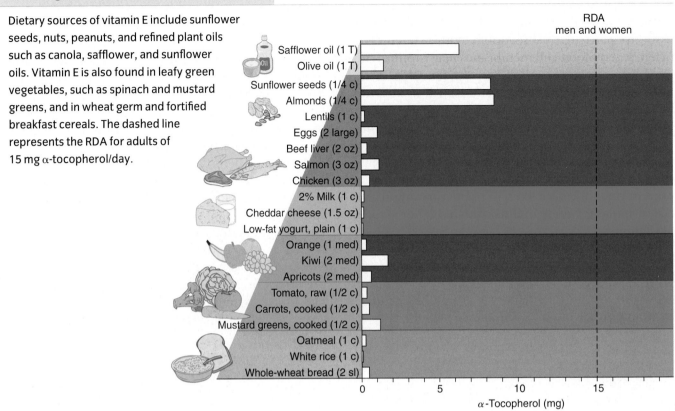

Dietary sources of vitamin E include sunflower seeds, nuts, peanuts, and refined plant oils such as canola, safflower, and sunflower oils. Vitamin E is also found in leafy green vegetables, such as spinach and mustard greens, and in wheat germ and fortified breakfast cereals. The dashed line represents the RDA for adults of 15 mg α-tocopherol/day.

Meeting vitamin E needs

Nuts, seeds, and plant oils are the best sources of vitamin E; fortified products such as breakfast cereals also make a significant contribution to our vitamin E intake (FIGURE 7.31). The need for vitamin E increases as polyunsaturated fat intake increases because polyunsaturated fats are particularly susceptible to oxidative damage; fortunately, polyunsaturated oils are one of the best sources of dietary vitamin E. However, because vitamin E is sensitive to destruction by oxygen, metals, light, and heat, when vegetable oils are repeatedly used for deep-fat frying, most of the vitamin E in them is destroyed.

The chemical name for vitamin E is **tocopherol**. Several forms of vitamin E occur naturally in food, but the body can use only the **alpha-tocopherol (α-tocopherol)** form to meet vitamin E requirements. Therefore, the RDA is expressed as mg α-tocopherol. Synthetic α-tocopherol used in supplements and fortified foods provides only half as much vitamin E activity as the natural form. Supplement labels often express vitamin E content in IUs (International Units). Appendix J contains information for converting IUs into mg α-tocopherol.

There is no evidence of adverse effects from consuming large amounts of vitamin E naturally present in foods. The amounts typically contained in supplements are also safe for most people; however, large doses can interfere with blood clotting, so individuals taking blood-thinning medications should not take vitamin E supplements. The UL is 1000 mg/day from supplemental sources.

VITAMIN K

Blood is a fluid that flows easily through your blood vessels, but when you cut yourself, blood must solidify or clot to stop your bleeding. **Vitamin K** is needed for the production of several blood proteins, called clotting factors, that cause blood to clot (FIGURE 7.32). The *K* in vitamin K comes from the Danish word for coagulation, *koagulation*, which means "blood clotting." Abnormal blood coagulation is the major symptom of vitamin K deficiency. Without vitamin K, even a bruise or small scratch could cause you to bleed to death (see *What a Scientist Sees*).

Vitamin K and blood clotting FIGURE 7.32

Blood clotting requires a series of reactions that result in the formation of a fibrous protein called **fibrin**. Fibrin fibers form a net that traps platelets and blood cells and forms the structure of a blood clot. With a vitamin K deficiency, several of the clotting factors, including **prothrombin**, are not made correctly, and the blood will not clot.

DAMAGED TISSUE

Series of reactions involving clotting factors, several of which require vitamin K for formation

PROTHROMBIN → THROMBIN

(Requires vitamin K for formation)

FIBRINOGEN → FIBRIN

Fibrin threads that form the webbing of a blood clot

Anticoagulants Take Lives and Save Them

Consumers see using warfarin as way to eliminate some unwanted houseguests. A scientist sees that this rat poison can also be used to save lives. Warfarin is an anticoagulant, which means it prevents blood from clotting. It acts by blocking the activation of vitamin K. When rats eat warfarin, minor bumps and scrapes cause them to bleed to death. Dicoumarol, a derivative of warfarin, was first isolated from moldy clover hay in 1940. At that time, cows across the Midwest were bleeding to death because they were being fed such hay.

Blood clot formation is essential to survival, but blood clots in the arteries cause heart attacks and strokes and are responsible for killing about half a million Americans annually. Scientists have taken advantage of what they learned about dicoumarol and vitamin K and used it to save human lives. Dicoumarol was the first anticoagulant used in humans that could be taken orally rather than by injection. In the 1950s the more potent anticoagulant warfarin, also known by the brand name Coumadin, was developed. It was used to treat President Eisenhower when he had a heart attack in 1955, and this "rat poison" is still used to treat heart attack patients today. Why might patients taking warfarin need to avoid vitamin K supplements?

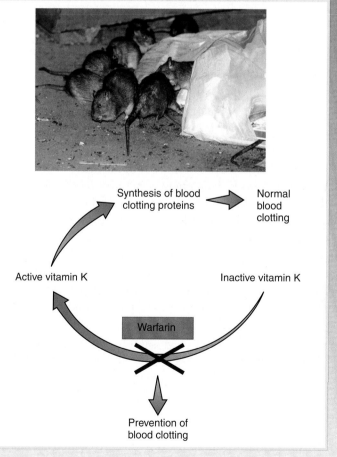

Synthesis of blood clotting proteins → Normal blood clotting

Active vitamin K   Inactive vitamin K

Warfarin

Prevention of blood clotting

Leafy green vegetables, such as spinach, broccoli, Brussels sprouts, kale, and turnip greens, and some vegetable oils are good sources of vitamin K. The dashed lines indicate the AI for adult men and women, which are 120 µg/day and 90 µg/day, respectively.

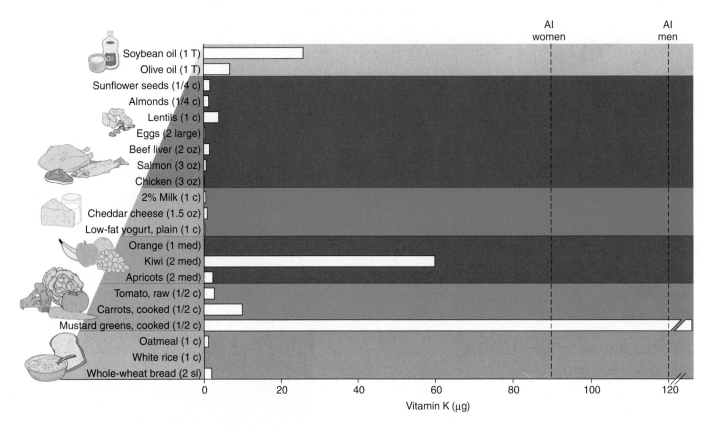

Vitamin K is also needed for the synthesis of several proteins involved in bone formation and breakdown. With a vitamin K deficiency, bone mineral density is reduced, and the risk of fractures increases.[39] Therefore, adequate vitamin K may be important for the prevention or treatment of osteoporosis.[40]

Unlike other fat-soluble vitamins, the body uses vitamin K rapidly, so a constant supply is necessary. Although only a small number of foods provide a significant amount of vitamin K, typical intakes in North America meet recommendations, and deficiency is very rare in the healthy adult population (FIGURE 7.33).[21] Another source of vitamin K is synthesis by bacteria in the intestine. Deficiency can be precipitated by long-term antibiotic use, which kills the bacteria in the gastrointestinal tract that synthesize the vitamin. Newborns are also at risk of deficiency because when a baby is born, no bacteria are present in the gut to synthesize vitamin K. The facts that little vitamin K is transferred to the baby from the mother before birth and that breast milk is a poor source of this vitamin also put newborns at risk. To ensure normal blood clotting, infants are typically given a vitamin K injection within six hours of birth.

A summary of the fat-soluble vitamins is provided in TABLE 7.4.

A summary of the fat-soluble vitamins TABLE 7.4

Vitamin	Sources	Recommended intake for adults	Major functions	Deficiency diseases and symptoms	Groups at risk of deficiency	Toxicity	UL
Vitamin A (retinol, retinal, retinoic acid, vitamin A acetate, vitamin A palmitate, retinyl palmitate, provitamin A, carotene, ß-carotene, carotenoids)	Retinol: liver, fish, fortified milk and margarine, butter, eggs; carotenoids: carrots, leafy greens, sweet potatoes, broccoli, apricots, cantaloupe	700–900 µg/day	Vision, health of of cornea and other epithelial tissue, cell differentiation, reproduction, immune function	Night blindness, xerophthalmia, poor growth, dry skin, impaired immune function	People living in poverty (particularly children and pregnant women), people who consume very low-fat or low-protein diets	Headache, vomiting, hair loss, liver damage, skin changes, bone pain, fractures, birth defects	3000 µg/day of preformed vitamin A
Vitamin D (calciferol, cholecalciferol, calcitriol, ergocalciferol, dihydroxy vitamin D)	Egg yolk, liver, fish oils, tuna, salmon, fortified milk, synthesis from sunlight	5–15 µg/day	Absorption of calcium and phosphorus, maintenance of bone	Rickets in children: abnormal growth, misshapen bones, bowed legs, soft bones; osteomalacia in adults: weak bones and bone and muscle pain	Some breast-fed infants; children and elderly people (especially those with dark skin and little exposure to sunlight); people with kidney disease	Calcium deposits in soft tissues, growth retardation, kidney damage	50 µg/day
Vitamin E (tocopherol, alpha-tocopherol)	Vegetable oils, leafy greens, seeds, nuts, peanuts	15 mg/day	Antioxidant, protects cell membranes	Broken red blood cells, nerve damage	People with poor fat absorption, premature infants	Inhibition of vitamin K activity	1000 mg/day from supplemental sources
Vitamin K (phylloquinones, menaquinone)	Vegetable oils, leafy greens, synthesis by intestinal bacteria	90–120 µg/day	Synthesis of blood-clotting proteins and proteins in bone	Hemorrhage	Newborns (especially premature), people on long-term antibiotics	Anemia, brain damage	ND

Note: UL, Tolerable Upper Intake Level; ND, not determined due to insufficient evidence

---

CONCEPT CHECK STOP

How does vitamin A help us see in the dark?

Why is vitamin D called the sunshine vitamin?

How does vitamin E protect membranes?

What is the main symptom of vitamin K deficiency?

Meeting Needs with Dietary Supplements

LEARNING OBJECTIVES

List some population groups that may benefit from vitamin and mineral supplements.

Discuss the benefits and risks of herbal supplements.

Explain how the safety of dietary supplements is monitored.

Currently about half of all adult Americans take some form of dietary supplement on a daily basis, and about 80% take them occasionally.[41] We take them for a variety of reasons—to energize ourselves, to protect ourselves from disease, to cure illnesses, to lose weight, to enhance what we obtain from the foods we eat, and simply to ensure against deficiencies. These products may be beneficial and even necessary under some circumstances for some people, but they also have the potential to cause harm.

Some dietary supplements contain vitamins and minerals, some contain herbs and other plant-derived substances, and some contain compounds that are found in the body but are not essential in the diet.[42] While supplements can help us obtain adequate amounts of specific nutrients, they do not provide all the benefits of foods. A pill that meets a person's vitamin needs does not provide the energy, protein, minerals, fiber, or phytochemicals supplied by food sources of these vitamins.

WHO NEEDS VITAMIN/MINERAL SUPPLEMENTS?

Eating a variety of foods is the best way to meet nutrient needs, and most healthy adults who consume a reasonably good diet do not need supplements. In fact, an argument against the use of supplements is that supplement use gives people a false sense of security, causing them to pay less attention to the nutrient content of the foods they choose. For some people, however, taking supplements may be the only way to meet certain nutrient needs because of low intakes, increased needs, or excess losses (**TABLE 7.5**).

Groups for whom dietary supplements are recommended TABLE 7.5

Group	Recommendation
Dieters	People who consume fewer than 1600 Calories/day should take a multivitamin/multimineral supplement.[43]
Vegans and those who eliminate all dairy foods	To obtain adequate vitamin B_{12}, people who do not eat animal products need to take supplements or consume vitamin B_{12}-fortified foods. Because dairy products are an important source of calcium and vitamin D, vegetarians and others who do not consume dairy products due to lactose intolerance or milk allergies or for other reasons, may benefit from taking supplements that provide calcium and vitamin D.
Infants and children	Supplemental fluoride, vitamin D, and iron are recommended under certain circumstances.
Young women and pregnant women	Women of childbearing age should consume 400 μg of folic acid daily from either fortified foods or supplements. Supplements of iron and folic acid are recommended for pregnant women, and multivitamin/multimineral supplements are usually prescribed during pregnancy.
Older adults	Because of the high incidence of atrophic gastritis in adults over 50, vitamin B_{12} supplements or fortified foods are recommended. It may also be difficult for older adults to meet the AI for vitamin D and calcium, so supplements of these nutrients are often recommended.
Individuals with dark skin pigmentation	People with dark skin may be unable to synthesize enough vitamin D to meet their needs for this vitamin and may therefore benefit from supplementation.
Individuals with restricted diets	Individuals with health conditions that affect what foods they eat or how nutrients are used may require vitamin and mineral supplements.
People taking medications	Medications may interfere with the body's use of certain nutrients.
Cigarette smokers and alcohol users	People who smoke heavily require more vitamin C and possibly vitamin E than do nonsmokers.[4,44] Alcohol consumption inhibits the absorption of B vitamins and may interfere with B vitamin metabolism.

HERBAL SUPPLEMENTS

Technically, an herb is a nonwoody, seed-producing plant that dies at the end of the growing season. However, the term *herb* is generally used to refer to any botanical or plant-derived substance. Throughout history, folk medicine has used herbs to prevent and treat disease. Today, herbs and herbal supplements are still popular (**FIGURE 7.34**). They are readily available and relatively inexpensive, and they can be purchased without a trip to the doc-

Popular herbal supplements FIGURE 7.34

▲ *Ginkgo biloba*, also called "maidenhair," is one of the top-selling herbal medicinal supplement in the United States.[45] It is marketed to enhance memory and to treat a variety of circulatory ailments,[46] but supplements have not been found to benefit memory or other aspects of cognitive function in healthy adults.[47] Taking *Ginkgo biloba* may cause side effects that include headaches and gastrointestinal symptoms.[45] *Ginkgo biloba* also interacts with a number of medications. It can cause bleeding when combined with warfarin or aspirin, elevated blood pressure when combined with a thiazide diuretic, and coma when combined with the antidepressant trazodone.[48]

▲ St. John's wort, taken to promote mental well-being, contains low doses of the chemical found in the antidepressant drug fluoxetine (Prozac). The results of some clinical trials suggest that it is effective for the treatment of depression. Side effects include nausea and allergic reactions. St John's wort should not be used in conjunction with prescription antidepressant drugs, and it has been found to interact with anticoagulants, heart medications, birth control pills, and medications used to treat HIV infection.[45,49,50]

▲ Ginseng has been used in Asia for centuries for its energizing, stress-reducing, and aphrodisiac properties. Today it is popular for its effects on cardiovascular, central nervous system, endocrine, and sexual function. Despite claims, there is little evidence that ginseng benefits health, and it may not be safe for everyone.[51,52] It can cause diarrhea, headache, insomnia, and changes in blood pressure and interacts with other medications.[45,48,52]

▲ Hippocrates recommended garlic for treating pneumonia and other infections, as well as cancer and digestive disorders. Although it is no longer recommended for those purposes, recent research has shown that garlic may lower blood cholesterol.[53] Even though we often spice our food with garlic, garlic supplements are not safe for everyone. They could be harmful for people undergoing treatment for HIV infection,[50] and could lead to bleeding in those taking the anticoagulant drug warfarin.[48]

▲ Native Americans used petals of the echinacea plant as a treatment for colds, flu, and infections. Today, the plant's root is typically used, and it is a popular herbal cold remedy. Echinacea is believed to act as an immune system stimulant, but there is little evidence that it is beneficial in either preventing or treating the common cold.[54] Although side effects have not been reported, allergies are possible.[45]

tor or a prescription. Although these features are appealing to consumers who want to manage their own health, they may also cause problems. When a drug is prescribed by a physician, we are assured that it is an established treatment for our ailment, that each dose will contain the same amount of the drug, that the physician or pharmacist has considered other medications we are taking and other medical conditions that may alter the effectiveness of the drug, and that the drug itself will not cause a severe side effect. These assumptions cannot be made with herbs. Some herbs may be toxic, either alone or in combination with other drugs and herbs (TABLE 7.6). Some may contain bacteria or other contaminants. And it is difficult to know what dose of an herb you are taking. Even

Potential benefits and side effects of common herbal ingredients TABLE 7.6

Product	Suggested benefit	Side effects
Astragalus (Huang ch')	Immune stimulant	Low blood pressure, dizziness, fatigue
Cat's Claw (uña de gato)	Relieves arthritis and indigestion, immune stimulant	Headache, dizziness, vomiting. Should not be taken by individuals who are pregnant
Chamomile	Aids indigestion, promotes relaxation	Allergy possible
Chaparral*	Cancer cure, acne treatment, antioxidant	Liver damage, possibly irreversible
Comfrey (borage)*	As a poultice for wounds and sore joints, as a tea for digestive disorders	Do not take orally, even as tea; obstruction of blood flow to liver resulting in liver failure and possibly death
Dong Quai	Increases energy	May cause birth defects
Echinacea (purple coneflower, snake root, Indian head)	Topically for wound healing, internally as an immune stimulant, cold remedy	Allergy possible, adverse effects in pregnant women and people with autoimmune disorders
Ephedra (Ma Huang, Chinese ephedra, epitonin)*	Relieves cold symptoms, weight loss	High blood pressure, irregular heartbeat, heart attack, stroke, death; banned by the FDA
Ginger	Relieves motion sickness and nausea	Irregular heartbeat with large doses
Ginkgo biloba (maidenhair)	Improves memory and mental function, improves circulation	GI distress, headache, allergic skin reactions
Ginseng	Enhances immunity, improves sexual function	Diarrhea, headache, insomnia, low or high blood pressure
Germander	Weight loss	Liver disease, possibly death
Kava	Relieves anxiety and stress	Visual disturbances, dizziness, GI discomfort, hepatitis
Kombucha tea (mushroom tea, kvass tea, kwassan, kargasck)	General well-being	GI upset, liver damage, possibly death
Lobelia (Indian tobacco)*	Relaxation, respiratory remedy	Breathing problems, rapid heartbeat, low blood pressure, convulsions, coma, death
Milk thistle	Protects against liver disease	May decrease effectiveness of some medications
Saw palmetto	Improves urinary flow with enlarged prostate	Constipation, diarrhea, headache, high blood pressure, nausea, urine retention, decreased libido
St. John's wort (hypericum)	Promotes mental well-being	Contains similar ingredients as the antidepressant drug fluoxetine (Prozac) and should not be used by people taking antidepressants, allergic reactions
Stephania (magnolia)*	Weight loss	Kidney damage, including kidney failure resulting in transplant or dialysis
Valerian	Mild sedative	GI upset, headache, restlessness
Willow bark*	Pain and fever relief	Reye's syndrome, allergies
Wormwood*	Relieves digestive ailments	Numbness or paralysis of legs, delirium, paralysis
Yohimbe	Aphrodisiac	Tremors, anxiety, high blood pressure, rapid heart beat, psychosis, paralysis

* Has been shown to have serious side effects and should be avoided.

herbs that have been pressed and packaged into pills may not provide the same dose in each pill. Also, because consumers decide what conditions to treat with herbal remedies, these remedies can be used inappropriately or instead of necessary medical intervention.[45]

CHOOSE SUPPLEMENTS WITH CARE

Using dietary supplements can be part of an effective strategy to promote good health, but supplements are not a substitute for a healthy diet, and they are not without risks of their own. The Dietary Supplement Health and Education Act (DSHEA) of 1994 defined the term *dietary supplement* and created standards for labeling these products (see Chapter 2). However, it left most of the responsibility for manufacturing practices and safety in the hands of manufacturers. To help ensure that these products contain the right ingredients and the right amount per dose, the FDA established dietary supplement "current Good Manufacturing Practice" (cGMP) regulations. These require manufacturers to test their products to ensure identity, purity, strength, and composition.[55] However, because the DSHEA gives supplement manufacturers the responsibility for ensuring that their products are safe, the FDA does not approve the safety and effectiveness of supplements before they are marketed. If a problem arises with a specific product, the FDA must prove that the supplement represents a risk before it can require the manufacturer to remove the supplement from the market. The exception to this rule is products that contain new ingredients. Prior to marketing a supplement containing an ingredient that was not sold in the United States before October 15, 1994, the manufacturer must provide the FDA with safety data. Ingredients sold prior to this date are presumed to be safe, based on their history of use by humans.

Because supplements are not regulated as strictly as drugs, consumers need to use care and caution when choosing dietary supplements. If you choose to use dietary supplements, a safe option is a multivitamin/multimineral supplement that does not exceed 100% of the RDAs. Although there is little evidence that the average person benefits from such a supplement, there is also little evidence of harm. Here are a number of suggestions that will help you when choosing or using dietary supplements:

- **Consider why you want it.** If you are taking it to ensure good health, does it provide both vitamins and minerals? If you want to supplement specific nutrients, are they contained in the product?

- **Compare product costs.** Just as more isn't always better, more expensive is not always better either.

- **Read the label.** Does the supplement contain potentially toxic levels of any nutrient? Are you taking the amount recommended on the label? For any nutrients that exceed 100% of the Daily Value, check to see if they exceed the UL (see Appendix A) (**FIGURE 7.35**). Does it contain any nonvitamin/nonmineral ingredients? If so, have any of them been shown to be toxic to someone like you?

Check the Supplement Facts

FIGURE 7.35

This Supplement Facts panel is from a supplement marketed to reduce appetite and therefore promote weight loss. Would you recommend it? Why or why not?

Supplement Facts		
Serving Size: 2 Capsules		
Servings Per Container: 60		
	Amount Per Serving	**DV%**
Vitamin C (as ascorbic acid)	60mg	100%
Pantothenic Acid (as calcium, pantothenate)	20mg	200%
Vitamin B-6 (as pyridoxine hcl)	8mg	400%
Niacin	5mg	25%
Folate (as folic acid)	100mcg	25%
Zinc (as zinc gluconate)	5mg	33%
Copper (as copper gluconate)	500mcg	25%
NADH (Nicotinamide Adenine Dinucleotide)	1000mcg	*
Hoodia Gordonii Extract (20:1 Extract- Equal to 2000 mg of whole plant)	100mg	*
5-Hydroxytryptophan (Griffonia Simplicifolia)	25mg	*
N, N Dimethylglycine	50mg	*
Trimethylglycine	75mg	*
L-Phenylalanine	600mg	*
Decaffinated Green Tea Extract (Total Catechins 130mg, Epigaliocatechin Galiate (EGCG 70mg))	175mg	*
Salvia Scalarea Extract	50mg	*
Choline (as bitartrate)	75mg	*

This supplement contains more than 100% of the Daily Value for vitamin B$_6$. Does this amount exceed the UL?

This product contains a number of ingredients that are not vitamins or minerals and therefore have no Daily Value or UL. Are they safe?

*Daily Value (DV, not established)

Recommended Use: As a dietary supplement take two capsules before breakfast on a empty stomach (or before exercise) and two capsules at mid afternoon preferably with 8 oz of water.

231

- **Check the expiration date.** Some nutrients degrade over time, so expired products will have a lower nutrient content than is shown on the label. This is particularly true if the product has not been stored properly.

- **Consider your medical history.** Do you have a medical condition that recommends against certain nutrients or other ingredients? Are you taking prescription medication that an ingredient in the supplement may interact with? Check with a physician, dietitian, or pharmacist to help identify these interactions.

- **Approach herbal supplements with caution.** If you are ill or taking medications, consult your physician before taking herbs. Do not take herbs if you are pregnant, and do not give them to children. Do not take combinations of herbs. Do not use herbs for long periods. Stop taking any product that causes side effects.

- **Report harmful effects.** If you suffer a harmful effect or an illness that you think is related to the use of a supplement, seek medical attention and go to the FDA Reporting Web site, at www.fda.gov/safety/medwatch/howtoreport/ucm053074.htm, for information about how to proceed.

CONCEPT CHECK **STOP**

Why is it recommended that vegans and older adults take vitamin B$_{12}$ supplements?

Why is it important to tell your physician if you are taking an herbal supplement?

How does the DSHEA influence the safety of dietary supplements?

SUMMARY

1 A Vitamin Primer

1. **Vitamins** are essential organic nutrients that do not provide energy and are required in small quantities in the diet to maintain health. Vitamins are classified by their solubility in either water or fat. Vitamins are present naturally in foods and added through fortification and enrichment.

2. Vitamin **bioavailability** is affected by the composition of the diet, conditions in the digestive tract, and the ability to transport and activate the vitamin once it has been absorbed.

3. Vitamins promote and regulate body activities. The B vitamins act as **coenzymes**. Some vitamins are **antioxidants**, which protect the body from **oxidative damage** by **free radicals**.

4. In developing countries, vitamin deficiencies remain a major public health problem. They are less common in industrialized countries due to fortification and a more varied food supply.

Fat-soluble vitamins

Water-soluble vitamins

Blood

Lymph

2 The Water-Soluble Vitamins

1. **Thiamin** is a coenzyme that is particularly important for glucose metabolism and **neurotransmitter** synthesis; a deficiency of thiamin, called **beriberi**, causes nervous system abnormalities. Thiamin is found in whole and enriched grains.

2. **Riboflavin** coenzymes are needed for ATP production and for the utilization of several other vitamins. Milk is one of the best food sources of riboflavin.

3. **Niacin** coenzymes are needed for the breakdown of carbohydrate, fat, and protein and for the synthesis of fatty acids and cholesterol. A deficiency results in **pellagra**, which is characterized by dermatitis, diarrhea, and dementia. The amino acid tryptophan can be converted into niacin. High doses lower blood cholesterol but can cause toxicity symptoms.

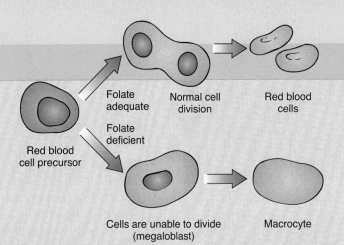

Red blood cell precursor

Folate adequate → Normal cell division → Red blood cells

Folate deficient → Cells are unable to divide (megaloblast) → Macrocyte

4. **Biotin** is needed for the synthesis of glucose and fatty acids, as well as for the metabolism of certain amino acids. Some of our biotin need is met by bacterial synthesis in the gastrointestinal tract.

5. **Pantothenic acid** is part of coenzyme A, required for the production of ATP from carbohydrate, fat, and protein and the synthesis of cholesterol and fat. It is widespread in the food supply.

6. **Vitamin B$_6$** is particularly important for amino acid and protein metabolism. Deficiency causes numbness and tingling and may increase the risk of heart disease because it is needed to keep levels of homocysteine low. Food sources include meats and whole grains. Large doses of vitamin B$_6$ can cause nervous system abnormalities.

7. **Folate** is necessary for the synthesis of DNA, so it is especially important for rapidly dividing cells. Folate deficiency results in **macrocytic anemia**. Low

levels of folate before and during early pregnancy are associated with an increased incidence of **neural tube defects**. Food sources include liver, legumes, oranges, leafy green vegetables, and fortified grains. A high intake of folate can mask some of the symptoms of vitamin B$_{12}$ deficiency.

8. Absorption of **vitamin B$_{12}$** requires stomach acid and **intrinsic factor**. Without intrinsic factor, only tiny amounts are absorbed, and **pernicious anemia** occurs. Vitamin B$_{12}$ is needed for the metabolism of folate and fatty acids and to maintain **myelin**.

Deficiency results in macrocytic anemia and nerve damage. Vitamin B$_{12}$ is found almost exclusively in animal products. Deficiency is a concern in vegans and in older individuals with **atrophic gastritis**.

9. **Vitamin C** is necessary for the synthesis of **collagen**, hormones, and neurotransmitters. Vitamin C deficiency, called **scurvy**, is characterized by poor wound healing, bleeding, and other symptoms related to the improper formation and maintenance of collagen. Vitamin C is also a water-soluble antioxidant. The best food sources are citrus fruits.

3 The Fat-Soluble Vitamins

1. **Vitamin A** is a fat-soluble vitamin needed in the visual cycle and for growth and cell **differentiation**. Its role in **gene expression** makes it essential for maintenance of epithelial tissue, reproduction, and immune function. Vitamin A deficiency causes blindness and death. Preformed vitamin A **retinoids** are found in liver, eggs, fish, and fortified dairy products. High intakes are toxic and have been linked to birth defects and bone loss. Provitamin A **carotenoids**, such as **β-carotene**, are found in yellow-orange fruits and vegetables such as mangoes, carrots, and apricots, as well as leafy greens. Some carotenoids are antioxidants. Carotenoids are not toxic, but a high intake can give the skin a yellow-orange appearance.

2. **Vitamin D** can be made in the skin by exposure to sunlight, so dietary needs vary depending on the amount synthesized. Vitamin D is found in fish oils and fortified milk. It is essential for maintaining proper levels of calcium and phosphorus in the body. A deficiency in children results in **rickets**; in adults, vitamin D deficiency causes **osteomalacia**. Adequate vitamin D is associated with reduced incidence of certain cancers.

3. **Vitamin E** functions primarily as a fat-soluble antioxidant. It is necessary for reproduction and protects cell membranes from oxidative damage. It is found in nuts, plant oils, green vegetables, and fortified cereals.

4. **Vitamin K** is essential for blood clotting. Because vitamin K deficiency is a problem in newborns, they are routinely given vitamin K injections

at birth. Warfarin, a substance that inhibits vitamin K activity, is used medically as an anticoagulant. Vitamin K is found in plants and is synthesized by bacteria in the gastrointestinal tract.

Ultraviolet light

Vitamin D (inactive) in food

Vitamin D precursor

Vitamin D (inactive)

Liver

4 Meeting Needs with Dietary Supplements

1. About half the adult population in the United States takes some type of dietary supplement. Vitamin and mineral supplements are recommended for dieters, vegetarians, pregnant women and women of childbearing age, older adults, and other nutritionally vulnerable groups.

2. Herbal supplements are currently popular. These products may have beneficial physiological actions, but their dosage is not regulated and they can be toxic either on their own or in combination with other herbs, medications, or medical conditions.

3. Manufacturers are responsible for the consistency and safety of supplements before they are marketed. The FDA regulates dietary supplement labeling and can monitor their safety once they are being sold. When choosing a dietary supplement, it is important to carefully consider both the potential risks and benefits of the product.

KEY TERMS

CRITICAL AND CREATIVE THINKING QUESTIONS

1. Anna is 28 years old. She and her husband plan to start a family soon. Because Anna is overweight and knows she will put on more weight if she has a baby, she begins a low-carbohydrate diet to slim down before she gets pregnant. She eliminates breads, grains, legumes, starchy vegetables, and fruit from her diet. What nutrient that is important early in pregnancy would be lacking in this diet? What could Anna add to her diet to increase her intake of this nutrient? Will taking a prenatal vitamin supplement prescribed at her first prenatal visit be enough to reduce the risk of neural tube defects?

2. The following dietary supplement products are on sale at a local nutrition store:

   Pyridoxine: 100 mg
   Stress tabs: pyridoxine, 35 mg; thiamin, 1 mg; riboflavin, 1.1 mg; niacin, 30 mg; choline, 500 mg
   Folic acid: 800 µg

   Do any of these supplements pose a risk for toxicity at the dose listed above? Which ones and why? What would happen if a consumer took twice the recommended dose? Would you recommend them for everyone? for a specific group? Why or why not?

3. Sam is a fast-food fanatic. For breakfast, he stops for coffee and doughnuts. Lunch is an iced tea, a ham-and-cheese sub with lettuce and mayonnaise, and a cookie. Dinner is a soft drink, burger, and fries. Name two vitamins likely to be lacking in Sam's diet if he eats like this every day. Why are these vitamins likely to be deficient?

4. Why might someone with kidney failure develop a vitamin D deficiency?

5. Explain why a dark-skinned Nigerian exchange student living in Buffalo, New York, is at risk for vitamin D deficiency.

6. Explain why a deficiency either of vitamin B_{12} or of folate causes red blood cells to be larger than normal.

7. Explain why infections are more common and immunization programs are less successful in regions where vitamin A deficiency is prevalent.

What is happening in this picture ?

These children, who live in Russia, are being exposed to UV radiation to prevent vitamin D deficiency.

- Why does this treatment help them meet their need for vitamin D?

- Why are children in Russia at risk for vitamin D deficiency?

- What else could be done to ensure that they get adequate amounts of vitamin D?

SELF-TEST

(Check your answers in Appendix L.)

1. Which of the following vitamins is *not* added to grains during enrichment?

   a. thiamin
   b. riboflavin
   c. niacin
   d. vitamin B_6
   e. folate

2. Which vitamin is needed for the reaction labeled with the letter A?

   a. thiamin
   b. vitamin C
   c. vitamin B_6
   d. vitamin A
   e. vitamin K

3. Which of the following descriptions of the water-soluble vitamins is false?

   a. niacin—a deficiency causes pellagra
   b. thiamin—can be synthesized from tryptophan
   c. pantothenic acid—found in most foods
   d. vitamin C—needed for the cross-linking of collagen
   e. vitamin B_6—needed for amino acid metabolism

4. Which of the following statements is true of all the B vitamins?

   a. They are all electron carriers.
   b. They are all needed for DNA synthesis.
   c. They are all coenzymes.
   d. They all contain energy that is used to fuel body activities.
   e. They are all fat soluble.

5. Which of the following nutrients is *not* essential in the diet when sun exposure is adequate?

   a. riboflavin
   b. vitamin E
   c. vitamin K
   d. vitamin D

6. Which of the following statements about folate is false?

   a. Adequate amounts decrease the incidence of neural tube defect–affected pregnancies.
   b. It is needed for DNA synthesis.
   c. A deficiency causes macrocytic anemia.
   d. It can be made in the body from methionine.
   e. Enriched grain products are fortified with folate.

7. The disease scurvy is due to a deficiency of _____.

   a. vitamin K
   b. vitamin D
   c. vitamin C
   d. vitamin A
   e. thiamin

8. A deficiency of vitamin K leads to _____.

   a. rickets
   b. blindness
   c. scurvy
   d. pellagra
   e. decreased blood clotting

9. Which of the following is a poor source of ß-carotene?

   a. milk
   b. carrots
   c. sweet potatoes
   d. spinach
   e. apricots

10. The food sources of _____ are illustrated by this graph.

a. vitamin C
b. folate
c. vitamin B$_{12}$
d. thiamin
e. vitamin B$_6$

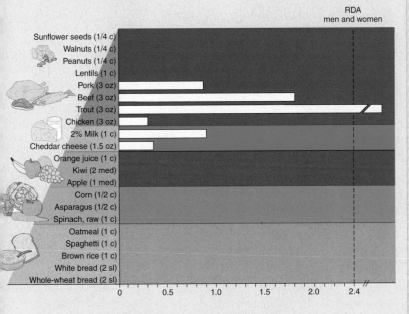

RDA
men and women

Sunflower seeds (1/4 c)
Walnuts (1/4 c)
Peanuts (1/4 c)
Lentils (1 c)
Pork (3 oz)
Beef (3 oz)
Trout (3 oz)
Chicken (3 oz)
2% Milk (1 c)
Cheddar cheese (1.5 oz)
Orange juice (1 c)
Kiwi (2 med)
Apple (1 med)
Corn (1/2 c)
Asparagus (1/2 c)
Spinach, raw (1 c)
Oatmeal (1 c)
Spaghetti (1 c)
Brown rice (1 c)
White bread (2 sl)
Whole-wheat bread (2 sl)

0   0.5   1.0   1.5   2.0   2.4

11. The actions of _____ are illustrated here.

a. vitamin C
b. vitamin D
c. vitamin B$_6$
d. vitamin K
e. vitamin E

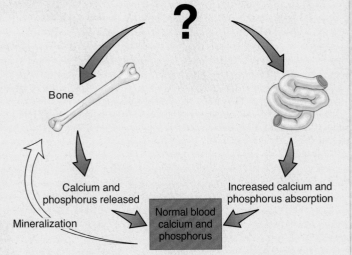

?

Bone

Calcium and
phosphorus released

Mineralization

Increased calcium and
phosphorus absorption

Normal blood
calcium and
phosphorus

12. It is recommended that older adults get their vitamin B$_{12}$ from fortified foods and supplements because _____.

a. they eat a poor diet
b. their requirement for B$_{12}$ is higher than that of younger people
c. many have atrophic gastritis and are not able to absorb the vitamin B$_{12}$ found in foods
d. they have higher vitamin B$_{12}$ losses than other groups

13. Vitamin A deficiency causes the eye condition illustrated here because _____.

a. the visual pigment rhodopsin cannot be synthesized.
b. collagen is not made correctly
c. there is insufficient antioxidant protection
d. bone development is abnormal.
e. mucus-secreting cells do not differentiate normally

14. Which of the following statements is true of vitamin E?

a. It is needed in energy metabolism.
b. It protects cell membranes from oxidative damage.
c. Deficiency is a common problem in North America.
d. Supplements increase fertility even in people with adequate vitamin E status.
e. It is needed for night vision.

15. Elevated blood homocysteine has been associated with an increased risk of cardiovascular disease. Deficiencies of _____ may increase levels of homocysteine in the blood.

a. pantothenic acid, riboflavin, and vitamin C
b. biotin, thiamin, and vitamin B$_6$
c. vitamin B$_6$, folate, and vitamin B$_{12}$
d. thiamin, riboflavin, and niacin

Water and Minerals

Throughout human history, cultures have flourished along the banks of rivers and streams, where fresh water is easily accessible. With adequate water, humanity thrived. In order for each of us to stay healthy, we too need a sufficient supply of clean, fresh water.

It is in the water of Earth's first seas that scientists propose life itself originally appeared. These primitive seas were not plain water but rather a complex mixture of minerals and water. Over time, as simple organisms developed greater complexity, many left this mineral-rich external marine environment behind. To survive, they needed to bring with them a similar internal environment. Within our bodies today, minerals and water make up an "internal sea" that allows the chemistry of life to function.

Getting the right amounts of minerals and water remains essential to survival. Inadequate and excessive intakes of certain minerals are world health problems contributing to such conditions as high blood pressure, bone fractures, anemia, and increased risk of infection. Today, getting enough water may prove to be an even greater challenge to human survival than meeting mineral needs. Pollution and population growth are making fresh water an increasingly rare commodity: India must rely more and more on bottled water for its burgeoning populations; great swaths of Africa and eastern Europe face similar challenges; even the huge aquifers beneath the United States are diminishing. The water crisis may make shrinking oil supplies seem like a minor inconvenience for the simple reason that without water, we die.

Water

Have you ever felt nauseated, light-headed, or dizzy while exercising on a hot day? If so, you might have been suffering from **dehydration**. Lack of sufficient water in the body causes deficiency symptoms more rapidly than does a deficiency of any other nutrient. These symptoms can be alleviated almost as rapidly as they appeared by drinking enough water to restore your body's water balance.

dehydration
A state that occurs when not enough water is present to meet the body's needs.

THE DISTRIBUTION OF WATER IN THE BODY

In adults, water accounts for about 60% of body weight. Water is found in different proportions in different tissues, with about 75% of muscle consisting of water, for example, and about 25% of bone. Water is found both inside cells (intracellular) and outside cells (extracellular) in the blood, the lymph, and the spaces between cells (FIGURE 8.1A). The cell membranes that separate the intracellular and extracellular spaces are not watertight; water can pass right through them.

Water distribution FIGURE 8.1

A About one-third of the water in the body is intracellular, located inside the cells. The other two-thirds is extracellular, located outside the cells. The extracellular portion includes the water in the blood and lymph, the water between cells, and the water in the digestive tract, eyes, joints, and spinal cord.

B The amount of water in blood and tissues is affected by blood pressure and the force generated by osmosis. In the capillaries, blood pressure pushes water out of the blood, while osmosis moves water into or out of the blood to equalize the concentration of dissolved particles.

Fluid between cells   Fluid in blood   Blood vessel   Red blood cells   Intracellular fluid

Extracellular fluid

Osmosis causes fluid to move into and out of cells in response to the concentration of dissolved substances inside and outside the cell.

Higher blood pressure at the arterial side of the capillaries forces water from the blood into the tissues.   Capillary blood vessel   Lower blood pressure and differences in solute concentration at the venous side draw fluid back into the capillaries by osmosis.

Water balance FIGURE 8.2

A To maintain water balance, intake must equal output. A typical man who is in water balance loses and consumes almost 3 liters of water daily. This figure approximates the amounts of water that enter the body from food, drink, and metabolism and the amounts lost in urine and feces, as well as through evaporation in an adult who is not sweating. Increasing water consumption proportionately increases excretion of water in urine. ▼

Water intake

Food 625 ml

Drink 1875 ml

Metabolism 250 ml

Water output

Feces 200 ml

Urine 1450 ml

Evaporation 1100 ml

▲

B Dehydration due to diarrhea is a major cause of child death in the developing world. Replacing fluids and electrolytes in the right combinations can save lives. In some cases oral rehydration therapy is sufficient. Drinking mixtures made by simply dissolving a large pinch of table salt and a fistful of sugar in a jug of clean water can restore the body's water balance by promoting the absorption of water and sodium. In severe cases of diarrhea administration of intravenous fluids, as seen in this hospital in Bangladesh, is needed to restore hydration.

The distribution of water between various intra- and extracellular spaces depends on differences in the concentrations of dissolved substances, or **solutes**, such as proteins, sodium, potassium, and other small molecules. These concentration differences drive *osmosis*, the diffusion of water in a direction that equalizes the concentration of dissolved substances on either side of a membrane (see Chapter 3). Water is also moved by **blood pressure**, which forces water from the capillary blood vessels into the spaces between the cells of the surrounding tissues. When blood pressure is lower than the pressure created by osmosis, water is drawn back into the capillaries (**FIGURE 8.1B**). The body regulates the amount of water in cells and in different extracellular spaces by adjusting the concentration of dissolved particles and relying on osmosis to move the water.

> **blood pressure**
> The amount of force exerted by the blood against the walls of arteries.

WATER BALANCE

The amount of water in the body remains relatively constant over time. Because water cannot be stored in the body, water intake and output must be balanced to maintain the right amount. Most of the water we consume comes from water and other liquids that we drink. Solid foods also provide water; most fruits and vegetables are over 80% water, and even roast beef is about 50% water. A small amount of water is also produced in the body as a by-product of metabolic reactions. We lose water from our bodies in urine and feces, through evaporation from the lungs and skin, and in sweat (**FIGURE 8.2A**).

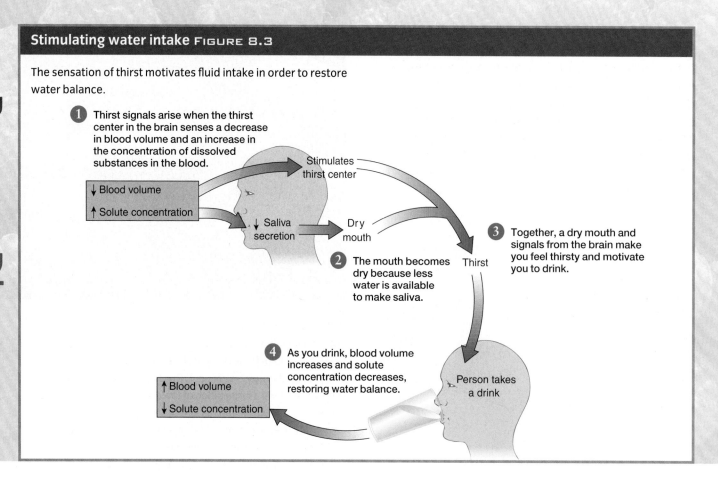

Stimulating water intake FIGURE 8.3

The sensation of thirst motivates fluid intake in order to restore water balance.

1 Thirst signals arise when the thirst center in the brain senses a decrease in blood volume and an increase in the concentration of dissolved substances in the blood.

↓ Blood volume
↑ Solute concentration

Stimulates thirst center

↓ Saliva secretion → Dry mouth

2 The mouth becomes dry because less water is available to make saliva.

Thirst

3 Together, a dry mouth and signals from the brain make you feel thirsty and motivate you to drink.

Person takes a drink

4 As you drink, blood volume increases and solute concentration decreases, restoring water balance.

↑ Blood volume
↓ Solute concentration

Under most circumstances, the majority of water losses occur in the urine. In a healthy person, only a small amount of water is lost in the feces, usually less than a cup per day. This is remarkable because every day about 9 L of fluid enters the gastrointestinal tract, but more than 95% of this is absorbed before the feces are eliminated. However, in cases of severe diarrhea, large amounts of water can be lost via this route. If the lost fluid is not replaced quickly, the individual may become severely dehydrated (**FIGURE 8.2B**).

We are continuously losing water from the skin and respiratory tract due to evaporation. The amount of water lost through evaporation varies greatly, depending on activity, temperature, humidity, and body size. In a temperate climate, an inactive person loses about 1 L/day; the amount increases with increases in activity, environmental temperature, and body size, as well as when humidity is low.

In addition to being lost through evaporation, water is lost through sweat when you exercise or when the environment is hot. More sweat is produced as exercise intensity increases and as the environment becomes hotter and more humid. An individual doing light work at a temperature of 84°F will lose about 2 to 3 L of sweat/day. Strenuous exercise in a hot environment can increase this to 2 to 4 L in an hour.[1] Clothing that permits the evaporation of sweat helps keep the body cool and therefore decreases the amount of sweat produced.

Regulating water intake
When water losses increase, intake must increase to keep body water at a healthy level. The need to consume water is signaled by the sensation of **thirst**. Thirst is caused by dryness in the mouth as well as by signals from the brain (**FIGURE 8.3**). It is a powerful urge but often lags behind the need for water, and we don't or can't always drink when we are thirsty. Therefore, thirst alone cannot be relied on to maintain water balance.

Not drinking enough to replace water losses can be a problem for athletes exercising in hot weather. They lose water rapidly in sweat but do not feel thirsty until they have lost so much body water that their performance is compromised.[2] To maintain water balance, it is recommended that athletes drink at a rate that closely matches the rate of water loss due to sweating.[3]

Regulating water loss: The kidneys

To maintain water balance, the kidneys regulate water loss in urine. The kidneys typically produce about 1 to 2 L of urine/day, but urine production varies, depending on the amount of water consumed and the amount of waste that needs to be excreted.

The kidneys function like a filter. As blood flows through them, water molecules and other small molecules move through the filter and out of the blood, while blood cells and large molecules are retained in the blood. Some of the water and other molecules that are filtered out are reabsorbed into the blood, and the rest are excreted in the urine.

The amount of water that is reabsorbed into the blood rather than excreted in the urine depends on conditions in the body. When the solute concentration in the blood is high, as it would be in an athlete who has not consumed enough water, a hormone called **antidiuretic hormone (ADH)** signals the kidneys to reabsorb water, reducing the amount lost in the urine (**FIGURE 8.4**). This reabsorbed water is returned to the blood, preventing the concentration of dissolved particles from increasing further. When the solute concentration in the blood is low, as it might be after the athlete has guzzled several glasses of water, ADH levels decrease. Now the kidneys reabsorb less water, and more water is excreted in the urine, allowing the solute concentration in the blood to increase to its normal level.

The amount of water lost from the kidneys can also be affected by regulating the amount of sodium and other substances dissolved in the blood (as discussed later in the chapter).

Even though the kidneys work to control how much water is lost, their ability to concentrate urine is limited because there is a minimum amount of water that must be lost as dissolved wastes are excreted. If there are a lot of wastes to be excreted, more water must be lost. Wastes that must be eliminated in the urine include urea and other nitrogen-containing molecules (produced by protein breakdown), ketones (from incomplete fat breakdown), sodium, and other minerals.

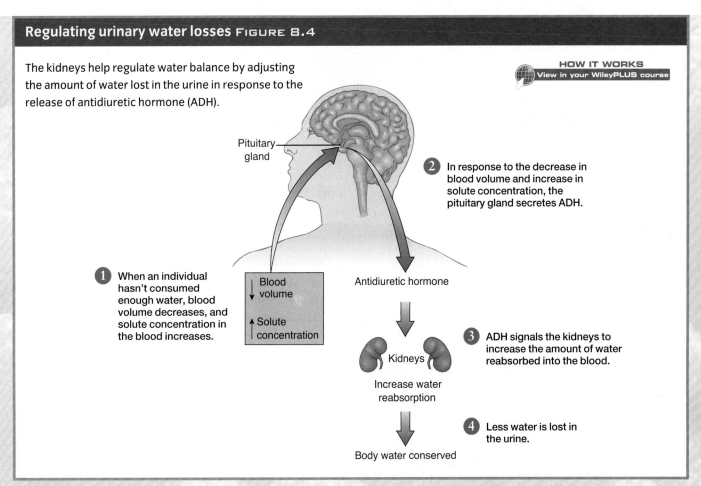

Regulating urinary water losses FIGURE 8.4

The kidneys help regulate water balance by adjusting the amount of water lost in the urine in response to the release of antidiuretic hormone (ADH).

HOW IT WORKS
View in your WileyPLUS course

Pituitary gland

1. When an individual hasn't consumed enough water, blood volume decreases, and solute concentration in the blood increases.

↓ Blood volume
↑ Solute concentration

2. In response to the decrease in blood volume and increase in solute concentration, the pituitary gland secretes ADH.

Antidiuretic hormone

Kidneys
Increase water reabsorption

3. ADH signals the kidneys to increase the amount of water reabsorbed into the blood.

4. Less water is lost in the urine.

Body water conserved

Process Diagram

Increased blood flow at the surface of the body causes the skin to become red in hot weather and during strenuous activity. Shunting blood to the skin allows heat to be transferred from the blood to the surroundings. Evaporation of sweat cools the skin and the blood near the surface of the skin.

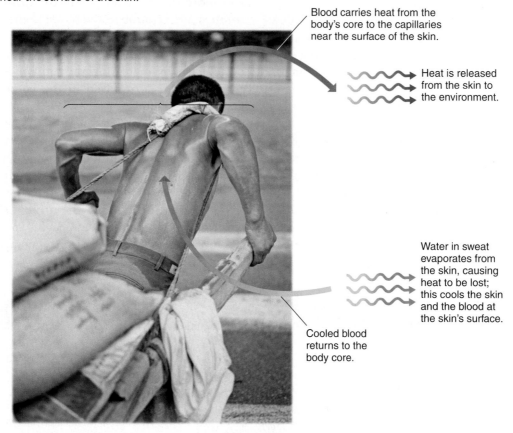

Blood carries heat from the body's core to the capillaries near the surface of the skin.

Heat is released from the skin to the environment.

Water in sweat evaporates from the skin, causing heat to be lost; this cools the skin and the blood at the skin's surface.

Cooled blood returns to the body core.

THE FUNCTIONS OF WATER

Water doesn't provide energy, but it is essential to life. Water in the body serves as a medium for and participant in metabolic reactions, helps regulate acid base balance, transports nutrients and wastes, provides protection, and helps regulate temperature.

Water in metabolism and transport Water is an excellent **solvent**; glucose, amino acids, minerals, proteins, and many other substances that are needed by body cells dissolve in water. The chemical reactions of metabolism that support life take place in water. Water also participates in a number of reactions that join small molecules together or break apart large ones. Some of the reactions in which water participates help maintain the proper level of acidity in the body. Water is the primary constituent of blood, which flows through our bodies, delivering oxygen and nutrients to cells and delivering waste products to the lungs and kidneys for excretion.

Water as protection Water bathes the cells of the body and lubricates and cleanses internal and external body surfaces. Water in tears lubricates the eyes and washes away dirt; water in synovial fluid lubricates the joints; and water in saliva lubricates the mouth, helping us chew and swallow food. Because water resists compression, it cushions the joints and other parts of the body against shock. The cushioning effect of water in the amniotic sac protects the fetus as it grows inside the uterus.

Water and body temperature The fact that water holds heat and changes temperature slowly helps keep body temperature constant, but water is also actively involved in temperature regulation (**FIGURE 8.5**). The water in blood helps regulate body temperature by

Urine color is an indication of whether you are drinking enough. Pale yellow urine indicates you are well hydrated. The darker the urine the greater level of dehydration.

Well hydrated

Mild dehydration

Severe dehydration

increasing or decreasing the amount of heat lost at the surface of the body. When body temperature starts to rise, the blood vessels in the skin dilate, causing more blood to flow close to the surface, where it can release some of the heat to the surrounding air. Cooling is aided by the production of sweat. When body temperature increases, the brain triggers the sweat glands in the skin to produce sweat, which is mostly water. As sweat evaporates from the skin, additional heat is lost, cooling the body.

WATER IN HEALTH AND DISEASE

Without food, you could probably survive for about eight weeks, but without water, you would last only a few days. Too much water can also be a problem if it changes the osmotic balance, disrupting the distribution of water within the body.

Dehydration Dehydration occurs when water loss exceeds water intake. It causes a reduction in blood volume, which impairs the ability to deliver oxygen and nutrients to cells and remove waste products. Early symptoms of dehydration include thirst, headache, fatigue, loss of appetite, dry eyes and mouth, and dark-colored urine (FIGURE 8.6). Dehydration affects physical and cognitive performance. As dehydration worsens, it causes nausea, difficulty concentrating, confusion, and disorientation. The milder symptoms of dehydration disappear quickly after water or some other beverage is consumed, but if left untreated, dehydration can become severe enough to require medical attention. A water loss amounting to about 10% to 20% of body weight can be fatal. Athletes are at risk for dehydration because they may lose large amounts of water in sweat. Elderly people and infants are also at risk for dehydration (FIGURE 8.7).

Groups at risk for dehydration FIGURE 8.7

Older adults are at risk for dehydration because the thirst mechanism becomes less sensitive with age. Infants are at risk because their body surface area relative to their weight is much greater than that of adults, so they lose proportionately more water through evaporation; also, their kidneys cannot concentrate urine efficiently, so they lose more water in urine. In addition, they cannot tell us they are thirsty.

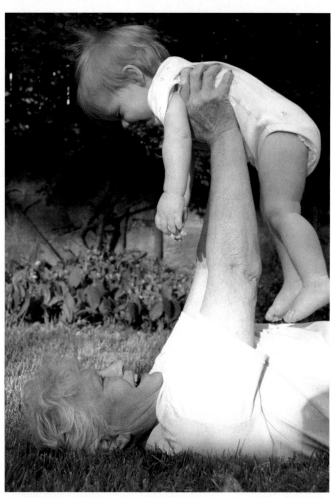

Water intoxication It is difficult to consume too much water under normal circumstances. However, overhydration, or **water intoxication**, can occur under some conditions. When there is too much water relative to the amount of sodium in the body, the concentration of sodium in the blood drops, a condition called **hyponatremia** (FIGURE 8.8). When this occurs, water moves out of the blood vessels into the tissues by osmosis, causing them to swell. Swelling in the brain can cause disorientation, convulsions, coma, and death. The early symptoms of water intoxication may be similar to those of dehydration: nausea, muscle cramps, disorientation, slurred speech, and confusion. It is important to determine whether the symptoms are due to dehydration or water intoxication because while drinking water will alleviate dehydration, it will worsen the symptoms of water intoxication.

> **water intoxication** A condition that occurs when a person drinks enough water to significantly lower the concentration of sodium in the blood.

MEETING WATER NEEDS

We need more water than any other nutrient. The DRIs recommend 3.7 L (3700 grams)/day for men and 2.7 L (2700 g)/day for women.[4] However, the actual amount you need each day varies depending on your activity level, the environmental temperature and humidity, and your diet. Activity increases water needs because it increases the amount of water lost in sweat; such losses are greater in a hot, humid environment. Diet affects water needs by changing the amount of waste that needs to be excreted in the urine or the amount of water lost in the feces. A low-calorie diet increases water needs because as body fat and protein are broken down to fuel the body, ketones and urea are produced and must be excreted in the urine. A high-salt diet increases water losses because the excess must be excreted in the urine. A high-fiber diet increases water needs because more water is held in the intestines and excreted in the feces.

Most beverages, whether water, milk, juice, or soda, help meet the overall need for water (see *What a Scientist Sees*). Beverages containing caffeine, such as coffee, tea, and cola, increase water losses for a short period because caffeine is a **diuretic**. Over the course of a day, however, the increase in water loss is small, so the net amount of water that caffeinated beverages add to the body is similar to the amount contributed by noncaffeinated beverages. Alcohol is also a diuretic; the overall effect it has on water balance depends on the relative amounts of water and alcohol in the beverages being consumed.[4]

> **diuretic** A substance that increases the amount of urine passed from the body.

Too much water FIGURE 8.8

Water and salts, primarily sodium, are lost in sweat. Drinking plain water after excessive sweating can therefore dilute the salts remaining in the blood. To help prevent this, athletes exercising for more than an hour should consume beverages, such as sports drinks, that contain dilute solutions of sodium and other salts as well as sugar. (discussed further in Chapter 10.)

Normal blood sodium concentration

Water and sodium lost in sweat

Replacing just water dilutes sodium (hyponatremia)

Is Bottled Water Better?

Many Americans see bottled water as safer and better than tap water. What a scientist sees is that the jug at the water cooler and the expensive bottled water that you guzzle at the gym are not really much different from tap water. The purity standards for bottled water set by the FDA are comparable to the minimum standards set by the EPA for municipal water systems.

By definition, bottled water doesn't have to be anything special; it can be any water as long as it has no added ingredients except safe and suitable antimicrobial agents. About 25% of the bottled water sold in the United States is actually the same water that comes from municipal water supplies.[5] Bottled water that comes from a tap must be clearly labeled as such. However, water that has been taken from a municipal water supply and then treated—for example, filtered or disinfected—need not indicate that it is tap water. "Distilled water" and "purified water" are examples of water that has been taken from municipal water supplies and then treated. Artesian water, spring water, well water, and mineral water come from underground sources rather than from municipal sources.

Bottled water costs more than tap water (As much as $10.00/gallon for some bottled water versus less than $0.01/gallon for tap water), generates 1.5 million tons of plastic waste per year, and consumes oil, which is used to produce the bottles. Do you think bottled water is worth the price?

EPA and FDA water regulations

Contaminant	Maximum level allowed in tap water (EPA)	Maximum level allowed in bottled water (FDA)
Arsenic	0.01 mg/L	0.01 mg/L
Asbestos	7 million fibers/L	7 million fibers/L
Cyanide	0.2 mg/L	0.2 mg/L
Lead	0.015 mg/L	0.005 mg/L
Mercury	0.002 mg/L	0.002 mg/L
Nitrate	10 mg/L	10 mg/L

The Food and Drug Administration (FDA) has adopted most of the Environmental Protection Agency's (EPA's) tap water standards as standards for bottled water. As a result, standards for contaminants in tap water and bottled water are very similar. This table lists a few of the toxic chemicals that are regulated by the EPA and the FDA. The regulations also include maximum allowances for disease-causing microorganisms and radioactive compounds.

CONCEPT CHECK **STOP**

How does osmosis affect the distribution of water in the body?

What is the role of antidiuretic hormone?

How does water help cool the body?

What happens to the body if water losses exceed intake?

An Overview of Minerals

Minerals are found in the ground on which we walk, the jewels we wear on our fingers, and even some of the makeup we wear on our faces, but perhaps their most significant impact on our lives comes from their importance in our diet. There are more than 20 **minerals** that you need to consume in your food to stay healthy. Some of these make up a significant portion of your body weight; others are found in minute quantities. If more than 100 milligrams of a mineral/day is required in the diet, an amount equivalent in weight to about two drops of water, the mineral is considered a **major mineral**; these include sodium, potassium, chloride, calcium, phosphorus, magnesium, and sulfur. Minerals that are needed in smaller amounts are referred to as **trace minerals**; these include iron, copper, zinc, selenium, iodine, chromium, fluoride, manganese, molybdenum, and others. Just because you need more of the major minerals than of the trace minerals doesn't mean that one group is more important than the other. A deficiency of a trace mineral is just as damaging to your health as a deficiency of a major mineral.

minerals
In nutrition, elements needed by the body in small amounts to maintain structure and regulate chemical reactions and body processes.

major minerals
Minerals required in the diet in amounts greater than 100 mg/day or present in the body in amounts greater than 0.01% of body weight.

trace minerals
Minerals required in the diet in amounts of 100 mg or less/day or present in the body in amounts of 0.01% of body weight or less.

Minerals in MyPyramid FIGURE 8.9

Minerals are found in all the MyPyramid food groups, but some groups are particularly good sources of specific minerals. Eating a variety of foods, including fresh fruits, vegetables, nuts, legumes, whole grains and cereals, milk, seafood, and lean meats can maximize your diet's mineral content.

GRAINS	VEGETABLES	FRUITS	MILK	MEAT & BEANS
Iron, Zinc, Selenium, Copper, Magnesium, Chromium, Sulfur, Manganese, Sodium, Potassium, Phosphorus	Iron, Calcium, Potassium, Magnesium, Molybdenum	Iron, Potassium	Calcium, Zinc, Phosphorus, Potassium, Iodine, Molybdenum	Iron, Zinc, Magnesium, Potassium, Chromium, Sulfur, Iodine, Selenium, Phosphorus, Copper, Manganese, Fluoride

Plant foods such as these contain substances that can reduce mineral absorption when consumed in large amounts.

Oxalates, found in spinach, rhubarb, beet greens, and chocolate, have been found to interfere with the absorption of calcium and iron.

Phytic acid, or phytate, found in whole grains, bran, and soy products, binds calcium, zinc, iron, and magnesium, limiting the absorption of these minerals. Phytic acid can be broken down by yeast, so the bioavailability of minerals is higher in yeast-leavened foods such as breads.

Tannins, found in tea and some grains, can interfere with the absorption of iron.

MINERALS IN OUR FOOD

Minerals in the diet come from both plant and animal sources (FIGURE 8.9). Some minerals are present as functioning components of the plant or animal and are therefore present in consistent amounts. For instance, the iron content of beef is predictable because iron is part of the muscle protein that gives beef its red color. In other foods, minerals are present as contaminants from the soil or from processing. For example, plants grown in an area where the soil is high in selenium are higher in selenium than plants grown in other areas, and milk from dairies that use sterilizing solutions that contain iodine is a source of iodine. Minerals are also added to food intentionally during processing. Sodium is added to soups and crackers as a flavor enhancer; iron is added to enriched grain products; and calcium, iron, and other minerals are typically added to fortified breakfast cereals.

Processing can also remove minerals from foods. For example, when vegetables are cooked, the cells are broken down, and potassium is lost in the cooking water. When the skins of fruits and vegetables or the bran and germ of grains are detached, magnesium, iron, selenium, zinc, and copper are lost.

MINERAL BIOAVAILABILITY

The *bioavailability* of the minerals that we consume in foods varies. For some minerals, such as sodium, we absorb almost all that is present in our food, but for others we absorb only a small percentage. Calcium absorption is typically about 25%, for instance, and iron absorption may be as low as 5%. How much of a particular mineral is absorbed may vary from food to food, meal to meal, and person to person.

In general, the minerals in animal products are better absorbed than those in plant foods. The difference in absorption is due in part to the fact that plants contain substances such as phytic acid, tannins, oxalates, and fiber that bind minerals in the gastrointestinal tract and can reduce absorption (FIGURE 8.10). The North American diet generally does not contain enough of any of these components to cause a mineral deficiency, but diets in developing countries may. For example, in some populations, the phytate content of the diet is high enough to cause a zinc deficiency.

Selenium, sulfur, zinc, copper, and manganese are needed for the functioning of antioxidant enzymes and molecules that can defend the body against damaging chemicals.

Sodium, potassium, and chloride help regulate fluid balance. ▼

Zinc, iodine, and calcium are needed for normal growth and development.

Iron, magnesium, ▶ zinc, chromium, selenium, iodine, phosphorus, and calcium are needed to provide energy for physical activity and to regulate metabolism.

◀ Calcium, sodium, potassium, and chloride are needed for the transmission of nerve impulses and for muscle contraction.

◀ Iron, copper, calcium, zinc, selenium, and magnesium are needed to keep blood healthy and immune function strong.

Calcium, phosphorus, magnesium, and fluoride are needed to maintain the health of bones and teeth. ▶

NATIONAL GEOGRAPHIC

Cofactors FIGURE 8.12

The binding of a cofactor to an enzyme activates the enzyme. Coenzymes, discussed in Chapter 7, are a type of cofactor.

HOW IT WORKS
View in your WileyPLUS course

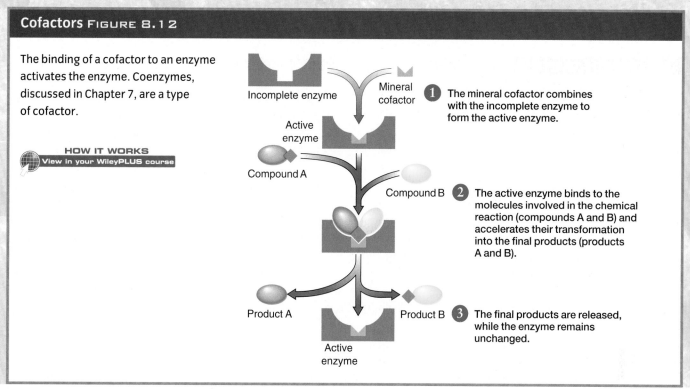

Incomplete enzyme

Mineral cofactor

1 The mineral cofactor combines with the incomplete enzyme to form the active enzyme.

Active enzyme

Compound A

Compound B

2 The active enzyme binds to the molecules involved in the chemical reaction (compounds A and B) and accelerates their transformation into the final products (products A and B).

Product A

Product B

3 The final products are released, while the enzyme remains unchanged.

Active enzyme

---

ion An atom or a group of atoms that carries an electrical charge.

The presence of one mineral can also interfere with the absorption of another. For example, mineral **ions** that carry the same charge compete for absorption in the gastrointestinal tract. Calcium, magnesium, zinc, copper, and iron all carry a 2+ charge, so a high intake of one may reduce the absorption of another. Although generally not a problem when whole foods are consumed, a large dose of one mineral from a dietary supplement may interfere with the absorption of other minerals.

The body's need for a mineral may also affect how much of that mineral is absorbed. For instance, if plenty of iron is stored in your body, you will absorb less of the iron you consume. Life stage can also affect absorption; for example, calcium absorption doubles during pregnancy, when the body's needs are high.

MINERAL FUNCTIONS

Minerals contribute to the body's structure and help regulate body processes (**FIGURE 8.11**). Many serve more than one function. For example, we need calcium to keep our bones strong as well as to maintain normal blood pressure, allow muscles to contract, and transmit nerve signals from cell to cell. Some minerals help regulate water balance, others help regulate energy production, and some affect growth and development through their role in the expression of certain genes. Many minerals act as **cofactors** needed for enzyme activity (**FIGURE 8.12**). None of the minerals we require acts in isolation. Instead, they interact with each other as well as with other nutrients and other components of the diet.

cofactor
An inorganic ion or coenzyme that is required for enzyme activity.

CONCEPT CHECK STOP

HOW do minerals and vitamins differ?

HOW do phytates, oxalates, and tannins decrease mineral bioavailability?

What is the function of a cofactor?

Electrolytes: Sodium, Potassium, and Chloride

W e think of **electrolytes** as the things we get by guzzling a sports drink. But what exactly are they, and why do we need them? Electrolytes are negatively or positively charged ions. Although many substances in the body are electrolytes, in nutrition, and in sports drinks, the term *electrolyte* refers to the three principal electrolytes in body fluids: sodium, potassium, and chloride. These electrolytes are important in maintaining fluid balance and allowing nerve impulses to travel throughout our bodies, signaling the activities that are essential for life.

electrolytes
Positively and negatively charged ions that conduct an electrical current in solution. Commonly refers to sodium, potassium, and chloride.

ELECTROLYTES IN THE BODY

Sodium and potassium carry a positive charge, and chloride carries a negative charge. Sodium is most commonly found combined with chloride as **sodium chloride**, what we call either "salt" or "table salt." The concentrations of sodium, potassium, and chloride inside a cell differ dramatically from those outside the cell. Potassium is the principal positively charged intracellular ion, sodium is the most abundant positively charged extracellular ion, and chloride is the principal negatively charged extracellular ion.

Functions of electrolytes Electrolytes help regulate fluid balance; the distribution of water throughout the body depends on the concentration of electrolytes and other solutes. Water moves by osmosis in response to differences in concentration. So, for example, if the concentration of sodium in the blood increases, water will move into the blood from intracellular and other extracellular spaces to equalize the concentration of sodium and other dissolved substances (**FIGURE 8.13A**).

Electrolyte functions FIGURE 8.13

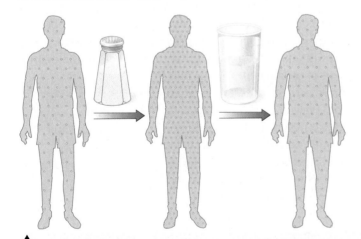

▲ A Have you ever noticed that you weigh a few extra pounds the morning after eating a salty dinner? The salt you consume in such a meal increases your blood sodium concentration and stimulates you to drink enough to dilute it. The extra pounds you see on the scale reflect the extra water you have temporarily stowed away.

B You feel a pinprick because it stimulates nerves beneath the surface of the skin. This stimulation increases the permeability of the nerve cell membrane to sodium and then to potassium. The sodium rushes in (shown here), initiating a nerve impulse. Potassium then rushes out to restore the electrical charge across the membrane. The increase in sodium permeability at one spot triggers an increase on the adjacent patch of membrane, spreading the nerve impulse along the nerve to the brain. Once the impulse has passed, the original ion concentrations inside and outside the membrane are restored by a sodium/potassium pump in the membrane so that a new nerve signal can be triggered. ▼

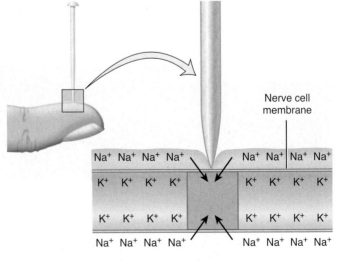

Nerve cell membrane

Regulation of blood pressure Figure 8.14

A drop in blood pressure triggers events that cause blood vessels to constrict and the kidneys to retain water. An increase in blood pressure inhibits these events so that blood pressure does not continue to rise.

Low blood pressure

Kidneys

1 A decrease in blood pressure triggers the kidneys to release the enzyme renin.

Renin helps form angiotensin II

2 Renin converts angiotensin into angiotensin I, which is activated to angiotensin II.

4 Angiotensin II stimulates release of the hormone **aldosterone** from the adrenal gland.

Release of aldosterone

Blood vessels constrict

3 Angiotensin II increases blood pressure by constricting the walls of blood vessels.

5 Aldosterone increases sodium reabsorption by the kidneys. Water follows the sodium, helping to maintain blood volume and blood pressure.

Kidneys retain sodium and water

Normal blood pressure

Sodium, potassium, and chloride are also essential for generating and conducting nerve impulses. Nerve impulses are created by the movement of sodium and potassium ions across the nerve cell membrane. When a nerve cell is at rest, potassium is concentrated inside the nerve cell, and sodium stays outside the cell. Sodium and potassium ions cannot pass freely across the cell membrane. But when a nerve is stimulated, the cell membrane becomes more permeable to sodium, allowing sodium ions to rush into the nerve cell, which initiates a nerve impulse (**Figure 8.13B**).

Regulating electrolyte balance

Our bodies are efficient at regulating the concentration of electrolytes, even when dietary intake varies dramatically. Sodium and chloride balance is regulated to some extent by the intake of both salt and water. When salt intake is high, thirst is stimulated in order to increase water intake. Very low salt intake stimulates a "salt appetite" that causes you to crave salt. The craving that triggers your desire to plunge into a bag of salty chips, however, is not due to this salt appetite. It is a learned preference, not a physiological drive. If you cut back on your salt intake, you will find that your taste buds become more sensitive to the presence of salt, and foods taste saltier.

Thirst and salt appetite help ensure that appropriate proportions of salt and water are taken in, but the kidneys are the primary regulator of sodium, potassium,

and chloride concentrations in the body. Excretion of these electrolytes in the urine is decreased when intake is low and increased when intake is high.

Because water follows sodium by osmosis, the ability of the kidneys to conserve sodium provides a mechanism for conserving water in the body. This mechanism also helps regulate blood pressure. When the concentration of sodium in the blood increases, water follows, causing an increase in blood volume. Changes in blood volume can change blood pressure. Changes in blood pressure, in turn, trigger the production and release of proteins and hormones that affect the amount of sodium, and hence water, retained by the kidneys (**Figure 8.14**).

Regulation of blood potassium levels is also important. Even a small increase can be dangerous. If blood potassium levels begin to rise, body cells are stimulated to take up potassium. This short-term regulation prevents the amount of potassium in the extracellular fluid from getting lethally high. Long-term regulation of potassium balance depends on the release of proteins that cause the kidney to excrete potassium and retain sodium.

ELECTROLYTES IN HEALTH AND DISEASE

Electrolyte deficiencies are uncommon in healthy people. Sodium, potassium, and chloride are plentiful in most diets, and the kidneys of healthy individuals are efficient

hypertension
Blood pressure that is consistently elevated to 140/90 mm mercury or greater.

at regulating the amounts of these electrolytes in the body. Acute deficiencies and excesses can occur due to illness or extreme conditions. The health problem most commonly associated with electrolyte imbalance is **hypertension**, or high blood pressure. Hypertension is a serious public health concern in the United States; about 25% of adult Americans and more than half of those over age 60 years have hypertension.[4] Of these, 30% don't know they have it.

Electrolyte deficiency

Deficiencies of any of the electrolytes can lead to electrolyte imbalance, which can cause disturbances in acid–base balance, poor appetite, muscle cramps, confusion, apathy, constipation, and, eventually, irregular heartbeat. For example, the sudden death that can occur as a result of fasting, anorexia nervosa, or starvation may be due to heart failure caused by potassium deficiency. Sodium, chloride, and potassium depletion can occur when losses of these electrolytes are increased by heavy and persistent sweating, chronic diarrhea or vomiting, or kidney disorders that lead to excessive excretion. Medications can also interfere with electrolyte balance. For example, certain diuretic medications that are used to treat high blood pressure cause potassium loss.

Electrolyte toxicity

It is not possible for healthy people to consume too much potassium from foods. If, however, supplements are consumed in excess or kidney function is compromised, blood levels of potassium can increase and potentially cause death due to an irregular heartbeat. A high oral dose of potassium generally causes vomiting, but if too much potassium enters the blood, it can cause the heart to stop.

It is difficult to consume more sodium than the body can handle because we usually drink more water when we consume more sodium. Though rare, elevation of blood sodium can result from massive ingestion of salt, such as may occur from drinking seawater or consuming salt tablets. The most common cause of high blood sodium is dehydration and the symptoms are similar to those of dehydration.

Hypertension

Hypertension, or high blood pressure, has been called "the silent killer" because it has no outward symptoms but can lead to atherosclerosis, heart attack, stroke, kidney disease, and early death. It is caused by an increase in blood volume or a narrowing of the blood vessels. Hypertension is a complex disorder resulting from disturbances in one or more of the mechanisms that control body fluid and electrolyte balance.

Elevated blood pressure is treated with diet, exercise, and medication. To allow early treatment and avoid the potentially lethal side effects of elevated blood pressure, people should have their blood pressure monitored regularly. A healthy blood pressure is 120/80 mm of mercury or less. Blood pressure between 120/80 and 139/89 is referred to as **prehypertension**, and blood pressure that is consistently 140/90 mm of mercury or greater indicates hypertension (see Appendix C).[6]

Some of the risk of developing hypertension is genetic; your risk is increased if you have a family history of the disease. It is more common in African Americans than in Mexican Americans or non-Hispanic whites.[7] Whether you are genetically predisposed to hypertension or not, your risk of developing high blood pressure increases as you grow older and is higher if you are overweight, particularly if your excess fat is in your abdominal region. Lack of physical activity, heavy alcohol consumption, and stress can also increase blood pressure.[8] Regular exercise can prevent or delay the onset of hypertension, and weight loss can help reduce blood pressure in obese individuals. Your risk of developing high blood pressure can also be increased or decreased by your dietary choices.

Diet and blood pressure

Dietary intake of sodium, chloride, potassium, calcium, and magnesium can affect your blood pressure and your risk of hypertension. Diets that are high in salt (sodium chloride) are associated with an increased incidence of hypertension, whereas diets that are high in potassium, calcium, and magnesium are associated with a lower average blood pressure.[9,10] Other components of the diet, such as the amount of fiber and the type and amount of fat, may also affect your risk of developing hypertension. Although changing any one of these dietary factors has only a minor impact on blood pressure, a dietary pattern that incorporates the recommended amounts of each of these can have a significant impact on blood pressure. The **DASH (Dietary Approaches to Stop Hypertension) diet** does just that.

The DASH diet provides moderate amounts of sodium and plenty of fiber, potassium, magnesium, and calcium; it is low in total fat, saturated fat, and cholesterol (see Appendix D). Following the DASH diet lowers blood pressure in individuals with elevated blood pressure. Reductions in blood pressure are even greater when the DASH diet is combined with a reduction in sodium intake (**FIGURE 8.15**).[11,12]

Visualizing

The effect of diet on blood pressure FIGURE 8.15

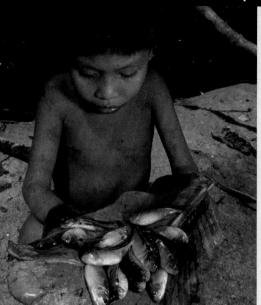

This Yanomami Indian boy lives in the rainforests of Brazil. The Yanomami diet consists of locally grown crops, nuts, insects, fish, and game. It contains less than a gram of salt a day, the lowest salt intake recorded for any population. The Yanomami have very low average blood pressure and no hypertension. Studying the salt intake and blood pressure of the Yanomami and 51 other populations around the world helped to establish a relationship between salt intake and hypertension; diets that are high in salt are associated with an increased incidence of hypertension.[9]

A diet that is high in fruits and vegetables, which are good sources of potassium, magnesium, and fiber, reduces blood pressure compared to a similar diet containing fewer fruits and vegetables. The amounts in the measuring cups shown here, about 2 cups of fruit and 2½ cups of vegetables, represent the amount recommended for a 2000-Calorie DASH diet.[13]

The original DASH diet provided about 3000 mg of sodium/day, an amount only slightly less than the typical intake in the United States. When the sodium content of this diet was lowered, there was an even greater reduction in blood pressure. Lowering sodium also reduced blood pressure in the group consuming a typical American diet.[12]

A blood pressure measurement is two numbers: systolic over diastolic

120/80

Systolic is the maximum pressure in the arteries →

Diastolic is the minimum pressure in the arteries →

Systolic blood pressure (mm mercury)

- Typical American diet
- DASH diet

Diastolic blood pressure (mm mercury)

Dietary sodium level — Intermediate / Low

DASH diet recommendations for a 2000–calorie diet

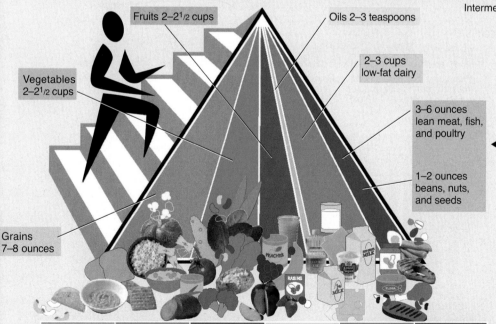

Fruits 2–2½ cups

Oils 2–3 teaspoons

2–3 cups low-fat dairy

3–6 ounces lean meat, fish, and poultry

1–2 ounces beans, nuts, and seeds

Vegetables 2–2½ cups

Grains 7–8 ounces

The DASH diet (upper portion of the figure) is abundant in fruits and vegetables; includes low-fat dairy products, whole grains, legumes, and nuts, and incorporates moderate amounts of lean meat. These recommendations are similar to those of MyPyramid: (bottom of figure) Choose whole grains; eat plenty of fruits and vegetables; have beans, nuts, and seeds more often; and keep discretionary calories low by choosing lean meats and low-fat dairy products.

GRAINS	VEGETABLES	FRUITS	OILS	MILK	MEAT & BEANS
6 ounces	2½ cups	2 cups	6 teaspoons	3 cups	5½ ounces

My Pyramid recommendations for 2000–calorie diet

NATIONAL GEOGRAPHIC

Use iProfile to compare the sodium content of fresh vegetables with that of canned vegetables.

WHAT SHOULD I EAT? Water and Electrolytes

Stay hydrated
- Drink before, during, and after you exercise.
- Guzzle two extra glasses of water when you are out on a hot day.
- Bring a bottle of water with you in your car.

Boost your potassium intake
- Double your vegetable serving at dinner.
- Take two pieces of fruit for lunch.
- Drink orange juice instead of soda or punch.

Reduce your sodium intake
- Choose more unprocessed foods.
- Do not add salt to the water when cooking rice, pasta, and cereals.
- Flavor foods with lemon juice, onions, garlic, pepper, curry, basil, oregano, or thyme rather than with salt.
- Limit salty snacks such as potato chips, salted nuts, salted popcorn, and crackers.
- Limit condiments such as soy sauce, barbecue sauce, ketchup, and mustard; they are high in sodium.

MEETING ELECTROLYTE NEEDS

Most people in the United States need to reduce their salt intake and increase their potassium intake to meet recommendations for a healthy diet (see *What Should I Eat?*). The recommended salt intake is 3800 mg/day for adults ages 19 to 50. Because salt is 40% sodium and 60% chloride by weight, this represents 1500 mg of sodium and 2300 mg of chloride. The Daily Value for sodium is somewhat higher—no more than 2400 mg of sodium/day. The UL for sodium, which is based on the increase in blood pressure seen with higher sodium

Processing adds sodium
FIGURE 8.16

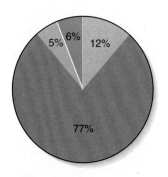

- Home cooking
- Salt shaker at the table
- Naturally present in foods
- Added to processed food

▲ A About 77% of the salt we eat comes from processed foods. Only about 12% comes from salt found naturally in food, while 11% comes from salt added in cooking and at the table.[14]

B Processed foods are generally higher in sodium and may also be lower in potassium than unprocessed foods. Some of the sodium in processed foods comes from salt added for flavoring; some is added as a preservative to inhibit microbial growth. In addition to sodium chloride, sodium bicarbonate, sodium citrate, and sodium glutamate are added to preserve and flavor foods. ▼

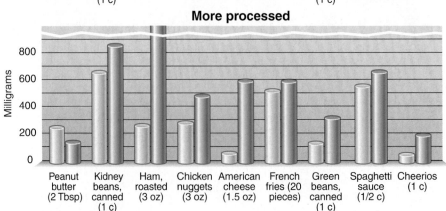

intakes, is only 2300 mg/day. The typical daily intake of sodium in the U.S. diet is between 2400 and 4800 mg of sodium.

The DRIs recommend a potassium intake of 4700 mg/day; the Daily Value is at least 3500 mg/day for adults. This amount is significantly higher than the typical 2000 to 3000 mg consumed by most Americans. No UL has been set for potassium.

One of the reasons our diet is high in salt (sodium chloride) and low in potassium is that we eat a lot of processed foods, which are high in sodium and chloride, and too few fresh unprocessed foods, such as fruits, vegetables, whole grains, and fresh meats, which are high in potassium. Over three-quarters of the salt we eat is from foods that have had salt added during processing and manufacturing (FIGURE 8.16).

You can lower the amount of sodium in your diet by limiting your intake of processed foods and cutting down on the amount of salt added in cooking and at the table. A diet that is high in fruits and vegetables will easily meet potassium intake recommendations; daily intakes of 8000 to 11,000 mg are not uncommon.[4] Food labels can help identify low-sodium foods (FIGURE 8.17). Some medications can also contribute a significant amount of sodium. Drug facts labels on over-the-counter medications can help identify those that contain large amounts of sodium.

TABLE 8.1, on the next page, summarizes information about water, sodium, chloride, and potassium.

Sodium on food labels FIGURE 8.17

Food labels are an important source of information about the sodium content of packaged foods. In addition to the information illustrated here, a food that meets the definition for *low-sodium* and provides 20% or less of the Daily Value for fat, saturated fat, and cholesterol per serving can include on the label the health claim that diets that are low in sodium may reduce the risk of high blood pressure.

Nutrition Facts
Serving Size 1/2 cup (125g)
Servings Per Container about 3½

Amount Per Serving		
Calories 50	Calories from Fat 10	
		%Daily Value**
Total Fat 1g		**2%**
Saturated Fat 0g		**0%**
Cholesterol 0mg		**0%**
Sodium 250mg		**10%**
Potassium 530mg		**15%**
Total Carbohydrate 9g		**3%**
Dietary Fiber 1g		**4%**
Sugars 7g		
Protein 2g		

Vitamin A 10%	•	Vitamin C 25%
Calcium 2%	•	Iron 10%

*Percent Daily Values are based on a 2,000 calorie diet. Your daily values may be higher or lower depending on your calorie needs.

	Calories:	2,000	2,500
Total Fat	Less than	65g	80g
Sat Fat	Less than	20g	25g
Cholesterol	Less than	300mg	300mg
Sodium	Less than	2,400mg	2,400mg
Potassium		3,500mg	3,500mg
Total Carbohydrate		300g	375g
Dietary Fiber		25g	30g

The Nutrition Facts section lists the total amount of sodium per serving and the percentage of the Daily Value this amount represents.

The Daily Value for sodium for a 2000-Calorie diet is given at the bottom of the label.

Light Spaghetti Sauce, 250 milligrams (mg) per serving
Regular Spaghetti Sauce, 500mg per serving

SPAGHETTI SAUCE
LIGHT IN SODIUM
50% Less Sodium than our regular spaghetti sauce (See side panel for nutrition information.)

"Light in sodium" means that this food contains 50% less sodium than regular spaghetti sauce. "Sodium free" means that a food contains less than 5 mg of sodium per serving, "low sodium" means that a food contains 140 mg or less of sodium per serving, and "reduced sodium" means that a food contains at least 25% less sodium than a reference food.

A summary of water and the electrolytes TABLE 8.1

Nutrient	Sources	Recommended intake for adults	Major functions	Deficiency diseases and symptoms	Groups at risk of deficiency	Toxicity	UL
Water	Drinking water, other beverages, and food	2.7–3.7 L/day	Solvent, reactant, protector, transporter, regulator of temperature and pH	Thirst, weakness, poor endurance, confusion, disorientation	Infants, people with fever and diarrhea, elderly individuals, athletes	Confusion, coma, convulsions	ND
Sodium	Table salt, processed foods	<2300 mg; ideally 1500 mg/day	Major positive extracellular ion, nerve transmission, muscle contraction, fluid balance	Muscle cramps	People consuming a severely sodium-restricted diet, those who sweat excessively	High blood pressure in sensitive people	2300 mg/day
Potassium	Fresh fruits and vegetables, legumes, whole grains, milk, meat	4700 mg/day or more	Major positive intracellular ion, nerve transmission, muscle contraction, fluid balance	Irregular heartbeat, fatigue, muscle cramps	People consuming poor diets high in processed foods, those taking thiazide diuretics	Abnormal heartbeat	ND
Chloride	Table salt, processed foods	<3600 mg/day; ideally 2300 mg/day	Major negative extracellular ion, fluid balance	Unlikely	None	None likely	3600 mg/day

Note: UL, Tolerable Upper Intake Level; ND, not determined.

CONCEPT CHECK STOP

Why does eating a salty meal cause your weight to increase temporarily?

Why is hypertension called "the silent killer"?

What is the DASH diet?

Which types of foods contribute the most sodium to the American diet?

Major Minerals and Bone Health

LEARNING OBJECTIVES

Describe factors that affect peak bone mass and the rate of bone loss.

Explain how blood calcium levels are regulated.

List foods that are good sources of calcium.

Describe functions of calcium, phosphorus, and magnesium that are unrelated to their role in bone.

Bones are the hardest, strongest structures in the human body. They support our weight, whether we are stepping off a curb or jumping rope. Age, however, heralds a loss of bone strength. For many people, the loss is so great that the force of stepping off a curb is enough to cause their bones to fracture.

Bone is strong because it is composed of a protein framework, or matrix, that is hardened by deposits of minerals. This matrix consists primarily of the protein collagen.

The mineral portion of bone is composed mainly of calcium associated with phosphorus, but it also contains magnesium, sodium, fluoride, and a number of other minerals. Healthy bone requires adequate dietary protein and vitamin C to maintain the collagen and a sufficient supply of calcium and other minerals to ensure solidity. Adequate vitamin D (discussed in Chapter 7) is needed to maintain appropriate levels of calcium and phosphorus. There is also growing evidence of the importance of vitamin K for bone health.[15]

bone remodeling

A continuous process in which small amounts of bone are removed and replaced by new bone.

BONE IN HEALTH AND DISEASE

Like other tissues in the body, bone is alive, and it is constantly being broken down and re-formed through a process called **bone remodeling**. Most bone is formed early in life. During childhood, bones grow larger; even after growth stops, bone mass continues to increase into young adulthood (FIGURE 8.18A). The maximum amount of bone that you have in

Visualizing

Bone mass and osteoporosis FIGURE 8.18

A Changes in the balance between bone formation and bone breakdown cause bone mass to increase in children and adolescents and decrease in adults as they grow older. ▼

Both men and women lose bone slowly after about age 35.

In growing children, total bone mass increases as the bones grow larger.

Men achieve a higher peak bone mass than do women.

In women, bone loss is accelerated for about 5 years after menopause.

— Males
— Females

During puberty, bone mass increases rapidly, and sex differences in bone mass appear.

Bone mass / Age (years) 0 10 20 30 40 50 60 70 80

Bone weakened by osteoporosis   Normal bone

▲

B Osteoporosis, shown here compared to normal bone, is a major public health problem in the United States and elsewhere around the world. In the United States, about 10 million people over age 50 have osteoporosis, and another 34 million are at risk due to low bone mass, called **osteopenia**.[16]

C Osteoporosis leads to 1.5 million fractures annually, which account for $18 billion per year in direct medical costs.[16] Spinal compression fractures, shown here, are common and may result in loss of height and a stooped posture (called a "dowager's hump"). ▶

Normal spine   Osteoporotic spine

When weakened by osteoporosis, the front edge of the vertebrae collapses more than the back edge, so the spine bends forward.

NATIONAL GEOGRAPHIC

peak bone mass
The maximum bone density attained at any time in life, usually occurring in young adulthood.

osteoporosis
A bone disorder characterized by reduced bone mass, increased bone fragility, and increased risk of fractures.

your lifetime, called **peak bone mass**, is achieved somewhere between the ages of 16 and 30. Up to this point, bone formation occurs more rapidly than breakdown, so the total amount of bone increases. After about age 35 to 45, the amount of bone that is broken down begins to exceed the amount that is formed, so total bone mass decreases. Over time, if enough bone is lost, the skeleton is weakened, and fractures occur more easily, a condition referred to as **osteoporosis** (Figure 8.18b, c).

Factors affecting the risk of osteoporosis

The risk of developing osteoporosis depends on the level of peak bone mass and the rate at which bone is lost. These variables are affected by genetics, gender, age, hormone levels, and lifestyle factors such as smoking, alcohol consumption, exercise, and diet (Table 8.2).

Women have a higher risk of osteoporosis because they have less bone than men and lose it faster as they age. **Age-related bone loss** occurs in

age-related bone loss The bone loss that occurs in both men and women as they advance in age.

both men and women, but women lose additional bone for about five years after **menopause**. This **postmenopausal bone loss** is related to the decline in estrogen level, which affects bone cells and decreases the amount of calcium absorbed in the intestines. A low calcium intake is the most significant dietary factor contributing to osteoporosis (see *What a Scientist Sees*). The effect of diet on bone mass is discussed in more depth later in the chapter.

A factor that is associated with a reduced risk of osteoporosis is excess body weight.[18] Having greater body weight, whether that weight is due to an increase in muscle mass or to excess body fat, increases bone mass because it increases the amount of weight the bones must support. In other words, stressing the bones makes them grow stronger. A similar effect is seen in people of all body weights who engage in weight-bearing exercise. In postmenopausal women, excess body fat may also reduce risk because adipose tissue is an important source of estrogen, which helps maintain bone mass and enhances calcium absorption.

menopause
The time in a woman's life when the menstrual cycle ends.

postmenopausal bone loss
The accelerated bone loss that occurs in women for about five years after the menstrual cycle stops.

Factors affecting the risk of osteoporosis TABLE 8.2

Risk factor	How it affects risk
Gender	Fractures due to osteoporosis are about twice as common in women as in men. Men are larger and heavier than women and therefore have a greater peak bone mass. Women lose more bone than men due to postmenopausal bone loss.
Age	Bone loss is a normal part of aging, and risk increases with age.
Race	African Americans have denser bones than do Caucasians and Southeast Asians, so their risk of osteoporosis is lower.[16]
Family history	Having a family member with osteoporosis increases risk.
Body size	Individuals who are thin and light have an increased risk because they have less bone mass.
Smoking	Tobacco use weakens bones.
Exercise	Weight-bearing exercise, such as walking and jogging, throughout life strengthens bone, and increasing weight-bearing exercise at any age can increase your bone density.
Alcohol abuse	Long-term alcohol abuse reduces bone formation and interferes with the body's ability to absorb calcium.
Diet	A diet that is lacking in calcium and vitamin D plays a major role in the development of osteoporosis. Low calcium intake during the years of bone formation results in a lower peak bone mass, and low calcium intake in adulthood can accelerate bone loss.

Soda Versus Milk

Carbonated beverages have become a part of American culture. The average woman in her 20s drinks two 12-ounce sodas a day; teenage boys drink about two and a half.[17] When you grab a can of soda from a vending machine, convenience store, fast-food

	Low–fat milk	Cola soft drink
Serving size (oz)	8	12
Energy (kcal)	102	150
Protein (g)	8	0
Calcium (mg)	300	0
Phosphorus (mg)	235	45
Riboflavin (mg)	0.4	0
Vitamin A (mg)	144	0
Vitamin D (mg)	2.5	0
Caffeine (mg)	0	40

restaurant, or grocery store, you see a cold, delicious beverage . What a scientist sees is the beverage's nutritional impact. A 12-ounce can of soda contains about 10 teaspoons of sugar and few other nutrients. Replacing an 8-ounce glass of milk with a 12-ounce soda increases the amount of added sugar in the diet by about 40 grams and reduces protein, calcium, vitamin A, vitamin D, and riboflavin intake.

Teenage boys and girls today drink twice as much soda as milk, whereas 20 years ago, boys drank more than twice as much milk as soda, and girls drank 50% more milk than soda.[17] Milk is the major source of calcium in the U.S. diet, so as milk is being replaced by soda, the reduction in calcium intake is of great concern. Teenage girls consume only 60% of the recommended amount of calcium, with soda drinkers consuming almost one-fifth less calcium than those who don't drink soda.[17] Osteoporosis is a major problem among older adults today, and when these adults were children, they drank twice as much milk as kids do today. How do you think the trend away from milk consumption will affect the incidence of osteoporosis 30 years from now?

Preventing and treating osteoporosis You can't feel your bones weakening, so people with osteoporosis may not know that their bone mass is dangerously low until they are in their 50s or 60s and experience a bone fracture. Once osteoporosis has developed, it is difficult to restore lost bone. Therefore, the best treatment for osteoporosis is to prevent it by achieving a high peak bone mass and slowing the rate of bone loss. A diet that contains adequate amounts of calcium and vitamin D produces greater peak bone mass and slows bone loss. Higher intakes of zinc, magnesium, potassium, fiber, and vitamin C—nutrients that are plentiful in fruits and vegetables—are also associated with greater bone mass.[19] Maintaining an active lifestyle that includes weight-bearing exercise and limits smoking and alcohol consumption will further increase and maintain bone density.

Risk of osteoporosis can be increased by high intakes of phytate, oxalates, and tannins, which reduce calcium absorption, and by high dietary sodium intake, which increases calcium loss in the urine.[20] High protein intake also increases urinary calcium losses, but high levels of protein do not have a negative effect on bone mass when calcium intake is adequate.[21]

Osteoporosis is commonly treated with estrogen to reduce bone breakdown and increase calcium absorption, along with supplements of calcium and vitamin D and regular weight-bearing exercise. Treatments also include other hormones and drugs, called bisphosphonates that inhibit the activity of cells that break down bone. Bisphosphonates have been shown to prevent postmenopausal bone loss, increase bone mineral density, and reduce the risk of fractures. Their effectiveness is enhanced by calcium supplementation.[22]

CALCIUM

In an average person, about 1.5% of body weight is due to calcium, and 99% of this is found in the bones and teeth. The remaining calcium is located in body cells and fluids, where it is needed for muscle contraction, release of neurotransmitters, blood pressure regulation, cell communication, blood clotting, and other essential functions. Neurotransmitter release is critical to nerve function because neurotransmitters relay nerve impulses from one nerve to another and from nerves to other cells. Calcium in muscle cells is essential for muscle contraction because it allows the muscle proteins actin and myosin to interact. Calcium may help regulate blood pressure by controlling the contraction of muscles in the blood vessel walls and signaling the secretion of substances that regulate blood pressure.

Calcium in health and disease
The various roles of calcium are so vital to survival that powerful regulatory mechanisms maintain calcium concentrations both inside and outside cells. Slight changes in blood calcium levels trigger the release of hormones that work to keep calcium levels constant. When calcium levels drop, *parathyroid hormone (PTH)* is released (see Chapter 7). PTH acts in a number of tissues to increase blood calcium levels (**FIGURE 8.19**). If blood calcium levels become too high, PTH secretion stops, and **calcitonin** is released. Calcitonin is a hormone that acts primarily on bone to inhibit the release of calcium into the blood.

When too little calcium is consumed, the body maintains normal blood levels by breaking down bone to release calcium, a process called **bone resorption**. This process provides a steady supply of calcium and causes no short-term symptoms. Over time, however, a calcium deficiency can reduce bone mass. Low calcium intake during the years of bone formation results in lower peak bone mass. If calcium intake is low after peak bone mass has been achieved, the rate of bone loss may be increased and, along with it, the risk of osteoporosis.

Too much calcium can also affect health. Elevated blood calcium levels can cause symptoms such as loss of appetite, nausea, vomiting, constipation, abdominal pain, thirst, and frequent urination. Severe elevation may

Raising blood calcium levels FIGURE 8.19

Low blood calcium triggers the secretion of parathyroid hormone (PTH) from the parathyroid gland. PTH stimulates the release of calcium from bone and causes the kidneys to reduce calcium loss in the urine and to activate vitamin D. Activated vitamin D increases the absorption of calcium from the gastrointestinal tract and acts with PTH to stimulate calcium release from the bone. The overall effect of PTH is to rapidly restore blood calcium levels to normal.

Low blood calcium

Parathyroid hormone

Stimulates calcium release from bone

Reduces calcium lost in urine

Activates vitamin D

Increases intestinal calcium absorption

Normal blood calcium

Dairy products are an important source of calcium. Fish, such as sardines, that are consumed with the bones are also a good source, as are legumes, almonds, and some green vegetables, such as kale and broccoli. Grains are a moderate source, but because we consume them in large quantities, they make a significant contribution to our calcium intake.

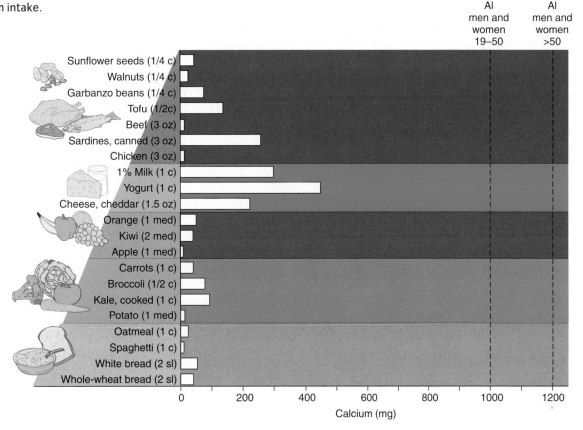

cause confusion, delirium, coma, and even death. Because the level of calcium in the blood is finely regulated, elevated blood calcium is rare and is most often caused by cancer and by disorders that increase the secretion of PTH. It can also result from increases in intestinal calcium absorption due to excessive vitamin D intake or high intakes of calcium in combination with antacids.

High calcium intake from supplements can interfere with the availability of iron, zinc, magnesium, and phosphorus and may promote the formation of kidney stones in some individuals.[22] Based on the occurrence of kidney stones and elevated blood calcium, as well as the potential for decreased absorption of other essential minerals, the UL for calcium in adults has been set at 2500 mg/day.

Meeting calcium needs
For adults ages 19 to 50, recommended calcium intake is 1000 mg/day. The recommended intake is higher in older adults because

their calcium absorption is decreased due to lower blood levels of the active form of vitamin D and a decrease in responsiveness to vitamin D.[23] An additional drop in calcium absorption occurs in women after menopause due to the decrease in estrogen levels. Calcium absorption is higher at times when the body's need for calcium is greater. In young adults, about 25% of dietary calcium is absorbed; during pregnancy, when the fetal skeleton is forming, the rate of absorption increases to over 50%; and during infancy, about 60% of dietary calcium is absorbed.

The main source of calcium in the North American diet is dairy products (FIGURE 8.20). Individuals who do not consume dairy products can meet their calcium needs by consuming leafy dark green vegetables, fish consumed with bones, foods processed with calcium, and foods fortified with calcium, such as juices and breakfast cereals.

Individuals who do not meet their calcium needs through their diet alone can benefit from calcium supplements (FIGURE 8.21). In young individuals, supplemental calcium can increase peak bone mass. In postmenopausal women, calcium supplements are not effective at increasing bone mass, but they can help reduce the rate of bone loss.

Whether your calcium comes from foods or from supplements, bioavailability must be considered. Vitamin D is the nutrient that has the most significant impact on calcium absorption. When calcium intake is high, calcium is absorbed by diffusion, but when intake is low to moderate, as it typically is, absorption depends on the active form of vitamin D. When vitamin D is deficient, less than 10% of dietary calcium may be absorbed, compared to the typical 25% when it is present. Other dietary components that affect calcium absorption include acidic foods, lactose, and fat, which increase calcium absorption, and oxalates, phytates, tannins, and fiber, which inhibit calcium absorption. For example, spinach is a high-calcium vegetable, but only about 5% of its calcium is absorbed; the rest is bound by oxalates and excreted in the feces.[24] Vegetables such as kale, collard greens, turnip greens, mustard greens, and Chinese cabbage are low in oxalates, so their calcium is more readily absorbed.

Chocolate also contains oxalates, but chocolate milk is still a good source of calcium because the amount of oxalates from the chocolate added to a glass of milk is small.

PHOSPHORUS

Most of the phosphorus in your body is associated with calcium as part of the hard mineral crystals in bones and teeth. The smaller amount of phosphorus in soft tissues performs an essential role as a structural component of phospholipids, DNA and RNA, and ATP. It is also important in regulating the activity of enzymes and maintaining the proper level of acidity in cells (FIGURE 8.22).

Phosphorus in health and disease Blood levels of phosphorus are not controlled as strictly as calcium levels, but the kidneys help maintain phosphorus levels in a ratio with calcium that allows minerals to be deposited into bone. A deficiency of phosphorus can lead to bone loss, weakness, and loss of appetite. Inadequate phosphorus intake is rare because phosphorus is widely distributed in food. Marginal phosphorus status may be caused by losses due to chronic diarrhea or poor absorption due to overuse of aluminum-containing antacids.

Calcium supplements FIGURE 8.21

If you are not getting enough calcium from foods, a supplement that contains a calcium compound alone or calcium with vitamin D can help you meet your calcium needs. A multivitamin/ multimineral supplement will provide only a small amount of the calcium you need. Use the Supplement Facts label to choose an appropriate supplement.

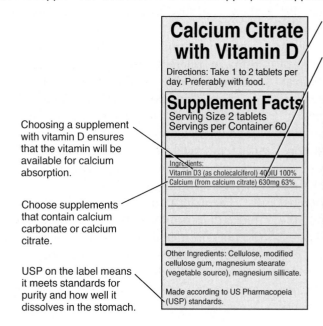

500 mg taken twice a day provides 100% of the AI for adults ages 19 to 50.

Calcium is absorbed best when taken in doses of 500 mg or less.

Choosing a supplement with vitamin D ensures that the vitamin will be available for calcium absorption.

Choose supplements that contain calcium carbonate or calcium citrate.

USP on the label means it meets standards for purity and how well it dissolves in the stomach.

Calcium Citrate with Vitamin D
Directions: Take 1 to 2 tablets per day. Preferably with food.

Supplement Facts
Serving Size 2 tablets
Servings per Container 60

Ingredients:
Vitamin D3 (as cholecalciferol) 400IU 100%
Calcium (from calcium citrate) 630mg 63%

Other Ingredients: Cellulose, modified cellulose gum, magnesium stearate (vegetable source), magnesium sillicate.

Made according to US Pharmacopeia (USP) standards.

Some antacids are also sources of calcium. These are over-the-counter medications, so they carry a Drug Facts panel rather than a Supplement Facts panel.

Most of the phosphorus in the body helps form the structure of bones and teeth. Phosphorus also plays an important role in a host of cellular activities.

Phosphorus is important in energy metabolism because the high-energy bonds of ATP are formed between phosphate groups.

Phosphorus is a component of phospholipids, which form the structure of cell membranes.

Phosphorus is involved in regulating enzyme activity; the addition of a phosphorus-containing group to certain enzymes can activate or inactivate them.

Phosphorus is a major constituent of DNA and RNA, which orchestrate the synthesis of proteins.

Phosphorus is part of a compound that can prevent changes in acidity so that chemical reactions inside the cell can proceed normally.

Mitochondria   Cell membrane   Nucleus   Cytoplasm

Excessive phosphorus intake can lead to bone loss. Although current levels of phosphorus intake in the United States are not believed to contribute to osteoporosis as long as calcium intake is adequate, there is concern that the increased use of food additives that contain phosphorus, particularly in soft drinks, which often replace milk, may affect bone health.[25] The UL for phosphorus is 4000 mg/day for adults.[22]

Meeting phosphorus needs

Dairy products such as milk, yogurt, and cheese, as well as meat, cereals, bran, eggs, nuts, and fish, are good sources of phosphorus. Food additives used in baked goods, cheese, processed meats, and soft drinks also provide phosphorus. Most diets meet the RDA of 700 mg/day for adults.[22]

MAGNESIUM

Magnesium is far less abundant in the body than are calcium and phosphorus, but it is still essential for healthy bones. About 50% to 60% of the magnesium in the body is in bone, where it helps maintain bone structure. The rest of the magnesium is found in cells and fluids throughout the body. Magnesium is involved in regulating calcium homeostasis and is needed for the action of vitamin D and many hormones, including PTH. Magnesium is important for the regulation of blood pressure and may play a role in maintaining cardiovascular health. In addition, magnesium forms a complex with ATP that stabilizes ATP's structure. It is therefore needed in every metabolic reaction that generates or uses ATP. This includes reactions needed for the release of energy from carbohydrate, fat, and protein; the functioning of the nerves and muscles; and the synthesis of DNA, RNA, and protein, making it particularly important for dividing, growing cells.

Magnesium in health and disease

Although overt magnesium deficiency is rare, the typical intake of magnesium in the United States is below the RDA. Low intakes of magnesium have been associated with a number of chronic diseases, including osteoporosis.[26] Magnesium deficiency can cause nausea, muscle weakness and cramping, irritability, mental derangement, and changes in blood pressure and heartbeat. As discussed earlier, dietary patterns that are high in magnesium are associated with lower blood pressure, and epidemiological evidence suggests that the risk of atherosclerosis is lower for people with adequate magnesium intake than for those with less magnesium in their diet.[27] Areas with "hard" water, which is high in calcium and magnesium, tend to have lower rates of death from cardiovascular disease. Low blood magnesium levels affect levels of blood calcium and

Sources of magnesium

FIGURE 8.23

Magnesium is a component of the green pigment chlorophyll, so leafy greens such as spinach and kale are good sources of this mineral. Nuts, seeds, legumes, bananas, and the germ and bran of whole grains are also good sources of magnesium. The dashed lines represent the RDA of 420 and 320 mg/day for adult men and women over age 30, respectively.[22]

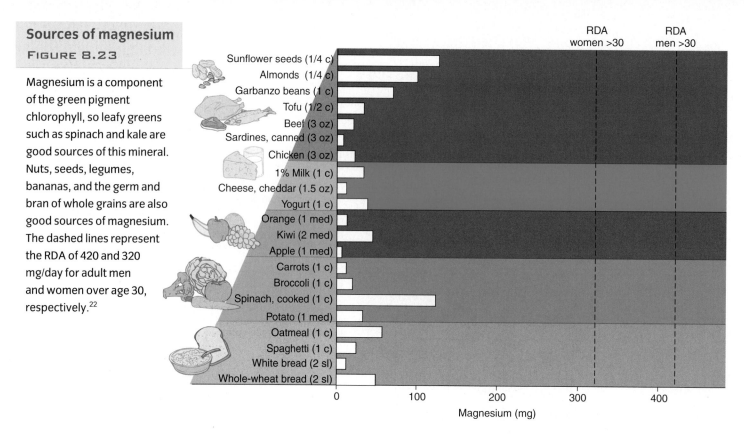

potassium; therefore, some of the symptoms of magnesium deficiency may be due to alterations in the levels of these other minerals.

No adverse effects have been observed from magnesium consumed in foods, but toxicity may occur from drugs containing magnesium, such as milk of magnesia and supplements that include magnesium. Magnesium toxicity causes nausea, vomiting, low blood pressure, and other cardiovascular changes. The UL for adults and adolescents over age 9 is 350 mg of magnesium from supplements or medications.[22]

Meeting magnesium needs
Magnesium is found in many foods but in small amounts, so you can't get all you need from a single food (**FIGURE 8.23** and *What Should I Eat?*). Enriched grain products are poor sources because magnesium is lost in processing, and it is not added back by enrichment. For example, removing the bran and germ

WHAT SHOULD I EAT? | **Calcium, Phosphorus, and Magnesium**

Use iProfile to find a nondairy source of calcium.

Get calcium into your body and your bones
- Have three servings of dairy a day: milk, yogurt, cheese.
- Bone up on calcium by eating sardines or canned salmon, which are eaten with the bones.
- Choose leafy greens—they are a vegetable source of calcium.
- Walk, jog, or jump up and down—weight-bearing exercises build up bone.

Don't fret about phosphorus—it's in almost everything you eat.

Maximize your magnesium
- Choose whole grains.
- Sprinkle nuts and seeds on your salad, cereal, and stir-fry.
- Go for the green—whenever you eat green, you are eating magnesium; most greens contain calcium, too.

from wheat kernels reduces the magnesium content of a cup of white flour to only 28 mg, compared with the 166 mg in a cup of whole-wheat flour. Magnesium absorption is enhanced by the active form of vitamin D and decreased by the presence of phytates and calcium.

SULFUR

Sulfur is part of the proteins in bones and other parts of the body because the amino acids methionine and cysteine, needed for protein synthesis, contain sulfur. Cysteine is also part of glutathione, a molecule that plays an important role in detoxifying drugs and protecting cells from oxidative damage. The vitamins thiamin and biotin, which are essential for energy metabolism, also contain sulfur, and sulfur-containing ions are important in regulating acidity in the body.

We consume sulfur as a part of dietary proteins and the sulfur-containing vitamins. Sulfur is also found in some food preservatives, such as sulfur dioxide, sodium sulfite, and sodium and potassium bisulfite. There is no recommended intake for sulfur, and no deficiencies are known when protein needs are met.

TABLE 8.3 provides a summary of the sources and functions of calcium, phosphorus, magnesium, and sulfur.

A summary of calcium, phosphorus, magnesium, and sulfur TABLE 8.3

Mineral	Sources	Recommended intake for adults	Major functions	Deficiency diseases and symptoms	Groups at risk of deficiency	Toxicity	UL
Calcium	Dairy products, fish consumed with bones, leafy green vegetables, fortified foods	1000–1200 mg/day	Bone and tooth structure, nerve transmission, muscle contraction, blood clotting, blood pressure regulation, hormone secretion	Increased risk of osteoporosis	Postmenopausal women; elderly people; those who consume a vegan diet, are lactose intolerant, or have kidney disease	Elevated blood calcium, kidney stones, and other problems in susceptible individuals	2500 mg/day from food and supplements
Phosphorus	Meat, dairy, cereals, baked goods	700 mg/day	Structure of bones and teeth, membranes, ATP, and DNA; acid–base balance	Bone loss, weakness, lack of appetite	Premature infants, alcoholics, elderly people	Calcium resorption from bone	4000 mg/day
Magnesium	Greens, whole grains, legumes, nuts, seeds	310-420 mg/day	Bone structure, ATP stabilization, enzyme activity, nerve and muscle function	Nausea, vomiting, weakness, muscle pain, heart changes	Alcoholics, individuals with kidney and gastro-intestinal disease	Nausea, vomiting, low blood pressure	350 mg/day from nonfood sources
Sulfur	Protein foods, preservatives	None specified	Part of amino acids, vitamins, acid–base balance	None when protein needs are met	None	None likely	ND

Note: UL, Tolerable Upper Intake Level; ND, not determined.

CONCEPT CHECK STOP

Why are women at greater risk for osteoporosis than are men?

What happens when blood calcium levels decrease?

How can vegans meet their calcium needs?

What is the relationship between magnesium and ATP?

Trace Minerals

J ust as the best cooks know that a pinch of this or a dash of that can enhance the flavor of a special dish, the presence of minute quantities of certain minerals can boost the nutritional impact of a person's diet. The trace minerals, so called because they are needed in extremely small amounts, are essential to health. For some trace minerals, the amount in food is affected by where the food is grown and/or how it is handled. When modern transportation systems make available foods produced in many locations, these variations balance each other and are unlikely to affect an individual's mineral status. In countries where the diet consists predominantly of locally grown foods, trace mineral deficiencies and excesses are more likely to occur.

IRON

In the 1800s, iron tablets were used to treat young women whose blood lacked "coloring matter." Today we know that the "coloring matter" is the iron-containing protein **hemoglobin**. The hemoglobin in red blood cells transports oxygen to body cells and carries carbon dioxide away from them for elimination by the lungs. Most of the iron in the body is part of hemoglobin, but iron is also needed for the production of other iron-containing proteins. It is part of **myoglobin**, a protein found in muscle that enhances the amount of oxygen available for use in muscle contraction. Iron is essential for ATP production because it is a part of several proteins needed in aerobic metabolism. Iron-containing proteins are also involved in drug metabolism and immune function.

Iron absorption, uses, and loss FIGURE 8.24

The amount of iron available to the body depends on both the amount absorbed into the mucosal cells of the small intestine and the amount transported to the rest of the body. The iron that is transported may be used to synthesize iron-containing proteins, such as hemoglobin needed for red blood cell formation, or increase iron stores in the liver or spleen.

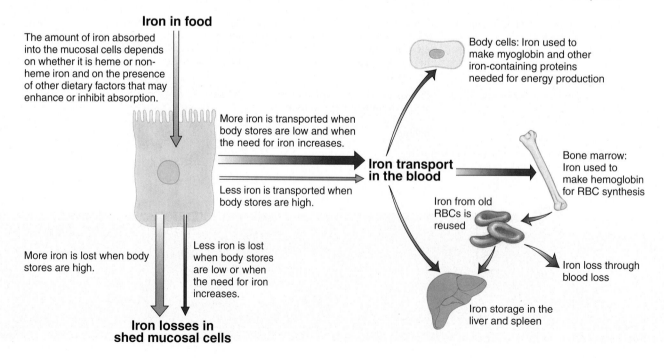

Iron in food

The amount of iron absorbed into the mucosal cells depends on whether it is heme or non-heme iron and on the presence of other dietary factors that may enhance or inhibit absorption.

More iron is transported when body stores are low and when the need for iron increases.

Less iron is transported when body stores are high.

More iron is lost when body stores are high.

Less iron is lost when body stores are low or when the need for iron increases.

Iron losses in shed mucosal cells

Body cells: Iron used to make myoglobin and other iron-containing proteins needed for energy production

Iron transport in the blood

Bone marrow: Iron used to make hemoglobin for RBC synthesis

Iron from old RBCs is reused

Iron loss through blood loss

Iron storage in the liver and spleen

Sources of iron FIGURE 8.25

The best sources of highly absorbable heme iron are red meats and organ meats such as liver and kidney. Legumes, leafy greens, and whole grains are good sources of nonheme iron; enriched grains are also good sources of nonheme iron because it is added during enrichment. The RDA for adult men and postmenopausal women is 8 mg/day. Due to menstrual losses, the RDA for women of childbearing age is set much higher, 15 mg/day for young women 14 to 18 years and 18 mg/day for women 19 to 50.

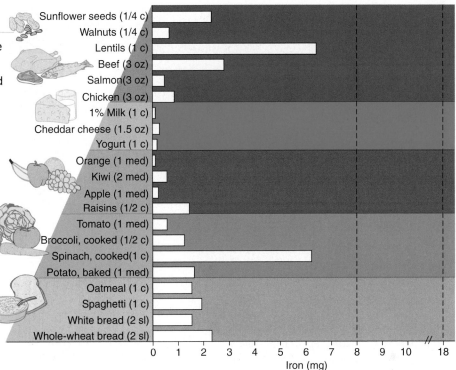

Iron absorption and transport

The amount of iron absorbed from the intestine depends on the form of the iron and on the dietary components consumed along with it. Much of the iron in meats is **heme iron**— iron that is part of a chemical complex found in proteins such as hemoglobin and myoglobin. Heme iron is absorbed more than twice as efficiently as the nonheme iron found in plant sources such as leafy green vegetables, legumes, and grains. The amount of nonheme iron absorbed can be enhanced or reduced by the foods and nutrients consumed in the same meal.

> **heme iron** A readily absorbable form of iron found in meat, fish, and poultry that is chemically associated with certain proteins.

Once iron is absorbed, the amount that is delivered to the cells of the body depends to some extent on the body's needs. When the body's iron status is high, less iron is transported in the blood for storage or delivery to cells and more is left in the mucosal cells of the intestine and lost when the cells die and are sloughed into the intestinal lumen. When iron status is low, more iron is transported out of the mucosal cells for use by the body (**FIGURE 8.24**). This regulation is important because iron that leaves the mucosal cells is not easily eliminated. Even when red blood cells die, the iron in their hemoglobin is not lost from the body; instead, it is recycled and can be incorporated into new red blood cells. Even in healthy individuals, most iron loss occurs through blood loss, including blood lost during menstruation and the small amounts lost from the gastrointestinal tract. Some iron is also lost through the shedding of cells from the intestine, skin, and urinary tract.

Meeting iron needs

Iron in the diet comes from both plant and animal sources (**FIGURE 8.25**). Animal products provide both heme and nonheme iron, but only the less readily absorbed nonheme iron is found in plants. Nonheme iron absorption can be enhanced as much as sixfold if it is consumed along with foods that are rich in vitamin C. Consuming beef, fish, or poultry in the same meal as nonheme iron also increases absorption. For example, a small amount of hamburger in a pot of chili will enhance the body's absorption of iron from the beans. If the pot is made of iron, it increases iron intake because the iron leaches into food. Iron absorption is decreased by fiber, phytates, tannins, and oxalates, which bind iron in the gastrointestinal tract. The presence of other minerals with the same charge, such as calcium, may also decrease iron absorption.

The RDA for iron assumes that the diet contains both plant and animal sources of iron.[28] A separate RDA category has been created for vegetarians. These recommendations are higher, to take into account lower iron absorption from plant sources. People who do not eat meat can increase their iron intake by consuming foods fortified with iron.

Normal red blood cells

Iron deficiency anemia

Iron deficiency anemia occurs when there is too little iron to synthesize adequate amounts of hemoglobin. It results in red blood cells that are small and pale.

Iron deficiency anemia is the final stage of iron deficiency. Inadequate iron intake first causes a decrease in the amount of stored iron, followed by low iron levels in the blood plasma. It is only after plasma levels drop that there is no longer enough iron to maintain hemoglobin in red blood cells.

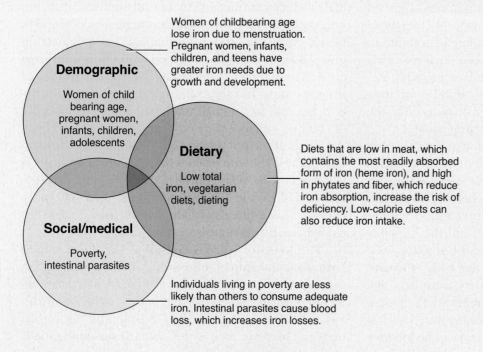

Demographic

Women of child bearing age, pregnant women, infants, children, adolescents

Dietary

Low total iron, vegetarian diets, dieting

Social/medical

Poverty, intestinal parasites

Women of childbearing age lose iron due to menstruation. Pregnant women, infants, children, and teens have greater iron needs due to growth and development.

Diets that are low in meat, which contains the most readily absorbed form of iron (heme iron), and high in phytates and fiber, which reduce iron absorption, increase the risk of deficiency. Low-calorie diets can also reduce iron intake.

Individuals living in poverty are less likely than others to consume adequate iron. Intestinal parasites cause blood loss, which increases iron losses.

The risk of iron deficiency is highest among individuals with greater iron losses, those with greater needs due to growth and development, and those who are unable to obtain adequate dietary iron. In the United States, it affects 3% of adolescent girls and women of childbearing age and 2% of children between the ages of 1 and 2 years.[31] The incidence is greatest among low-income and minority women and children.

iron deficiency anemia An iron deficiency disease that occurs when the oxygen-carrying capacity of the blood is decreased because there is insufficient iron to make hemoglobin.

Iron in health and disease

When there is too little iron in the body, hemoglobin cannot be produced. When sufficient hemoglobin is not available, the red blood cells that are formed are small and pale, and they are unable to deliver adequate oxygen to the tissues. This condition is known as **iron deficiency anemia** (FIGURE 8.26). Symptoms of iron deficiency anemia include fatigue, weakness, headache, decreased work capacity, inability to maintain body temperature in a cold environment, changes in behavior, decreased resistance to infection, impaired development in infants, and increased risk of lead poisoning in young children. Anemia is the last stage of iron deficiency. Earlier stages have no symptoms because they do not affect the amount of iron in red blood cells, but levels of iron in the blood plasma and in body stores are low (see the *Case Study*). Iron deficiency anemia is the most common nutritional deficiency; more than 2 billion people, or over 30% of the world's population, suffer from iron deficiency anemia.[29,30]

CASE STUDY

AVOIDING ANEMIA

Hanna is a 23-year-old graduate student from South Carolina. She has been working long hours and is always tired. She tries to eat a healthy diet; she has been a lacto-ovo vegetarian for the past six months.

What puts Hanna at risk for iron deficiency anemia?

▼

Your answer:

Hanna goes to the health center to see if there is a medical reason for her tiredness. They draw her blood to check her for anemia. The results of Hanna's blood work are summarized in the figure at right.

Iron stores

Iron in plasma

Iron in RBCs

Normal iron status | Hanna's iron status

What does the blood test reveal about Hanna's iron status? Is her tiredness due to iron deficiency anemia? Why or why not?

▼

Your answer:

Hanna meets with a dietitian. A diet analysis reveals that because she consumes no meat, most of her protein comes from dairy products. She consumes about eight servings of whole grains, three fresh fruits, and about a cup of cooked vegetables daily. She drinks four glasses of iced tea daily. Her average iron intake is about 12 mg/day.

Name three dietary factors that put Hanna at risk for iron deficiency.

▼

Your answer:

How could Hanna increase her iron intake?

She could use an iron-fortified breakfast cereal, eat more leafy greens, add dried fruits, and include legumes in her diet more often. She could also exchange her stainless-steel cookware for an iron skillet.

What could Hanna do to increase the absorption of the nonheme iron in her diet?

▼

Your answer:

(Check your answers in Appendix K.)

To protect children, the labels of iron-containing drugs and supplements are required to display this warning. Iron-containing products should be stored out of the reach of children or other individuals who might consume them in excess.[32]

WARNING: CLOSE TIGHTLY AND KEEP OUT OF REACH OF CHILDREN. CONTAINS IRON, WHICH CAN BE HARMFUL OR FATAL TO CHILDREN IN LARGE DOSES. IN CASE OF ACCIDENTAL OVERDOSE, SEEK PROFESSIONAL ASSISTANCE OR CONTACT A POISON CONTROL CENTER IMMEDIATELY.

Iron also causes health problems if too much is consumed. Acute iron toxicity caused by excessive consumption of iron-containing supplements is one of the most common forms of poisoning among children under age 6. Iron poisoning may cause damage to the lining of the intestine, abnormalities in body acidity, shock, and liver failure. Even a single large dose can be fatal (**FIGURE 8.27**). A UL has been set at 45 mg/day from all sources.[28]

Accumulation of iron in the body over time, referred to as **iron overload**, is most commonly due to an inherited condition called **hemochromatosis**, which permits increased iron absorption.[33] Hemochromatosis afflicts about 1 in 200 to 1 in 500 Americans, making it one of the most common genetic disorders in the United States.[34] It has no symptoms early in life, but in middle age, nonspecific symptoms such as weight loss, fatigue, weakness, and abdominal pain develop. If allowed to progress, the accumulation of excess iron can damage the heart and liver and increase the risk of diabetes and cancer. The treatment for hemochromatosis is simple: regular blood withdrawal. Iron loss through blood withdrawal will prevent the complications of iron overload, but to be effective, the treatment must be initiated before organs have been damaged. Therefore, genetic screening is essential to identify and treat individuals before any damage occurs.

> **hemochromatosis**
> An inherited disorder that results in increased iron absorption.

COPPER

It is logical that consuming too little iron will cause iron deficiency anemia, but consuming too little copper can also cause this problem. Iron status and copper status are interrelated because a copper-containing protein is needed for iron to be transported from the intestinal cells.

Even if iron intake is adequate, iron can't get to tissues if copper is not present. Thus copper deficiency results in iron deficiency that may lead to anemia. Copper also functions as a component of a number of important proteins and enzymes that are involved in connective tissue synthesis, lipid metabolism, maintenance of heart muscle, and function of the immune and central nervous systems.[28]

We consume copper in seafood, nuts and seeds, whole-grain breads and cereals, and chocolate; the richest dietary sources of copper are organ meats such as liver and kidney. As with many other trace minerals, soil content affects the amount of copper in plant foods. The RDA for copper for adults is 900 micrograms (μg)/day.

When there is too little copper in the body, the protein collagen does not form normally, resulting in skeletal changes similar to those seen in vitamin C deficiency. Copper deficiency also causes elevated blood cholesterol, reflecting copper's role in cholesterol metabolism. Copper deficiency has been associated with impaired growth, degeneration of the heart muscle and the nervous system, and changes in hair color and structure. Because copper is needed to maintain the immune system, a diet that is low in copper increases the incidence of infections. Also, because copper is an essential component of one form of the antioxidant enzyme superoxide dismutase (SOD), a copper deficiency will weaken antioxidant defenses.

Severe copper deficiency is relatively rare, although it may occur in premature infants. It can also occur if zinc intake is high because high dietary zinc interferes with the absorption of copper. Copper toxicity from dietary sources is also rare but has occurred as a result of drinking from contaminated water supplies or consuming acidic foods or beverages that have been stored in copper containers. Toxicity is more likely to occur from supplements containing copper. Excessive copper intake causes abdominal pain, vomiting, and diarrhea. The UL has been set at 10 mg of copper/day.[28]

One of zinc's most important roles is in gene expression. Zinc-containing DNA-binding proteins allow vitamin A, vitamin D, and a number of hormones to interact with DNA. The zinc forms "fingers" in the protein structure. When a vitamin or hormone binds to the protein, the zinc fingers bind to DNA, turning on genes and, thus, the synthesis of the proteins for which they code. Without zinc, these vitamins and hormones cannot function properly.

ZINC

Zinc, the most abundant intracellular trace mineral, is involved in the functioning of approximately 100 different enzymes, including a form of SOD, which is vital for protecting cells from free-radical damage. Zinc is needed to maintain adequate levels of metal binding proteins, which also scavenge free radicals.[35] Zinc is needed by enzymes that function in the synthesis of DNA and RNA, in carbohydrate metabolism, in acid–base balance, and in a reaction that is necessary for the absorption of folate from food. Zinc plays a role in the storage and release of insulin, the mobilization of vitamin A from the liver, and the stabilization of cell membranes. It influences hormonal regulation of cell division and is therefore needed for the growth and repair of tissues, the activity of the immune system, and the development of sex organs and bone. Some of the functions of zinc can be traced to its role in gene expression (Figure 8.28).

Zinc transport from the mucosal cells of the intestine into the blood is regulated. When zinc intake is high, more zinc is held in the mucosal cells and lost in the feces when these cells die. When zinc intake is low, more dietary zinc passes into the blood for delivery to tissues.

Meeting zinc needs We consume zinc in red meat, liver, eggs, dairy products, vegetables, and seafood (Figure 8.29). Because many plant foods are high in substances that bind zinc, it is absorbed better from animal sources than from plant sources.

Meat, seafood, dairy products, legumes, and seeds are good sources of zinc. Refined grains are not because zinc is lost in milling and not added back. Yeast-leavened grain products are better sources of zinc than are unleavened products because yeast leavening reduces phytate content. The dashed lines represent the RDA for adult men and women, which are 11 and 8 mg/day, respectively.

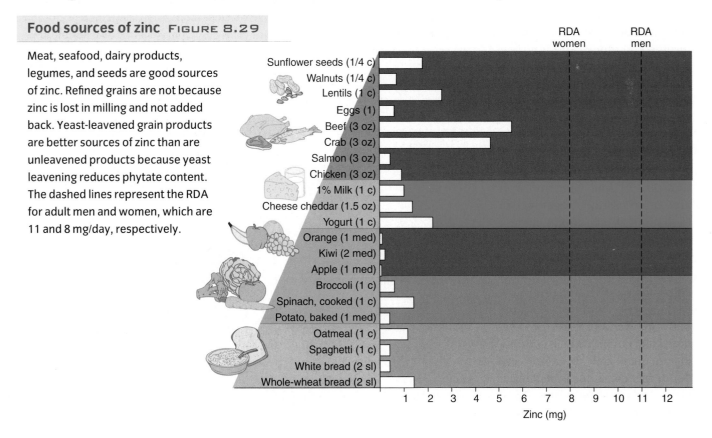

Zinc in health and disease

Symptomatic zinc deficiency is relatively uncommon in North America, but in developing countries, it has important health and developmental consequences. Zinc deficiency interferes with growth and development, impairs immune function, and causes skin rashes and diarrhea. Diminished immune function is a concern even when zinc deficiency is mild. Because zinc is needed for the proper functioning of vitamins A and D and the activity of numerous enzymes, deficiency symptoms can resemble those of other essential nutrient deficiencies.

The risk of zinc deficiency is greater in areas where the diet is high in phytate, fiber, tannins, and oxalates, which limit zinc absorption. In the 1960s, a syndrome of growth depression and delayed sexual development was observed in Iranian and Egyptian men consuming a diet based on plant protein. The diet was not low in zinc, but it was high in grains containing phytates, which interfered with zinc absorption, thus causing the deficiency.

It is difficult to consume a toxic amount of zinc from food. However, high doses from supplements can cause toxicity symptoms. A single dose of 1 to 2 g can cause gastrointestinal irritation, vomiting, loss of appetite, diarrhea, abdominal cramps, and headaches. High intakes have been shown to decrease immune function, reduce concentrations of HDL cholesterol in the blood, and interfere with the absorption of copper. High doses of zinc can also interfere with iron absorption because iron and zinc are transported through the blood by the same protein. The converse is also true: Too much iron can limit the transport of zinc. Zinc and iron are often found together in foods, but food sources do not contain large enough amounts of either to cause imbalances.

Zinc supplements are marketed to improve immune function, enhance fertility and sexual performance, and cure the common cold. For individuals consuming adequate zinc, there is no evidence that extra zinc is beneficial. Supplements have not been shown to improve sexual function, and there is little evidence that zinc lozenges, promoted to reduce the duration and severity of cold symptoms, are effective.[36] However, in individuals with a mild zinc deficiency, supplementation may result in improved wound healing, immunity, and appetite; in children, it can result in improved growth and learning, and in older adults it can improve immune response.[37] A UL has been set at 40 mg/day from all sources.[28]

SELENIUM

The amount of selenium in food varies greatly, depending on the concentration of selenium in the soil where the food is produced. In regions of China with low soil selenium levels, a form of heart disease called **Keshan disease** occurs in children and young women. This disease can be prevented and cured with selenium supplements. In contrast, people living in regions of China with very high selenium in the soil may develop symptoms of selenium toxicity (**FIGURE 8.30**).

Soil selenium and health FIGURE 8.30

The amount of selenium in the soil varies widely from one region of China to another. When the diet consists primarily of locally grown food, these differences affect selenium intake and, therefore, health. When the diet includes foods from many different locations, the high selenium content of foods grown in one geographic region is offset by the low selenium content of foods from other regions.

Hair and nail brittleness and loss occur in people living in regions of China with high selenium levels in the soil (intake of 5 mg/day). Other toxicity symptoms include nausea, diarrhea, abdominal pain, nervous system abnormalities, fatigue, and irritability.

Selenium deficiency causes muscular discomfort, weakness, and in some cases Keshan disease. However, Keshan disease is not caused entirely by selenium deficiency. It is believed to be due to a combination of selenium deficiency and a viral infection.[38]

Soil selenium
- Deficient
- Low
- Normal
- High
- Very high
- Not investigated

Selenium is incorporated into the structure of certain proteins. One of these proteins is the antioxidant enzyme **glutathione peroxidase**. Glutathione peroxidase neutralizes peroxides before they can form free radicals, which cause oxidative damage (**FIGURE 8.31**). In addition to its antioxidant role in glutathione peroxidase, selenium is part of a protein needed for the synthesis of the **thyroid hormones**, which regulate metabolic rate.

Meeting selenium needs

Selenium deficiencies and excesses are not a concern in the United States because the foods we consume come from many different locations around the country and around the world. The RDA for selenium for adults is 55 µg/day.[39] The average intake in the United States meets, or nearly meets, this recommendation for all age groups. Seafood, kidney, liver, and eggs are excellent sources of selenium. Grains, nuts, and seeds can be good sources, depending on the selenium content of the soil in which they were grown. Fruits, vegetables, and drinking water are generally poor sources. The UL for adults is 400 µg/day from diet and supplements.[39]

Selenium and cancer

An increased incidence of cancer has been observed in regions where selenium intake is low, suggesting that selenium plays a role in preventing cancer. In 1996, a study investigating the effect of selenium supplements on people with a history of skin cancer found that the supplement had no effect on the recurrence of skin cancer but that the incidence of lung, prostate, and colon cancer decreased in the selenium-supplemented group.[40] This result caused speculation that selenium supplements could reduce the risk of cancer. Continued study, however, has led to the conclusion that the reduction in the incidence of lung and prostate cancer seen in the 1996 study occurred primarily in people who began the study with low levels of selenium. It appears that an adequate level of selenium is necessary to prevent cancer, but the role of supplemental selenium in preventing cancer is still under investigation.[41]

IODINE

About three-fourths of the iodine in the body is found in a small gland in the neck called the **thyroid gland**. The reason iodine is concentrated in this gland is that it is an es-

Glutathione peroxidase FIGURE 8.31

Glutathione peroxidase is a selenium-containing enzyme that neutralizes peroxides before they can form free radicals. Selenium therefore can reduce the body's need for vitamin E, which neutralizes free radicals.

sential component of the thyroid hormones, which are produced here. Thyroid hormones regulate metabolic rate, growth, and development, and they promote protein synthesis.

Iodine in health and disease

Thyroid hormone levels are carefully regulated. If blood levels drop, **thyroid-stimulating hormone** is released. This hormone signals the thyroid gland to take up iodine and synthesize more thyroid hormones. When the supply of iodine is adequate, thyroid hormones can be produced, and the return of thyroid hormones to normal levels turns off the synthesis of thyroid-stimulating hormone. If iodine is

Visualizing

Iodine deficiency disorders FIGURE 8.32

NATIONAL GEOGRAPHIC

Anterior pituitary

When thyroid hormone levels drop too low, ▶ thyroid-stimulating hormone stimulates the thyroid gland to take up iodine and synthesize more hormones. If iodine is not available, thyroid hormones cannot be made, and the stimulation continues, causing the thyroid gland to enlarge.

Thyroid-stimulating hormone

Thyroid gland

Decrease in thyroid hormones

Thyroid hormones made

Thyroid gland enlarges (goiter)

Iodine available

Iodine deficient

NATIONAL GEOGRAPHIC

Cretinism is ▶ characterized by symptoms that include impaired mental development, deaf mutism, and growth failure. Unlike with goiter, the damage is permanent.

A goiter, which is an enlarged thyroid ▶ gland, can be seen as a swelling in the neck. In milder cases of goiter, treatment with iodine causes the thyroid gland to return to its normal size, but it may remain enlarged in more severe cases.

Although iodine ▶ deficiency remains a global health issue, its incidence has declined dramatically since universal salt iodization was adopted in 1993. UNICEF estimates that 66% of all households now have access to iodized salt.[42]

Degree of public health significance of iodine nutrition based on median urinary iodine

Severe iodine deficiency (<20 µg/l)

Moderate iodine deficiency (20–49 µg/l)

Mild iodine deficiency (50–99 µg/l)

Optimal iodine status (100–199 µg/l)

Risk of iodine-induced hyperthyroidism (200–299 µg/l)

Risk of adverse health consequences (>300 µg/l)

No data

Source: de Benoist B et al., eds. Iodine status worldwide. WHO Global Database on Iodine Deficiency. Geneva, World Health Organization, 2004.
Data was produced by WHO using the best available evidence and do not necessarily correspond to the official statistics of Member States.

deficient, thyroid hormones cannot be synthesized (Figure 8.32). Without sufficient thyroid hormones, metabolic rate slows, causing fatigue and weight gain.

The most obvious outward sign of iodine deficiency is an enlarged thyroid gland, called a **goiter**, but because of the importance of the thyroid hormones for growth and development, other iodine deficiency disorders are also prevalent (see Figure 8.32). If iodine is deficient during pregnancy, the risk of stillbirth and spontaneous abortion increases; insufficient iodine during pregnancy can cause a condition called **cretinism** in the child. Iodine deficiency impairs mental function and reduces intellectual capacity in children and adolescents. Though easily prevented, it is the world's most prevalent cause of brain damage.[42]

Iodine deficiency is most common in regions where the soil is low in iodine and there is little access to fish and seafood. The risk of iodine deficiency is also increased by the consumption of foods that contain **goitrogens**, substances that interfere with iodine utilization or with thyroid function. Goitrogens are found in turnips, rutabaga, cabbage, millet, and cassava. When these foods are boiled, the goitrogen content is reduced because some of these compounds leach into the cooking water. Goitrogens are primarily a problem in African countries where cassava is a dietary staple. Goitrogens are not a problem in the U.S. because the typical diet does not include large amounts of foods containing them.

Chronically high intakes or a sudden increase in iodine intake can also cause an enlargement of the thyroid gland. For example, in a person with a marginal intake, a large dose from supplements could cause thyroid enlargement even at levels that would not be toxic in a healthy person. The UL for adults is 1100 µg of iodine/day from all sources.[28]

Meeting iodine needs The iodine content of food varies, depending on the soil in which plants are grown or where animals graze. When Earth was formed, all soils were high in iodine, but today mountainous areas and river valleys have little iodine left in the soil because it has been washed out by glaciers, snow, rain, and floodwaters. The iodine washed from the soil has accumulated in the oceans. Therefore, foods from the sea, such as fish, seafood, and seaweed, are the best sources of iodine.

Today most of the iodine in the North American diet comes from **iodized salt** (Figure 8.33). Iodine deficiency is rare in North America, and typical iodine intake meets or exceeds the RDA of 150 µg/day for adult men and women.[28]

We also obtain iodine from contaminants and other additives in foods. Iodine-containing additives used in cattle feed and disinfectants used on milking machines and milk storage tanks increase the iodine content of dairy products. Iodine-containing sterilizing agents are also used in fast-food restaurants, and iodine is used in dough conditioners and some food colorings. Despite our intake of iodine from iodized salt and contaminants, toxicity is rare in the United States.

CHROMIUM

Chromium is the key component of what has been called the "glucose tolerance factor," a small peptide required to maintain normal blood glucose levels. It is believed to act by enhancing the effects of insulin.[43] Insulin facilitates the entry of glucose into cells and stimulates the synthesis of proteins, lipids, and glycogen. When chromium is deficient, more insulin is required to produce the same effect. A deficiency of chromium therefore affects the body's ability to regulate blood glucose, causing diabetes-like symptoms such as elevated blood glucose levels and increased insulin levels.[43]

Iodized salt Figure 8.33

Iodized salt was first introduced in Switzerland in the 1920s as a way to combat iodine deficiency. Salt was chosen because it is readily available, inexpensive, and consumed in regular amounts throughout the year. It takes only about half a teaspoon of iodized salt to provide the recommended amount of iodine. Iodized salt should not be confused with sea salt, which is a poor source of iodine because its iodine is lost in the drying process.

Chromium picolinate supplements

FIGURE 8.34

Because chromium is needed for insulin action and insulin promotes protein synthesis, it is likely that adequate chromium is necessary to increase lean body mass. However, studies of chromium picolinate and other chromium supplements in healthy human subjects have not found them to have beneficial effects on muscle strength, body composition, or weight loss.[44]

Dietary sources of chromium include liver, brewer's yeast, nuts, and whole grains. Milk, vegetables, and fruits are poor sources. Refined carbohydrates such as white breads, pasta, and white rice are also poor sources because chromium is lost in milling and not added back in the enrichment process. Chromium intake can be increased by cooking in stainless-steel cookware because chromium leaches from the steel into the food. The recommended intake for chromium is 35 µg/day for men age 19 to 50 and 25 µg/day for women age 19 to 50.[28]

Overt chromium deficiency is not a problem in the United States; nevertheless, chromium, in the form of chromium picolinate, is a common dietary supplement. It is popular with athletes and dieters because it is thought to reduce body fat and increase muscle mass (**FIGURE 8.34**). Toxicity is always a concern with nutrient supplements, but in the case of chromium, there is little evidence of dietary toxicity in humans. The DRI committee concluded that there was insufficient data to establish a UL for chromium.[28]

FLUORIDE

Fluoride helps prevent **dental caries** (cavities) in both children and adults. During tooth formation, fluoride is incorporated into the crystals that make up tooth enamel. These fluoride-containing crystals are more resistant to acid than are crystals formed when fluoride is not present. Fluoride therefore helps protect the teeth from the cavity-causing acids produced by bacteria in the mouth. Adequate fluoride has its greatest effect during the period of maximum tooth development (up to age 13), but it continues to have benefits throughout life. In addition to making tooth enamel more acid resistant, fluoride in saliva prevents cavities by reducing the amount of acid produced by bacteria, inhibiting the dissolution of tooth enamel by acid, and increasing enamel re-mineralization after acid exposure.

Fluoride is also incorporated into the mineral crystals in bone. There is evidence that fluoride stimulates bone formation and therefore might strengthen bones in adults who have osteoporosis. Slow-release fluoride supplements have been shown to increase bone mass and prevent new fractures.[45]

Meeting fluoride needs Fluoride is present in small amounts in almost all soil, water, plants, and animals. The richest dietary sources of fluoride are toothpaste, tea, marine fish consumed with their bones, and fluoridated water (see *What Should I Eat?*). Because food readily absorbs the fluoride in cooking water, the fluoride content of food can be significantly increased when it is handled and prepared using water that contains fluoride. Cooking utensils also affect the fluoride content of foods. Foods cooked with Teflon utensils can pick up fluoride from the Teflon, whereas aluminum cookware can decrease the fluoride content of foods. Bottled water usually does not

---

WHAT SHOULD I EAT? Trace Minerals

Use iProfile to find the trace element content of a cup of pinto beans.

Add more iron
- Eat red meat, poultry, or fish—they are all good sources of heme iron.
- Add raisins to your oatmeal.
- Fortify your breakfast by eating iron-fortified cereal.
- Dust off the iron skillet.
- Have some beans—they are a good vegetarian source of iron.

Increase iron absorption
- Have orange juice with your iron-fortified cereal.
- Don't take your calcium supplement with your iron sources.

Think zinc
- Scramble some eggs.
- Beef up your zinc by having a few ounces of meat.
- Eat whole grains, but make sure they are yeast leavened.

Trace down your minerals
- Check to see if your water is fluoridated.
- See if your salt is iodized.
- Replace refined grains with whole grains to increase your chromium intake.
- Have some seafood to add selenium to your diet.

This graph illustrates that the incidence of dental caries in children increases when the concentration of fluoride in the water supply is lower. If the fluoride concentration of the water is too high, it increases the risk of fluorosis.

Too little fluoride makes teeth more susceptible to dental caries.

The optimal amount of fluoride makes teeth resistant to decay and does not cause fluorosis.

Too much fluoride (intakes of 2 to 8 mg/day or greater in children) causes teeth to appear mottled, a condition called fluorosis.

contain fluoride, so people who habitually drink bottled water need to obtain fluoride from other sources.

The recommended intake for fluoride for people 6 months of age and older is 0.05 mg/kg/day. This is equivalent to about 3.8 mg/day for a 76-kg man and 3.1 mg/day for a 61-kg woman. Fluoridated water provides about 0.7 to 1.2 mg of fluoride/liter. The American Academy of Pediatrics suggests a fluoride supplement of 0.25 mg/day for children 6 months to 3 years of age, 0.5 mg/day for children ages 3 to 6 years, and 1.0 mg/day for those ages 6 to 16 years who are receiving less than 0.3 mg/liter of fluoride in the water supply. These supplements are available by prescription for children living in areas with low fluoride concentrations in the water supply.

Fluoridation of water
To promote dental health, fluoride is added to public water supplies in many communities. Currently about 66% of people served by public water systems receive fluoridated water.[46] When fluoride intake is low, tooth decay is more frequent (FIGURE 8.35). Water fluoridation is a safe, inexpensive way to prevent dental caries, but some people still believe that the added fluoride increases the risk of cancer and other diseases. These beliefs are not supported by scientific facts;

fluorosis
A condition caused by chronic overconsumption of fluoride, characterized by black and brown stains and cracking and pitting of the teeth.

the small amounts of fluoride consumed in drinking water promote dental health and do not pose a risk for health problems such as cancer, kidney failure, or bone disease.[47]

Although the levels of fluoride included in public water supplies are safe, too much fluoride can be toxic. In children, too much fluoride causes **fluorosis** (see Figure 8.35). Recently, there has been an increase in fluorosis in the United States due to chronic ingestion of fluoride-containing toothpaste. The fluoride in toothpaste is good for your teeth, but swallowing it can increase fluoride intake to dangerous levels. Swallowed toothpaste is estimated to contribute about 0.6 mg per day of fluoride in young children. Due to concern over excess fluoride intake, the following warning is now required on all fluoride-containing toothpastes: "If you accidentally swallow more than used for brushing, seek professional help or contact a poison control center immediately."

In adults, doses of 20 to 80 mg of fluoride/day can result in changes in bone health that may be crippling, as well as changes in kidney function and possibly nerve and muscle function. Death has been reported in cases involving an intake of 5 to 10 g/day. The UL for fluoride is set at 0.1 mg/kg/day for infants and children less than 9 years of age and at 10 mg/day for those between 9 and 70 years.[22]

MANGANESE, MOLYBDENUM, AND OTHER TRACE MINERALS

In addition to the seven we have just examined, there are many other trace minerals in the human body. DRI recommendations have been set for two of them: manganese and molybdenum.[28]

Manganese is a constituent of some enzymes and an activator of others. Enzymes that require manganese are involved in carbohydrate, and cholesterol metabolism; bone formation; synthesis of urea; and prevention of oxidative damage because manganese is a component of a form of superoxide dismutase. The recommended intake for manganese is 2.3 mg/day for adult men and 1.8 mg/day for adult women. The best dietary sources of manganese are whole grains, nuts, legumes, and leafy green vegetables.

Molybdenum is also needed to activate enzymes. It functions in the metabolism of sulfur-containing amino acids and nitrogen-containing compounds that are present in DNA and RNA; in the production of a waste product called uric acid; and in the oxidation and detoxification of various other compounds. The recommended intake for molybdenum is 45 μg/day for adult men and women. The molybdenum content of food varies with the molybdenum content of the soil in the regions where the food is produced. The most reliable sources include milk and milk products, organ meats, breads, cereals, and legumes. Molybdenum is readily absorbed from foods; the amount in the body is regulated by excretion in the urine and bile.

A summary of the trace minerals TABLE 8.4

Mineral	Sources	Recommended intake for adults	Major functions	Deficiency diseases and symptoms	Groups at risk of deficiency	Toxicity	UL
Iron	Red meats, leafy greens, dried fruit, legumes, whole and enriched grains	8–18 mg/day	Part of hemoglobin (which delivers oxygen to cells), myoglobin (which holds oxygen in muscle), and proteins needed for ATP production; needed for immune function	Iron deficiency anemia: fatigue; weakness; small, pale red blood cells; low hemoglobin levels; inability to maintain normal body temperature	Infants and preschool children, adolescents, women of childbearing age, pregnant women, athletes, vegetarians	Gastrointestinal upset, liver damage	45 mg/day
Zinc	Meat, seafood, whole grains, dairy products, legumes, nuts	8–11 mg/day	Regulates protein synthesis; functions in growth, development, wound healing, immunity, and antioxidant enzymes	Poor growth and development, skin rashes, decreased immune function	Vegetarians, low-income children, elderly people	Decreased copper absorption, depressed immune function	40 mg/day
Copper	Organ meats, nuts, seeds, whole grains, seafood, cocoa	900 μg/day	A component of proteins needed for iron absorption, lipid metabolism, collagen synthesis, nerve and immune function, and protection against oxidative damage	Anemia, poor growth, bone abnormalities	People who consume excessive amounts of zinc in supplements	Vomiting, abdominal pain, diarrhea, liver damage	10 mg/day

(continued)

Mineral	Sources	Recommended intake for adults	Major functions	Deficiency diseases and symptoms	Groups at risk of deficiency	Toxicity	UL
Manganese	Nuts, legumes, whole grains, tea, leafy vegetables	1.8–2.3 mg/day	Functions in carbohydrate and cholesterol metabolism and antioxidant enzymes	Growth retardation	None	Nerve damage	11 mg/day
Selenium	Meats, seafood, eggs, whole grains, nuts, seeds	55 µg/day	Antioxidant as part of glutathione peroxidase, synthesis of thyroid hormones; spares vitamin E	Muscle pain, weakness, Keshan disease	Populations in areas where the soil is low in selenium	Nausea, diarrhea, vomiting, fatigue, changes in hair and nails	400 µg/day
Iodine	Iodized salt, saltwater fish, seafood, seaweed, dairy products	150 µg/day	Needed for synthesis of thyroid hormones	Goiter, cretinism, impaired brain function, growth and developmental abnormalities	Populations in areas where the soil is low in iodine and iodized salt is not used	Enlarged thyroid	1110 µg/day
Chromium	Brewer's yeast, nuts, whole grains, meat, mushrooms	25–35 µg/day	Enhances insulin action	High blood glucose	Malnourished children	None reported	ND
Fluoride	Fluoridated water, tea, fish, toothpaste	3–4 mg/day	Strengthens tooth enamel, enhances re-mineralization of tooth enamel, reduces acid production by bacteria in the mouth	Increased risk of dental caries	Populations in areas with unfluoridated, water, those who drink mostly bottled water	Fluorosis: mottled teeth, kidney damage, bone abnormalities	10 mg/day
Molybdenum	Milk, organ meats, grains, legumes	45 µg/day	Cofactor for a number of enzymes	Unknown in humans	None	Arthritis and joint inflammation	2 mg/day

Note: UL, Tolerable Upper Intake Level; ND, not determined.

There is evidence that arsenic, boron, nickel, silicon, and vanadium play a role in human health. The DRI committee reviewed the need for and functions of these minerals, but there was insufficient data to establish a recommended intake for any of them. Other trace minerals that are believed to play a physiological role in human health include aluminum, bromine, cadmium, germanium, lead, lithium, rubidium, and tin. Their specific functions have not been defined, and they have not been evaluated by the DRI committee. All the minerals, both those that are known to be essential and those that are still being assessed for their role in human health, can be obtained by choosing a variety of foods from each of the MyPyramid food groups.

TABLE 8.4 provides a summary of the trace minerals.

CONCEPT CHECK STOP

Why does iron deficiency cause fatigue?

What is the function of iodine?

How does selenium reduce the body's need for vitamin E?

How does fluoride protect the teeth?

SUMMARY

1 Water

1. Water, which is found intracellularly and extracellularly, accounts for about 60% of adult body weight. The amount of water in the blood is a balance between the forces of **blood pressure** and osmosis.

2. Because water isn't stored in the body, intake from fluids and foods must replace losses in urine, feces, and sweat, as well as from evaporation. Water intake is stimulated by the sensation of **thirst**. The kidneys regulate urinary water losses.

3. In the body, water is a **solvent** where chemical reactions occur; it also transports nutrients and wastes,

provides protection, helps regulate temperature, and participates in chemical reactions and acid–base balance.

4. **Dehydration** occurs when there is too little water in the body. **Water intoxication** causes **hyponatremia**, which can result in abnormal fluid accumulation in body tissues.

5. The recommended intake of water is 2.7 L/day for women and 3.7 L/day for men; needs vary depending on environmental conditions and activity level.

2 An Overview of Minerals

1. **Major minerals** and **trace minerals** are distinguished by the amounts needed in the diet and found in the body. Both plant and animal foods are good sources of minerals.

2. Mineral bioavailability is affected by the food source of the mineral, the body's need, and interactions with other minerals, vitamins, and dietary components such as fiber, phytates, oxalates, and tannins.

3. Minerals are needed to provide structure and to regulate biochemical reactions, often as **cofactors**.

3 Electrolytes: Sodium, Potassium, and Chloride

1. The minerals sodium, potassium, and chloride are **electrolytes** that are important in the maintenance of fluid balance and the functioning of nerves and muscles. The kidneys are the primary regulator of electrolyte and fluid balance.

2. Sodium, potassium, and chloride depletion can occur when losses are increased by heavy and persistent sweating, chronic diarrhea, or vomiting. Diets high in sodium and low in potassium are associated with an increased risk of **hypertension**. The **DASH diet**—a dietary pattern moderate in sodium; high in potassium, magnesium, calcium, and fiber; and low in fat, saturated fat, and cholesterol— lowers blood pressure.

3. The U.S. diet is abundant in sodium and chloride from processed foods and table salt but generally low in potassium, which is high in unprocessed foods such as fresh fruits and vegetables. Recommendations for health suggest that we increase our intake of potassium and consume less sodium.

Normal spine Osteoporotic spine

4 Major Minerals and Bone Health

1. Bone is a living tissue that is constantly remodeled. **Peak bone mass** occurs in young adulthood. **Age-related bone loss** occurs in adults when more bone is broken down than is made. Bone loss is accelerated in women after **menopause**. **Osteoporosis** occurs when bone mass is so low that it increases the risk of bone fractures.

2. Most of the calcium in the body is found in bone, but calcium is also needed for essential functions such as nerve transmission, muscle contraction, blood clotting, and blood pressure regulation. Good sources of calcium in the U.S. diet include dairy products, fish consumed with bones, and leafy green vegetables. Low blood calcium causes the release of **parathyroid hormone (PTH)**, which affects the amount of calcium excreted in the urine, absorbed from the diet, and released from bone. When blood calcium is high, **calcitonin** blocks calcium release from bone.

3. Phosphorus is widely distributed in foods. It plays an important structural role in bones and teeth. Phosphorus helps prevent changes in acidity and is an essential component of phospholipids, ATP, DNA, and RNA.

4. Magnesium is important for bone health and blood pressure regulation, and it is needed as a cofactor and to stabilize ATP. The best dietary sources are whole grains and green vegetables.

5. Sulfur is found in protein and is part of the structure of certain vitamins and of glutathione, which protects cells from oxidative damage.

5 Trace Minerals

1. Iron functions as part of **hemoglobin, myoglobin**, and proteins in energy metabolism. The amount of iron absorbed depends on the form of iron and other dietary components. **Heme iron**, found in meats, is more absorbable than nonheme iron, which is the only form found in plant foods. **Iron deficiency anemia** causes fatigue and decreased work capacity. The amount of iron transported from the intestinal cells to body cells depends on the amount needed. If too much iron is absorbed, as in **hemochromatosis**, the heart and liver can be damaged, and diabetes and cancer are more likely. A single large dose of iron is toxic and can be fatal.

2. Copper functions in proteins that affect iron and lipid metabolism, synthesis of connective tissue, antioxidant capacity, and iron transport. High levels of zinc can cause a copper deficiency. A copper deficiency can result in anemia and bone abnormalities. Seafood, nuts, seeds, and whole-grain breads and cereals are good sources of copper.

3. Zinc is needed for the activity of many enzymes, and zinc-containing proteins are needed for gene expression. Good sources of zinc include red meats, eggs, dairy products, and whole grains. The amount of zinc in the body is regulated primarily by the amount absorbed and lost through the small intestine. Zinc deficiency depresses immunity. Too much zinc depresses immune function and contributes to copper and iron deficiency.

4. Selenium is part of the antioxidant enzyme **glutathione peroxidase** and is needed for the synthesis of **thyroid hormones**. Dietary sources include seafood, eggs, organ meats, and plant foods grown in selenium-rich soils. Selenium deficiency causes muscle discomfort and weakness and is associated with **Keshan disease**. Low selenium intake has been linked to increased cancer risk.

5. Iodine is an essential component of thyroid hormones. The best sources of iodine are seafood, foods grown near the sea, and **iodized salt**. When iodine is deficient, the **thyroid gland** enlarges, forming a **goiter**. Iodine deficiency also affects growth and development. The use of iodized salt has reduced the incidence of iodine deficiency worldwide.

6. Chromium is needed for normal insulin action and glucose utilization. It is found in liver, brewer's yeast, nuts, and whole grains.

7. Fluoride is necessary for the maintenance of bones and teeth and the prevention of **dental caries**. Dietary sources of fluoride include fluoridated drinking water, toothpaste, tea, and marine fish consumed with bones. Too much fluoride causes **fluorosis** in children.

Normal red blood cells

Iron deficiency anemia

KEY TERMS

- dehydration p. 240
- solutes p. 241
- blood pressure p. 241
- thirst p. 242
- antidiuretic hormone (ADH) p. 243
- solvent p. 244
- water intoxication p. 246
- hyponatremia p. 246
- diuretic p. 246
- minerals p. 248
- major minerals p. 248
- trace minerals p. 248
- ion p. 251
- cofactor p. 251
- electrolytes p. 252
- sodium chloride p. 252

- aldosterone p. 253
- hypertension p. 254
- prehypertension p. 254
- DASH (Dietary Approaches to Stop Hypertension) diet p. 254
- osteopenia p. 259
- bone remodeling p. 259
- peak bone mass p. 260
- osteoporosis p. 260
- age-related bone loss p. 260
- menopause p. 260
- postmenopausal bone loss p. 260
- calcitonin p. 262
- bone resorption p. 262
- hemoglobin p. 268
- myoglobin p. 268

- heme iron p. 269
- iron deficiency anemia p. 271
- iron overload p. 272
- hemochromatosis p. 272
- Keshan disease p. 274
- glutathione peroxidase p. 275
- thyroid hormones p. 275
- thyroid gland p. 275
- thyroid-stimulating hormone p. 275
- goiter p. 277
- cretinism p. 277
- goitrogens p. 277
- iodized salt p. 277
- dental caries p. 278
- fluorosis p. 279

CRITICAL AND CREATIVE THINKING QUESTIONS

1. Why might a thirsty sailor who drank sea water die of dehydration?

2. Virginia works at a desk. The only exercise she gets is when she takes care of her nieces and nephews one weekend a month. Her typical diet includes a breakfast of cereal, tomato juice, and coffee. She has a snack of donuts and coffee at work, and for lunch she joins coworkers for a fast-food cheeseburger, fries, and a milkshake. When she gets home, she snacks on a soda and peanuts or chips. Dinner is usually a TV dinner with milk. A recent physical exam indicated that her blood pressure is elevated. What dietary and lifestyle changes would you recommend to help Virginia lower her blood pressure?

3. Use food labels to identify three processed foods you commonly eat that contain more than 10% of the Daily Value for sodium per serving. What less-processed choices might you substitute for these? If you typically consumed a serving of each of these processed foods per day, by how much would these substitutions lower your sodium intake?

4. Many people in the United States must limit milk consumption due to lactose intolerance. What foods can they include in their diets to help meet their calcium needs?

5. This table shows the incidence of hip fractures in different groups within a population of older adults. Use your knowledge of bone physiology to explain the differences observed among white women, white men, black women, and black men.

Population group	Annual incidence of hip fracture per 1000
Caucasian women	30
Caucasian men	13
African American women	11
African American men	7

6. A researcher asked his new technician to prepare a diet for his laboratory animals. The technician is interrupted several times while mixing the diet and is unfamiliar with the scale he is using to weigh the diet ingredients. After the diet is fed to the animals for several months, they begin to show signs of anemia. An error in diet preparation is suspected. Use the diet ingredients listed below to suggest which trace mineral deficiencies or excesses could cause anemia. What vitamin deficiencies can cause anemia?

Diet Ingredients

Starch, Sucrose, Casein (protein), Corn oil, Mixed plant fibers, Vitamin A, Vitamin D, Vitamin E, Vitamin K, B vitamin mix, Calcium, Sodium, Potassium, Magnesium, Chloride, Zinc, Iron, Iodine, Selenium, Copper, Manganese, Chromium, Molybdenum

7. Mary Beth has just been diagnosed with anemia that is believed to be due to a deficiency in her diet. The total amount of hemoglobin in her blood is low, as is her hematocrit (the percentage of her blood that is made up or red blood cells). What other information can help determine what nutrient deficiency is the cause?

8. Evaluate your risk of developing osteoporosis based on your age, ethnicity, gender, diet, and lifestyle.

What is happening in this picture ?

This photo shows astronaut Pete Conrad riding a stationary bike during his 28-day stay aboard Skylab in 1973. Weight-bearing exercise and adequate nutrient intake are important for the maintenance of bone.

Why is scheduled exercise even more important for bone health in space than it is on Earth?

What nutrients other than calcium might be of particular concern for bone health in an astronaut? Why?

SELF-TEST

(Check your answers in Appendix L.)

1. In a sedentary individual, most water is lost via _____.

   a. evaporation from the skin and lungs
   b. sweat
   c. saliva
   d. urine
   e. feces

2. _____ will increase water needs.

   a. A high-salt diet
   b. A high-protein diet
   c. A high-fiber diet
   d. A very low-calorie diet
   e. All of the above

3. If the concentration of solutes in your blood increases (i.e., the blood is more concentrated), which one of the following is most likely to occur?

   a. You will lose more water in the urine.
   b. Antidiuretic hormone will be released.
   c. You will begin to sweat.
   d. Your body temperature will go up.
   e. You will feel hungry.

4. The risk of high blood pressure is increased by _____.

   a. obesity
   b. family history
   c. high salt diet
   d. sedentary lifestyle
   e. all of the above

5. Which one of the following is occurring at the point labeled with the arrow?

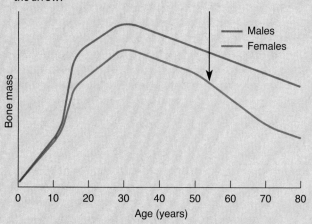

   a. Bone formation is occurring more rapidly than bone breakdown.
   b. Peak bone mass has been reached.
   c. Bone breakdown exceeds bone formation due to normal aging.
   d. Bone loss is accelerated after menopause.

6. Which of the following statements about iron is false?

   a. When iron levels are high, more is eliminated from the body in the urine.
   b. Heme iron is better absorbed than nonheme iron.
   c. Iron is a part of the oxygen-carrying protein hemoglobin.
   d. Iron is a part of the oxygen-storage protein myoglobin.
   e. Red meat is a good source of heme iron.

7. Hemochromatosis is treated with iron supplements.

   a. True
   b. False

8. Which of the following does not occur when blood calcium levels drop too low?

   a. More calcium is excreted in the urine.
   b. Bone is broken down, releasing calcium into the blood.
   c. Vitamin D is activated by the kidney.
   d. Parathyroid hormone is released.
   e. Intestinal absorption of calcium increases.

9. Which of the following is a function of iodine?

   a. It is an antioxidant.
   b. It is needed for insulin action.
   c. It is a component of the thyroid hormones.
   d. It is a component of superoxide dismutase.
   e. It is needed to cross-link collagen.

10. Women of childbearing age need more iron than men of the same age because they _____.

   a. are more active
   b. are growing
   c. lose more iron in the digestive tract
   d. have more muscle mass
   e. lose iron through menstruation

11. Which of the following statements about zinc is false?

   a. The amount that moves from the intestinal cells into the blood is regulated.
   b. Phytates present in grain products enhance zinc absorption.
   c. Zinc is involved in regulating protein synthesis.
   d. Zinc is part of the protein that allows vitamin A to affect gene expression.
   e. Zinc is absorbed better from meat than from plant foods.

12. Which of the following statements about selenium is false?

   a. It is part of the antioxidant enzyme glutathione peroxidase.
   b. It reduces some of the need for vitamin E.
   c. The amount in grain depends on the selenium content of the soil where it is grown.
   d. Low intakes are linked to a type of heart disease called Keshan disease.
   e. It is needed for the mineralization of bones and teeth.

13. The woman shown here has a deficiency of which of the following minerals?

   a. calcium
   b. iodine
   c. iron
   d. chromium
   e. magnesium

14. Chromium increases the effectiveness of _____.

   a. insulin
   b. thyroid hormone
   c. thyroid stimulating hormone
   d. antidiuretic hormone
   e. parathyroid hormone

15. Which of the following is most likely to have caused the condition shown here?

   a. living in a community that does not have fluoridated water
   b. taking calcium supplements
   c. swallowing toothpaste
   d. absorbing too much iron

Energy Balance and Weight Management

"**D**ieting is hard work!" This statement can be an excuse, a plea, a motivator, or a come-on, but whatever its context, to many people it is an undeniable truth. Responsible weight management is a challenge. It involves choosing the right amount of food and exercise to keep weight in the healthy range. And it often means doing so in the face of an endless array of affordable foods.

Food producers and sellers urge us to buy, eat, upsize, and supersize. In response, we consume food in larger amounts than we need to sustain health, and often the result is obesity, unfitness, and disease. Meanwhile, the weight-loss and diet industries—and "experts"—urge us to buy the latest device, diet plan, superfood, power shake, or diet book; consume less food at each meal; and exercise more.

As other nations strive for Western patterns of consumption, weight problems manifest themselves in their populations as well. Even people on a subsistence diet find themselves confronting societal pressure to improve their "standard of living." The irony is that many lack the resources—but not the desire—to do so. Sadly, vast numbers of humans still lack the wherewithal to maintain a minimum dietary standard and hence are subject to afflictions ranging from vitamin deficiencies to starvation. For them, weight management may mean simply having enough food to meet the body's energy demands.

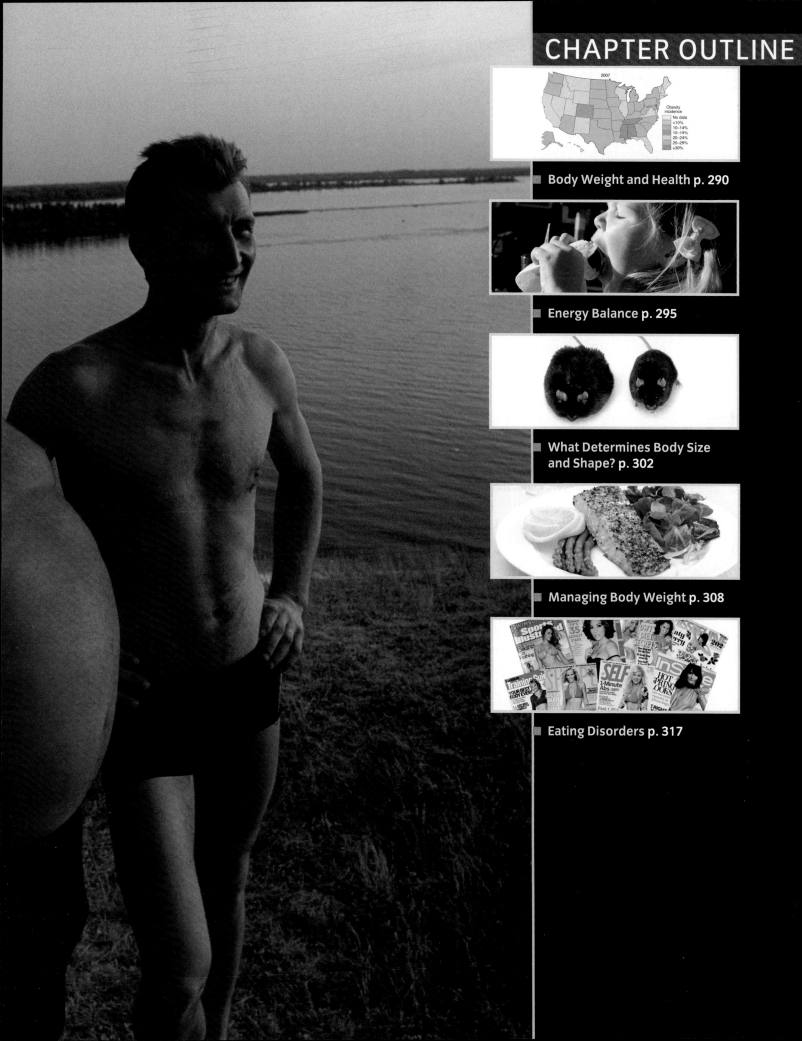

CHAPTER OUTLINE

Body Weight and Health

I n the United States today, a staggering 66% of adults are either **overweight** or **obese**.[1] The numbers have increased dramatically over the past 40 to 50 years (**FIGURE 9.1**). In 1960, only 13.4% of American adults were obese. By 1990, about 23% were obese, and today, only two decades later, 32% are obese. Obesity affects both men and women and all racial and eth- nic groups. Obesity rates for minorities often exceed those in the general population: Among African Americans,

obese Having excess body fat. Obesity is defined as having a body mass index (ratio of weight to height squared) of 30 kg/m² or greater.

overweight Being too heavy for one's height, usually due to an excess of body fat. Overweight is defined as having a body mass index (ratio of weight to height squared) of 25 to 29.9 kilograms/meter² (kg/m²).

34% of men and 54% of women are obese; among Mexican Americans, about 32% of men and over 42% of women are obese.[1]

Obesity is a growing concern world-wide. It is such an important trend that the word *globesity* has been coined to reflect the escalation of global obesity and over-weight. Around the world, approximately 1.6 billion adults are overweight, and 400 million are obese. The World Health Orga-nization projects that by 2015, approxi-mately 2.3 billion adults will be overweight and more than 700 million will be obese.[2] Once considered a problem only in high-income coun-tries, overweight and obesity are now on the rise in low- and middle-income countries, particularly in urban settings.

Obesity on the rise FIGURE 9.1

These maps show the percentage of the adult population classified as obese in each state in 1990 and 2007. The dramatic rise in overweight and obesity in the United States over the past few decades has led medical and public health officials to label the situation an epidemic.

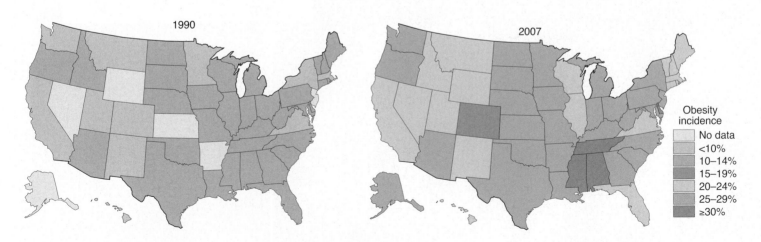

1990

2007

Obesity incidence
- No data
- <10%
- 10–14%
- 15–19%
- 20–24%
- 25–29%
- ≥30%

Obesity-related health complications have reached epidemic proportions in the United States and elsewhere around the world. On this graph a risk value of 1 represents the risk of having each disease if your weight is in the healthy range. A value of 2 indicates that the risk is doubled.

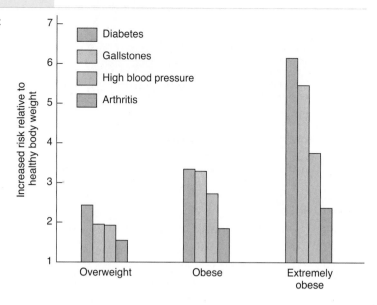

WHAT'S WRONG WITH HAVING TOO MUCH BODY FAT?

Having too much body fat increases a person's risk of developing a host of chronic health problems, including high blood pressure, heart disease, high blood cholesterol, diabetes, gallbladder disease, arthritis, sleep disorders, respiratory problems, menstrual irregularities, and cancers of the breast, uterus, prostate, and colon (**FIGURE 9.2**). Obesity also increases the incidence and severity of infectious disease and has been linked to poor wound healing and surgical complications. The more excess body fat you have, the greater your health risks. The longer you carry excess fat, the greater the risks; individuals who gain excess weight at a young age and remain overweight throughout life face the greatest health risks.

Being overweight also has psychological and social consequences. Overweight and obese individuals of any age are more likely to experience depression, negative self-image, and feelings of inadequacy.[3] They may also be discriminated against in college admissions, in the workplace, and even on public transportation. The physical health consequences of excess body fat may not manifest themselves as disease for years, but the psychological and social problems are experienced every day.

Because obesity increases health problems, it increases health care costs. Estimates suggest that obesity "costs" about $117 billion per year—more than the health care costs incurred by daily smokers and heavy drinkers.[4] The greater the number of obese people, the higher the nation's health care expenses and the higher the cost to society as a whole in terms of lost wages and productivity.

WHAT IS A HEALTHY WEIGHT?

A healthy weight is a weight that minimizes health risks. Your body weight is the sum of the weight of your fat and your **lean body mass**. Some body fat is essential for health, but too much increases your risk for a number of chronic health problems. How much weight and fat is too much depends on your age, gender, and lifestyle and where your fat is located.

> **lean body mass**
> Body mass attributed to nonfat body components such as bone, muscle, and internal organs; also called *fat-free mass*.

Body mass index (BMI) The current standard for assessing the healthfulness of body weight is **body mass index (BMI)**, which is determined by dividing body weight (in kilograms) by height (in meters) squared. A healthy BMI for adults is between 18.5 and 24.9 kg/m^2. People with a BMI in this range have the lowest health risks. Although BMI is not

> **body mass index (BMI)** A measure of body weight relative to height that is used to compare body size with a standard.

Underweight is associated with increased risk of early death, but this does not mean that all thin people are at risk.[7] People who are naturally lean have a lower incidence of certain chronic diseases and do not face increased health risks due to their low body weight. However, low body fat due to starvation, eating disorders, or a disease process decreases energy reserves and the ability of the immune system to fight disease.

What's your BMI? FIGURE 9.3

To find your BMI, locate your height in the leftmost column and read across to your weight. Follow the column containing your weight up to the top line to find your BMI. A BMI < 18.5 kg/m² is classified as **underweight**, a BMI ≥ 25 and < 30 kg/m² is classified as overweight, and a BMI of ≥ 30 kg/m² is classified as obese. A BMI ≥ 40 kg/m² is considered **extreme obesity**, or **morbid obesity**.

Height (feet/inches)	UNDER-WEIGHT		NORMAL						OVERWEIGHT					OBESE										EXTREME OBESITY		
BMI	17	18	19	20	21	22	23	24	25	26	27	28	29	30	31	32	33	34	35	36	37	38	39	40	41	42
	Body Weight (pounds)																									
4'10"	81	86	91	96	100	105	110	115	119	124	129	134	138	143	148	153	158	162	167	172	177	181	186	191	196	201
4'11"	84	89	94	99	104	109	114	119	124	128	133	138	143	148	153	158	163	168	173	178	183	188	193	198	203	208
5'0"	87	92	97	102	107	112	118	123	128	133	138	143	148	153	158	163	168	174	179	184	189	194	199	204	209	215
5'1"	90	95	100	106	111	116	122	127	132	137	143	148	153	158	164	169	174	180	185	190	195	201	206	211	217	222
5'2"	93	98	104	109	115	120	126	131	136	142	147	153	158	164	169	175	180	186	191	196	202	207	213	218	224	229
5'3"	96	102	107	113	118	124	130	135	141	146	152	158	163	169	175	180	186	191	197	203	208	214	220	225	231	237
5'4"	99	105	110	116	122	128	134	140	145	151	157	163	169	174	180	186	192	197	204	209	215	221	227	232	238	244
5'5"	102	108	114	120	126	132	138	144	150	156	162	168	174	180	186	192	198	204	210	216	222	228	234	240	246	252
5'6"	105	112	118	124	130	136	142	148	155	161	167	173	179	186	192	198	204	210	216	223	229	235	241	247	253	260
5'7"	108	115	121	127	134	140	146	153	159	166	172	178	185	191	198	204	211	217	223	230	236	242	249	255	261	268
5'8"	112	119	125	131	138	144	151	158	164	171	177	184	190	197	203	210	216	223	230	236	243	249	256	262	269	276
5'9"	115	122	128	135	142	149	155	162	169	176	182	189	196	203	209	216	223	230	236	243	250	257	263	270	277	284
5'10"	119	126	132	139	146	153	160	167	174	181	188	195	202	209	216	222	229	236	243	250	257	264	271	278	285	292
5'11"	122	129	136	143	150	157	165	172	179	186	193	200	208	215	222	229	236	243	250	257	265	272	279	286	293	301
6'0"	125	133	140	147	154	162	169	177	184	191	199	206	213	221	228	235	242	250	258	265	272	279	287	294	302	309
6'1"	129	137	144	151	159	166	174	182	189	197	204	212	219	227	235	242	250	257	265	272	280	288	295	302	310	318
6'2"	132	140	148	155	163	171	179	186	194	202	210	218	225	233	241	249	256	264	272	280	287	295	303	311	319	326
6'3"	136	144	152	160	168	176	184	192	200	208	216	224	232	240	248	256	264	272	279	287	295	303	311	319	327	335
6'4"	140	148	156	164	172	180	189	197	205	213	221	230	238	246	254	263	271	279	287	295	304	312	320	328	336	344

Source: Adapted from National Institutes of Health, National Heart, Lung, and Blood Institute, 2000.

Although BMI can be a useful tool, other information is also needed to determine health risks. For example, someone who is overweight based on BMI but consumes a healthy diet and exercises regularly may be more fit and at lower risk for chronic diseases than someone with a BMI in the healthy range who is sedentary and eats a poor diet.

A high BMI may be caused by either too much body fat or a large amount of muscle. Therefore, in muscular athletes, BMI does not provide an accurate estimate of health risk. Both of these individuals have a BMI of 33, but only the man on the right has excess body fat. The high body weight of the man on the left is due to his large muscle mass. His body fat, and hence disease risk, is low.

actually a measure of body fat, it is recommended as a way to assess body fatness that is better than measuring weight alone.[5,6] You can use FIGURE 9.3 to determine your BMI or calculate it according to either of these equations:

$$BMI = Weight\ in\ kilograms/(Height\ in\ meters)^2$$
or
$$BMI = [Weight\ in\ pounds/(Height\ in\ inches)^2] \times 703$$

Body composition **Body composition**, which refers to the relative proportions of fat and lean tissue that make up the body, affects the risks associated with excess body weight. Having more than the recommended percentage of body fat increases health risks, whereas having more lean body mass does not. In general, women store more body fat than men do, so the level that is healthy for women is somewhat higher than the level that is healthy for men. A healthy level of body fat for a young adult female is between 21 and 32% of total weight; for young adult males, it is between 8 and 19%.[8] With aging, lean body mass decreases and body fat increases, even if body weight remains the same. Some of this change may be prevented through exercise. Body composition can be measured using a variety of techniques (FIGURE 9.4).

Techniques for measuring body composition FIGURE 9.4

Skinfold thickness. Skinfold thickness uses calipers to measure the thickness of the fat layer under the skin at several locations. This technique assumes that the amount of fat under the skin is representative of total body fat. It is fast, easy, and inexpensive but can be inaccurate if not performed by a trained professional.

Underwater weighing. Underwater weighing relies on the fact that lean tissue is denser than fat tissue. The difference between a person's weight on land and his or her weight underwater is used to calculate body density; the higher a person's body density, the less fat he or she has. Underwater weighing is accurate but can't be used for small children or for ill or frail adults.

Air displacement. The BOD POD measures the amount of air displaced by the body in a closed chamber and uses this along with body weight to determine body density, which is related to body fat mass. This method is accurate and easy for the subject but expensive and not readily available.

Bioelectric impedance. Bioelectric impedance analysis measures an electric current traveling through the body. It is based on the fact that current moves easily through lean tissue, which is high in water, but is slowed by fat, which resists current flow. Bioelectric impedance measurements are fast, easy, and painless but can be inaccurate if the amount of body water is higher or lower than typical. For example, in someone who has been sweating heavily, the estimate of percent body fat obtained using bioelectric impedance will be artificially high.

Dual energy X-ray absorptiometry (DXA). DXA distinguishes among various body tissues by measuring differences in levels of X-ray absorption. A single investigation can accurately determine total body mass, bone mineral mass, and body fat percentage, but the apparatus is expensive and not readily available.

A People who carry their excess fat around and above the waist have more visceral fat. Those who carry their extra fat below the waist, in the hips and thighs, have more subcutaneous fat. In the popular literature, these body types have been dubbed "apples" and "pears," respectively.

Visceral fat

Abdominal muscle layer

Subcutaneous fat

B Waist circumference is indicative of the amount of visceral fat, the type of fat that is associated with increased health risk. Waist measurements along with BMI are used to estimate the health risk associated with excess body fat. These waist circumference "cutpoints" are not useful in patients with a BMI of 35 kg/m² or greater.

In men a BMI of 25 to 34.9 kg/m² and a waist circumference >40 inches indicates visceral fat storage.

In women a BMI of 25 to 34.9 kg/m² and a waist circumference >35 inches indicates visceral fat storage.

NATIONAL GEOGRAPHIC

Location of body fat The location of body fat stores affects the risks associated with having too much fat (**FIGURE 9.5**). Excess **subcutaneous fat**, which is adipose tissue located under the skin, does not increase health risk as much as does excess **visceral fat**, which is adipose tissue located around the organs in the abdomen. Generally, fat in the hips and lower body is subcutaneous, whereas fat in the abdominal region is primarily visceral. Visceral fat is more metabolically active than subcutaneous fat, releasing dozens of biologically active substances that can contribute to disease.[9] An increase in visceral fat is associated with a higher incidence of heart disease, high blood cholesterol, high blood pressure, stroke, diabetes, and breast cancer.

Where your extra fat is deposited is determined primarily by your genes.[10] Visceral fat storage is more common in men than in women, but after menopause, the amount of visceral fat in women increases. Age and environment also influence where fat is stored.[11] Visceral fat storage increases with age. Stress, tobacco use, and alcohol consumption predispose people to visceral fat deposition, whereas weight loss and exercise reduce the amount of visceral fat.

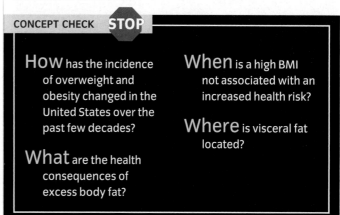

CONCEPT CHECK STOP

HOW has the incidence of overweight and obesity changed in the United States over the past few decades?

What are the health consequences of excess body fat?

When is a high BMI not associated with an increased health risk?

Where is visceral fat located?

Energy Balance

LEARNING OBJECTIVES

Identify lifestyle factors that have led to weight gain among Americans.

Explain the principle of energy balance.

Describe the components of energy expenditure.

Calculate your EER at various levels of activity.

Americans' **energy balance** is out of balance, and as a result we are gaining weight. According to the principle of energy balance, if you consume the same amount of energy—or calories—as you expend, your body weight will remain the same. If you consume more energy than you expend, you will gain weight, and if you expend more energy than you consume, you will lose weight. In the United States today, our energy intake is exceeding our energy expenditure. Bringing it back into balance requires an understanding of how many calories we need and how we use energy.

energy balance
The amount of energy consumed in the diet compared with the amount expended by the body over a given period.

AMERICA'S ENERGY IMBALANCE

Over the past 40 years, changes in environmental and social factors have affected what we eat, how much we eat, and how much exercise we get. Simply put, more Americans are overweight than ever before because we are eating more and burning fewer calories than we did 40 years ago.[12] Food is plentiful and continuously available, and little activity is required in our daily lives.[13]

Eating more In America today, supermarkets, fast-food restaurants, and convenience marts make palatable, affordable food readily available to the majority of the population 24 hours a day. We are constantly bombarded with cues to eat: Advertisements entice us with tasty, inexpensive foods, and convenience stores, food courts, and vending machines tempt us with the sights and smells of fatty, sweet, high-calorie snacks. The accessibility of tempting treats stimulates **appetite**. Because appetite is triggered by external cues such as the sight or smell of food, it is usually appetite, and not **hunger**,

appetite A desire to consume specific foods that is independent of hunger.

hunger A desire to consume food that is triggered by internal physiological signals.

40 years ago   Today

Soft drinks
62%

French fries
57%

Cheeseburgers
24%

Percent increase in portion size

Portion distortion FIGURE 9.6

The burgers and French fries served in fast-food restaurants today are two to five times larger than they were when fast food first appeared about 40 years ago. Soft-drink serving sizes have also escalated. A large fast-food soft drink today contains 32 ounces, providing about 300 Calories, and 20-oz bottles have replaced 12-oz cans in many vending machines.

that makes us stop for an ice cream cone on a summer afternoon or give in to the smell of freshly baked chocolate chip cookies while strolling through the mall.

In addition to having more enticing choices available to us, we consume more calories today because portion sizes have increased (FIGURE 9.6).[14] The more food that is put in front of people, the more they eat.[15] People tend to eat in units, such as one cookie, one sandwich, or one bag of chips, regardless of the size of the unit. So if we are presented with larger units, we eat more.

Social changes over the past few decades have also contributed to the increase in the number of calories Americans consume. Busy schedules and an increase in the number of single-parent households and households with two working parents mean that families are often too rushed to cook meals at home. As a result, prepackaged, convenience, and fast-food meals have become

mainstays. These foods are typically higher in fat and energy than foods prepared at home.

Moving less
Along with America's rising energy intake, there has been a decline in the amount of energy Americans expend, both at work and at play (FIGURE 9.7). Fewer American adults today work in jobs that require physical labor. People drive to work rather than walk or bike, take elevators instead of stairs, use dryers rather than hang clothes outside, and cut the lawn with riding mowers rather than with push mowers. All these simple changes reduce the amount of energy expended daily. Americans are also less active during their leisure time because busy schedules and long days at work and commuting leave little time for active recreation. Instead, at the end of the day, people tend to sit in front of television sets, video games, and computers.

Inactivity is also contributing to excess body weight among children. In the 1960s, schools provided daily physical education classes, and children spent their after-school hours playing outdoors; today, they are more likely to spend their afternoons indoors with televisions, video games, and computers. As a result, they burn fewer calories, snack more, and consequently gain weight. Sixteen percent of U.S. children and adolescents ages 2 through 19 are obese.[17]

Inactivity contributes to obesity FIGURE 9.7

A typical office worker today walks only about 3000 to 5000 steps per day (2000 steps = approximately 1 mile). In contrast, in the Amish community—where automobiles and other modern conveniences are not allowed—a typical adult takes 14,000 to 18,000 steps a day. The overall incidence of obesity among the Amish is only 4%.[16]

BALANCING ENERGY INTAKE AND EXPENDITURE

The energy needed to fuel your body comes from the food you eat and the energy stored in your body. You use this energy to stay alive, process your food, move, and grow.

Energy intake The amount of energy you consume depends on what and how much you eat and drink. The carbohydrate, fat, protein, and alcohol consumed in food and drink all contribute energy: 4, 9, 4, and 7 Calories/gram, respectively (**FIGURE 9.8A** on the next page). Vitamins, minerals, and water, though essential nutrients, do not provide energy. You can determine your calorie intake by using food labels or looking up values in a food composition table or database (**FIGURE 9.8B**).

Energy expenditure The total amount of energy used by the body each day is called **total energy expenditure**. It includes the energy needed to maintain basic body functions as well as that needed to fuel physical activity and process food. In individuals who are growing or pregnant, total energy expenditure also includes the energy used to deposit new tissues. In women who are lactating, it includes the energy used to produce milk. A small amount of energy is also used to maintain body temperature in a cold environment.

For most people, about 60 to 75% of total energy expenditure is used for **basal metabolism**. Basal metabolism includes all the essential metabolic reactions and life-sustaining functions needed to keep you alive, such as breathing, circulating blood, regulating body temperature, synthesizing tissues, removing waste products, and sending nerve signals. The rate at which energy is used for these basic functions is the **basal metabolic rate (BMR)**. The energy expended for basal metabolism does *not* include the energy needed for physical activity or for the digestion and absorption of food (**FIGURE 9.8C**).

BMR increases with increasing body weight and is affected by body composition because it takes more energy to maintain lean tissue than to maintain body fat (see Figure 9.8C). BMR is generally higher in men than in women because men have a greater amount of lean body mass. BMR decreases with age, partly because of the decrease in lean body mass that occurs as we get older. BMR is also lower when calorie intake is consistently below the body's needs.[20] This drop in BMR reduces the amount of energy needed to maintain body weight. It is a beneficial adaptation in someone who is starving, but in someone who is trying to lose weight it is frustrating because it makes weight loss more difficult.

Physical activity is the second major component of total energy expenditure. In most people, physical activity accounts for a smaller proportion of total energy expenditure than basal metabolism does, about 15 to 30% of energy requirements (**FIGURE 9.8D**). The energy we expend in physical activity includes both planned exercise and daily activities such as walking to work, typing, performing yard work, work-related activities, and even fidgeting. This **nonexercise activity thermogenesis (NEAT)** includes the energy expended for everything that is not sleeping, eating, or sports-like exercise. It accounts for the majority of the energy expended for activity and varies enormously, depending on an individual's occupation and daily movements.

The amount of energy used for activity depends on the size of the person, how strenuous the activity is, and the length of time it is performed. Because it takes more energy to move a heavier object, the amount of energy expended for many activities increases as body weight increases. More strenuous activities, such as jogging, use more energy than do less strenuous activities, such as walking, but if you walk for an hour, you will probably burn as many calories as you would jogging for 30 minutes (Appendix I).

We also use energy to digest food and to absorb, metabolize, and store the nutrients from this food. The energy used for these processes is called either the **thermic effect of food (TEF)** or **diet-induced thermogenesis**. This energy expenditure causes body temperature to rise slightly for several hours after a person has eaten. The energy required for TEF is estimated to be about 10% of energy intake but can vary, depending on the amounts and types of nutrients consumed (**FIGURE 9.8E**).

basal metabolism The energy expended to maintain an awake, resting body that is not digesting food.

basal metabolic rate (BMR) The rate of energy expenditure under resting conditions. It is measured after 12 hours without food or exercise.

nonexercise activity thermogenesis (NEAT) The energy expended for everything we do other than sleeping, eating, or sports-like exercise.

thermic effect of food (TEF) or **diet-induced thermogenesis** The energy required for the digestion of food and absorption, metabolism, and storage of nutrients.

What you weigh is determined by the balance between how much energy you take in and how much energy you expend.

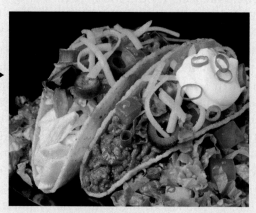

A The number of calories in a food depends on how much carbohydrate, fat, and protein it contains. This taco contains 9 g of protein, 16 g of carbohydrate, and 13 g of fat. Its energy content is (9 g × 4 Cal/g protein) + (16 g × 4 Cal/g carbohydrate) + (13 g × 9 Cal/g fat) = 217 Cal

Nutrition Facts

Serving Size 8 fl oz (240mL)
Servings Per Container 2

Amount Per Serving

Calories 100

	%Daily Value*
Total Fat 0g	0%
Sodium 10 mg	0%
Total Carb 26g	9%
Sugars 25g	
Protein 0g	

Percent daily values are based on a 2,000 calorie diet.

This iced tea provides 100 Calories per serving. One bottle contains two servings. Finishing the whole bottle will add 200 Calories to your intake for the day, mostly in the form of added sugars.

B The Nutrition Facts panel shows the Calories per serving, but to know how many Calories your portion contains, you need to check the serving size. Often the portions of foods and beverages that people consume are larger than the servings listed on the label. As a result, they consume more Calories than they think they do.

Energy in

C Aerobic metabolism uses oxygen and produces carbon dioxide. Therefore, measures of these gases in expired air can be used to estimate energy expenditure. If measures are taken in the morning, in a warm room, before rising, and at least 12 hours after food intake or activity, they can be used to estimate the energy expended for basal metabolism. For convenience, measurements are often made after only 5 to 6 hours without food or exercise. This measurement, called the **resting metabolic rate (RMR)**, yields values about 10 to 20% higher than BMR values.[18] ▼

Factors that increase basal metabolism
Higher lean body mass
Greater height and weight
Male gender
Pregnancy
Lactation
Growth
Fever
Elevated thyroid hormone levels
Stimulant drugs such as caffeine and tobacco
Exercise

E The amount of energy used to process the food we eat varies with the size and composition of the meal. A bigger meal produces a greater thermic effect of food (TEF). A high-fat meal yields a lower TEF than one high in carbohydrate or protein because dietary fat can be used and stored more efficiently.[19]

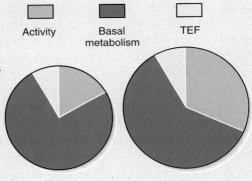

Activity Basal metabolism TEF

D Adding physical activity to your day increases the total number of calories you must consume to maintain your weight. Some athletes and laborers use more energy to fuel activity than they do for basal metabolism. ▶

Sedentary person (1800 Cal/day)

Physically active person (2200 Cal/day)

Energy out

Excess energy consumed as dietary fat is easily stored as body fat. Excess energy consumed as dietary carbohydrate is stored as glycogen or converted into fat. Excess energy consumed as dietary protein is converted into body fat. When you eat less than you need, you retrieve energy from these stores. Liver glycogen and a small amount of body protein are broken down to supply glucose, and triglycerides in adipose tissue are broken down to supply fatty acids for energy.

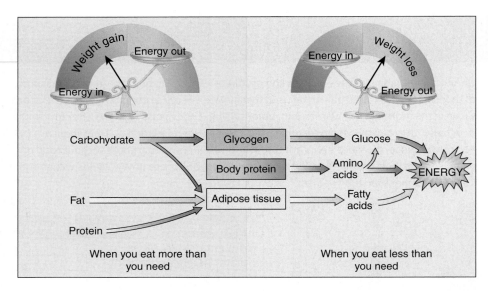

The basics of weight gain and weight loss

If you consume more energy than you expend, the excess energy is stored for later use (FIGURE 9.9). A small amount of energy is stored as glycogen in liver and muscle, but most is stored as fat in **adipocytes**, which make up adipose tissue. Adipocytes contain large fat droplets (see Figure 5.10B). The cells increase in size as they accumulate more fat, and they shrink as fat is removed. If intake exceeds needs over the long term, adipocytes enlarge, and the amount of body fat increases, causing weight gain. The larger the number of adipocytes, the greater the body's ability to store fat. Most adipocytes are formed during infancy and adolescence, but excessive weight gain can cause the formation of new adipocytes at any time of life.

adipocytes
Cells that store fat.

Stored energy is used when energy intake is reduced, both in the short term, such as when you haven't eaten a meal for a few hours, and in the long term, such as when you are trying to lose weight. To maintain a steady supply of blood glucose, liver glycogen is broken down (see Figure 9.9). Glucose is also supplied by the breakdown of small amounts of body protein, primarily muscle protein, to yield amino acids. These amino acids can then be used to make glucose or produce ATP. Energy for tissues that don't require glucose is provided by the breakdown of stored fat. Nutrients consumed in the next meal replenish these stores, but with prolonged energy restriction, fat and protein are lost, and body weight is reduced. It is estimated that an energy deficit of about 3500 Calories results in the loss of a pound of adipose tissue.

ESTIMATED ENERGY REQUIREMENTS

The current recommendation for energy intake in the United States is the *estimated energy requirement* (*EER*; see Chapter 2), the number of calories needed for a healthy individual to maintain his or her weight.[18] It is calculated using equations that take into account gender, age, height, weight, activity level, and life stage, all of which affect calorie needs.

To calculate your EER, you must first determine your physical activity level.[18] Do this by keeping a daily log of your activities, recording the amount of time spent at each. Use FIGURE 9.10 to help translate the amount of time you spend engaged in moderate-intensity or vigorous activity into an activity level (sedentary, low active, active, or high active). Each activity level corresponds to a numerical physical activity (PA) value that can be used to calculate your EER. For example, if you spend about an hour a day walking (a moderate-intensity activity) or about 45 minutes jogging (a vigorous activity), you are in the active category and should use the active PA value corresponding to your age and gender when calculating your EER.

Activity level has a significant effect on calorie needs. For example, a 22-year-old man who is 6 feet tall and weighs 185 pounds needs about 2770 Calories/day if he is at a sedentary activity level but almost 600 more if he is at an active level.

Once you have determined your physical activity level, calculate your EER by entering your age, weight, height, and PA value (see Figure 9.10) into the appropriate EER prediction equation. TABLE 9.1 provides equations for normal-weight adults and children age 9 and older. Equations for other groups are in Appendix A.

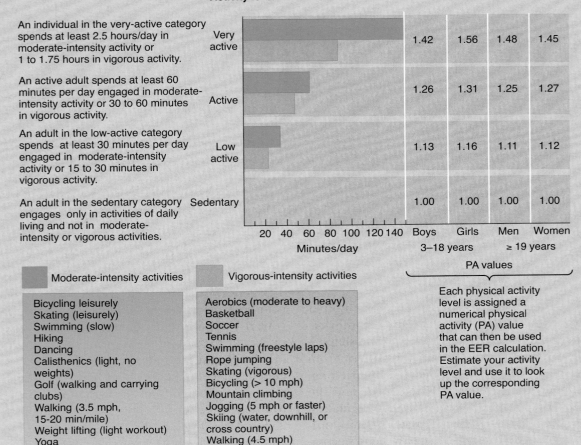

Activity level

An individual in the very-active category spends at least 2.5 hours/day in moderate-intensity activity or 1 to 1.75 hours in vigorous activity.

An active adult spends at least 60 minutes per day engaged in moderate-intensity activity or 30 to 60 minutes in vigorous activity.

An adult in the low-active category spends at least 30 minutes per day engaged in moderate-intensity activity or 15 to 30 minutes in vigorous activity.

An adult in the sedentary category engages only in activities of daily living and not in moderate-intensity or vigorous activities.

Activity level	Boys 3–18 years	Girls 3–18 years	Men ≥ 19 years	Women ≥ 19 years
Very active	1.42	1.56	1.48	1.45
Active	1.26	1.31	1.25	1.27
Low active	1.13	1.16	1.11	1.12
Sedentary	1.00	1.00	1.00	1.00

Minutes/day: 20 40 60 80 100 120 140

PA values

Each physical activity level is assigned a numerical physical activity (PA) value that can then be used in the EER calculation. Estimate your activity level and use it to look up the corresponding PA value.

Moderate-intensity activities

Bicycling leisurely
Skating (leisurely)
Swimming (slow)
Hiking
Dancing
Calisthenics (light, no weights)
Golf (walking and carrying clubs)
Walking (3.5 mph, 15-20 min/mile)
Weight lifting (light workout)
Yoga

Vigorous-intensity activities

Aerobics (moderate to heavy)
Basketball
Soccer
Tennis
Swimming (freestyle laps)
Rope jumping
Skating (vigorous)
Bicycling (> 10 mph)
Mountain climbing
Jogging (5 mph or faster)
Skiing (water, downhill, or cross country)
Walking (4.5 mph)

What are your physical activity level and PA value? FIGURE 9.10

A sedentary person spends about 2.5 hours per day engaged in the activities of daily living, such as housework, homework, yard work, and gardening. Adding either moderate-intensity or vigorous activity, or a combination of the two, will put him or her in the low-active, active, or very-active category, depending on the amount of additional energy expended. Compared to moderate-intensity activity, vigorous activity will burn the same number of calories in less time.

EER prediction equations TABLE 9.1

Life stage	EER prediction equation*
Boys 9–18 years	$EER = 88.5 - (61.9 \times \text{Age in yrs}) + PA\,[(26.7 \times \text{Weight in kg}) + (903 \times \text{Height in m})] + 25$
Girls 9–18 years	$EER = 135.3 - (30.8 \times \text{Age in yrs}) + PA\,[(10.0 \times \text{Weight in kg}) + (934 \times \text{Height in m})] + 25$
Men ≥19 years	$EER = 662 - (9.53 \times \text{Age in yrs}) + PA\,[(15.91 \times \text{Weight in kg}) + (539.6 \times \text{Height in m})]$
Women ≥19 years	$EER = 354 - (6.91 \times \text{Age in yrs}) + PA\,[(9.36 \times \text{Weight in kg}) + (726 \times \text{Height in m})]$

For example, if you are an active 19-year-old male who weighs 72.7 kg and is 1.75 m tall,
$EER = 662 - (9.53 \times 19\,\text{yrs}) + 1.25([15.91 \times 72.7\,\text{kg}] + [539.6 \times 1.75\,\text{m}]) = 3107\,\text{Cal/day}$

*These equations are appropriate for determining EERs in normal weight individuals. Equations that predict the amount of energy needed for weight maintenance in overweight and obese individuals are also available (see Appendix A).

CONCEPT CHECK STOP

Why are more Americans obese today compared to 40 years ago?

Where in the body is most energy stored when intake exceeds expenditure?

Which component of energy expenditure is easiest to modify?

What is your EER?

What Determines Body Size and Shape?

LEARNING OBJECTIVES

Discuss genetic and environmental factors that affect body weight.

List four physiological signals that determine whether you feel hungry or full.

Describe how hormones regulate body fat levels.

Discuss factors that cause some people to gain weight more easily than others.

You are probably shaped like your mother or your father. This is because the information that determines body size and shape is contained in the genes you inherit from your parents (**FIGURE 9.11**). Some of us inherit long, lean bodies, and others inherit huskier builds and the tendency to put on pounds. Genes involved in regulating body weight have been called **obesity genes** because variations in these genes determine the likelihood of becoming obese. More than 300 genes and regions of human chromosomes have been linked to obesity.[21] These genes are responsible for the production of proteins that affect how much food you eat, how much energy you expend, and the way fat is stored in your body. But genes are not the only factor; regardless of your genetic background, the lifestyle choices you make play an important role in determining what you weigh.

GENES VS. ENVIRONMENT

The genes you inherit play a major role in determining your body weight. If one or both of your parents is obese, your risk of becoming obese is increased by a factor of 2 or 3, and the risk increases with the magnitude of the obesity. By studying identical twins, who have the same genetic makeup, researchers have been able to determine that about 75% of the variation in BMI can be attributed to genes.[22,23] This means that the remaining 25% is determined by the environment in which you live and the lifestyle choices you make (see the *Case Study*).

Genes determine body shape FIGURE 9.11

The genes we inherit from our parents are important determinants of our body size and shape. The boy on the left inherited his father's long, lean body, whereas the boy on the right has his father's huskier build and will likely have a tendency to be overweight throughout his life.

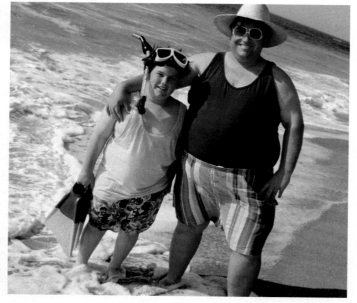

BALANCING ENERGY: GENETICS AND LIFESTYLE

Aysha was a chubby baby. Into her teens, she continued to be slightly overweight. Because her parents are both obese, no one was surprised by Aysha's size. During her freshman year at college, she gained 10 lbs and became resigned to the inevitability that she would be fat like her parents. Then she noticed that the choices many of her thin friends made—both in the foods they ate and how they spent their free time—were different from the choices she made. She decided to make some changes.

Aysha, now 23 years old, is 5 feet 4 inches tall and weighs 155 lbs.

What is her BMI? Is it in the healthy range?

▼

Your answer:

By recording and analyzing her food intake for three days, Aysha determines that she consumes about 2450 Calories/day. By keeping an activity log, she estimates that a typical day includes 30 minutes of walking rapidly around campus—a moderate-intensity activity.

What is her EER?

▼

Your answer:

How does Aysha's EER compare with her intake? Is she in energy balance?

▼

Your answer:

Aysha decides to start exercising more and to cut down on her portions at meals and make healthier choices. Meal A, shown below, used to be her typical lunch, and Meal B is her new lunch.

How can Meal B have fewer calories even though it looks like more food?

▼

Your answer:

Why might Meal B satisfy hunger just as well as or better than Meal A?

▼

Your answer:

If Aysha adds an additional 30 minutes of moderate-intensity exercise every day, by how much will her EER increase?

▼

Your answer:

Do you think Aysha is destined to be overweight? Explain your answer.

▼

Your answer:

(Check your answers in Appendix K.)

A B

When individuals who are genetically susceptible to weight gain find themselves in an environment where food is appealing and plentiful and physical activity is easily avoided, obesity is a likely outcome but not the only possible one. If you inherit genes that predispose you to being overweight but carefully monitor your diet and exercise regularly, you can maintain a healthy weight. It is also possible for individuals with no genetic tendency toward obesity to end up overweight if they consume a high-calorie diet and get little exercise. The interplay between genetics and lifestyle is illustrated by the higher incidence of obesity in Pima Indians living in Arizona than in a genetically similar group of Pima Indians living in Mexico (**FIGURE 9.12**).[24]

REGULATION OF FOOD INTAKE AND BODY WEIGHT

What we eat and how much we exercise vary from day to day, but body weight tends to stay relatively constant for long periods. The body compensates for variations in diet and exercise by adjusting energy intake and expenditure to keep weight at a particular level, or **set point**. This set point, which is believed to be determined in part by genes, explains why your weight remains fairly constant, despite the added activity of a weekend hiking trip, or why most people gain back the weight they lose when they follow a weight-loss diet.[27]

To regulate weight and fatness at a constant level, the body must be able to respond both to short-term changes in food intake and to long-term changes in the amount of stored body fat. Signals related to food intake affect hunger and **satiety** over a short period—from meal to meal—whereas signals from adipose tissue trigger the brain to adjust both food intake and energy expenditure for long-term weight regulation.

satiety The feeling of fullness and satisfaction caused by food consumption that eliminates the desire to eat.

Genes vs. environment FIGURE 9.12

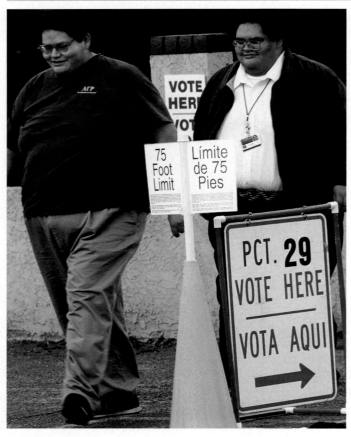

◀ **A** Genetic analysis of the Pima Indian population living in Arizona has identified a number of genes that may be responsible for this group's tendency to store excess body fat.[25] When this genetic susceptibility is combined with a lifestyle that includes lots of high-calorie foods and demands little physical activity, the outcome is the strikingly high incidence of obesity seen in this population.

B The Pima Indians of Mexico have the same genetic susceptibility to obesity as the Arizona Pimas but are farmers who work in the fields and consume the food they grow.[26] They still have higher rates of obesity than would be predicted from their diet and exercise patterns, suggesting that they possess genes that favor fat storage, but they are significantly less obese than the Arizona Pimas.[24] ▼

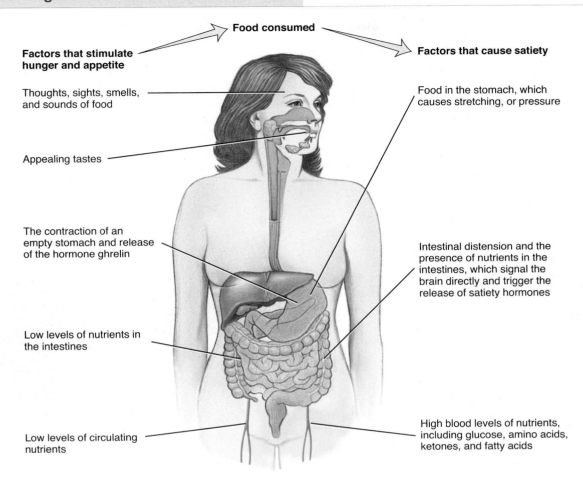

Food consumed

Factors that stimulate hunger and appetite

Thoughts, sights, smells, and sounds of food

Appealing tastes

The contraction of an empty stomach and release of the hormone ghrelin

Low levels of nutrients in the intestines

Low levels of circulating nutrients

Factors that cause satiety

Food in the stomach, which causes stretching, or pressure

Intestinal distension and the presence of nutrients in the intestines, which signal the brain directly and trigger the release of satiety hormones

High blood levels of nutrients, including glucose, amino acids, ketones, and fatty acids

Regulating how much we eat at each meal

How do you know how much to eat for breakfast or when it is time to eat lunch? The physical sensations of hunger or satiety that determine how much you eat at each meal are triggered by signals from the gastrointestinal tract, levels of nutrients and hormones circulating in the blood, and messages from the brain.[28] Some signals are sent before you eat to tell you that you are hungry, some are sent while food is in the gastrointestinal tract, and some occur when nutrients are circulating in the bloodstream (**FIGURE 9.13**).

The hormone **ghrelin** may cause you to feel hungry around lunchtime, regardless of when and how much you ate for breakfast. Ghrelin, which is produced by the stomach, is believed to stimulate the desire to eat at usual mealtimes. Blood levels of ghrelin rise an hour or two before a meal and drop very low after a meal. Another hor-

mone, peptide PYY, causes a reduction in appetite. It is released from the gastrointestinal tract after a meal, and the amount released is proportional to the number of calories in the meal.[29]

Psychological factors can also affect hunger and satiety. Some people eat for comfort and to relieve stress. Others lose their appetite when they experience these emotions. Psychological distress can alter the mechanisms that regulate food intake.

Regulating how much we weigh over the long term

Sometimes we don't pay attention to how full we are after a meal, and we make room for dessert anyway. If this happens often enough, it can cause an increase in body weight and fatness. To return fatness to a set level, the body must be able to monitor how much fat is present. Some of this information comes from hormones.

Leptin is a good example of a hormone that can affect body weight. Leptin is produced by the adipocytes. The amount produced is proportional to the size of the adipocytes, and the effect of leptin on energy intake and expenditure depends on the amount released (see *What a Scientist Sees*). Unfortunately, leptin regulation, like other regulatory mechanisms, is much better at preventing weight loss than at preventing weight gain. Obese individuals generally have high levels of leptin, but these levels are not effective at reducing calorie intake and increasing energy expenditure.[30]

Despite regulatory mechanisms that act to keep our weight stable, changes in physiological, psychological, and environmental circumstances cause the level at which body weight is maintained to change, usually increasing it over time. This supports the hypothesis that the mechanisms that defend against weight loss are stronger than those that prevent weight gain.[31]

Leptin and Body Fat

The average person looking at this picture sees a normal mouse and a very fat mouse. A scientist sees an explanation for obesity. In a normal mouse, leptin acts in the hypothalamus to help maintain body fat at a normal level. As shown in the diagram, the effect of leptin depends on how much of it is present. If the mouse loses weight, fat is lost from adipocytes, and less leptin is released, causing an increase in food intake and a decrease in energy expenditure. If the mouse gains weight, the adipocytes accumulate fat, and more leptin is released, triggering events that decrease food intake and increase energy expenditure.

The mouse on the left inherited a defective leptin gene, so it produces no leptin. Even when the adipocytes enlarge, leptin levels do not increase. The lack of leptin continues to signal the mouse to eat more and expend less energy. The mouse on the right also inherited a defective leptin gene, but treatment with leptin injections returned its weight to normal. What might happen to a mouse with a defect that causes overproduction of leptin?

Increased energy intake and decreased energy expenditure

Decreased leptin

Increased leptin

No increase in leptin

Decreased energy intake and increased energy expenditure

Normal mice

Genetically obese mice

Weight loss

Weight gain

Hypothalamus

Adipocytes at set point size

NEAT difference between obese and lean people FIGURE 9.14

Sedentary obese individuals were found to stand and walk less than sedentary lean individuals and therefore expended about 350 Calories/day fewer than their lean counterparts. This difference remained even when the obese subjects lost weight and the lean subjects gained weight.[33]

WHY DO SOME PEOPLE GAIN WEIGHT MORE EASILY THAN OTHERS?

A few cases of human obesity have been linked directly to defects in specific genes,[32] but mutations in single genes are not responsible for most human obesity. Rather, variations in many genes interact with one another and affect metabolic rate, food intake, fat storage, and activity level. These in turn affect body weight, determining why some of us stay lean and others put on pounds.

Some people, such as the Pima Indians discussed earlier, may gain weight more easily because they inherited genes that make them more efficient at using energy and storing fat. Throughout human history, starvation has threatened survival. Over time, the human body has evolved ways to conserve body fat stores and prevent weight loss. Individuals with the "thriftiest" metabolism would have been more likely to survive. In the United States today, however, food is abundant, so people who inherited these "thrifty genes" are more likely to be obese.

Some people may gain weight more easily because they inherit a tendency to expend less energy on activity. Even if they spend the same amount of time exercising as a lean person, their total energy expenditure may be lower because they expend less energy for NEAT activities, such as housework, walking between classes, fidgeting, and moving to maintain posture (FIGURE 9.14).

CONCEPT CHECK **STOP**

What is the role of genes in regulating body weight?

Why do we feel hungry at about the same times every day?

What happens to leptin levels when you lose weight?

Why are some of us fat and some of us lean?

Managing Body Weight

LEARNING OBJECTIVES

Evaluate an individual's weight and medical history to determine whether weight loss is recommended.

Discuss the recommendations for the rate and amount of weight loss.

Distinguish between a good weight management program and a fad diet.

Explain how medications and surgery can promote weight loss.

 anaging your body weight to keep it in the healthy range requires maintaining a balance between energy intake and energy expenditure. For some people, weight man-

agement may mean avoiding weight gain as they age by making healthy food choices, controlling portion size, and maintaining an active lifestyle. For others, it may mean making major lifestyle changes in order to reduce their weight into the healthy range and keep it there.

WHO SHOULD LOSE WEIGHT?

These days, just about everybody wants to lose a few pounds or more, but not everyone who is concerned about their weight needs to lose weight in order to be healthy. The risks associated with carrying excess weight are related to the degree of the excess, the location of the excess fat, and the presence of other diseases or risk factors that often accompany excess body fat (**FIGURE 9.15**).

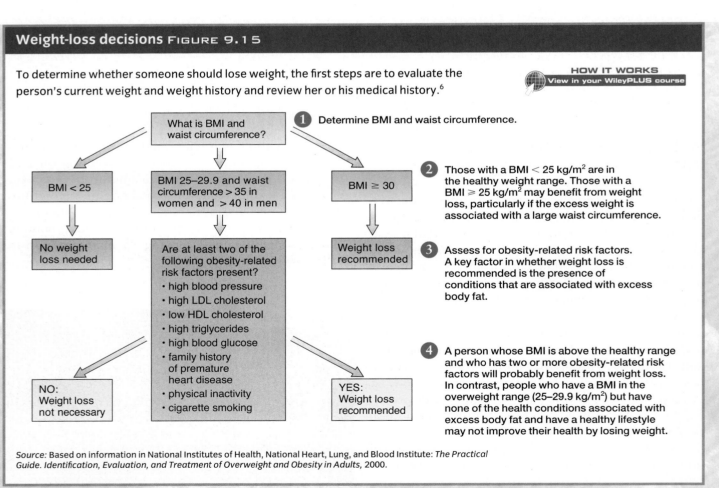

Weight-loss decisions FIGURE 9.15

Process Diagram

To determine whether someone should lose weight, the first steps are to evaluate the person's current weight and weight history and review her or his medical history.[6]

HOW IT WORKS
View in your WileyPLUS course

What is BMI and waist circumference?

1 Determine BMI and waist circumference.

BMI < 25 → No weight loss needed

BMI 25–29.9 and waist circumference > 35 in women and > 40 in men

BMI ≥ 30 → Weight loss recommended

2 Those with a BMI < 25 kg/m² are in the healthy weight range. Those with a BMI ≥ 25 kg/m² may benefit from weight loss, particularly if the excess weight is associated with a large waist circumference.

Are at least two of the following obesity-related risk factors present?
- high blood pressure
- high LDL cholesterol
- low HDL cholesterol
- high triglycerides
- high blood glucose
- family history of premature heart disease
- physical inactivity
- cigarette smoking

NO: Weight loss not necessary

YES: Weight loss recommended

3 Assess for obesity-related risk factors. A key factor in whether weight loss is recommended is the presence of conditions that are associated with excess body fat.

4 A person whose BMI is above the healthy range and who has two or more obesity-related risk factors will probably benefit from weight loss. In contrast, people who have a BMI in the overweight range (25–29.9 kg/m²) but have none of the health conditions associated with excess body fat and have a healthy lifestyle may not improve their health by losing weight.

Source: Based on information in National Institutes of Health, National Heart, Lung, and Blood Institute: *The Practical Guide. Identification, Evaluation, and Treatment of Overweight and Obesity in Adults,* 2000.

Repeated cycles of weight loss and gain, referred to as *weight cycling*, or *yo-yo dieting*, decrease the likelihood that future attempts at weight loss will be successful.[34]

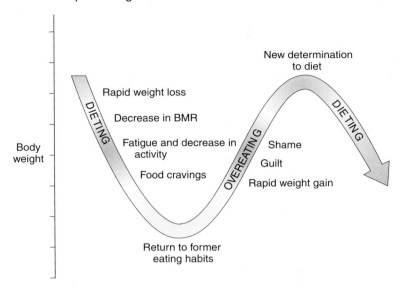

WEIGHT-LOSS GOALS AND GUIDELINES

Losing weight requires tipping the energy balance scale by eating less, exercising more, or some combination of the two. A pound of adipose tissue provides about 3500 Calories. Therefore, to lose a pound of fat, you need to decrease your intake and/or increase your expenditure by this amount. To lose a pound in a week, you would need to tip your energy balance by about 500 Calories/day.

The medical goal for weight loss in an overweight person is to reduce the health risks associated with being overweight. For most people, a loss of 5% to 15% of body weight will significantly reduce disease risk.[6] Losing weight slowly, at a rate of 1/2 to 2 lbs/week, helps ensure that most of what is lost is fat and not lean tissue. The more severe energy restriction needed for rapid weight loss leads to greater losses of water and protein and causes a more significant drop in BMR. People who lose weight rapidly are more likely to regain the weight, leading to repeated cycles of weight loss and gain (FIGURE 9.16). Successful long-term weight management involves a combination of decreasing intake, increasing activity, and changing the behavior patterns that led to weight gain in the first place.

Decreasing energy intake For healthy weight loss, intake must be low in energy but high in nutrients in order to provide for all the body's nutrient needs (see *What Should I Eat?* on the next page). Even when choosing nutrient-dense foods, it is difficult to meet nutrient needs with an intake of fewer than 1200 Calories/day; therefore, dieters consuming less than this amount should take a multivitamin/ multimineral supplement. Medical supervision is recommended if intake is below 800 Calories/day.

Increasing physical activity Exercise increases energy expenditure and therefore makes weight loss easier. If food intake stays the same, adding enough exercise to expend 200 Calories five days a week will result in the loss of a pound in about three and a half weeks. Exercise also promotes muscle development, and because muscle is metabolically active tissue, increased muscle mass increases energy expenditure. In addition, physical activity improves overall fitness and relieves boredom and stress. Weight loss is maintained better when physical activity is included. The benefits of exercise are discussed more fully in Chapter 10.

The *Dietary Guidelines for Americans* recommend an hour of moderate to vigorous activity on most days to prevent gradual weight gain in adulthood.[5] For those who need to lose weight or have lost weight and want to keep it off, more than 60 minutes of moderate exercise per day may be necessary.

Watch your serving size
- Pour chips or crackers into a one-serving bowl rather than eating right from the bag or box.
- Check labels to see if your portion matches the serving size on the label.
- Don't supersize—choose a small drink and a small order of fries.
- Have a plain burger, not one with a special sauce or an extra-large patty.
- When you eat out, share an entrée with a friend or take some home for lunch the next day.

Cut down on high-calorie foods
- Have one scoop of ice cream rather than two.
- Have an apple with lunch instead of a candy bar.
- Bring your own lunch rather than eating out.
- Have water instead of soda.
- Switch to low-fat milk.

Balance intake with exercise
- Go for a bike ride.
- Try bowling or miniature golf instead of watching TV on Friday nights.
- Take a walk during your lunch break or after dinner.
- Play tennis; you don't have to be good to get plenty of exercise.
- Get off the bus one stop early.

Modifying behavior After people lose weight, they typically go off their "diet." When eating patterns return to what they were previously, these dieters then regain the weight they lost. To manage your weight at a healthy level, you need to establish a pattern of food intake and exercise that allows you to enjoy foods and activities you like and that you can maintain throughout your life without gaining weight. Changing food consumption and exercise patterns requires identifying behaviors that led to weight gain and replacing them with new ones that promote and maintain weight loss. This can be accomplished through **behavior modification** (FIGURE 9.17).

■ **behavior modification**
A process that is used to gradually and permanently change habitual behaviors.

Managing America's weight To become a thinner nation, we need strategies that can help all Americans improve their food choices, reduce serving sizes, and increase their physical activity.[35] Although successful weight management ultimately depends on an individual's choices, food manufacturers and restaurants can help us cut calories by offering healthier foods and packaging or serving foods in smaller portions. Communities can help increase activity by providing parks, bike paths, and other recreational facilities for people of all ages. Businesses and schools can contribute by offering more opportunities for physical activity at the workplace and during the school day.

Even small changes, if they are consistent, can arrest the increase in obesity in the population. It has been estimated that a population-wide shift in energy balance of only 100 Calories/day, the equivalent of walking a mile or cutting out a scoop of ice cream, would prevent further weight gain in 90% of the population.[36]

SUGGESTIONS FOR WEIGHT GAIN

As difficult as weight loss is for some people, weight gain can be equally elusive for underweight individuals. The first step toward weight gain is a medical evaluation to rule out medical reasons for low body weight. This is particularly important when weight loss occurs unexpectedly. If the low body weight is due to low energy intake or high energy expenditure, gradually increasing consumption of energy-dense foods is suggested. Energy intake can be increased by eating meals more frequently; adding healthy high-calorie snacks, such as nuts, peanut butter, or milkshakes, between meals; and replacing low-calorie drinks such as water and diet beverages with fruit juices and milk.

ABCs of behavior modification FIGURE 9.17

Behavior modification is based on the theory that behaviors involve three factors: antecedents or cues that lead to a behavior, the behavior itself, and the consequences of the behavior. These are referred to as the ABCs of behavior modification. The steps shown here can be used to identify and change undesirable behaviors.

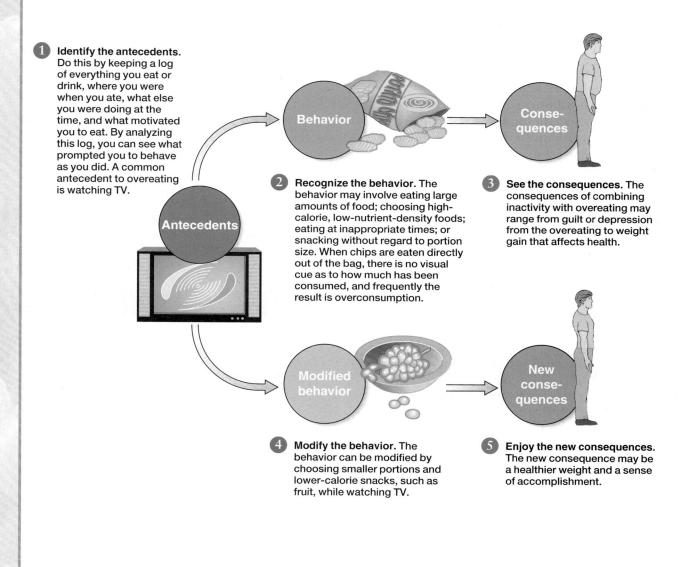

1 **Identify the antecedents.** Do this by keeping a log of everything you eat or drink, where you were when you ate, what else you were doing at the time, and what motivated you to eat. By analyzing this log, you can see what prompted you to behave as you did. A common antecedent to overeating is watching TV.

2 **Recognize the behavior.** The behavior may involve eating large amounts of food; choosing high-calorie, low-nutrient-density foods; eating at inappropriate times; or snacking without regard to portion size. When chips are eaten directly out of the bag, there is no visual cue as to how much has been consumed, and frequently the result is overconsumption.

3 **See the consequences.** The consequences of combining inactivity with overeating may range from guilt or depression from the overeating to weight gain that affects health.

4 **Modify the behavior.** The behavior can be modified by choosing smaller portions and lower-calorie snacks, such as fruit, while watching TV.

5 **Enjoy the new consequences.** The new consequence may be a healthier weight and a sense of accomplishment.

To encourage a gain in muscle rather than fat, strength-training exercise should be a component of any weight gain program. This approach requires extra calories to fuel the activity needed to build muscles. These recommendations apply to individuals who are naturally thin and have trouble gaining weight on the recommended energy intake. However, this dietary approach may not promote weight gain for those who limit intake because of an eating disorder.

DIETS AND FAD DIETS

Want to lose 10 lbs in just 5 days? What dieter wouldn't? People who are desperate to lose weight are prey to all sorts of diets that promise quick fixes. They willingly eat a single food for days at a time, select foods on the basis of special fat-burning qualities, and consume odd combinations at specific times of the day. Most diets, no matter how outlandish, will promote weight loss because they reduce energy intake. Even diets that focus on modifying fat or carbohydrate intake or promise to allow unlimited amounts of certain foods work because intake is reduced. The true test of the effectiveness of a weight-loss plan is whether it promotes weight loss that can be maintained over the long term.

People often don't recognize that if you lose weight, you need to eat less to stay at the lower weight. For example, an inactive 30-year-old 5'4" woman who weighs 170 lbs needs to consume about 2100 Calories/day to maintain her weight. If she loses 40 lbs but does not change her activity level, she will need to consume only about 1880 Calories to maintain her healthier reduced weight. If, once the weight is lost, she resumes her pre-weight-loss dietary pattern, eating 2100 Calories/day, she will regain all the lost weight.

Effective weight-management programs promote healthy weight-loss diets and encourage changes in the lifestyle patterns that led to weight gain. When selecting a program, look for one that is based on sound nutrition and exercise principles, suits your individual preferences in terms of food choices as well as time and costs, and promotes long-term lifestyle changes. Quick fixes are tempting, but if the program's approach is not one that can be followed for a lifetime, it is unlikely to promote successful weight management (TABLE 9.2).

Some of the most common methods for reducing calorie intake include using exchange lists for diet planning, eating pre-portioned meals or liquid meals, and reducing the fat or carbohydrate content of the diet (FIGURE 9.18). All these methods cause weight loss by limiting, in one way or another, the number of calories consumed.

Distinguishing between healthy diets and fad diets TABLE 9.2	
A healthy diet . . .	*A fad diet . . .*
Promotes a healthy dietary pattern that meets nutrient needs, includes a variety of foods, suits food preferences, and can be maintained throughout life.	Limits food selections to a few food groups or promotes rituals such as eating only specific food combinations. As a result, it may be limited in certain nutrients and in variety.
Promotes a reasonable weight loss of 0.5 to 2 lbs per week and does not restrict Calories to under 1200/day.	Promotes rapid weight loss of much more than 2 lbs/week.
Promotes or includes physical activity.	Advertises weight loss without the need to exercise.
Is flexible enough to be followed when eating out and includes foods that are easily obtained.	May require a rigid menu or avoidance of certain foods or may include "magic" foods that promise to burn fat or speed up metabolism.
Does not require costly supplements.	May require the purchase of special foods, weight-loss patches, expensive supplements, creams, or other products.
Promotes a change in behavior. Teaches new eating habits. Provides social support.	Does not recommend changes in activity and eating habits, recommends an eating pattern that is difficult to follow for life, or provides no support other than a book that must be purchased.
Is based on sound scientific principles and may include monitoring by qualified health professionals.	Makes outlandish and unscientific claims, does not support claims that it is clinically tested or scientifically proven, claims that it is new and improved or based on some new scientific discovery, or relies on testimonials from celebrities or connects the diet to trendy places such as Beverly Hills.

Common dieting methods FIGURE 9.18

| | | | |
| 1/3 cup rice | = | 1 slice bread | = | 1/2 medium potato, baked |

80 Calories
15 g carbohydrate
3 g protein
0–1 g fat

80 Calories
15 g carbohydrate
3 g protein
0–1 g fat

80 Calories
15 g carbohydrate
3 g protein
0–1 g fat

A Some diet plans regulate calories by recommending certain numbers of servings from specific food lists. Foods that are in the same Exchange list, such as rice, bread, and potatoes, are similar in their energy and macronutrient content, so they can be exchanged for one another (see Appendix E). These plans include a variety of foods and are likely to meet nutrient needs. They teach meal-planning skills that are easy to apply away from home and can be used over the long term.

B Pre-portioned meals or liquid formulas make it easier to eat less, but they are not practical when traveling or eating out, and they do not teach the food selection skills needed to make a long-term lifestyle change. Programs that rely exclusively on liquid formulas are not recommended without medical supervision.

C Because fat is high in calories, consuming a low-fat diet typically reduces calorie intake. Low-fat diets can include large quantities of fresh fruits and vegetables, which are low in fat and calories and high in nutrients and phytochemicals. But just because a food is low in fat does not mean it can be consumed in unlimited amounts. In the 1990s, low-fat cookies, crackers, and cakes flooded the market. These foods were low in fat but not in energy. When eaten in excess, they contribute to weight gain.

D Where are the rice and potatoes? Low-carbohydrate diets limit bread and grains, fruits, some vegetables, and milk while allowing unlimited quantities of meats and fats. Weight loss occurs on these diets because people eat less. This may be due to metabolic changes that suppress appetite, but intake is also reduced because of the monotony of the food choices.[37]

WEIGHT-LOSS DRUGS AND SUPPLEMENTS

Prescription drugs for the treatment of obesity include those that reduce appetite by affecting the activity of brain neurotransmitters (for example, sibutramine, brand name Meridia, and phentermine, trade name Adipex) and those that decrease the absorption of fat in the intestine (for example, orlistat, brand name Xenical). Medications such as these are recommended only for individuals whose health is seriously compromised by their body weight: obese individuals (BMI greater than 30 kg/m^2) and overweight individuals with a BMI greater than or equal to 27 kg/m^2 who have two or more obesity-related risk factors or diseases.[6] One of the major disad-vantages of drug treatment is that even if the drug promotes weight loss, the weight is usually regained when the drug is discontinued.

Like prescription drugs, over-the-counter weight-loss medications are regulated by the FDA and must adhere to strict guidelines regarding the dose per pill and the effectiveness of the ingredients. The FDA has approved only a limited number of substances for sale as nonprescription weight-loss medications. One of these is a nonprescription version of orlistat, which became available in 2007 (see *What a Scientist Sees*). As with prescription medications, any weight loss that occurs with over-the-counter weight-loss medications is usually regained when the product is no longer consumed.

Alli: Blocking Fat Absorption

Alli is an over-the-counter version of a prescription weight-loss drug. Consumers see using it as a way to lose weight without needing to watch food intake quite so carefully. Scientists see that it acts by disabling the enzyme lipase. Lipase breaks triglycerides into fatty acids, which are absorbed and can then be used or stored for energy. When Alli is present, the triglycerides are not broken down, so they cannot be absorbed. The undigested fat continues through the intestines and is eliminated in the feces. This cuts the number of calories that get into your body, but it is not without side effects. Fat in the colon may cause gas, diarrhea, and more frequent and hard-to-control bowel movements. Will Alli be an effective weight-loss aid for someone who does not exercise or try to reduce his or her energy intake?

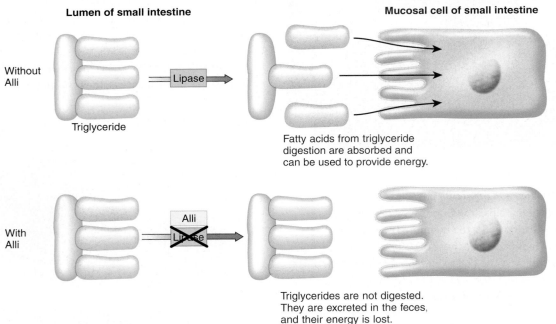

Lumen of small intestine

Mucosal cell of small intestine

Without Alli

Lipase

Triglyceride

Fatty acids from triglyceride digestion are absorbed and can be used to provide energy.

With Alli

Alli

Lipase

Triglycerides are not digested. They are excreted in the feces, and their energy is lost.

The dangers of fat burners FIGURE 9.19

In 2003, Baltimore Orioles pitcher Steve Bechler died of complications from heatstroke following a spring training workout. It was concluded that ephedra played a significant role in his death. Ephedra use is associated with serious side effects such as hypertension, arrhythmia, heart attack, stroke, and seizure.[45] Shortly after this episode, the FDA banned the sale of products containing ephedra. Although the legality of the ban was challenged, it was upheld, and the sale of ephedra-containing dietary supplements remains illegal in the United States.[46]

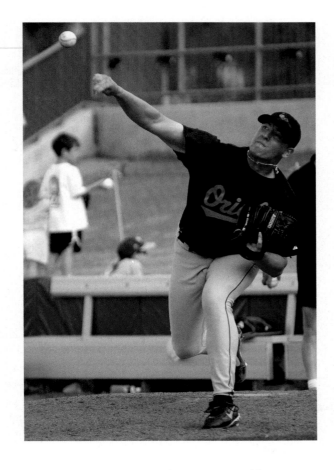

In addition to weight-loss drugs, there are hundreds of dietary supplements that claim to promote weight loss. As with other dietary supplements, weight-loss supplements are not strictly regulated by the FDA, so their safety and effectiveness may not have been carefully tested. Weight-loss supplements often include herbal sources of compounds contained in prescription medications. Some of these are powerful drugs with dangerous side effects. It cannot be assumed that a product is safe simply because it is labeled "herbal" or "all natural."

Weight-loss supplements that contain soluble fiber promise to reduce the amount you eat by filling up your stomach. Although they are safe, there is little evidence that they promote weight loss.[38] Hydroxycitric acid, conjugated linoleic acid, and chromium picolinate are weight-loss supplements that promise to enhance fat loss by altering metabolism so as to prevent the synthesis and deposition of fat. None of these has been shown to be effective for promoting weight loss in humans.[39–41] Supplements that boost energy expenditure, often called "fat burners," can be effective but have serious and potentially life-threatening side effects. One of the most popular and controversial herbal fat burners is ephedra,

a stimulant that increases blood pressure and heart rate and constricts blood vessels. Due to safety concerns, it was banned by the FDA in 2004 (FIGURE 9.19). After the ban was instituted, supplement manufacturers substituted other herbal products, such as bitter orange, which contain similar stimulants and therefore may have similar side effects.[42] Fat burners also typically contain guarana, an herbal source of caffeine. Green tea extract is another popular supplement used to boost metabolism and aid weight loss. It appears to be safe if used in appropriate amounts, but studies have not shown it to enhance weight loss.[43,44]

Taking some dietary supplements results in weight loss through water loss—either because these supplements are diuretics or because they cause diarrhea. Water loss decreases body weight but does not cause a decrease in body fat. Herbal laxatives found in weight-loss teas and supplements include senna, aloe, buckthorn, rhubarb root, cascara, and castor oil. Overuse of these substances can have serious side effects, including nausea, diarrhea, vomiting, stomach cramps, chronic constipation, fainting, and severe electrolyte imbalances, leading to cardiac arrhythmia and death.[47]

Gastric bypass and banding FIGURE 9.20

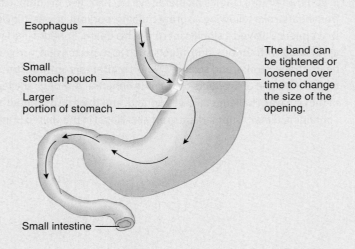

A Gastric bypass involves bypassing part of the stomach and small intestine by connecting the intestine to the upper portion of the stomach. Food intake is reduced because the stomach is smaller, and absorption is reduced because the small intestine is shortened. Gastric bypass entails short-term surgical risks and a long-term risk of nutrient deficiencies, particularly of vitamin B_{12}, folate, calcium, and iron, because absorption of these nutrients is reduced.[48]

B Gastric banding involves surgically placing an adjustable band around the upper part of the stomach, creating a small pouch. The narrow opening between the stomach pouch and the rest of the stomach slows the rate at which food leaves the pouch. This promotes weight loss by reducing the amount of food that can be consumed at one time and slowing digestion. Gastric banding entails less surgical risk and is more easily reversible than other types of weight-loss surgery.

gastric bypass
A surgical procedure that reduces the size of the stomach and bypasses a portion of the small intestine.

adjustable gastric banding
A surgical procedure in which an adjustable band is placed around the upper portion of the stomach to limit the volume that the stomach can hold and the rate of stomach emptying.

WEIGHT-LOSS SURGERY

A number of surgical procedures decrease body weight by altering the gastrointestinal tract so as to reduce food intake and absorption. These surgical approaches are recommended only in cases in which the risk of dying from the complications of obesity is great: individuals who fit the definition of extreme obesity (BMI ≥ 40 kg/m^2) and those with a BMI between 35 and 40 kg/m^2 who have other life-threatening conditions that could be remedied by weight loss.[6] At present, the most popular surgical approaches to treating obesity are **gastric bypass** and **adjustable gastric banding** (FIGURE 9.20).

Another popular surgical procedure for reducing body fat is **liposuction**. This procedure involves inserting a large hollow needle under the skin into a fat deposit and literally vacuuming out the fat. Liposuction is considered a cosmetic procedure and does not significantly reduce overall body weight.

CONCEPT CHECK STOP

Why is weight loss not recommended for everyone with a BMI above the healthy range?

What are some characteristics of a good weight-loss program?

How much weight loss per week is recommended?

How does gastric bypass cause weight loss?

◻ Significant weight loss is usually achieved 18 to 24 months after weight-loss surgery. NBC's *Today Show* weather anchor Al Roker lost 100 lbs after undergoing gastric bypass surgery. Some weight gain is common after 2 to 5 years. Even after surgery, it is necessary to limit the types and amounts of food consumed in order to maintain the lower weight.

Eating Disorders

LEARNING OBJECTIVES

Distinguish among anorexia, bulimia, and binge-eating disorder.

Describe demographic and psychological factors associated with an increased risk of developing an eating disorder.

Discuss how body ideal and the media affect the incidence of eating disorders.

Explain what is meant by the binge/purge cycle.

What and how much people eat varies depending on social occasions, emotions, time limitations, hunger, and the availability of food, but generally people eat when they are hungry, choose foods that they enjoy, and stop eating when they are satisfied. Abnormal or disordered eating occurs when a person is overly concerned with food, eating, and body size and shape. When the emotional aspects of food and eating overpower the role of food as nourishment, an **eating disorder** may develop. Eating disorders affect physical and nutritional health and psychosocial functioning. If untreated, they can be fatal.

eating disorder
A psychological illness characterized by specific abnormal eating behaviors, often intended to control weight.

Eating Disorders   317

Distinguishing among eating disorders TABLE 9.3

| Characteristic | Eating disorder | | |
	Anorexia nervosa	Bulimia nervosa	Binge-eating disorder
Body weight	Below normal (<85% of recommended)	Usually normal	Above normal
Binge eating	Possibly	Yes, at least twice a week for three months	Yes, at least twice a week for six months
Purging	Possibly	Yes, at least twice a week for three months	No
Restricts food intake	Yes	Yes	Yes
Body image	Dissatisfaction with body and distorted image of body size	Dissatisfaction with body and distorted image of body size	Dissatisfaction with body
Fear of being fat	Yes	Yes	Not excessive
Self-esteem	Low	Low	Low
Menstrual abnormalities	Absence of at least three consecutive periods	No	No
Typical age of onset	Preadolescence/adolescence	Adolescence/young adults	Adults of all ages

TYPES OF EATING DISORDERS

Mental health guidelines define three categories of eating disorders: **anorexia nervosa**, **bulimia nervosa**, and **eating disorders not otherwise specified (EDNOS)**, which includes **binge-eating disorder** and other abnormal eating behaviors that don't qualify as anorexia or bulimia (TABLE 9.3).

WHAT CAUSES EATING DISORDERS?

We do not completely understand what causes eating disorders, but we do know that genetic, psychological, and sociocultural factors contribute to their development (FIGURE 9.21). Eating disorders can be triggered by traumatic events such as sexual abuse or by day-to-day occurrences such as teasing or judgmental comments by a friend or a coach. Eating disorders occur in people of all ages, races, and socioeconomic backgrounds, but some groups are at greater risk than others. Women are more likely than men to develop eating disorders. In the United States, eating disorders affect about 3% of

anorexia nervosa An eating disorder characterized by self-starvation, a distorted body image, and abnormally low body weight.

bulimia nervosa An eating disorder characterized by the consumption of a large amount of food at one time (binge eating) followed by purging behaviors such as self-induced vomiting to prevent weight gain.

binge-eating disorder An eating disorder characterized by recurrent episodes of binge eating in the absence of purging behavior.

body image The way a person perceives and imagines his or her body.

girls and women between ages 18 and 30.[49] Professional dancers, models, and others who are concerned about maintaining a low body weight are most likely to develop eating disorders.[49] Eating disorders commonly begin in adolescence, when physical, psychological, and social development is occurring rapidly.

Psychological issues

People with eating disorders often have low self-esteem. *Self-esteem* refers to the judgments people make and maintain about themselves—a general attitude of approval or disapproval as to worth and capability. A poor **body image** contributes to low self-esteem. Eating disorders are characterized not only by dissatisfaction with one's body but also with a distorted body image. Someone with a distorted body image is unable to judge the size of his or her own body. Thus, even if a young woman achieves a body weight comparable to that of a fashion model, she may continue to see herself as fat and strive to lose more weight.

People with eating disorders are often perfectionists who set very high standards for themselves and strive to be in control of their bodies and their lives. Despite their many achievements, they feel inadequate,

Eating disorders are caused by a combination of genetic, psychological, and sociocultural factors. Although these disorders are not necessarily passed from parent to child, the genes that a person inherits contribute to personality traits and other psychological and biological characteristics that can predispose him or her to developing an eating disorder. When placed in the right sociocultural environment, an individual who carries such genes will be more likely than others to develop an eating disorder.

GENETIC
- Inherited personality traits
- Genes that affect hunger, satiety, and body weight

PSYCHOLOGICAL
- Low self-esteem
- Need for self-control
- Unhealthy body image

SOCIOCULTURAL
- Thin body ideal
- Influences from media, family, and friends
- Abundant food supply

defective, and worthless. They may use their relationship with food to gain control over their lives and boost their self-esteem. They believe that controlling their food intake and weight demonstrates their ability to control other aspects of their lives and solves other problems. Even if they feel insecure, helpless, or dissatisfied in other aspects of their lives, if they are in control of their food intake, weight, and body size, they can associate this control with success.

Sociocultural issues What is viewed as an "ideal" body differs across cultures and has changed throughout history (FIGURE 9.22 on the next page). Cultural ideals about body size are linked to body image and the incidence of eating disorders.[50] Eating disorders occur in societies where food is abundant and the body ideal is thin. They do not occur in societies where food is scarce and people must worry about where their next meal is coming from.

U.S. culture today is a culture of thinness. Messages about what society views as a perfect body—the ideal that we should strive for—are constantly delivered by television, movies, magazines, advertisements, and even toys. Tall, lean fashion models adorn billboards and magazine covers. Thinness is associated with beauty, success, intelligence, and vitality. A young woman facing a future in which she must be independent, have a prestigious job, maintain a successful love relationship, bear and nurture children, manage a household, and keep up with fashion trends can become overwhelmed. Unable to master all these roles, she may look for some aspect of her life that she can control. Food intake and body weight are natural choices because thinness is associated with success. These messages about how we should look are difficult to ignore and can create pressure to achieve this ideal body. But it is a standard that is very difficult to meet—a standard that is contributing to disturbances in body image and eating behavior.

Although men currently represent a small percentage of people with eating disorders, the numbers are increasing.[53] This is likely due to increasing pressure to achieve an ideal male body. Advertisements directed at men are showing more and more exposed skin, with a focus on well-defined abdominal and chest muscles.

Visualizing

Body ideal and body weight FIGURE 9.22

A A fuller figure is still desirable in many cultures. Young women in these cultures, such as the Zulu of South Africa, may struggle to gain weight in order to achieve what is viewed as the ideal female body. As television images of very thin western women become more accessible, the Zulu cultural view of plumpness as desirable may be changing.[51]

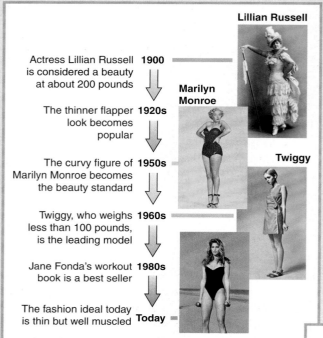

Actress Lillian Russell is considered a beauty at about 200 pounds — **1900**

Lillian Russell

The thinner flapper look becomes popular — **1920s**

Marilyn Monroe

The curvy figure of Marilyn Monroe becomes the beauty standard — **1950s**

Twiggy

Twiggy, who weighs less than 100 pounds, is the leading model — **1960s**

Jane Fonda's workout book is a best seller — **1980s**

The fashion ideal today is thin but well muscled — **Today**

B Thinness has not always been the beauty standard in the United States. This timeline shows how the female body ideal has changed over the years. As female models, actresses, and other cultural icons have become thinner over the past several decades, the incidence of eating disorders has increased.

C The fashion models whom women want to emulate are thinner than 98% of women in the United States. The average American woman is 5'4" tall and weighs 160 lbs. The average fashion model is 5'11" tall and weighs 117 lbs. And the difference between models and average women has been increasing over the years. Forty years ago, the average weight of a model was 8% lower than that of an average woman; today, the difference is over 25%.[52] ▼

D The toys that children play with set a cultural standard for body ideal. Little girls playing with Barbie dolls want to be like Barbie when they grow up, and boys playing with Superman, Batman, or GI Joe action figures want to be like them. This includes looking like them. Unfortunately, Barbie's measurements would be virtually unachievable if Barbie were life-sized. The same is true of the big chest, muscular arms and legs, and flat stomach with "six-pack" abs seen on male action figures.

ANOREXIA NERVOSA

Anorexia means lack of appetite, but in the case of the eating disorder anorexia nervosa it is a desire to be thin, rather than a lack of appetite, that causes individuals to decrease their food intake. Anorexia nervosa is characterized by severe weight loss, **amenorrhea**, constipation, and restlessness. It affects about 1% of female adolescents in the United States. The average age of onset is 17 years. There is a 5% death rate in the first two years, and the death rate can reach 20% in untreated individuals.[49]

amenorrhea
Delayed onset of menstruation or the absence of three or more consecutive menstrual cycles.

The psychological component of anorexia nervosa revolves around an overwhelming fear of gaining weight, even in individuals who are already underweight. It is not uncommon for individuals with anorexia to feel that they would rather be dead than fat. Anorexia is also characterized by disturbances in body image or perception of body size that prevent those with this disorder from seeing themselves as underweight even when they are dangerously thin. People with this disorder may use body weight and shape as a means of self-evaluation: "If I weren't so fat, everyone would like and respect me, and I wouldn't have other problems." However, no matter how much weight they lose, they do not gain self-respect, inner assurance, or the happiness they seek. Therefore, they continue to restrict their intake and use other behaviors to lose weight.

The most obvious behaviors associated with anorexia are those that contribute to the maintenance of a body weight that is 15% or more below normal. These behaviors include restriction of food intake, binge-eating and purging episodes in some patients, strange eating rituals, and excessive activity (**FIGURE 9.23**). For some individuals with anorexia, the increase in activity is surreptitious, such as going up and down stairs repeatedly or getting off the bus a few stops too early. For others, the activity takes the form of strenuous physical exercise. They may become fanatical athletes and feel guilty if they cannot exercise. They link exercise and eating, so a certain amount of exercise earns them the right to eat, and if they eat too much, they must pay the price by adding extra exercise. They do not stop when they are tired; instead, they train compulsively beyond reasonable endurance.

The first obvious physical manifestation of anorexia is weight loss. As weight loss becomes severe, symptoms of starvation begin to appear. Starvation affects mental function, causing the person to become apathetic, dull, exhausted, and depressed. Fat stores are depleted. Other symptoms that appear include muscle wasting, inflammation and swelling of the lips, flaking and peeling of skin, growth of fine hair (called lanugo) on the body, and dry, thin, brittle hair on the head. In females, estrogen levels drop, and menstruation becomes

A day in the life of an anorexic FIGURE 9.23

For individuals with anorexia, food and eating become an obsession. In addition to restricting the total amount of food they consume, anorexics develop personal diet rituals, limiting certain foods and eating them in specific ways. Although they do not consume very much food, they are preoccupied with food and spend an enormous amount of time thinking about it, talking about it, and preparing meals for others. Instead of eating, they move the food around the plate and cut it into tiny pieces.

Dear Diary,

For breakfast today I had a cup of tea. For lunch I ate some lettuce and a slice of tomato, but no dressing. I cooked dinner for my family. I love to cook, but it is hard not to taste. I tried a new chicken recipe and served it with rice and asparagus. I even made a chocolate cake for dessert but I didn't even lick the bowl from the frosting. When it came time to eat, I only took a little. I told my mom I nibbled while cooking. I pushed the food around on my plate so no one would notice that I only ate a few bites. I was good today – I kept my food intake under control. The scale says I have lost 20 pounds, but I still look fat.

A day in the life of a bulimic FIGURE 9.24

The amount of food consumed during a binge varies but is typically on the order of 3400 Calories, while a normal young woman may consume only about 2000 Calories in an entire day. Self-induced vomiting is the most common purging behavior. At first a physical maneuver such as sticking a finger down the throat is needed to induce vomiting, but patients eventually learn to vomit at will. Binging and purging are followed by intense feelings of guilt and shame.

Dear Diary,

Today started well. I stuck to my diet through breakfast, lunch, and dinner, but by 8 PM I was feeling depressed and bored. I thought food would make me feel better. Before I knew it I was at the convenience store buying two pints of ice cream, a large bag of chips, a one pound package of cookies, half dozen candy bars, and a quart of milk. I told the clerk I was having a party. But it was a party of one. Alone in my dorm room I started by eating the chips, then polished off the cookies and the candy bars, washing them down with milk and finishing with the ice cream. Luckily no one was around so I was able to vomit without anyone hearing. I feel weak and guilty but also relieved that I got rid of all those calories. Tomorrow, I will start a new diet.

irregular or stops. In males, testosterone levels decrease. In the final stages of starvation, the person experiences abnormalities in electrolyte and fluid balance and cardiac irregularities. Suppression of immune function leads to infection, which further increases nutritional needs.

The goal of treatment for anorexia nervosa is to help resolve the psychological and behavioral problems underlying it while providing for physical and nutritional rehabilitation. Treatment requires an interdisciplinary team of nutritional, psychological, and medical specialists and typically requires years of therapy. The goal of nutrition intervention is to promote weight gain by increasing energy intake and expanding dietary choices.[49] In more severe cases, anorexics are hospitalized, and their food intake and exercise behaviors are controlled. Intravenous nutrition may be necessary to keep an anorexic individual alive. Some anorexics make full recoveries, but about half have poor long-term outcomes—remaining irrationally concerned about weight gain and never achieving normal body weight. Some patients with anorexia also transition to bulimia nervosa.[54]

BULIMIA NERVOSA

Bulimia comes from the Greek *bous* ("ox") and *limos* ("hunger"), denoting hunger of such intensity that a person could eat an entire ox. The term *bulimia nervosa* was coined in 1979 by a British psychiatrist who suggested that bulimia consists of powerful urges to overeat in combination with a morbid fear of becoming fat and avoidance of the fattening effects of food by inducing vomiting and/or abusing purgatives.[55]

Like anorexia, bulimia is characterized by an intense fear of becoming fat and a negative body image, accompanied by a distorted perception of body size. Because self-esteem is highly tied to impressions of body shape and weight, people with bulimia may blame all their problems on their appearance. They are preoccupied with the fear that once they start eating, they will not be able to stop. They may engage in continuous dieting, which leads to a preoccupation with food. They are often socially isolated and may avoid situations that will expose them to food, such as going to parties or out to dinner; thus they become further isolated.

Bulimia typically begins with food restriction motivated by the desire to be thin. Overwhelming hunger may finally cause the dieting to be interrupted by a period of overeating. Eventually a pattern develops that consists of semi-starvation interrupted by periods of gorging. During a binge-eating episode, a bulimic experiences a sense of lack of control. Binges usually last less than 2 hours and occur in secrecy. Eating stops when the food runs out, or when pain, fatigue, or an interruption intervenes. The amount of food consumed in a binge may not always be enormous, but the bulimic individual perceives it as a binge episode (**FIGURE 9.24**).

After binge episodes, bulimics use various behaviors to eliminate the extra calories and prevent weight gain. Some use behaviors such as fasting or excessive exercise, but most use purging behaviors such as vomiting or taking laxatives, diuretics, or other medications. Self-induced vomiting does eliminate some of the food before the nutrients have been absorbed, preventing weight gain, but laxatives and diuretics cause only water loss. Nutrient absorption is almost complete before food enters the colon, where laxatives have their effect. The weight loss associated with laxative abuse is due to dehydration. Diuretics also cause water loss, but via the kidney rather than the GI tract. They do not cause fat loss.

It is the purging portion of the binge/purge cycle that is most hazardous to health. Vomiting brings stomach acid into the mouth. Frequent vomiting affects the gastrointestinal tract by causing tooth decay, sores in the mouth and on the lips, swelling of the jaw and salivary glands, irritation of the throat and esophagus, and changes in stomach capacity and the rate of stomach emptying.[49] It also causes broken blood vessels in the face due to the force of vomiting, as well as electrolyte imbalance, dehydration, muscle weakness, and menstrual irregularities. Laxative and diuretic abuse can also cause dehydration and electrolyte imbalance.

The overall goal of therapy for people with bulimia nervosa is to reduce or eliminate bingeing and purging behavior by separating the patients' eating behavior from their emotions and their perceptions of success and promoting eating in response to hunger and satiety. Psychological issues related to body image and a sense of lack of control over eating must be resolved. Nutritional therapy must address physiological imbalances caused by purging episodes as well as provide education on nutrient needs and how to meet them. Treatment has been found to speed recovery, especially if it is provided soon after symptoms begin, but for some women this disorder may remain a chronic problem throughout life.[56]

BINGE-EATING DISORDER

Binge-eating disorder is the most common eating disorder. Unlike anorexia and bulimia, binge-eating disorder is not uncommon in men, who account for about 40% of cases. It is most common in overweight individuals (FIGURE 9.25). Individuals with binge-eating disorder engage in recurrent episodes of binge eating but do not regularly engage in purging behaviors.

The major complications of binge-eating disorder are the health problems associated with obesity, which include diabetes, high blood pressure, high cholesterol levels, gallbladder disease, heart disease, and certain types of cancer. Treatment of binge-eating disorder involves counseling to improve body image and self-acceptance; a healthy, nutritious diet; and increased exercise to promote weight loss along with behavior therapy to reduce bingeing.

A day in the life of a binge eater FIGURE 9.25

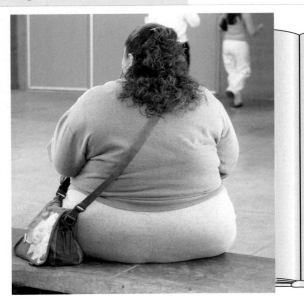

People with binge-eating disorder often seek help for their weight rather than for their disordered eating pattern. It is estimated that 10 to 15% of people enrolled in commercial weight-loss programs suffer from this disorder.[57]

Dear Diary,

I got on the scale today. What a mistake! My weight is up to 250 pounds. I hate myself for being so fat. Just seeing that I gained more weight made me feel ashamed – all I wanted to do was bury my feelings in a box of cookies or a carton of ice cream. Why do I always think the food will help? Once I started eating I couldn't stop. When I finally did I felt even more disgusted, depressed, and guilty. I am always on a diet but it is never long before I lose control and pig out. I know my eating and my weight are not healthy but I just can't seem to stop.

EATING DISORDERS IN SPECIAL GROUPS

Although anorexia and bulimia are most common in women in their teens and 20s, eating disorders occur in both genders and all age groups. Both male and female athletes are at high risk for eating disorders, with an incidence of 10 to 20%.[49,58] Eating disorders occur during pregnancy and are becoming more frequent among younger children due to social values about food and body weight. They also occur in individuals with diabetes.

A number of less common eating disorders appear in special groups within the general population (TABLE 9.4).

PREVENTING AND GETTING TREATMENT FOR EATING DISORDERS

Because eating disorders are often triggered by weight-related criticism, elimination of this type of behavior can have a major impact on prevention. Another important

Other eating disorders TABLE 9.4

Eating disorder	Who is affected	Characteristics and consequences
Anorexia athletica	Athletes in weight-dependent sports such as dance, figure skating, gymnastics, track and field, cycling, wrestling, and horse racing	Engaging in compulsive exercise to lose weight or maintain a very low body weight. Can lead to more serious eating disorders and serious health problems, including kidney failure, heart attack, and death.
Female athlete triad	Female athletes in weight-dependent sports	A triad of disordered eating, amenorrhea, and osteoporosis. The energy restriction, along with high levels of exercise, causes amenorrhea. Low estrogen levels then interfere with calcium balance, eventually causing reductions in bone mass and an increased risk of bone fractures (discussed further in Chapter 10).
Bigorexia (muscle dysmorphia or reverse anorexia)	Bodybuilders and avid gym-goers; more common in men than in women	An obsession with being small and underdeveloped. Those affected believe that their muscles are inadequate, even when they have good muscle mass. They become avid weight lifters and may experiment with steroids or other muscle-enhancing drugs.
Avoidance emotional disorder	Children	Similar to anorexia nervosa in that the child avoids eating and experiences weight loss and the other physical symptoms of anorexia. However, there is no distorted body image or fear of weight gain.
Selective eating disorder	Children	Children with this disorder will eat only a few foods, mostly carbohydrate. If the disorder continues for long periods, it increases the risk of malnutrition.
Night-eating syndrome	Obese adults and those experiencing stress	A disorder that involves consuming most of the day's calories late in the day or at night. People with this disorder—which contributes to weight gain—are tense, anxious, upset, or guilty while eating. A similar disorder, in which a person may eat while asleep and have no memory of the events, is called nocturnal sleep-related eating disorder (NSRED) and is considered a sleep disorder, not an eating disorder.
Pica	Pregnant women, children, people with psychiatric disturbances and developmental disabilities, people whose family or ethnic customs include eating certain nonfood substances, people who are hungry and try to ease hunger and cravings with nonfood substances	Craving and eating nonfood items such as dirt, clay, paint chips, plaster, chalk, laundry starch, coffee grounds, and ashes. Depending on the items consumed, pica can cause perforated intestines and contribute to mineral deficiencies or intestinal infections.
Insulin misuse (diabulimia)	People with type 1 diabetes	Type 1 diabetes is a disease that forces patients to focus on food portions and body weight. This may cause some to become preoccupied with their weight and to control it by withholding insulin.[59] Without insulin, glucose cannot enter cells to provide fuel, blood levels rise, and weight drops. Uncontrolled blood sugar can lead to blindness, kidney disease, heart disease, nerve damage, and amputations.

target for reducing the incidence of eating disorders is the media. If the unrealistically thin body ideal presented by the media could be altered, the incidence of eating disorders would likely decrease. Even with these interventions, however, eating disorders are unlikely to go away entirely. Education through schools and communities about the symptoms and complications of eating disorders can help people identify friends and family members who are at risk and persuade those with early symptoms to seek help.

The first step in preventing individuals from developing eating disorders is to recognize those who are at risk. Early intervention can help prevent at-risk individuals from developing serious eating disorders. Excessive concerns about body weight, having friends who are preoccupied with weight, being teased by peers about weight, and family problems all predispose a person to developing an eating disorder.

Once an eating disorder has developed, the person usually does not get better on his or her own. The actions of family members and friends can help people suffering from eating disorders get help before their health is impaired. But it is not always easy to persuade a friend or relative with an eating disorder to agree to seek help. People with eating disorders are good at hiding their behaviors and denying the problem, and often they do not want help. When confronted, one person might be relieved that you are concerned and willing to help, whereas another might be angry and defensive. When approaching someone about an eating disorder, it is important to make it clear that you are not forcing the person to do anything she or he doesn't want to do. Continued encouragement can help some people agree to seek professional help.

CONCEPT CHECK STOP

Which eating disorder is characterized by extreme weight loss? Which is characterized by excess weight?

What factors contribute to the higher incidence of eating disorders among women than among men?

What is meant by body image?

How does a food binge differ from "normal" overeating?

SUMMARY

1 Body Weight and Health

1. More Americans today are **overweight** and **obese** than ever before. Excess body fat increases the risk of chronic diseases such as diabetes, heart disease, high blood pressure, and certain types of cancer.

2. **Body mass index (BMI)** can be used to evaluate the health risks of a particular body weight and height. Measures of **body composition** can be used to determine the proportion of a person's weight that is due to fat. Excess **visceral fat** is a greater health risk than excess **subcutaneous fat**.

2 Energy Balance

1. Americans are getting fatter because they are consuming more calories due to poor food choices and larger portion sizes and moving less due to modern lifestyles in which computers, cars, and other conveniences reduce the amount of energy expended in work and play.

2. The principle of **energy balance** states that if energy intake equals energy expenditure, body weight will remain constant. Energy is provided to the body by the carbohydrate, fat, and protein in the food we eat. This energy is used to maintain **basal metabolic rate (BMR)**, to support activity, and for the **thermic effect of food (TEF)**. When excess energy is consumed, it is stored, primarily as fat in **adipocytes**, causing weight gain. When energy in the diet does not meet needs, energy stores in the body are used, and weight is lost.

3. The energy needs of healthy people can be predicted by calculating their estimated energy requirements (EER). EER depends on gender, age, life stage, height, weight, and level of physical activity.

3 What Determines Body Size and Shape?

1. The genes people inherit affect their body size and shape, but environmental factors and personal choices concerning the amount and type of food consumed and the amount and intensity of exercise performed also affect body weight.

2. **Hunger** and **satiety** from meal to meal are regulated by signals from the gastrointestinal tract, hormones, and levels of circulating nutrients. Signals from fat cells, such as the release of **leptin**, regulate long-term energy intake and expenditure.

3. Inheriting an efficient metabolism or expending less energy through **nonexercise activity thermogenesis (NEAT)** may contribute to obesity.

4 Managing Body Weight

1. Weight loss is recommended for those with a BMI above the healthy range who have excess body fat or a large waist circumference or who have health conditions associated with obesity.

2. Weight management involves adjusting energy intake and expenditure to lose or maintain weight and **behavior modification** to keep weight in a healthy range over the long term. To lose a pound of adipose tissue, energy expenditure must be increased or intake decreased by approximately 3500 Calories. Slow, steady weight loss of 1/2 to 2 lb/week is more likely to be maintained than rapid weight loss.

2. If **underweight** is not due to a medical condition, weight gain can be accomplished by increasing energy intake and lifting weights to increase muscle mass.

3. A good weight-loss program is one that promotes physical activity and a wide variety of nutrient-dense food choices, does not require the purchase and consumption of special foods or combinations of foods, and can be followed for life.

4. Drug therapy and surgery are recommended only for those whose health is seriously compromised by their body weight. Currently, the most popular surgical approaches to treating obesity are **gastric bypass** and **adjustable gastric banding**.

5 Eating Disorders

1. **Eating disorders** are psychological disorders that involve dissatisfaction with body weight. **Anorexia nervosa** involves self-starvation, resulting in an abnormally low body weight. **Bulimia nervosa** is characterized by repeated cycles of **binge eating** followed by **purging** and other behaviors to prevent weight gain. **Binge-eating disorder** is characterized by bingeing without purging. People with this disorder are typically overweight.

2. Eating disorders are caused by a combination of genetic, psychological, and sociocultural factors. The lean body ideal in the United States is believed to contribute to disturbances in **body image** that lead to eating disorders. Treatment involves medical, psychological, and nutritional intervention to stabilize health, change attitudes about body size, and improve eating habits while supplying an adequate diet.

CRITICAL AND CREATIVE THINKING QUESTIONS

1. If a race of humans evolved on an island where food was always abundant, how might this have affected the frequency of different types of genes that affect the regulation of body weight?

2. Use your knowledge of food intake regulation to explain why drinking a large glass of water would make you feel less hungry for a short time but not for more than an hour or so.

3. If you were invited to offer advice to your town's planning committee what recommendations would you have to help promote physical activity? What recommendations would you have for the middle school in order to encourage physical activity and healthy eating?

4. Why is leptin sometimes referred to as a *lipid thermostat*?

5. Design a weight loss plan for someone who is 40 years old and 40 lbs overweight.

6. A late-night TV advertisement promotes a diet pill that is supposed to cause a weight loss of 10 lbs in the first week. Assuming that you did not change your activity, how many Calories would you have to eliminate from your diet *each day* to lose 10 lbs of adipose tissue in a week? Based on your calculation, do you think it is possible to lose 10 lbs of fat in one week? Why or why not?

7. Beth is 22 years old and has a BMI in the healthy range. Discuss the steps she can take to prevent weight gain as she gets older.

8. Discuss how bulimia might affect each side of the energy balance equation.

What is happening in this picture ?

Sumo wrestlers train for many hours each day and eat huge quantities of food. The result is a high BMI and a large waist but surprisingly little visceral fat.

Why do these individuals have a low level of visceral fat?

Do you think they are at risk for diabetes and heart disease?

What type of fat is hanging over the belt of this wrestler?

What may happen if this wrestler retires and stops exercising but keeps eating large amounts of food?

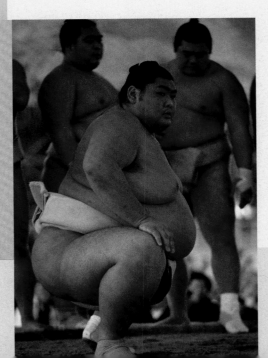

(Check your answers in Appendix L.)

1. Which statement about basal metabolic rate (BMR) is false?

   a. In an average person, it is the largest component of energy expenditure.
   b. It includes the energy needed for kidney function and heartbeat.
   c. It includes the energy needed for exercise.
   d. It is measured in a warm room before rising, after 12 hrs without food or exercise.
   e. It is the energy expended to keep an awake, resting body alive.

2. Excess body fat increases the risk of _____.

   a. diabetes
   b. high blood cholesterol
   c. certain cancers
   d. high blood pressure
   e. all of the above

3. In order to calculate a person's BMI, you need to know the person's _____.

   a. height and weight
   b. age and activity level
   c. lean body mass and waist circumference
   d. gender and weight
   e. gender and body composition

4. Which of the following has not contributed to the rising incidence of overweight and obesity in the United States?

   a. Americans use less energy in the activities of their daily lives than they used to.
   b. Portion sizes of our food have increased.
   c. We have ready access to food 24 hrs a day.
   d. Our genetics have changed.
   e. The number of people who work at jobs requiring strenuous physical labor has decreased.

5. The method of determining body composition shown here relies on what principle to determine the amount of body fat?

   a. Fat is less dense than water.
   b. Fat does not conduct electricity.
   c. The amount of subcutaneous fat is representative of total body fat.
   d. The extent to which X-rays penetrate fat is different from the extent to which they penetrate other tissues.

6. Which statement about EER is false?

   a. It is the amount of energy needed to maintain body weight.
   b. It is the amount of energy you expend daily.
   c. It increases if you lose weight.
   d. It decreases in adults as they get older.
   e. It increases if you exercise more.

7. Which statement about leptin is false?

    a. Someone with a defective leptin gene will most likely be obese.

    b. More leptin is released as adipocytes enlarge.

    c. Low leptin levels stimulate food intake and reduce energy expenditure.

    d. Most human obesity is due to abnormalities in the leptin gene.

    e. Leptin is better at defending against weight loss than against weight gain.

8. Long-term healthy weight loss is based on all of the following principles except _____.

    a. increasing physical activity

    b. adopting lifelong changes in eating habits

    c. eating specific combinations of foods that increase the number of calories burned

    d. keeping portion sizes moderate

    e. making nutrient-dense choices

9. Which statement about the type of body fat labeled by the letter A is false?

    a. This type of fat storage increases the risk of heart disease, diabetes, and high blood pressure.

    b. This type of fat storage can be reduced by eating grapefruit.

    c. This type of fat storage increase after menopause.

    d. This type of fat storage is more common in men than women.

    e. This type of fat storage can be reduced through exercise.

10. This chart most likely shows the distribution of energy expenditure in which of the following people?

    a. a cyclist who trains for 6 hrs a day

    b. an office worker who gets no exercise other than gardening

    c. a young adult who works out for 90 minutes a day

    d. an elderly man who is bedridden

11. True or false: It is possible for someone who is 50 lbs overweight to be in energy balance.

    a. True

    b. False

12. True or false: Everyone with a BMI in the overweight or obese range is at risk for weight-related health problems.

    a. True

    b. False

13. Which of the following is not a characteristic of anorexia nervosa?

    a. a fear of gaining weight

    b. a normal body weight

    c. a preoccupation with food

    d. an abnormal menstrual cycle

    e. a distorted body image

14. Which group is least likely to develop anorexia nervosa?

    a. ballet dancers

    b. fashion models

    c. female gymnasts

    d. actresses

    e. middle-aged men

15. Which eating disorder is characteristic of people who are overweight?

    a. anorexia

    b. bigorexia

    c. bulimia

    d. binge-eating disorder

Nutrition, Fitness, and Physical Activity

I n the 2008 Disney/Pixar film *WALL-E*, humans are enormously chubby couch potatoes, clad in infantile onesies. What produced such a body type? Microgravity, for one thing (these humans have lived on a gigantic spaceship for 700 years), but also, these humans don't *do anything* anymore. Everything is done for them by an army of compliant robots, holograms, and high-speed hover couches; even foods are pureed into shakes in a super-sized cup—no annoying chewing necessary for these space travelers going nowhere.

Technology is a means of simplifying tasks. Even animals use "tools" of one sort or another to minimize the expenditure of energy: Chimpanzees poke sticks into anthills to gather a meal rather than exhaustively dig into the hill; sea otters break open shellfish with rocks. As human technology has produced more and more labor-saving devices, physical exertion has lessened for larger and larger segments of the population. Concurrently—particularly in the developed world—the amount of food consumed per capita has increased. Simply put, we eat far beyond our energy requirements—and often eat foods that do not enhance our physical well-being.

Exercise and fitness are intimately linked with diet and nutrition. It may seem that, compared with earlier generations, we have to pay a lot more attention to what we eat and to how much activity we need to remain healthy. But if we do not, and simply let machines do the work, the future portrayed by *WALL-E* may not be all that fantastical.

NATIONAL GEOGRAPHIC

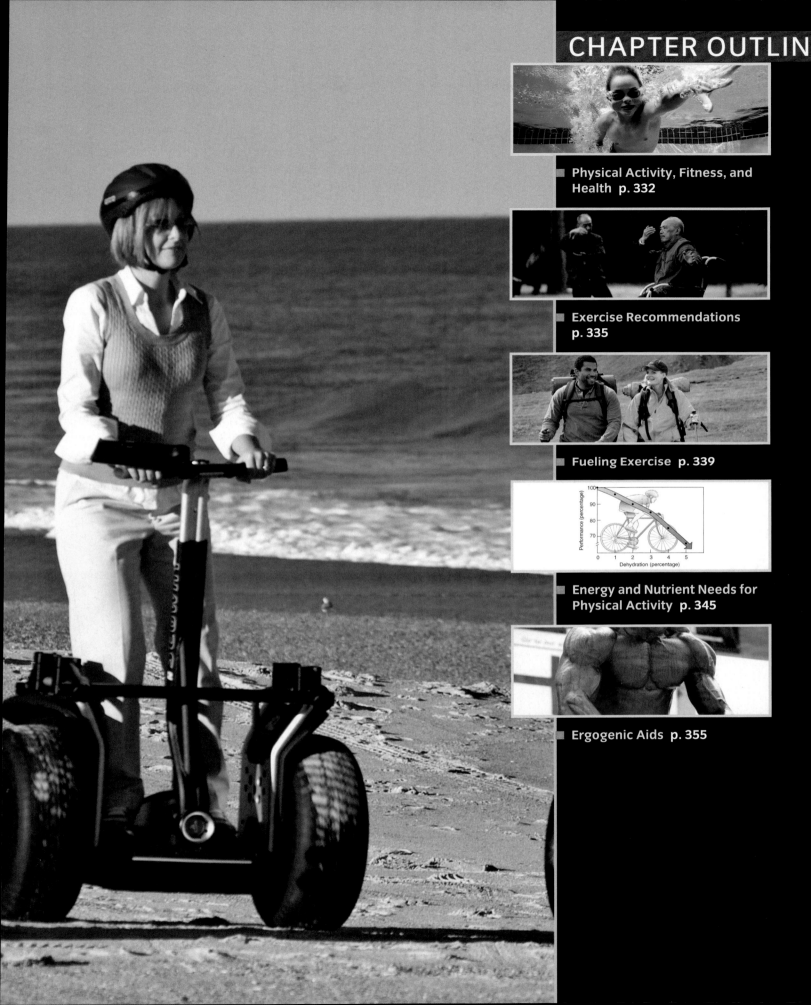

Physical Activity, Fitness, and Health

Exercise improves your **fitness** and overall health. This is true whether your fitness goal is to be able to walk around the block easily or to perform optimally in athletic competitions. Exercise, along with an adequate diet, is important in maintaining health and reducing the risk of chronic diseases such as cardiovascular disease and obesity.

> **fitness** A set of attributes related to the ability to perform routine physical activities without undue fatigue.

When you exercise, changes occur in your body: You breathe harder, your heart beats faster, and your muscles stretch and strain. If you exercise regularly, you adapt to the exercise you perform and as a result can continue for a few minutes longer, lift a heavier weight, or stretch a millimeter farther. This is known as the **overload principle**: The more you do, the more you are capable of doing. For example, if you run a given distance three times a week, in a few weeks you can run farther; if you lift heavy books for a few days, by the next week you have more muscle and can lift more books more easily. These adaptations improve your overall fitness.

> **overload principle** The concept that the body adapts to the stresses placed on it.

THE FOUR COMPONENTS OF FITNESS

A person's fitness is defined by his or her endurance, strength, flexibility, and body composition (**FIGURE 10.1**). A fit person can continue an activity for a longer period than an unfit person can before fatigue forces him or her to stop, but fitness is more than just stamina. Being fit also reduces the risk of chronic disease and makes weight management easier.

Cardiorespiratory endurance How long you can jog or ride your bike depends on the ability of your cardiovascular and respiratory systems, referred to jointly as the cardiorespiratory system, to deliver oxygen and

Visualizing

The components of fitness FIGURE 10.1

▲ **A** The cardiovascular and respiratory systems are strengthened by aerobic exercise, such as jogging, bicycling, and swimming. To be considered aerobic, an activity must be performed at an intensity that is low enough for you to carry on a conversation but high enough that you cannot sing while exercising.

B Weight lifting stresses the muscles, causing them to adapt by increasing in size and strength—a process called **hypertrophy**. The larger, stronger muscles can lift the same weight more easily. Muscles that are not used due to a lapse in weight training, injury, or illness become smaller and weaker. This process is called **atrophy**. Thus, there is truth to the saying "Use it or lose it."

cardiorespiratory endurance The efficiency with which the body delivers to cells the oxygen and nutrients needed for muscular activity and transports waste products from cells.

aerobic exercise Endurance exercise that increases heart rate and uses oxygen to provide energy as ATP.

aerobic capacity The maximum amount of oxygen that can be consumed by the tissues during exercise. Also called maximal oxygen consumption, or VO₂ max.

nutrients to your tissues and remove wastes. **Cardiorespiratory endurance** is enhanced by regular **aerobic exercise** (Figure 10.1A).

Regular aerobic exercise strengthens the heart muscle and increases the amount of blood pumped with each heartbeat. This in turn decreases **resting heart rate**, the rate at which the heart beats when the body is at rest to supply blood to the tissues. The more fit you are, the lower your resting heart rate and the more blood your heart can pump to your muscles during exercise. In addition to increasing the amount of oxygen-rich blood that is pumped to your muscles, regular aerobic exercise increases your muscles' ability to use oxygen to produce ATP. Your body's maximum ability to generate ATP using aerobic metabolism is called your **aerobic capacity**, or VO₂ max. Aerobic capacity is a function of the ability of the cardiorespiratory sys-

tem to deliver oxygen to the cells and the ability of the cells to use oxygen to produce ATP. The greater your aerobic capacity, the more intense activity you can perform before lack of oxygen affects your performance.

Muscle strength and endurance

Greater **muscle strength** enhances the ability to perform tasks such as pushing or lifting. In daily life, this could mean lifting a gallon of milk off the top shelf of the refrigerator with one hand, carrying a full trash can out to the curb, or moving a couch into your new apartment. Greater **muscle endurance** enhances your ability to continue repetitive muscle activity, such as shoveling snow or raking leaves. Muscle strength and endurance are increased by repeatedly using muscles in activities that require moving against a resisting force. This type of exercise is called either **strength-training exercise** or **resistance-training exercise** and includes activities such as weight lifting and calisthenics (Figure 10.1B).

muscle strength The amount of force that can be produced by a single contraction of a muscle.

muscle endurance The ability of a muscle group to continue muscle movement over time.

strength-training exercise or **resistance-training exercise** Activities that are specifically designed to increase muscle strength, endurance, and size.

▲ C Flexibility makes everyday tasks easier and can improve athletic performance. Too-tight muscles, tendons, and ligaments restrict motion at the joints, decreasing stride or stroke length and increasing the amount of energy needed to move the joints. Regularly moving limbs, the neck, and the torso through their full range of motion helps increase and maintain flexibility.

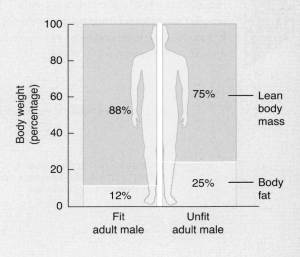

D A fit person ▶ has more muscle mass than an unfit person of the same height and weight. Engaging in aerobic exercise and resistance-training exercise has a positive impact on body composition, reducing body fat and increasing the proportion of lean tissue.

Body weight (percentage)

Fit adult male — 88%, 12%
Unfit adult male — 75%, 25%
Lean body mass / Body fat

Flexibility When you think of fitness, you may picture someone with bulging muscles, but fitness also involves flexibility. Flexibility determines your range of motion—how far you can bend and stretch muscles and ligaments. If your flexibility is poor, you cannot easily bend to tie your shoes or stretch to remove packages from the car. Improving flexibility improves performance in certain activities and may reduce your risk of injuries such as pulled muscles and strained tendons (**FIGURE 10.1C**).

Body composition Individuals who are physically fit have a greater proportion of muscle and a smaller proportion of fat than do unfit individuals of the same weight (**FIGURE 10.1D**). The amount of body fat a person has is also affected by gender and age. In general, women have more stored body fat than men. For young adult women, the desirable amount of body fat is 21 to 32% of total weight; in adult men, the desirable amount is 8 to 19%.[1]

EXERCISE AND THE RISK OF CHRONIC DISEASE

Regular exercise not only makes everyday tasks easier but can also prevent or delay the onset of chronic conditions such as cardiovascular disease, hypertension, type 2 diabetes, breast and colon cancer, and bone and joint disorders (**FIGURE 10.2**).[2] The health benefits of exercise are so great that they can even overcome some of the health risks of carrying excess body fat. Exercise reduces overall mortality, regardless of whether the person is lean, normal weight, or obese.[2] So even if you can't take off the pounds, you'll still get important benefits from continuing to exercise.

In addition to decreasing the risk of disease, exercise improves mood and self-esteem and increases vigor and overall well-being.[3] Exercise has also been shown to reduce depression and anxiety, as well as to improve the quality of life.[4] The mechanisms involved are not clear, but one hypothesis has to do with the production of **endorphins**. Exercise stimulates the release of these chemicals, which are thought to be natural mood enhancers that play a role in triggering what athletes describe as an "exercise high." In addition to causing this state of exercise euphoria, endorphins are thought to aid in relaxation, pain tolerance, and appetite control.

> **endorphins** Compounds that cause a natural euphoria and reduce the perception of pain under certain stressful conditions.

Health benefits of physical activity
FIGURE 10.2

Exercise improves strength and endurance, reduces the risk of chronic disease, aids weight management, reduces sleeplessness, improves self-image, and helps relieve stress, anxiety, and depression.

Exercise improves flexibility and balance.

Exercise increases the sensitivity of tissues to insulin and decreases the risk of developing type 2 diabetes.

Exercise reduces the risk of cardiovascular disease because it strengthens the heart muscle, lowers blood pressure, and increases HDL (good) cholesterol levels in the blood.

Regular exercise reduces the risk of colon cancer and breast cancer.

Exercise increases muscle mass, strength, and endurance.

Weight-bearing exercise stimulates bones to become denser and stronger and therefore reduces the risk of osteoporosis. The strength and flexibility promoted by exercise can help improve joint function.

EXERCISE AND WEIGHT MANAGEMENT

Exercise makes weight management easier because it increases both energy needs and lean body mass. During exercise, energy expenditure can rise well above the resting rate, and some of this increase persists for many hours after activity slows.[5] Over time, regular exercise increases lean body mass. Even at rest, lean tissue uses more energy than fat tissue; therefore, the increase in lean body mass increases basal energy expenditure. The combination of increased energy output during exercise, the rise in energy expenditure that persists for a period after exercise, and the increase in basal needs over the long term can have a major impact on total energy expenditure (**FIGURE 10.3**). The more energy you expend, the more food you can consume while maintaining a healthy weight. As discussed in Chapter 9, exercise is an essential component of any weight-reduction program: It increases energy needs, promotes loss of body fat, and slows the loss of lean tissue that occurs with energy restriction.

CONCEPT CHECK **STOP**

What distinguishes a fit person from an unfit one?

Why do your muscles get bigger when you lift weights?

How does exercise affect heart health?

How does exercise help with weight management?

Exercise increases energy expenditure
FIGURE 10.3

Total energy expenditure is the sum of the energy expended for basal metabolic rate (BMR), physical activity, and the thermic effect of food (TEF). Adding 30 minutes of exercise to your day increases energy expenditure by as much as 300 Calories. If the exercise is performed every day, it causes body composition to change, increasing muscle mass. Greater muscle mass increases BMR, which further increases total energy expenditure.

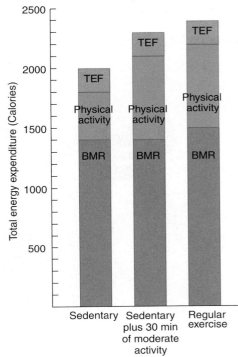

Exercise Recommendations

LEARNING OBJECTIVES

Describe the amounts and types of exercise recommended to improve health.

Classify activities as aerobic or anaerobic.

Plan a fitness program that can be integrated into your daily routine.

Explain overtraining syndrome.

 ost Americans do not exercise regularly, and 25% of American adults get no physical activity at all during their leisure time.[6] To reduce the risk of chronic disease, public health guidelines advise at least 150 minutes of moderate physical activity each week.[5,7,8] This is equivalent to 30 minutes of moderate exercise on most days.[7] Moderate exercise is the equivalent of walking or jogging a mile in 15 to 20 minutes.

Greater health benefits can be obtained by exercising more vigorously or for a longer duration.[8] To promote maintenance of a healthy body weight, an additional 30 minutes/day of exercise may be required, or a total of 60 minutes of moderate to vigorous exercise daily.[7] For those who have lost weight and want to keep it off, 60 to 90 minutes of moderate exercise daily is recommended.[7]

If you can't find the time or motivation to exercise for an hour a day, do not give up. Even a small amount of exercise is better than none.[8]

WHAT TO LOOK FOR IN A FITNESS PROGRAM

A complete fitness program includes aerobic exercise for cardiovascular conditioning, stretching exercises for flexibility, and resistance exercises to increase muscle strength and endurance and maintain or increase muscle mass.[8,9] The program should be integrated into an active lifestyle that includes a variety of everyday activities, enjoyable recreational activities, and a minimum amount of time spent in sedentary activities (FIGURE 10.4).

Moderate or vigorous aerobic exercise should be performed most days of the week. An activity is aerobic if

Exercise recommendations FIGURE 10.4

A Every day activities and aerobic exercise provide the base for an active lifestyle.

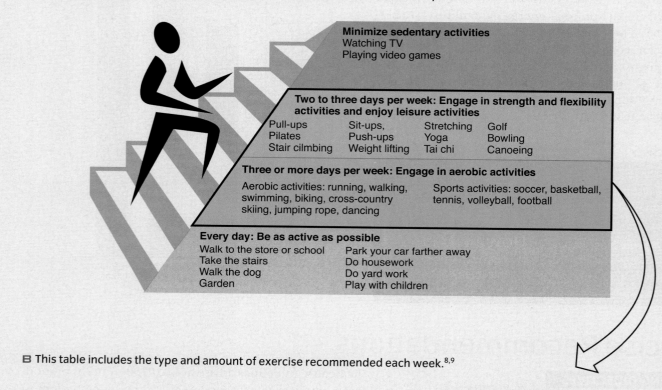

Minimize sedentary activities
Watching TV
Playing video games

Two to three days per week: Engage in strength and flexibility activities and enjoy leisure activities

Pull-ups	Sit-ups,	Stretching	Golf
Pilates	Push-ups	Yoga	Bowling
Stair cilmbing	Weight lifting	Tai chi	Canoeing

Three or more days per week: Engage in aerobic activities

Aerobic activities: running, walking, swimming, biking, cross-country skiing, jumping rope, dancing

Sports activities: soccer, basketball, tennis, volleyball, football

Every day: Be as active as possible

Walk to the store or school
Take the stairs
Walk the dog
Garden

Park your car farther away
Do housework
Do yard work
Play with children

B This table includes the type and amount of exercise recommended each week.[8,9]

	Recommendation	
	Intensity	**Frequency/Duration**
Flexibility	Extend to a position of mild discomfort	2 to 7 days/week hold each stretch for 10 to 30 seconds and repeat each stretch 3 to 5 times
Strength training	Use weights that are heavy enough for muscles to be near exhaustion after 10 to 12 repetitions	2 to 3 nonconsecutive days/week, 8 to 10 exercises for all major muscle groups, repeat each lift 8 to 12 times
Aerobic	Moderate: Raise heart rate to 60 to 69% of maximum	5 to 7 days/week for 30 to 60 minutes
	or	
	Vigorous: Raise heart rate to 70 to 85% of maximum	3 to 7 days/week for 25 to 60 minutes

maximum heart rate The maximum number of beats per minute that the heart can attain.

it raises your heart rate to 60 to 85% of your **maximum heart rate**; when you are exercising at an intensity in this range, you are said to be in your **aerobic zone** (FIGURE 10.5). For a sedentary individual who is beginning an exercise program, mild exercise such as walking can raise the heart rate into the aerobic zone. As fitness improves, an exerciser must perform more intense activity to raise the heart rate to this level.

Aerobic activities of different intensities can be combined to meet recommendations and achieve health benefits. The total amount of energy expended in physical activity depends on the intensity, duration, and frequency of the activity. Vigorous physical activity, such as jogging, that raises heart rate to the high end of the aerobic zone (70 to 85%) improves fitness more and burns more calories per unit of time than does moderate-intensity activity, such as walking, that raises heart rate only to the low end of the zone (60 to 69%).

Individuals should structure their fitness program based on their needs, goals, and abilities. For example, some people might prefer a short, intense workout such as 30 minutes of running, while others would rather work out for a longer time, at a lower intensity, such as a 1-hour walk. Some may choose to complete all their exercise during the same session, while others may spread their exercise throughout the day, in shorter bouts. Three short bouts of 10-minute duration can be as effective as a continuous bout of 30 minutes for reducing the risk of chronic disease.[9] A combination of intensities, such as a brisk 30-minute walk twice during the week in addition to a 20-minute jog on two other days, can meet recommendations.

Strength-training and stretching and can be performed less often than aerobic exercise. Strength training is needed only two to three days a week at the start of an exercise program and two days a week after the desired strength has been achieved. Strength training should not be done on consecutive days. The rest between sessions gives the muscles time to respond to the stress by getting stronger. Increasing the amount of weight lifted increases muscle strength, whereas increasing the number of repetitions improves muscle endurance. Flexibility exercises can be performed 2 to 7 days/week. Time spent stretching does not count towards meeting aerobic or strength training guidelines.

Calculating your aerobic zone FIGURE 10.5

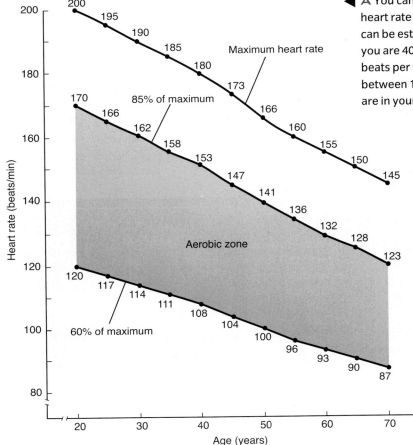

A You can calculate your aerobic zone by multiplying your maximum heart rate by 0.6 and 0.85. Maximum heart rate depends on age; it can be estimated by subtracting your age from 220. For example, if you are 40 years old, you have a maximum heart rate of 180 (220 − 40) beats per minute. If you exercise at a pace that keeps your heart rate between 108 (0.6 × 180) and 153 (0.85 × 180) beats per minute, you are in your aerobic zone.

B You can check your heart rate by feeling the pulse at the side of your neck, just below the jawbone. A pulse is caused by the heart beating and forcing blood through the arteries. The number of pulses per minute equals heart rate.

CREATING AN ACTIVE LIFESTYLE

Incorporating exercise into your day-to-day life may require a change in lifestyle, which is not always easy. Many people avoid exercise because they do not enjoy it, think it requires them to join an expensive health club, have little motivation to do it alone, or find it inconvenient and uncomfortable. Finding an exercise you enjoy, setting aside a time that is realistic and convenient, and finding a place that is appropriate and safe are important steps in starting and maintaining an exercise program (TABLE 10.1). Riding your bike to class or work rather than driving, taking a walk during your lunch break, and enjoying a game of catch or tag with your friends or family are all effective ways to increase your everyday activity level. The goal is to gradually make lifestyle changes that increase physical activity.

Before beginning an exercise program, check with your physician to be sure that your plans are appropriate for you, considering your medical history (FIGURE 10.6). If you choose to exercise outdoors rather than in a

Exercise is for everyone FIGURE 10.6

Almost anyone of any age can exercise, no matter where they live, how old they are, or what physical limitations they have.

gym, reduce or curtail exercise in hot, humid weather in order to avoid heat-related illness. In cold weather, wear clothing that allows for evaporation of sweat while providing protection from the cold. Start each exercise session with a warm-up, such as mild stretching or easy jogging, to increase blood flow to the muscles. End with a cool-down period, such as walking or stretching, to prevent muscle cramps and slowly reduce heart rate.

Don't overdo it. If you don't rest enough between exercise sessions, fitness and performance will not improve. During rest, the body replenishes energy stores, repairs damaged tissues, and builds and strengthens muscles. In athletes, excessive training without sufficient rest to allow for recovery can lead to **overtraining syndrome**. The most common symptom of this condition is fatigue that limits workouts and is felt even at rest. Some athletes experience decreased appetite, weight loss, muscle soreness, increased frequency of viral illnesses, and increased incidence of injuries. They may become moody, easily irritated, or depressed, experience altered sleep patterns, or lose their competitive desire and enthusiasm. Overtraining syndrome occurs only in serious athletes who are training extensively, but rest is essential for anyone who is working to increase fitness.

> **overtraining syndrome** A collection of emotional, behavioral, and physical symptoms that occurs when the amount and intensity of exercise exceeds an athlete's capacity to recover.

Suggestions for starting and maintaining an exercise program TABLE 10.1

- Start slowly. Set specific, attainable goals. Once you have met them, add more.
  - Walk around the block after dinner.
  - Get off the bus or subway one stop early.
  - Use half of your lunch break to exercise.
  - Do a few biceps curls each time you take the milk out of the refrigerator.
- Make your exercise fun and convenient.
  - Opt for activities you enjoy—bowling and dancing may be more fun for you than using a treadmill in the basement.
  - Find a partner to exercise with you.
  - Choose times that fit your schedule.
- Stay motivated.
  - Vary your routine—swim one day and mountain bike the next.
  - Challenge your strength or endurance once or twice a week and do moderate workouts on other days.
  - Track your progress by recording your activity.
  - Reward your success with a new book, movie, or workout clothes.
- Keep your exercise safe.
  - Warm up before you start.
  - Cool down when you are done.
  - Don't overdo it—alternate hard days with easy days, and take a day off when you need it.
  - Listen to your body and stop before an injury occurs.

CONCEPT CHECK STOP

How much aerobic exercise is recommended to reduce the risk of chronic disease?

What is your aerobic zone?

When does exercise fit best into your schedule?

Who is at risk for overtraining syndrome?

Fueling Exercise

The body runs on energy from the carbohydrate, fat, and protein in food and body stores. These fuels are needed whether you are writing a term paper, riding your bike to class, or running a marathon. Before they can be used to fuel activity, their energy must be converted into the high-energy compound ATP, the immediate source of energy for body functions. ATP can be generated both in the absence of oxygen, by **anaerobic metabolism**, and in the presence of oxygen, by **aerobic metabolism** (FIGURE 10.7). The type of metabolism that predominates during an activity determines how much carbohydrate, fat, and protein are used to fuel the activity.

Anaerobic vs. aerobic metabolism FIGURE 10.7

In the absence of oxygen, ATP can be produced only by anaerobic metabolism. Anaerobic metabolism can produce ATP very rapidly but must use glucose as a fuel. Anaerobic metabolism produces **lactic acid**, which can be used as a fuel for aerobic metabolism. When oxygen is present, the majority of ATP is produced by aerobic metabolism. Aerobic metabolism can use any fuel: carbohydrate, fat, or protein. It is slower but more efficient at generating ATP than anaerobic metabolism.

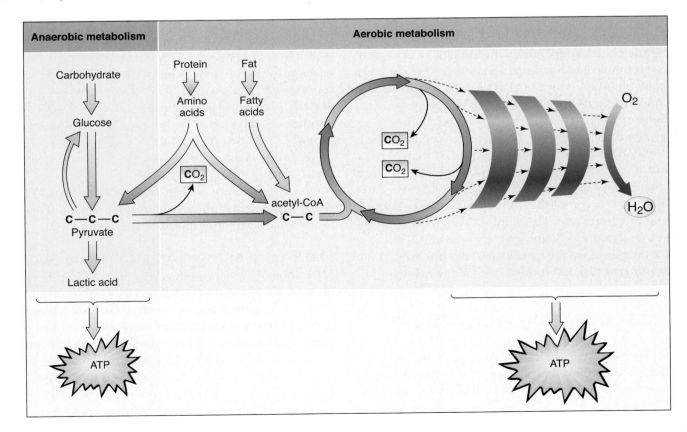

Increasing oxygen delivery FIGURE 10.8

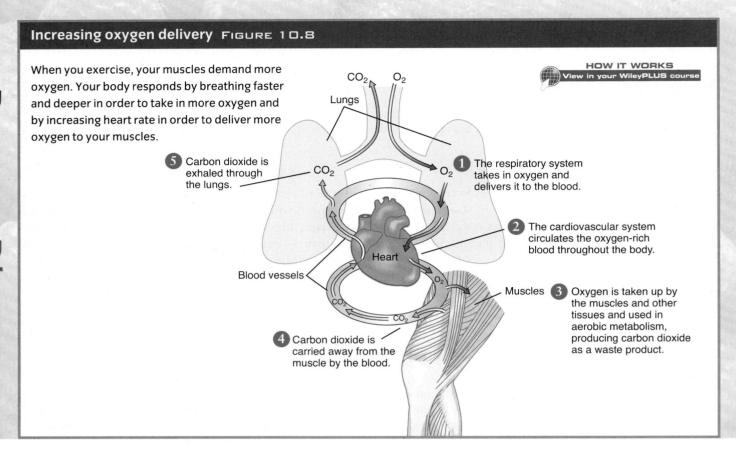

When you exercise, your muscles demand more oxygen. Your body responds by breathing faster and deeper in order to take in more oxygen and by increasing heart rate in order to deliver more oxygen to your muscles.

HOW IT WORKS
View in your WileyPLUS course

5 Carbon dioxide is exhaled through the lungs.

1 The respiratory system takes in oxygen and delivers it to the blood.

2 The cardiovascular system circulates the oxygen-rich blood throughout the body.

3 Oxygen is taken up by the muscles and other tissues and used in aerobic metabolism, producing carbon dioxide as a waste product.

4 Carbon dioxide is carried away from the muscle by the blood.

Lungs — CO_2 — O_2 — Blood vessels — Heart — Muscles

The amount of ATP produced by anaerobic versus aerobic metabolism depends on the availability of oxygen. Oxygen is inhaled by the lungs and delivered to the muscle by the blood (**FIGURE 10.8**). When you are at rest, your muscles do not need much energy, and your heart and lungs are able to deliver enough oxygen to meet your energy needs using aerobic metabolism. When you exercise, your muscles need more energy. To increase the amount of energy provided by aerobic metabolism, you must increase the amount of oxygen delivered to the muscles. Your body accomplishes this by increasing both heart rate and breathing rate. The ability of the circulatory and respiratory systems to deliver oxygen to tissues is affected by how long an activity is performed, the intensity of the activity, and the physical conditioning of the exerciser.

EXERCISE DURATION AND FUEL USE

When you take the first steps of your morning jog, your muscles increase their activity, but your heart and lungs have not had time to step up their delivery of oxygen to them. To get the energy they need, the muscles rely on the small amount of ATP that is stored in resting muscle. This is enough to sustain activity for a few seconds. As the stored ATP is used up, enzymes break down another high-energy compound, **creatine phosphate**, to convert ADP (adenosine diphosphate) to ATP, allowing your activity to continue. But, like the amount of ATP, the amount of creatine phosphate stored in the muscle at any time is small and soon runs out (**FIGURE 10.9**).

> **creatine phosphate**
> A compound stored in muscle that can be broken down quickly to make ATP.

Short-term energy: Anaerobic metabolism

After about 15 seconds of exercise, the ATP and creatine phosphate in your muscles are used up, but your heart rate and breathing have not increased enough to deliver more oxygen to the muscles. To get more energy at this point, your muscles must produce the additional ATP without oxygen (see Figure 10.7). This anaerobic metabolism can produce ATP very rapidly but can use only glucose as a fuel (**FIGURE 10.10**). The amount of glucose is limited, so anaerobic metabolism cannot continue indefinitely.

Changes in the source of ATP over time

FIGURE 10.9

The source of the ATP that fuels muscle contraction changes over the first few minutes of exercise.

During the first few seconds of exercise, the muscles get energy from stored ATP. Then, for the next 10 seconds or so, creatine phosphate stored in the muscles is broken down to form more ATP.

Anaerobic metabolism of glucose, obtained either from the blood or from muscle glycogen, becomes the predominant source of ATP when creatine phosphate stores have been depleted. Thirty seconds into the activity, anaerobic pathways are operating at full capacity.

After about two to three minutes, oxygen delivery to the muscles has increased enough to support aerobic metabolism, which uses fatty acids and glucose to produce ATP.

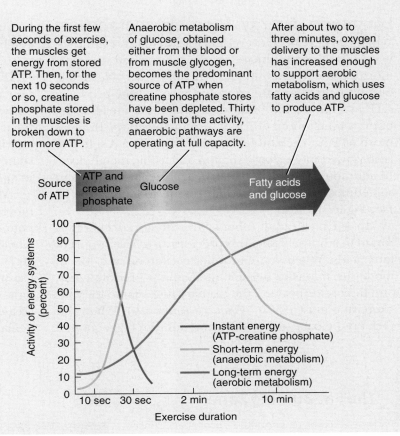

Fuels for anaerobic and aerobic metabolism

FIGURE 10.10

The glucose available to fuel muscle contraction comes from muscle glycogen breakdown or blood glucose. Blood glucose levels are maintained by the breakdown of liver glycogen, glucose synthesis by the liver, and carbohydrate consumed during exercise. Some of the fatty acids used as fuel come from triglycerides stored in the muscle, but most come from adipose tissue. The amino acids available to the body come from the digestion of dietary proteins and from the breakdown of body proteins.

Fueling Exercise 341

Long-term energy: Aerobic metabolism

When you have been exercising for two to three minutes, your breathing and heart rate have increased to supply more oxygen to your muscles. This allows aerobic metabolism to predominate. Aerobic metabolism produces ATP at a slower rate than does anaerobic metabolism, but it is much more efficient, producing about 18 times more ATP for each molecule of glucose. As a result, glucose is used more slowly than in anaerobic metabolism. In addition, aerobic metabolism can use fatty acids, and sometimes amino acids from protein, to generate ATP (see Figure 10.10).

In a typical adult, about 90% of stored energy is found in adipose tissue; this provides an ample supply of fatty acids. When you continue to exercise at a low to moderate intensity, aerobic metabolism predominates, and fatty acids become the primary fuel source for your exercising muscles (see *What a Scientist Sees*). When you pick up the pace, the relative amount of ATP generated by anaerobic versus aerobic metabolism and the fuels you burn will change.

Protein as a fuel for exercise

Although protein is not considered a major energy source for the body, even at rest, small amounts of amino acids are used for energy. The amount increases if your diet does not provide enough total energy to meet needs, if you consume more protein than you need, or if you are involved in endurance exercise (see Chapter 6).

When the nitrogen-containing amino group is removed from an amino acid, the remaining carbon compound can be broken down to produce ATP by aerobic metabolism or, in some cases, used to make glucose (see Figure 10.7). Exercise that continues for many hours increases the use of amino acids both as an energy source and as a raw material for glucose synthesis. Strength training does not increase the use of protein for energy, but it does increase the demand for amino acids for muscle building and repair.

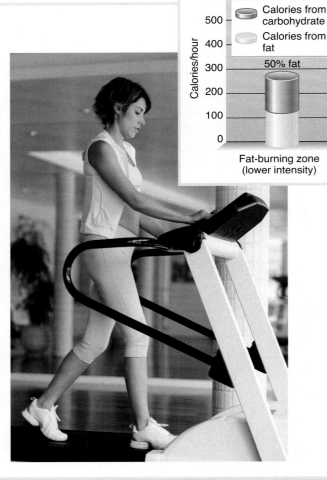

The Fat-Burning Zone

Have you ever jumped onto a treadmill and chosen the workout that puts you in the "fat-burning zone" rather than the one that puts you in the "cardio zone" because your goal was to lose weight? The fat-burning zone is a lower-intensity aerobic workout that keeps your heart rate between about 60 and 69% of maximum. The cardio zone is a higher-intensity aerobic workout that keeps heart rate between about 70 and 85% of maximum.

However, do you really burn more fat during a slow 30-minute jog in the fat-burning zone than during a vigorous 30-minute run in the cardio zone? A scientist sees that you do burn a higher percentage of calories from fat during a lower-intensity aerobic workout, but that's not the whole story. When you pick up the pace and exercise in what the treadmill calls the cardio zone, you continue to burn fat. The graph shows that 50% of the calories burned come from fat during the lower-intensity workout (that is, in the fat-burning zone) and only 40% come from fat during the higher-intensity workout. Looking at the actual numbers of calories burned, however, the scientist sees that at the higher intensity, you burn just as much fat (about 150 Calories/hour) but a much greater number of calories overall. Which workout will help you lose the most weight?

The effect of exercise intensity on fuel use FIGURE 10.11

Exercise intensity determines the contributions of carbohydrate, fat, and protein as fuels for ATP production. At rest and during low- to moderate-intensity exercise, aerobic metabolism predominates, so fatty acids are an important fuel source. As exercise intensity increases, the proportion of energy supplied by anaerobic metabolism increases, so glucose becomes the predominant fuel. Keep in mind, however, that during exercise, the total amount of energy expended is greater than the amount expended at rest.

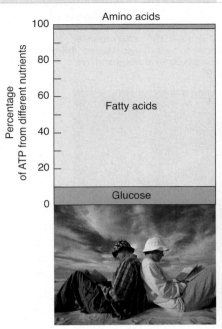

Rest | Moderate-intensity activity | High-intensity activity

EXERCISE INTENSITY AND FUEL USE

The energy contributions made by anaerobic and aerobic metabolism combine to ensure that your muscles get enough ATP to meet the demands you place on them. The relative contribution of each type of metabolism depends on how intense your activity is. With low-intensity activity, sufficient ATP can be produced by aerobic metabolism so that both glucose and fatty acids can be used by the muscles. With intense exercise, more ATP is needed, but oxygen delivery to and use by the muscles becomes limited, so the muscles must get the additional ATP they need by using anaerobic metabolism (FIGURE 10.11).

Lower-intensity exercise relies on aerobic metabolism, which is more efficient than anaerobic metabolism and uses both glucose and fatty acids for energy. The body's fat reserves are almost unlimited, so if fat is the fuel, exercise can theoretically continue for a very long time. For example, it is estimated that a 130-lb woman has enough energy stored as body fat to run 1000 miles.[10] However, even aerobic activity uses some glucose, which means that if exercise

fatigue Inability to continue an activity at an optimal level.

continues long enough, glycogen stores are eventually depleted, causing **fatigue**.

Fatigue occurs much more quickly with high-intensity exercise than with lower-intensity exercise because more intense exercise relies more on anaerobic metabolism, which can use only glucose for fuel. Glycogen stores thus are rapidly depleted (FIGURE 10.12). Anaerobic

Fatigue: "Hitting the wall" FIGURE 10.12

Glycogen depletion is a concern for athletes because the amount of stored glycogen available to produce glucose during exercise is limited. When athletes run out of glycogen, they experience a feeling of overwhelming fatigue that is sometimes referred to as "hitting the wall," or "bonking."

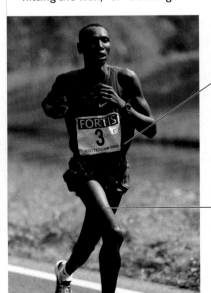

Between 60 and 120 grams of glycogen are stored in your liver; glycogen stores are highest just after a meal. Liver glycogen is used to maintain blood glucose between meals and during the night. Eating a high-carbohydrate breakfast will replenish the liver glycogen you used while you slept.

There are about 200 to 500 g of glycogen in the muscles of a 70-kg (154-lb) person. The glycogen in a muscle is used to fuel that muscle's activity.

Fueling Exercise 343

Aerobic training causes physiological changes in the cardiovascular system that increase the delivery of oxygen to cells. It also causes changes in the muscle cells that increase glycogen storage and the ability to use oxygen to generate ATP. ▼

▲ The total blood volume and number of red blood cells expands, increasing the amount of hemoglobin, so that more oxygen can be transported. The number of capillary blood vessels in the muscles increases so that blood is delivered to muscles more efficiently.

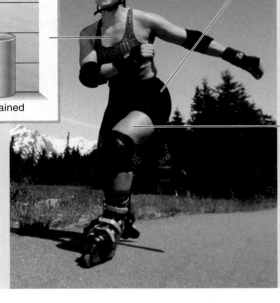

▲ The heart becomes larger and stronger so that the amount of blood pumped with each beat is increased. As shown here, the heart of a trained athlete can pump more blood per minute than can the heart of an untrained individual.

mitochondria

▲ In the muscle there is an increase in the ability to store glycogen and an increase in the number and size of muscle-cell mitochondria. Because aerobic metabolism occurs in the mitochondria, the greater size and number of mitochondria increases the cell's capacity to burn fatty acids to produce ATP.

metabolism also produces lactic acid. With low-intensity exercise, the small amounts of lactic acid produced are carried away from the muscles and used by other tissues as an energy source or converted back into glucose by the liver. During high-intensity exercise, the amount of lactic acid produced exceeds the amount that can be used by other tissues, and the lactic acid builds up in the muscle and subsequently in the blood. Until recently, it was assumed that lactic acid buildup was the cause of muscle fatigue, but we now know that although lactic acid buildup is associated with fatigue, it does not cause it.[11] Fatigue most likely has many causes, including glycogen depletion and changes in the muscle cells and the concentrations of molecules involved in muscle metabolism.

FITNESS TRAINING AND FUEL USE

When you exercise regularly to improve your fitness, the training causes physiological changes in your body. The changes caused by repeated bouts of aerobic exercise in-

crease the amount of oxygen that can be delivered to the muscles and the ability of the muscles to use oxygen to generate ATP by aerobic metabolism (FIGURE 10.13). This increased aerobic capacity allows fatty acids to be used for fuel so that glycogen is spared and the onset of fatigue is delayed. Training aerobically also increases the amount of glycogen stored in the muscles. Because trained athletes store more glycogen and use it more slowly, they can sustain aerobic exercise for longer periods at higher intensities than can untrained individuals.

CONCEPT CHECK STOP

What fuels are used in anaerobic metabolism?

What type of metabolism does a marathon runner rely on?

Why is a trained athlete able to perform at a higher intensity for a longer time than an untrained person?

Energy and Nutrient Needs for Physical Activity

Good nutrition is essential to performance, whether you are a marathon runner or a mall walker. Your diet must provide enough energy to fuel activity, enough protein to maintain muscle mass, sufficient micronutrients to permit utilization of the energy-yielding nutrients, and enough water to transport nutrients and cool your body. The major difference between the nutritional needs of a serious athlete and those of a casual exerciser is the amount of energy and water required.

ENERGY NEEDS

The amount of energy expended for any activity depends on the intensity, duration, and frequency of the activity and the weight of the exerciser (**FIGURE 10.14**). Whereas casual exercise may burn only 100 additional Calories a day, the training required for an endurance athlete, such as a marathon runner, may increase energy expenditure by 2000 to 3000 Calories/day. Some athletes require 6000 Calories a day to maintain their body weight. In general, the more intense the activity, the more energy it requires, and the more time is spent exercising, the more energy is expended (see Appendix I). Walking for 60 minutes, for instance, involves less work than running for the same amount of time and therefore requires less energy.

Gaining or losing weight
Body weight and composition can affect exercise performance. In sports such as football and weight lifting, having a large amount of muscle is advantageous, and athletes may try to build muscle and increase body weight. Healthy weight gain can be achieved through a combination of increased energy intake, adequate protein intake, and strength-training exercise to promote an increase in lean tissue rather than fat.

In sports such as ballet, gymnastics, and certain running events, small, light bodies offer an advantage, so athletes may restrict energy intake in order to maintain a low body weight. While a slightly leaner physique may be beneficial in these sports, dieting to maintain an unrealistically low weight may threaten health and performance. An athlete who needs to lose weight should do so in advance of the competitive season to prevent the calorie restriction from affecting performance. The general guidelines for healthy weight loss should be followed: Reduce energy intake by 200 to 500 Calories/day, increase activity, and change the behaviors that led to weight gain (see Chapter 9).

Unhealthy weight-loss practices
Successful athletes are vulnerable to eating disorders because their motivation and self-discipline make them more susceptible to the pressure to lose weight in order to optimize performance (see Chapter 9).[12] In athletes who develop anorexia nervosa, the restricted food intake can affect growth and maturation and impair exercise performance. In athletes who develop bulimia, purging can cause dehydration and electrolyte imbalance, which affect performance and put overall health at risk. In addition to using restricted food intake or purging to keep body weight low, athletes are more likely than nonathletes to engage in compulsive exercise behaviors in order to increase energy expenditure.

Factors affecting energy expenditure
FIGURE 10.14

This graph illustrates the impact of running pace and body weight on energy expenditure per hour. The longer an individual continues to run, the greater the amount of energy expended. Body weight affects energy needs because moving a heavier body requires more energy than moving a lighter one. Therefore, if the pace is the same, a 170-lb woman requires more energy to run for an hour than does a 125-lb woman.

Female athlete triad FIGURE 10.15

Women with female athlete triad typically have low body fat, do not menstruate regularly, and may experience multiple or recurrent stress fractures. Neither adequate dietary calcium nor the increase in bone mass caused by weight-bearing exercise can compensate for the bone loss caused by low estrogen levels. Treatment involves increasing energy intake and reducing activity so that menstrual cycles resume.[13]

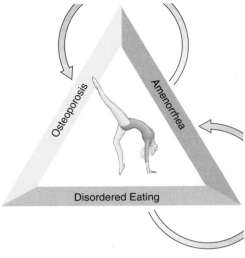

Estrogen is needed for calcium homeostasis in the bone and for calcium absorption in the intestines. Low levels lead to low peak bone mass, premature bone loss, and increased risk of stress fractures.

Osteoporosis

Amenorrhea

Disordered Eating

The extreme energy restriction of an eating disorder combined with exercise creates a physiological condition that is similar to starvation, which contributes to a drop in estrogen levels. Low estrogen causes amenorrhea.

In female athletes, the pressure to reduce body weight and fat in order to improve performance, achieve an ideal body image, and meet goals set by coaches, trainers, or parents may lead to a combination of symptoms referred to as the **female athlete triad.** This syndrome includes disordered eating patterns, amenorrhea, and disturbances in bone formation and breakdown that can lead to osteoporosis (**FIGURE 10.15**).

Athletes involved in sports that have weight classes, such as wrestling and boxing, are at particular risk for unhealthy weight-loss practices because they are under pressure to lose weight before a competition so that they can compete in a lower weight class. Competing at the high end of a weight class is thought to offer an advantage over smaller opponents. To lose weight rapidly, these athletes may use sporadic diets that severely restrict energy intake or dehydrate themselves through such practices as vigorous exercise, fluid restriction, wearing of vapor-impermeable suits, or use of hot environments such as saunas and steam rooms to increase sweat loss. They may also resort to even more extreme measures, such as vomiting and the use of diuretics and laxatives. These practices can be dangerous and even fatal (**FIGURE 10.16**). They may impair performance and can adversely affect heart and kidney function, temperature regulation, and electrolyte balance.

Making weight FIGURE 10.16

In 1997, three young wrestlers died while exercising in plastic suits in order to sweat off water.[14] As a result, wrestling weight classes were altered to eliminate the lightest class, plastic sweat suits were banned, weigh-ins were moved to one hour before competition, and mandatory weight-loss rules were instituted. The percentage of body fat can be no less than 5% for college wrestlers and 7% for high school wrestlers.

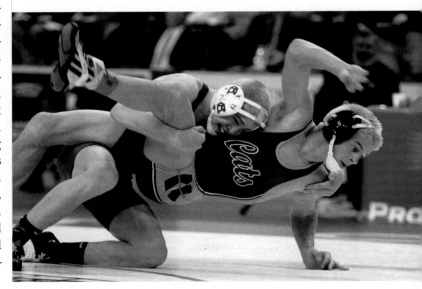

CARBOHYDRATE, FAT, AND PROTEIN NEEDS

The source of energy in an athlete's diet can be as important as the amount. To maximize glycogen stores and optimize performance, a diet providing about 6 to 10 g of carbohydrate/kg of body wt/day is recommended for physically active individuals (FIGURE 10.17).[15] The recommended amount of fat is the same as that for the general population—between 20 and 35% of energy.[15] To allow for enough carbohydrate, fat intakes at the lower end of this range may be needed for some athletes. Diets that are very low in fat (less than 20% of calories) do not benefit performance. Protein is not a significant energy source, accounting for only about 5% of energy expended, but dietary protein is needed to maintain and repair lean tissues, including muscle. A diet in which 15 to 20% of calories come from protein will meet the needs of most athletes.

As discussed in Chapter 6, competitive athletes participating in endurance or strength sports may require extra protein. In endurance events, such as marathons, protein is used for energy and to maintain blood glucose. Athletes participating in these events may benefit from 1.2 to 1.4 g of protein/kilogram of body weight/day. Athletes participating in strength events require amino acids to synthesize new muscle proteins and may benefit from 1.2 to 1.7 g/kg/day.[15] While this amount is greater than the RDA (0.8 g/kg/day), it is not greater than the amount of protein habitually consumed by athletes.[16]

VITAMIN AND MINERAL NEEDS

An adequate intake of vitamins and minerals is essential for optimal performance. These micronutrients are needed for energy production, oxygen delivery, protection against oxidative damage, and repair and maintenance of body structures.

Exercise increases the amounts of many vitamins and minerals used both in metabolism during exercise and in repairing tissues after exercise. In addition, exercise may increase losses of some micronutrients. Nevertheless, most athletes can meet their needs by consuming the amounts of vitamins and minerals recommended for the general population. Because athletes must eat more food to satisfy their higher energy needs, they consume extra vitamins and minerals with these foods, particularly if they choose nutrient-dense foods. Athletes who restrict their intake in order to maintain a low body weight may be at risk for vitamin and mineral deficiencies.

Antioxidants and oxidative damage
Exercise increases the amount of oxygen used by muscle and the rate of energy-producing metabolic reactions.[17] This increased oxygen use increases the production of free radicals, which can lead to oxidative damage and contribute to muscle fatigue.[18] To protect the body from oxidative damage, muscle cells contain antioxidant defenses, some of which may interact with dietary antioxidants such as vitamin C, vitamin E, β-carotene, and selenium. Despite the importance of antioxidants for health and performance, there is little evidence that supplementation with antioxidants improves human performance.[19]

Proportions of energy-yielding nutrients in an athlete's diet FIGURE 10.17

The proportions of carbohydrate, fat, and protein recommended for the diets of physically active individuals are within the ranges recommended to the general public: about 45 to 65% of total energy from carbohydrate, 20 to 35% of energy from fat, and 10 to 35% of energy from protein.

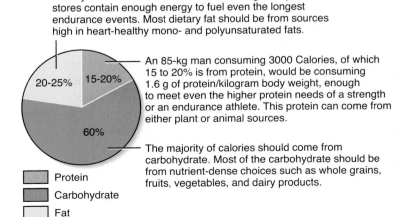

Dietary fat is essential for health even though body fat stores contain enough energy to fuel even the longest endurance events. Most dietary fat should be from sources high in heart-healthy mono- and polyunsaturated fats.

An 85-kg man consuming 3000 Calories, of which 15 to 20% is from protein, would be consuming 1.6 g of protein/kilogram body weight, enough to meet even the higher protein needs of a strength or an endurance athlete. This protein can come from either plant or animal sources.

The majority of calories should come from carbohydrate. Most of the carbohydrate should be from nutrient-dense choices such as whole grains, fruits, vegetables, and dairy products.

20-25% 15-20% 60%

Protein
Carbohydrate
Fat

Sports anemia FIGURE 10.18

Training causes blood volume to expand in order to increase oxygen delivery, but the synthesis of red blood cells lags behind the increase in blood volume. The result is a decrease in the percentage of blood volume that is red blood cells. However, the total number of red blood cells stays the same or increases slightly, so the transport of oxygen is not impaired. As training progresses, the number of red blood cells increases to catch up with the increase in total blood volume.

Normal

Sports anemia

Iron and anemia

The body requires iron to form hemoglobin, myoglobin, and a number of iron-containing proteins that are essential for the production of energy by aerobic metabolism. Exercise increases the need for a number of these proteins and may thereby increase iron needs. For example, exercise stimulates the production of red blood cells, so more iron is needed for hemoglobin synthesis. Prolonged training may also increase iron requirements because iron loss in feces, urine, and sweat increases.[15]

Another cause of iron loss is the breaking of red blood cells due to the contraction of large muscles or impact in events such as running. This type of red blood cell breakage is referred to as *foot-strike hemolysis.* It rarely causes anemia because most of the iron from these cells is recycled, and the breaking of red blood cells stimulates the production of new ones.

Reduced iron stores are not uncommon in athletes.[20] Female athletes are at particular risk; their needs are higher than those of male athletes because they need to replace the iron lost in menstrual blood.[21] In athletes of both sexes, inadequate iron intake often contributes to low iron stores. Iron intake may be low in athletes who are attempting to keep their body weight down and in those who do not eat meat, which is an excellent source of readily absorbable heme iron. If iron deficiency progresses to anemia, the body's ability both to transport oxygen and to provide energy by aerobic metabolism is reduced, impairing exercise performance as well as overall health.

Iron deficiency anemia (see Chapter 8) should not be confused with **sports anemia**, which is an adaptation to training that does not seem to impair the delivery of oxygen to tissues (FIGURE 10.18). Although a specific iron RDA has not been set for athletes, the DRIs acknowledge that the requirement may be 30 to 70% higher for athletes than for the general population.[22]

WATER NEEDS

Exercise increases water needs because it increases losses in sweat and from evaporation through the respiratory system. During exercise, most people drink only enough to assuage their thirst, but this amount typically is not enough to replace water losses. Therefore, they end their exercise session in a state of dehydration and must restore fluid balance during the remainder of the day.

The risk of dehydration is greater in hot than cold environments. However, dehydration may also occur when exercising in the cold because cold air tends to be dry, so evaporative losses from the lungs are greater. In addition, insulated clothing worn in cold weather may increase sweat loss, and fluid intake may be reduced because a chilled athlete may be reluctant to drink a cold beverage. Female athletes training in cold weather may also limit fluid intake in order to avoid the inconvenience of removing clothing in order to urinate.[15]

Even when fluids are consumed at regular intervals throughout exercise, it may not be possible to drink enough to compensate for losses. During exercise, water is needed to cool the body and to transport both oxygen and nutrients to the muscles and remove waste products from them. Not consuming enough water to replace losses can be hazardous to the performance and health of even the most casual exerciser (FIGURE 10.19).

Dehydration and heat-related illnesses

Dehydration occurs when water loss is great enough for blood volume to decrease, thereby reducing the ability of the circulatory system to deliver oxygen and nutrients to exercising muscles (see Chapter 8). A decrease in blood volume also reduces blood flow to the skin and the amount of sweat produced, thus limiting the body's ability to cool itself. As a result, core body temperature can increase, and with it the risk of various **heat-related illnesses**.

> **heat-related illnesses** Conditions, including heat cramps, heat exhaustion, and heat stroke, that can occur due to an unfavorable combination of exercise, hydration status, and climatic conditions.

Heat cramps are involuntary muscle spasms that occur during or after intense exercise, usually in the muscles involved in the exercise. They are a form of heat-related illness caused by an imbalance of electrolytes at the muscle cell membranes. They can occur when water and salt are lost during extended exercise.

Heat exhaustion occurs when water loss causes blood volume to decrease so much that it is not possible both to cool the body and to deliver oxygen to active muscles. It is a form of heat-related illness characterized by a rapid but weak pulse, low blood pressure, disorientation, profuse sweating, and fainting. A person who is experiencing symptoms of heat exhaustion should stop exercising and move to a cooler environment.

Heat exhaustion can progress to **heat stroke**, the most serious form of heat-related illness. It occurs when core body temperature rises above 105°F, causing the brain's temperature-regulatory center to fail. When this occurs, the individual does not sweat even though body temperature is rising. Heat stroke is characterized by elevated body temperature; hot, dry skin; extreme confusion; and unconsciousness. It requires immediate medical attention.

Exercising in hot, humid weather increases the risk of heat-related illnesses. As environmental temperature rises, the body has more difficulty dissipating heat, and as humidity rises, the body's ability to cool through evaporation decreases (FIGURE 10.20).

Dehydration and performance
FIGURE 10.19

As the severity of dehydration increases, exercise performance declines. Even mild dehydration—a water loss of 1 to 2% of body weight—can impair exercise performance. A 3% reduction in body weight can significantly reduce the amount of blood pumped with each heartbeat because the blood volume is decreased. This, in turn, reduces the circulatory system's ability to deliver oxygen and nutrients to cells and remove waste products.

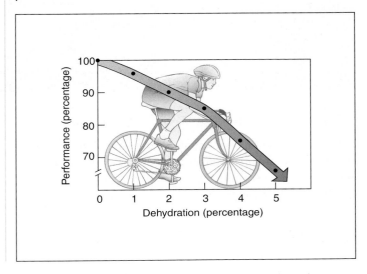

Heat index[23] FIGURE 10.20

Exercise in extreme conditions increases the risk of heat-related illness. *Heat index*, or *apparent temperature*, is a measure of how hot it feels when the relative humidity is added to the air temperature. To find the heat index, find the intersection of the temperature on the left side of the table and the relative humidity across the top. The colored zones correspond to heat index levels that may cause increasingly severe heat illnesses with continued exposure and/or physical activity.

Relative humidity (%)

°F	40	45	50	55	60	65	70	75	80	85	90	95	100
110	136												
108	130	137											
106	124	130	137										
104	119	124	131	137									
102	114	119	124	130	137								
100	109	114	118	124	129	136							
98	105	109	113	117	123	128	134						
96	101	104	108	112	116	121	126	132					
94	97	100	102	106	110	114	119	124	129	135			
92	94	96	99	101	105	108	112	116	121	126	131		
90	91	93	95	97	100	103	106	109	113	117	122	127	132
88	88	89	91	93	95	98	100	103	106	110	113	117	121
86	85	87	88	89	91	93	95	97	100	102	105	108	112
84	83	84	85	86	88	89	90	92	94	96	98	100	103
82	81	82	83	84	84	85	86	88	89	90	91	93	95
80	80	80	81	81	82	82	83	84	84	85	86	86	87

Air temperature

Heat index (apparent temperature)

With prolonged exposure and/or physical activity

Extreme danger
Heat stroke highly likely
Danger
Heat stroke, heat cramps, and/or heat exhaustion likely
Extreme caution
Heat stroke, heat cramps, and/or heat exhaustion possible
Caution
Fatigue possible

Hyponatremia in the Boston Marathon FIGURE 10.21

These discarded drinking cups along the route of the Boston Marathon indicate that runners are consuming a lot of fluid. But if the runners are drinking too much plain water, it can impair health by changing the proportion of water and sodium in the body. In 2002, a 28-year-old woman died after the Boston Marathon as a result of hyponatremia. A study done that year found that 13% of runners in the Boston Marathon had hyponatremia.[24]

Hyponatremia Sweating helps us stay cool. But if the water and sodium lost in sweat are not replaced in the right proportions, low blood sodium, or hyponatremia, may result (see Chapter 8). For most activities, sweat losses can be replaced with plain water, and lost electrolytes can be replaced during the meals following exercise. However, during endurance events such as marathons, when sweating continues for many hours, both water and sodium need to be replenished. If an athlete replaces the lost fluid with plain water, the sodium that remains in the blood is diluted, causing hyponatremia. As sodium concentrations in the blood decrease, fluid moves into body tissues by osmosis, causing swelling. Fluid accumulation in the lungs interferes with gas exchange, and fluid accumulation in the brain causes disorientation, seizure, coma, and death (FIGURE 10.21).

The risk of hyponatremia can be reduced by consuming a sodium-containing sports drink during long-distance events, increasing sodium intake several days prior to a competition, and avoiding Tylenol (acetaminophen), aspirin, ibuprofen, and other nonsteroidal anti-inflammatory drugs, which may contribute to the development of hyponatremia by interfering with kidney function. The early symptoms of hyponatremia may be similar to those of dehydration: nausea, muscle cramps, disorientation, slurred speech, and confusion. A proper diagnosis is important because drinking water alone will make the problem worse. Mild symptoms of hyponatremia can be treated by eating salty foods or drinking a sodium-containing beverage, such as a sports drink. More severe symptoms require medical attention.

Fluid recommendations for exercise Anyone who is exercising should consume extra fluids. Because thirst is not a reliable short-term indicator of the body's water needs, it is important to schedule regular fluid breaks. Typically, however, exercising individuals ingest amounts of fluids that are equal to only about one- to two-thirds of the amount lost in sweat.[25] To ensure hydration, adequate amounts of fluid should be consumed before, during, and after exercise.

Exercisers should drink generous amounts of fluid in the 24 hours before an exercise session and about 2 cups of fluid 4 hours before exercise. During exercise, whether casual or competitive, exercisers should try to drink enough fluid to prevent weight loss.[15] Drinking 6 to 12 ounces of fluid every 15 to 20 minutes for the duration of the exercise should maintain adequate hydration. To restore lost water after exercise, each pound of weight lost should be replaced with 16 to 24 oz (1 to 1.5 lbs) of fluid.[15]

The best type of beverage to consume during exercise depends on the duration of the exercise. For exercise lasting an hour or less, water is the only fluid needed, particularly if one of your exercise goals is weight management. A typical 16-ounce sports drink provides about 100 Calories, so it will replace about half of the calories expended during your 40-minutes ride on the stationary bicycle.

For exercise lasting more than 60 minutes, sports drinks or other beverages containing a small amount of carbohydrate (about 10 to 20 g of carbohydrate/cup) and electrolytes (around 150 milligrams of sodium in a cup) are recommended.[15] The carbohydrate is a source of glucose for the muscle and thus delays fatigue. Commercial sports drinks contain rapidly absorbed sources of carbohydrate such as glucose, sucrose, or glucose polymers (chains of glucose molecules). The right proportion of carbohydrate to water is important. If the concentration of carbohydrate is too low, it will not help performance; if it is too high, it will delay stomach emptying. Water and carbohydrate trapped in the stomach do not benefit the athlete and may cause stomach cramps. Because fruit juices and soft drinks contain twice as much sugar as sports drinks, they are not recommended unless they are diluted with an equal volume of water. The sodium in sports drinks helps prevent hyponatremia and also enhances intestinal absorption of water and glucose and stimulates thirst. Flavored beverages also tempt athletes to drink more, helping to ensure adequate hydration.

FOOD AND DRINK TO OPTIMIZE PERFORMANCE

For most of us, a trip to the gym requires no special nutritional planning, but for competitive athletes, when and what they eat before, during, and after competition are as important as a balanced overall diet. The type and amount of food eaten at these times may give or take away the extra seconds that can mean victory or defeat.

Maximizing glycogen stores

Glycogen stores are a source of glucose, and larger glycogen stores allow exercise to continue for longer periods. Glycogen stores and hence endurance are increased by increasing carbohydrate intake (**FIGURE 10.22**).

Serious endurance athletes who want to substantially increase their muscle glycogen stores before a competition may choose to follow a dietary regimen referred to as **glycogen supercompensation** or **carbohydrate loading**. This involves resting for one to three days before competition while consuming a very high-carbohydrate diet.[27,28] The diet should provide 10 to 12 g of carbohydrate/kilogram of body weight/day. For a 150-lb person, this is equivalent to about

> **glycogen super-compensation** or **carbohydrate loading**
> A regimen designed to increase muscle glycogen stores beyond their usual capacity.

Dietary carbohydrate and endurance FIGURE 10.22

The amount of carbohydrate consumed in the diet affects the level of muscle glycogen and hence an athlete's endurance. This graph shows endurance capacity during cycling exercise after three days of a low-carbohydrate diet (less than 5% carbohydrate), a normal diet (about 55% of energy from carbohydrate), and a high-carbohydrate diet (82% of energy from carbohydrate).[26]

700 g of carbohydrate per day. Having a stack of pancakes with syrup and a glass of juice for breakfast provides more than 200 g of carbohydrate. A number of commercial high-carbohydrate beverages (50 to 60 g of carbohydrate in 8 fluid oz) are available to help athletes consume the amount of carbohydrate recommended to maximize glycogen stores. (These should not be confused with sports drinks designed to be consumed during competition, which contain only about 10 to 20 g of carbohydrate in 8 fluid oz.) Trained athletes who follow a carbohydrate-loading regimen can double their muscle glycogen content.[28]

Although glycogen supercompensation is beneficial to endurance athletes, it provides no benefit, and even has some disadvantages, for those exercising for less than 90 min. For every gram of glycogen in the muscle, about 3 g of water are also deposited. This water will cause weight gain and may cause some muscle stiffness. As glycogen is used, the water is released. This can be an advantage when exercising in hot weather, but the extra weight is a disadvantage for individuals competing in short-duration events.

What to eat before exercise

Meals eaten before exercise should maximize glycogen stores and provide adequate hydration while minimizing digestion, hunger, and gastric distress. A pre-exercise meal should provide enough fluid to maintain hydration and should be high in carbohydrate (60 to 70% of calories). The carbohydrate will help maintain blood glucose and maximize glycogen stores. Muscle glycogen is depleted by activity, but liver glycogen is used to supply blood glucose and is depleted even during rest if no food is ingested.

This high-carbohydrate pre-exercise meal should contain about 300 Calories and be moderate in protein (10 to 20%) and low in fat (10 to 25%) and fiber in order to minimize gastrointestinal distress and bloating during competition (**Figure 10.23**). Spicy foods, which can cause heartburn, and large amounts of simple sugars, which can cause diarrhea, should also be avoided unless the athlete is accustomed to eating these foods.

What to eat during exercise

Most people don't need to eat while they exercise. If the activity lasts longer than an hour, however, it is important to consume carbohydrate during exercise in order to maintain glucose supplies. Carbohydrate consumption is particularly important for athletes who exercise in the morning, when liver glycogen levels are low.

Carbohydrate intake should begin shortly after exercise begins, and regular amounts should be consumed every 15 to 20 minutes during exercise. The carbohydrate should provide a combination of glucose and fructose. (Fructose alone is not as effective as the combination and may cause diarrhea.) This carbohydrate can be obtained from a sports drink, but consuming a solid-food snack or a carbohydrate gel with water is also appropriate. About 30 to 60 g of carbohydrate (the amount in a banana or an energy bar) each hour is recommended (see the *Case Study*).[15]

Snacks and sports drinks also provide sodium. Although the amounts of sodium lost in sweat during exercise lasting less than three to four hours are usually not enough to affect health or performance, a snack or beverage containing sodium is recommended for exercise lasting more than an hour in order to reduce the risk of hyponatremia, improve glucose and water absorption, and stimulate thirst.

The precompetition meal Figure 10.23

When we don't eat overnight liver glycogen stores are reduced, so eating is particularly important first thing on the morning of a competition. A high-carbohydrate meal, such as cereal, milk, and juice, two to four hours before competition will replenish liver glycogen stores. The effect of different foods should be tested during training, not during competition. In addition to providing nutritional clout, a meal that includes "lucky" foods may provide an added psychological advantage.

Mark enjoys long-distance cycling. On weekends, he often goes on a 40- or 50-mile ride, which takes him three to four hours. Despite the sports drink in his bike bottle, after about two hours, he gets hungry and fatigued, so he is looking for a snack that's easy to carry. He finds that some sports bars are high in protein and low in carbohydrate, some are high in carbohydrate and low in fat, and some have a more balanced ratio of carbohydrate, protein, and fat.

What type of bar will give Mark the energy he needs to continue his ride? Why?

Carbohydrate is the fuel that is depleted during prolonged exercise. So if Mark wants to have the energy to keep pedaling, he should choose a high-carbohydrate bar. These are often called *energy bars* or *endurance bars*. They contain the carbohydrate needed to prevent hunger and maintain blood glucose during a sporting event. Mark should use the Nutrition Facts panel to select a bar that provides about 45 g of carbohydrate and no more than about 8 g of fat and 16 g of protein. Bars that are higher in fat or protein or lower in carbohydrate will not give him the blood glucose boost he needs to continue riding.

What are the advantages and disadvantages of sports bars?

Your answer:

With flavors such as chocolate coconut, tropical crisp, and sesame raisin crunch, many sports bars don't sound too different from candy bars. For about half the cost, Mark can buy a candy bar to put in his bike bag.

Based on the labels shown here, how do sports bars differ from candy bars?

Your answer:

Suggest a snack for Mark that is nutritionally comparable to a sports bar but less expensive.

Your answer:

Nutrition Facts	Amount/Serving	% DV*	Amount/Serving	% DV*
Serving Size 1 bar (65g)	Total Fat 2g	3%	Total Carb 45g	15%
	Saturated Fat 0.5g	3%	Dietary Fiber 3g	12%
Calories 230	Trans Fat 0g		Sugars 14g	
Calories from Fat 20	Cholesterol 0mg	0%	Other Carb 28g	
Calories from Sat Fat 5	Sodium 90mg	4%		
*Percent Daily Values (DV) are based on a 2,000 calorie diet.	Potassium 145mg	4%	Protein 10g	

Vitamin A 0% • Vitamin C 100% • Calcium 30% • Iron 35% • Vitamin E 100%
Thiamin 100% • Riboflavin 100% • Niacin 100% • Vitamin B₆ 100%
Folate 100% • Vitamin B₁₂ 100% • Biotin 100% • Pantothenic Acid 100%
Phosphorus 35% • Magnesium 35% • Zinc 35% • Copper 35% • Chromium 20%

Nutrition Facts
Serving Size 1 bar (2 oz.) (57g)

Amount Per Serving	
Calories 271 Calories from Fat 122	
	% Daily Value*
Total Fat 14g	**21%**
Saturated Fat 5g	**26%**
Trans Fat 0g	
Cholesterol 5mg	**2%**
Sodium 140mg	**6%**
Total Carbohydrates 35g	**12%**
Dietery Fiber 1g	**5%**
Sugars 30g	
Protein 4g	

Vitamin A 2%	•	Vitamin C 0%
Calcium 5%	•	Iron 2%

*Based on a 2,000 calorie diet

(Check your answers in Appendix K.)

What to eat after exercise When you stop exercising, your body must shift from the task of breaking down glycogen, triglycerides, and muscle proteins for fuel to the job of restoring muscle and liver glycogen, depositing lipids, and synthesizing muscle proteins. Meals eaten after exercise should replenish lost fluid, electrolytes, and glycogen and provide protein for building and repairing muscle tissue.

After exercise, the first priority for all exercisers is to replace fluid losses. For serious athletes competing on consecutive days, glycogen replacement is also a priority. To maximize glycogen replacement, a high-carbohydrate meal or drink should be consumed within 30 minutes after the competition and again every two hours for about six hours.[15] Ideally, the meals or drinks should provide about 1.0 to 1.5 g of easily absorbed carbohydrate per kilogram of body weight, which is about 50 to 100 g of carbohydrate for a 70-kg (154-lb) person—the equivalent of 2 cups of pasta or 2 cups of chocolate milk.[29] Consuming foods such as these that contain both carbohydrate and protein, enhances glycogen synthesis even more than does consuming carbohydrate alone.[30] The protein in postexercise meals also provides the amino acids needed for muscle protein synthesis and repair (see *What Should I Eat?*).

The glycogen-restoring regimen just described can replenish muscle and liver glycogen within 24 hours of an athletic event and is critical for optimizing performance on the following day. Athletes who aren't competing again the next day can replenish their glycogen stores more slowly by consuming high-carbohydrate foods for the next day or so. About 600 g of carbohydrate, or about 8 to 10 g/kilogram of body weight, is recommended for the 24 hours after exercise.[15]

Most of us are not competitive athletes, so we don't need a special glycogen replacement strategy to ensure that our glycogen stores are replenished before our next visit to the gym. If your routine includes 30 to 60 minutes at the gym, a typical diet that provides about 55% of calories from carbohydrate will replace the glycogen used so that you will be ready for a workout again the next day.

CONCEPT CHECK ⬣ STOP

Why might a low-carbohydrate diet be a poor choice for an endurance athlete?

How much of what fluid should you drink during a two-hour bike ride?

Why are female athletes at particular risk for iron deficiency?

What should an athlete eat as a precompetition meal and why?

WHAT SHOULD I EAT?   Before, During, and After Exercise

Use iProfile to plan a precompetition meal that provides at least 50 g of carbohydrate.

Before You Exercise
- Fill a water bottle four hours before exercise and finish it before you start.
- Plan to have pasta but pass on the cream sauce.
- Have a pancake breakfast.
- Fix a bowl of cereal with low-fat milk.

During your short workouts (≤60 min)
- Fill your water bottle with water.
- Take a swallow of water every 15 min.

During your long workouts (>60 min)
- Fill your water bottle with a sports drink.
- Take a sip of fluid at every sign or intersection to make sure you consume at least 6 oz of fluid every 15 min.
- Carry an apple and a bagel to snack on.
- Bring a bar that's high in carbohydrates.

When you are finished
- Restore fluid losses after exercise—16 to 24 oz for each pound of weight lost.
- Refuel with a sandwich or a plate of pasta and a glass of chocolate milk.

Ergogenic Aids

LEARNING OBJECTIVES

Assess the health risks associated with anabolic steroids.

Explain why creatine supplements affect sprint performance.

Describe one way in which a supplement might improve endurance.

Citius, altius, fortius—faster, higher, stronger—is the motto of the Olympic Games. For as long as there have been competitions, athletes have yearned for anything that would give them a competitive edge. Everything from bee pollen and high-dose vitamins to ancient herbs and hormones has been used as an **ergogenic aid**.

ergogenic aid
A substance, appliance, or procedure that improves athletic performance.

Athletes are willing to go to great lengths to improve performance and are therefore susceptible to the lures of ergogenic supplements. Many of the vitamins, minerals, and other substances in these supplements are involved in providing energy for exercise or promoting recovery from exercise. A few are beneficial for certain types of activities, but many carry more risks than benefits (**FIGURE 10.24**). When considering whether to use an ergogenic supplement, or any other type of supplement, wise consumers weigh the health risks against the potential benefits (see Figure 7.35).

VITAMIN AND MINERAL SUPPLEMENTS

Many of the promises made to athletes about the benefits of vitamin and mineral supplements are extrapolated from the biochemical functions of these micronutrients. For example, B vitamin supplements are promoted to enhance ATP production because of their roles in muscle energy metabolism. Vitamin B_6, vitamin B_{12}, and folic acid are promoted for aerobic exercise because they are involved in the transport of oxygen to exercising muscle. These vitamins are indeed needed for energy metabolism, and a deficiency of one or more of them will interfere with ATP production and impair athletic performance. But providing more than the recommended amount does not deliver more oxygen to the muscle, cause more ATP to be produced, or enhance athletic performance.

Supplements of vitamin E, vitamin C, and selenium are promoted to athletes because of their antioxidant functions. As discussed earlier, exercise increases oxidative processes and therefore increases the production of free radicals, which cause cellular damage and have been associated with fatigue. However, antioxidant supplements have not been found to improve performance.[19]

Supplements of chromium (chromium picolinate), and vanadium (vanadyl sulfate), are marketed to increase lean body mass and decrease body fat. Chromium is needed for insulin action, and insulin promotes protein synthesis. However, studies have not consistently demonstrated that supplemental chromium has any effect on muscle strength, body composition, or other aspects of health (see Chapter 8).[31] Vanadium is also believed to assist the action of insulin, but there is no evidence that supplemental vanadium increases lean body mass.[32]

The impact of diet and supplements on performance FIGURE 10.24

This pyramid illustrates the relative impact of various nutrition strategies on exercise performance. Along with talent and hard work, the most significant benefit is achieved by eating a healthy overall diet. Foods and beverages used to supply energy and ensure hydration during an event can provide additional benefits, whereas most ergogenic supplements provide little or no performance boost.

A few specific supplements are beneficial in some cases

Sports foods and beverages used to refuel and rehydrate

An overall healthy diet

SUPPLEMENTS TO BUILD MUSCLE

Protein supplements are often marketed to athletes with the promise of enhancing muscle growth or improving performance. Adequate protein is necessary for muscle growth, but consuming extra protein, either as food or as supplements, does not increase muscle growth or strength.[32] Muscles enlarge in response to exercise stress. The protein provided by expensive supplements will not meet an athlete's needs any better than the protein found in a balanced diet. If an athlete's diet provides enough energy, it usually provides enough protein without a supplement.

Growth hormone is appealing to athletes because it increases muscle protein synthesis. Despite this physiological effect, however, it has not been shown to have ergogenic benefits.[33] Prolonged use of growth hormone can cause heart dysfunction, high blood pressure, and excessive growth of some body parts, such as hands, feet, and facial features. Growth hormone is on the World Anti-Doping Agency's list of banned substances.

Supplements of the amino acids ornithine, arginine, and lysine are marketed with the promise that they will stimulate the release of growth hormone and, in turn, enhance the growth of muscles. Large doses of these amino acids have been shown to stimulate the release of growth hormone. However, growth hormone levels in the blood of athletes taking these amino acids are no greater than levels typically resulting from exercise alone. Also, supplements of these amino acid have not been found to cause greater increases in muscle mass and strength than those achieved through strength-training exercise alone.[34,35]

What a Scientist Sees

Anabolic Steroids

Athletes looking at this photograph see the bulging muscles and enhanced performance that can be achieved with anabolic steroid use. A scientist sees that these are not the only effects that anabolic steroids have. These drugs make the body think natural testosterone is being produced, and therefore, as shown in the diagram, the body shuts down its own testosterone production. Natural testosterone stimulates and maintains the male sexual organs and promotes the development of bones and muscles and the growth of skin and hair. The synthetic testosterone in anabolic steroids has a greater effect on muscle, bone, skin, and hair than it does on sexual organs. Without natural testosterone, the sexual organs are not maintained; this leads to shrinkage of the testicles and a decrease in sperm production.[39]

In adolescents, the use of anabolic steroids causes cessation of bone growth and stunted height. Anabolic steroid use may also cause oily skin and acne, water retention in the tissues, yellowing of the eyes and skin, coronary artery disease, liver disease, and sometimes death. Users may experience psychological and behavioral side effects such as violent outbursts and depression, possibly leading to suicide.[39] Why do you think anabolic steroid use promotes muscle development but causes the testes to shrink?

◀ Despite the risks, between 1 million and 3 million athletes in the United States have used anabolic steroids.[38] Anabolic steroids are controlled substances and are banned by the International Olympic Committee, the National Collegiate Athletic Association (NCAA), and most other sporting organizations.[36]

When testosterone levels are low, the hypothalamus releases a ▶ hormone that stimulates the anterior pituitary to release a hormone that increases the production of testosterone by the testes. High levels of either natural or synthetic testosterone inhibit the release of the stimulatory hormone from the hypothalamus, shutting down the synthesis of natural testosterone.

anabolic steroids Synthetic fat-soluble hormones that mimic testosterone and are used to increase muscle strength and mass.

Anabolic steroids accelerate protein synthesis. When taken in conjunction with exercise and an adequate diet, they cause increases in muscle size and strength. However, they have extremely dangerous side effects (see *What a Scientist Sees*). Anabolic steroids are regulated as controlled substances. **Steroid precursors**, which are compounds that can be converted into steroid hormones in the body, are also classified as controlled substances.[36] The best known of these is androstenedione, often referred to as "andro." It was launched to public prominence when professional baseball player Mark McGwire announced his use of it during the 1998 major league baseball season, when he hit 70 home runs, breaking the league's single-season home-run record. Contrary to marketing claims, the use of andro or other steroid precursors has not been found to increase testosterone levels or produce any ergogenic effects, and they may cause some of the same side effects as anabolic steroids.[37]

SUPPLEMENTS TO ENHANCE PERFORMANCE IN SHORT, INTENSE ACTIVITIES

A number of supplements are marketed to athletes who seek to improve performance in activities that depend on quick bursts of intense activity. Supplements of β-hydroxy-β-methylbutyrate, known as HMB, are hypothesized to increase strength and lean body mass by decreasing muscle breakdown and speeding muscle repair. Early studies found that oral HMB supplements decreased muscle damage and increased muscle strength in response to resistance training.[40] However, more recent studies have not found these supplements to have an ergogenic effect on muscular strength, size, or endurance.[41]

Bicarbonate may provide some advantage for intense activities. Because bicarbonate acts as a buffer in the body, supplementing it is thought to neutralize acid and thus delay fatigue and allow improved performance. Taking sodium bicarbonate, which is just baking soda from the kitchen cupboard, before exercise has been found to improve performance and delay exhaustion in sports, such as sprint cycling, that entail intense exercise lasting only one to seven minutes, but it is of no benefit for lower-intensity aerobic exercise.[42] Just because baking soda is an ingredient in your cookies does not mean that it is risk free. Many people experience abdominal cramps and diarrhea after taking sodium bicarbonate, and other possible side effects have not been carefully researched.

One of the most popular ergogenic supplements is **creatine**. This nitrogen-containing compound is found primarily in muscle, where it is used to make creatine phosphate (**FIGURE 10.25**). Higher levels of creatine and creatine phosphate provide more quick energy for short-term maximal exercise. Creatine supplementation has been shown to improve performance in high-intensity exercise lasting 30 seconds or less.[43,44] It is therefore beneficial for exercise that requires explosive bursts of energy, such as sprinting and weight lifting, but not for long-term endurance activities, such as marathons.

Athletes also take creatine supplements to increase muscle mass and strength. Some of the increase in lean body mass is believed to be due to water retention related to creatine uptake in the muscle. In addition, an increase in muscle mass and strength may occur in response to the greater amount and intensity of training that may be achieved: Increased muscle creatine permits greater training intensity, which leads to greater muscle hypertrophy.[43,46]

Creatine boosts creatine phosphate
FIGURE 10.25

Creatine can be synthesized in the liver and kidneys and is also provided by meat and milk consumed in the diet. The more creatine consumed, the greater the amount of creatine stored in the muscles. Increasing creatine intake through supplement use has been shown to increase levels of muscle creatine and creatine phosphate, which is made from it.[45] During short bursts of intense activity, the creatine phosphate can be converted back into creatine, transforming ADP to ATP for muscle contraction.

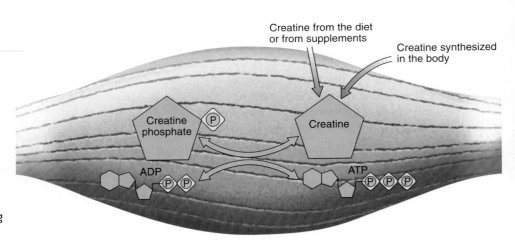

Long-term creatine supplementation appears to be safe at intakes of up to 5 g per day, but the safety of higher doses over the long term has not been established.[47] Ingestion of creatine before or during exercise is not recommended, and the FDA has advised consumers to consult a physician before using creatine.

SUPPLEMENTS TO ENHANCE ENDURANCE

Sprinters and weight lifters can benefit from increases in creatine phosphate levels, but endurance athletes are more concerned about running out of glycogen. Glycogen is spared when fat is used as an energy source, allowing exercise to continue for a longer time before glycogen is depleted and fatigue sets in. Supplements that increase the amount of fat or oxygen available to the muscle cell are used to increase endurance.

Carnitine supplements are marketed as fat burners—substances that increase the utilization of fat during exercise. Carnitine is needed to transport fatty acids into the mitochondria, where they are used to produce ATP by aerobic metabolism. However, enough carnitine is made in the body to ensure efficient use of fatty acids. Carnitine supplements have not been shown to increase endurance.[48]

Medium-chain triglycerides (MCT) are composed of fatty acids with medium-length carbon chains (8 to 10 carbons). These fatty acids can be absorbed directly into the blood without first being incorporated into chylomicrons. They are therefore absorbed quickly, causing blood fatty acids levels to rise and thereby increasing the availability of fat as a fuel for exercise. Nevertheless, research has not found that supplementation with MCT increases endurance, spares glycogen, or enhances performance.[49,50]

Caffeine, the stimulant found in coffee, tea, and some soft drinks, is the only fat burner that has been shown to enhance performance and endurance.[51] Drinking 2.5 cups of percolated coffee up to an hour before exercising has been shown to improve endurance. Caffeine enhances the release of fatty acids. When fatty acids are used as a fuel source, less glycogen is used, and the onset of fatigue is delayed. Athletes who are unaccustomed to caffeine respond better than those who consume it routinely. Caffeine also improves concentration and enhances alertness, but in some athletes, it may impair performance by causing GI upset.

Caffeine may be effective but consuming excess caffeine before a competition is illegal. The International Olympic Committee prohibits athletes from competing when caffeine levels in the urine are 12 µg/milliliter or greater. For urine caffeine to reach this level, an individual would need to drink six to eight cups of coffee in a two-hour period. Caffeine is also found in pill form; NoDoz contains about 100 mg of caffeine/tablet—about the same amount as in a cup of coffee.

Athletes have also used the hormone erythropoietin, known as EPO, to enhance endurance. Natural erythropoietin is produced by the kidneys and stimulates cells in the bone marrow to differentiate into red blood cells. EPO can enhance endurance by increasing the ability to transport oxygen to the muscles. It therefore increases aerobic capacity and spares glycogen. However, too much EPO can cause production of too many red blood cells, which can lead to excessive blood clotting, heart attacks, and strokes.[39] EPO was banned in 1990, after it was linked to the deaths of more than a dozen cyclists.[52]

OTHER SUPPLEMENTS

In addition to the supplements discussed thus far, hundreds of other products are marketed to athletes. Most have no effect on performance. For example, brewer's yeast is a source of B vitamins and some minerals but has not been found to have any ergogenic properties. Likewise, there is no evidence to support claims that bee pollen or wheat germ oil enhance performance. Royal jelly is a substance that worker bees produce to help the queen bee grow larger and live longer, but it does not appear to enhance athletic capacity in humans. Supplements of DNA and RNA are marketed to aid in tissue regeneration. DNA and RNA are needed to synthesize proteins, but they are not required in the diet, and supplements do not help replace damaged cells.

Herbal products are also marketed to athletes. Most have not been studied extensively for their ergogenic effects, so the only evidence of their benefits is anecdotal. Many can harm health as well as performance, so athletes should consider the risks before using these products.

CONCEPT CHECK **STOP**

How do anabolic hormones affect the production of testosterone?

Why are creatine supplements not helpful for endurance athletes?

How does EPO affect performance?

SUMMARY

1 Physical Activity, Fitness, and Health

1. Regular exercise improves **fitness**. How fit an individual is depends on his or her **cardiorespiratory endurance**, **muscle strength**, **muscle endurance**, flexibility, and body composition.

2. Regular exercise can reduce the risk of chronic diseases such as obesity, heart disease, diabetes, and osteoporosis. It can reduce overall mortality even in obese individuals.

3. Exercise helps manage body weight by increasing energy expenditure and by increasing the proportion of body weight that is lean tissue.

2 Exercise Recommendations

1. To reduce the risk of chronic disease, a minimum of 30 minutes of moderate-intensity exercise on most days is recommended. A well-designed fitness program involves aerobic exercise, stretching, and strength-training exercises.

2. An exercise program should include activities that are enjoyable, convenient, and safe. Rest is important to allow the body to recover and rebuild. In serious athletes, inadequate rest can lead to **overtraining syndrome**.

3 Fueling Exercise

1. During the first 10 to 15 seconds of exercise, ATP and **creatine phosphate** stored in the muscle provide energy to fuel activity. During the next 2 to 3 minutes, the amount of oxygen at the muscle remains limited, so ATP is generated by the **anaerobic metabolism** of glucose. After a few minutes, the delivery of oxygen at the muscle increases, and ATP can be generated by **aerobic metabolism**. Aerobic metabolism is more efficient than anaerobic metabolism and can utilize glucose, fatty acids, and amino acids as energy sources. The use of protein as an energy source increases when exercise continues for many hours.

2. For short-term, high-intensity activity, ATP is generated primarily from the anaerobic metabolism of glucose from glycogen stores. Anaerobic metabolism uses glucose more rapidly and produces **lactic acid**. Both of these factors are associated with the onset of **fatigue**. For lower-intensity exercise of longer duration, aerobic metabolism predominates, and both glucose and fatty acids are important fuel sources.

3. Fitness training causes changes in the cardiovascular system and muscles that improve oxygen delivery and utilization, allowing aerobic exercise to be sustained for longer periods at higher intensity.

4 Energy and Nutrient Needs for Physical Activity

1. The diet of an active individual should provide sufficient energy to fuel activity. The pressure to compete and maintain a body weight that is optimal for their sport puts some athletes at risk for eating disorders. A combination of excessive exercise and energy restriction puts female athletes at risk for the **female athlete triad**.

2. To maximize glycogen stores, optimize performance, and maintain and repair lean tissue, a diet providing about 60% of energy from carbohydrate, 20 to 25% of energy from fat, and about 15 to 20% of energy from protein is recommended.

(continued)

3. Sufficient vitamins and minerals are needed to generate ATP from macronutrients, to maintain and repair tissues, and to transport oxygen and wastes to and from the cells. Most athletes who consume a varied diet that meets their energy needs also meet their vitamin and mineral needs. Those who restrict their food intake may be at risk for deficiencies. Increased iron needs and greater iron losses due to fitness training put athletes, particularly female athletes, at risk for iron deficiency.

4. Water is needed to ensure that the body can be cooled and that nutrients and oxygen can be delivered to body tissues. If water intake is inadequate, dehydration can lead to a decline in exercise performance and increase the risk of **heat-related illness**. Adequate fluid intake before exercise ensures that athletes begin exercise well hydrated. Fluid intake during and after exercise must replace water lost in sweat and from evaporation through the lungs. Plain water is an appropriate fluid to consume for most exercise. Beverages containing carbohydrate and sodium are recommended for exercise lasting more than an hour. Drinking plain water during extended exercise increases the risk of hyponatremia.

5. Competitive endurance athletes may benefit from **glycogen supercompensation (carbohydrate loading)**, which maximizes glycogen stores before an event. Meals eaten before competition should help ensure adequate hydration, provide moderate amounts of protein, be high enough in carbohydrate to maximize glycogen stores, be low in fat and fiber to speed gastric emptying, and satisfy the psychological needs of the athlete. During exercise, athletes need beverages and food to replace lost fluid and provide carbohydrate and sodium. Postcompetition meals should replace lost fluids and electrolytes, provide carbohydrate to restore muscle and liver glycogen, and provide protein for muscle protein synthesis and repair.

5 Ergogenic Aids

1. Many types of **ergogenic aids** are marketed to improve athletic performance. Some are beneficial for certain types of activity, but many offer little or no benefit. An individual risk–benefit analysis should be used to determine whether a supplement is appropriate for you.

2. **Anabolic steroids** combined with resistance-training exercise increase muscle size and strength, but these supplements are illegal and have dangerous side effects.

3. **Creatine** supplementation has been shown to improve performance in short-duration, high-intensity exercise. Caffeine use can improve performance in endurance activities, but high doses are illegal during athletic competitions.

KEY TERMS

1. On the way to an out-of-town soccer match, Max's team stops at a fast-food restaurant. It is only about an hour before game time. Most of the boys have burgers, fries, and a soft drink. How might this affect their performance in the game? What would you recommend they do differently for the next match?

2. Evaluate your weekly physical activity. Does it meet the current exercise recommendations? Would you classify yourself as sedentary, low active, active, or very active? Do you include activities to enhance your strength, endurance, and flexibility? Can each of these activities be performed year-round? If not, suggest alternative activities and locations for inclement weather. How could you improve on what you are currently doing?

3. Given that aerobic metabolism depends on the availability of oxygen, suggest an experiment that could determine an athlete's aerobic capacity.

4. Using your knowledge of energy production and body energy stores, explain why during exercise cells rely more on glucose and fat for energy than on protein.

5. Two friends are running a marathon together. One has participated in an intensive training program. The other was too busy and trained only a few hours a week. After about 5 minutes of running the marathon, they have settled into a slow, steady pace and are able to carry on a conversation. After an hour, the well-trained individual is feeling good and so increases her pace. The untrained person tries to keep up but is no longer able to talk, and after about 15 minutes is fatigued and needs to stop. Why does the untrained person tire faster?

6. David is beginning an exercise program. He plans to run before lunch and then play racquetball every night after dinner. When he begins his exercise program, he finds that he feels lethargic and hungry before his late-morning run. After running, he doesn't have much of an appetite, so he saves his lunch until midafternoon. He is still hungry enough to eat dinner at home with his family but finds that he is getting stomach cramps and is too full when he goes to play racquetball. His typical diet is

   > Breakfast: Orange juice, coffee
   > Lunch: Ham and cheese sandwich, potato chips, soft drink, cookies
   > Dinner: Steak, baked potato with sour cream and butter, green beans in butter sauce, salad with Italian dressing, whole milk

   How might David change his diet to make it better suited to his exercise program? Do you think David will be able to stick with this exercise program? Why or why not? Suggest some changes that would make David's exercise program more convenient and more balanced.

7. Do a risk–benefit analysis of an ergogenic aid. (A quick way to do this is to use the Internet to collect information.) List the risks and benefits and then write a conclusion, stating why you would or would not take this substance.

What is happening in this picture ?

During competitive events, cyclists often spend six or more hours a day riding their bikes. This rider is collecting water bottles from his team's car. He will carry these ahead and deliver them to the other cyclists on his team.

▪ How much might someone need to drink during six hours of cycling?

▪ What type of fluid do you think is in the water bottles? Why?

▪ What type of food might the riders want to pick up from their team car?

(Check your answerns in Appendix L.)

1. Which bar indicates the proportion of energy obtained from glucose, fatty acids, and amino acids that would be used as fuel while studying for an exam?

a. A
b. B
c. C

2. Which of the following statements about aerobic exercise is false?

a. It increases heart rate.
b. It requires oxygen in metabolism.
c. It can use fat as a fuel.
d. It is performed at an intensity low enough to carry on a conversation.
e. It includes activities such as weight lifting and sprinting.

3. If an athlete loses a lot of water and salt in sweat but drinks only water, he is at risk for _____.

a. hypertension
b. hypodermic
c. hyperactivity
d. hyponatremia
e. dehydration

4. Andreas is 30 years old. He would like to exercise at an intensity that ensures he is in his aerobic zone. Use this graph to determine the heart rate range that is appropriate for Andreas.

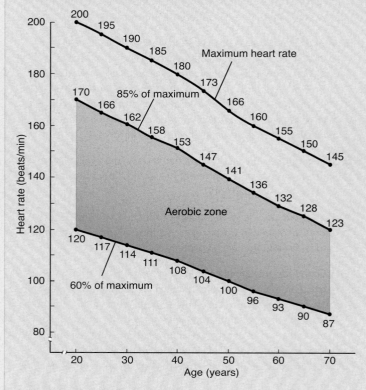

a. 114 to 162
b. 114 to 190
c. 120 to 170
d. 87 to 120
e. 123 to 170

5. The source of fuel in the first few seconds of exercise is

_____.

a. ATP and creatine phosphate
b. stored glycogen
c. glucose made by the liver
d. fatty acids
e. protein

6. Which statement is true of the energy system indicated by the arrow?

a. It provides energy for the first 10 to 15 seconds of activity.
b. It can use glucose, amino acids, and fatty acids to produce ATP.
c. It produces ATP rapidly but inefficiently.
d. It can only use glucose to generate ATP.

7. Which nutrient can be used to produce energy in the absence of oxygen?

a. protein
b. fatty acids
c. glucose
d. B vitamins
e. lactic acid

8. The female athlete triad consists of _____.

a. iron deficiency anemia, disordered eating, and excess menstrual blood loss
b. disordered eating, amenorrhea, and osteoporosis
c. dieting, excessive exercise, and folate deficiency
d. iron, calcium, and zinc deficiency

9. Which of the following statements about carbohydrate loading is false?

a. It provides a competitive advantage for sprinters and weight lifters.
b. It causes short-term weight gain.
c. It involves manipulating diet and activity patterns before an event.
d. It can enhance endurance.

10. Which of the following is a goal of precompetition meals?

a. maximize fat stores
b. increase muscle mass
c. keep the stomach full
d. maximize glycogen stores

11. True or false: A fit person will have a higher percentage of lean tissue than an unfit person of the same body weight.

a. True
b. False

12. The best fluid to consume during a marathon is _____.

a. plain water
b. fruit juice
c. a sports drink containing glucose and sodium
d. a protein shake

13. Amy lives in Connecticut, where the summer temperature and humidity can vary dramatically from day to day. On Monday, it is 88°F, with a relative humidity of 90%. On Tuesday, the temperature goes up to 96°F, but the humidity drops to 60%. By Wednesday, the temperature has dropped slightly to 92°F, but the humidity has increased to 65%. On Thursday, the temperature drops to 90°F, and the humidity climbs to 85%. Use the table shown here to determine which day has the lowest heat index.

Relative humidity (%)

°F	40	45	50	55	60	65	70	75	80	85	90	95	100
110	136												
108	130	137											
106	124	130	137										
104	119	124	131	137									
102	114	119	124	130	137								
100	109	114	118	124	129	136							
98	105	109	113	117	123	128	134						
96	101	104	108	112	116	121	126	132					
94	97	100	102	106	110	114	119	124	129	135			
92	94	96	99	101	105	108	112	116	121	126	131		
90	91	93	95	97	100	103	106	109	113	117	122	127	132
88	88	89	91	93	95	98	100	103	106	110	113	117	121
86	85	87	88	89	91	93	95	97	100	102	105	108	112
84	83	84	85	86	88	89	90	92	94	96	98	100	103
82	81	82	83	84	84	85	86	88	89	90	91	93	95
80	80	80	81	81	82	82	83	84	84	85	86	86	87

Air temperature

Heat index (apparent temperature)

With prolonged exposure and/or physical activity

Extreme danger
Heat stroke highly likely

Danger
Heat stroke, heat cramps, and/or heat exhaustion likely

Extreme caution
Heat stroke, heat cramps, and/or heat exhaustion possible

Caution
Fatigue possible

a. Monday
b. Tuesday
c. Wednesday
d. Thursday

14. Which best describes how creatine supplements might enhance performance?

a. They increase the amount of creatine phosphate in the muscle.
b. They increase the transport of fatty acids into the mitochondria.
c. They increase delivery of oxygen to the muscle.
d. They eliminate free radicals.

15. How much and how often should athletes drink during exercise?

a. as much as they can
b. enough to prevent weight loss
c. a cup every hour
d. nothing unless exercise lasts more than 60 minutes

Nutrition During Pregnancy and Infancy

A pregnant woman is responsible for providing adequate nutrition for herself and her developing child—hence the saying "You're eating for two now!" Optimal nutrition for the mother can help ensure the birth of a healthy baby. Inadequate nutrition during pregnancy produces an undernourished infant who may never catch up with healthy counterparts. Overnutrition during pregnancy may result in a larger baby, posing risks to both mother and child during birth.

Low maternal weight gain, lack of prenatal visits, obesity, and the presence of major chronic illnesses in the mother are factors that can compromise fetal nutrition. A fetus may also be subject to dangerous effects from deficiencies or excesses of vitamins and minerals. For example, lack of sufficient iodine during pregnancy has been linked to brain damage in the baby, insufficient iron creates an increased risk of anemia for an infant, and too much vitamin A causes an increased risk of birth defects of the head, face, heart, and brain.

The responsibility of the mother does not stop when the infant is born. The 40 weeks of a pregnancy produce a helpless newborn who requires a lengthy period of care. Breast milk provides optimal nutrition for a growing infant, and a breast-feeding mother's diet continues to affect the nutrition of her child. In addition, the quality of infant nutrition can affect both growth in the early years and the potential for developing chronic diseases later in life. Healthier pregnancies yield babies who become healthier children and ultimately healthier adults.

Changes in the Body During Pregnancy

LEARNING OBJECTIVES

Describe how the embryo and fetus are nourished.

Discuss why appropriate weight gain is important during pregnancy.

Explain why morning sickness, heartburn, and constipation are common during pregnancy.

Assess the risks associated with pregnancy-induced hypertension and gestational diabetes.

hether you end up 6 feet 4 inches or 5 feet 3 inches, you begin as a single cell that arises from the union of a sperm and an egg. Over the course of 40 weeks, this cell grows and develops into a fully formed human baby. Prenatal growth and development are carefully orchestrated processes that require adequate supplies of all the essential nutrients in order to progress normally.

In the days after **fertilization**, the single cell divides rapidly to form a ball of cells (**FIGURE 11.1**). The cells then begin to differentiate and move to form body structures. During these early steps in development, this ball of cells, obtains the nutrients it needs from the fluids around it. About a week

fertilization
The union of a sperm and an egg.

Process Diagram

Prenatal development FIGURE 11.1

This cross-section shows the path of the egg and developing embryo from the ovary, where the egg is produced, through the oviduct to the uterus, where most prenatal development occurs.

HOW IT WORKS
View in your WileyPLUS course

2 Fertilization occurs in the oviduct 12 to 24 hours after ovulation.

3 About 30 hours after fertilization, the fertilized egg has completed its first cell division.

4 About 3 or 4 days after fertilization, the developing embryo is a ball of about 100 cells.

1 Ovulation releases an egg from the woman's ovary.

Ovulation

Ovary

Uterine cavity

5 About 6 days after fertilization, the developing embryo begins to implant itself in the uterine lining. Implantation is complete by 14 days after fertilization.

Uterus

Frontal section through uterus, uterine tube, and ovary

6 During the embryonic stage of development, from 2 to 8 weeks after fertilization, cells differentiate and arrange themselves in the proper locations to form the major organ systems. The embryo shown here is about 5 to 6 weeks old and less than 3 cm long. The organ systems and external body structures are not fully developed. ▼

7 The fetal stage of development begins at 9 weeks after fertilization and continues until birth. During this time, the fetus grows, and internal and external body structures continue to develop. This fetus is about 16 weeks old and about 16 cm long. ▼

The placenta FIGURE 11.2

The placenta is made up of branchlike projections that extend from the embryo into the uterine lining, placing maternal and fetal blood in close proximity. The placenta allows nutrients and oxygen to pass from maternal blood to fetal blood and waste products to be transferred from fetal blood to maternal blood. Fetal blood travels to and from the placenta via the umbilical cord.

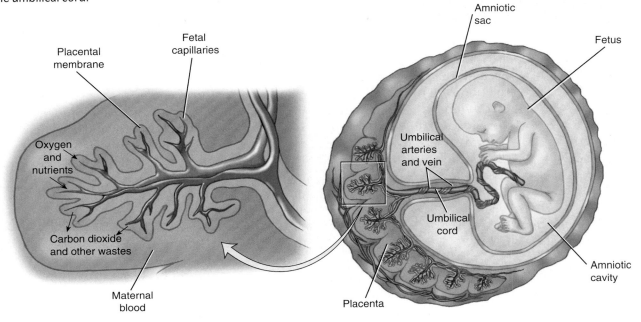

implantation
The process through which a developing embryo embeds itself in the uterine lining.

embryo
The developing human from two through eight weeks after fertilization.

after fertilization, the developing embryo begins burrowing into the lining of the uterus, and by two weeks, **implantation** is complete and it is now an **embryo**.

NOURISHING THE EMBRYO AND FETUS

The embryonic stage of development lasts until the eighth week after fertilization. During this time, the cells differentiate to form the multitude of specialized cell types that make up the human body. At the end of this stage, the embryo is about 3 centimeters long and has a beating heart. The rudiments of all major external and internal body structures have been formed.

The early embryo gets its nourishment by breaking down the lining of the uterus, but soon this source is inadequate to meet its growing needs. After about 5 weeks, the

placenta takes over the role of nourishing the embryo (FIG-URE 11.2). The placenta also secretes hormones that are necessary to maintain pregnancy.

From the ninth week on, the developing offspring is a **fetus**. During the fetal period, structures formed during the embryonic period grow and mature. The placenta continues to nourish the fetus until birth. During this time, the length of the fetus increases from about 3 cm to around 50 cm. The fetal period usually ends after 40 weeks with the birth of an infant weighing 3 to 4 kilograms (6.5 to 9 pounds).[1]

Infants who are born on time but have failed to grow well in the uterus are said to be **small for gestational age**. Those born before 37 weeks of gestation

placenta
An organ produced from maternal and embryonic tissues. It secretes hormones, transfers nutrients and oxygen from the mother's blood to the fetus, and removes metabolic wastes.

fetus A developing human from the ninth week after fertilization to birth.

Low-birth-weight infants FIGURE 11.3

Low-birth-weight and very-low-birth-weight infants require special care and a special diet in order to continue to grow and develop. Today, with advances in medical and nutritional care, infants born as early as 25 weeks of gestation and those weighing as little as 1 kg (2.2 lbs) can survive.

low birth weight A birth weight less than 2.5 kg (5.5 lbs).

very low birth weight A birth weight less than 1.5 kg (3.3 lbs).

are said to be **preterm**, or **premature**. Whether born too soon or too small, **low-birth-weight** infants and **very-low-birth-weight** infants are at increased risk for illness and early death (**FIGURE 11.3**).[2]

MATERNAL WEIGHT GAIN DURING PREGNANCY

During pregnancy, a woman's body undergoes many changes to support the growth and development of her child. Her blood volume increases by 50%. The placenta develops in order to allow nutrients to be delivered to the fetus and produce hormones that orchestrate other changes in the mother's body. The amount of body fat increases to provide the energy needed late in pregnancy. The uterus enlarges, muscles and ligaments relax to accommodate the growing fetus and allow for childbirth, and the breasts develop in preparation for **lactation**. All these changes naturally result in weight gain (**FIGURE 11.4A**).

lactation Production and secretion of milk.

A healthy, normal-weight woman should gain 11 to 16 kg (25 to 35 lbs) during pregnancy.[1] The rate of weight gain is as important as the amount gained. Little gain is expected in the first 3 months, or **trimester**—usually about 1 to 2 kg (2 to 4 lbs). In the second and third trimesters, the recommended maternal weight gain is about 0.5 kg (1 lb)/week. Women who are underweight and women who are overweight or obese at conception should also gain weight at a slow, steady rate, but the total amount of weight gain recommended is higher and lower than for normal-weight women, respectively (**FIGURE 11.4B**).[1,3]

Being underweight by 10% or more at the onset of pregnancy or gaining too little weight during pregnancy increases the risk of producing a low-birth-weight baby.[4] Excess weight, whether present before conception or gained during pregnancy, can also compromise pregnancy outcome. The mother's risks for high blood pressure, diabetes, a difficult delivery, and need for a **cesarean section** are increased by excess weight, as is the risk of having a **large-for-gestational-age** baby.[5] Excessive prenatal weight gain also increases the mother's long-term risk for obesity, and there is evidence that it may increase the risk that the baby will be overweight in childhood.[6,7] However, dieting during pregnancy is not advised, even for obese women. If possible, excess weight should be lost before the pregnancy begins or, alternatively, after the child has been born and weaned.

large for gestational age Weighing more than 4 kg (8.8 lbs) at birth.

PHYSICAL ACTIVITY DURING PREGNANCY

During pregnancy, women weigh more and carry that weight in the front of the body, where it can interfere with balance and put stress on bones, joints, and muscles, increasing the risk of exercise-related injury. However, this doesn't mean that a pregnant woman must give up her regular exercise routines. Physical activity during pregnancy can improve digestion; prevent excess weight gain, low back pain, and constipation; reduce the risk of diabetes and high blood pressure; and speed recovery from childbirth. Guidelines have been developed to maximize the benefits of exercise during pregnancy and minimize the risks of injury to mother and fetus. In general, women who were physically active before becoming pregnant can continue a program of about 30 minutes of carefully chosen moderate exercise per day.[4,8] Women who weren't active before pregnancy should slowly add low-intensity, low-impact activities.[8] Because intense exercise can limit the delivery of oxygen and nutrients to the fetus, intense exercise should be limited (**TABLE 11.1**).

Rate and composition of weight gain during pregnancy FIGURE 11.4

Total	25-35 lbs
Fetus	7-8 lbs
Amniotic fluid	2 lbs
Placenta	1-2 lbs
Uterus	2 lbs
Maternal blood	3-4 lbs
Breast tissue	2 lbs
Extracellular fluids	4 lbs
Maternal fat	4-11 lbs

◀ A The weight of an infant at birth accounts for about 25% of total weight gain during pregnancy. The placenta, amniotic fluid, and changes in maternal tissues, including enlargement of the uterus and breasts, expansion of the volume of blood and other extracellular fluids, and increased fat stores, account for the rest.

B A similar pattern of weight gain is recommended ▶ for women who are normal weight, underweight, overweight, or obese at the start of pregnancy, but the recommendations for total weight gain are different.[1]

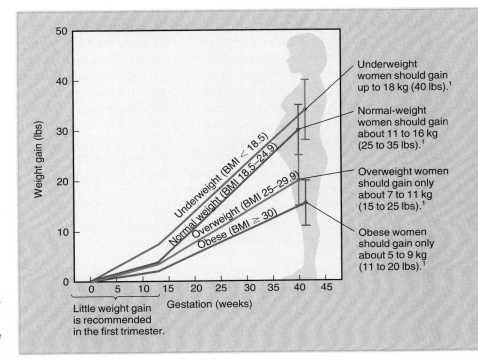

Underweight women should gain up to 18 kg (40 lbs).[1]

Normal-weight women should gain about 11 to 16 kg (25 to 35 lbs).[1]

Overweight women should gain only about 7 to 11 kg (15 to 25 lbs).[1]

Obese women should gain only about 5 to 9 kg (11 to 20 lbs).[1]

Little weight gain is recommended in the first trimester.

Weight gain (lbs) vs Gestation (weeks) — Underweight (BMI < 18.5), Normal weight (BMI 18.5–24.9), Overweight (BMI 25–29.9), Obese (BMI ≥ 30)

Guidelines for physical activity during pregnancy TABLE 11.1

Do . . .

Obtain permission from a health care provider before beginning an exercise program.

Increase activity gradually if you were inactive before pregnancy.

Exercise regularly rather than intermittently.

Stop exercising when fatigued.

Choose non-weight-bearing activities, such as swimming, that entail minimal risk of falls or abdominal injury.

Drink plenty of fluids before, during, and after exercise.

Don't . . .

Exercise strenuously during the first trimester; during the second and third trimesters, do not exercise strenuously for more than 15 minutes at a time.

Exercise to the point of exhaustion.

Scuba dive or engage in activities that entail risk of abdominal trauma, falls, or joint stress.

Exercise lying on your back after the first trimester.

Exercise in hot or humid environments.

DISCOMFORTS OF PREGNANCY

The physiological changes that occur during pregnancy can cause uncomfortable side effects. For example, the expansion in blood volume necessary to nourish the fetus often causes an accumulation of extracellular fluid in the tissues, a condition known as **edema**. Edema can be uncomfortable but does not increase medical risks unless it is accompanied by a rise in blood pressure.

Many women experience nausea and vomiting during the first trimester of pregnancy. This is referred to as **morning sickness**, but symptoms can occur at any time during the day or night. Morning sickness is thought to be related to hormones that are released early in pregnancy. The symptoms may be alleviated by eating small, frequent snacks of dry, starchy foods such as plain crackers or bread. In most women, the symptoms of morning sickness decrease significantly after the first trimester, but in some they last for the entire pregnancy and, in severe cases, may require intravenous nutrition.

The hormones produced during pregnancy to relax uterine muscles also relax the muscles of the gastrointestinal tract. This relaxation, along with crowding of the organs by the growing baby, can cause heartburn and constipation (**FIGURE 11.5**). Heartburn can be reduced by limiting high-fat foods, which leave the stomach slowly; avoiding substances, such as caffeine and chocolate, that are known to cause heartburn; eating small, frequent meals; and remaining upright after eating. Constipation can be prevented by maintaining a moderate level of physical activity and consuming plenty of fluids and high-fiber foods. Hemorrhoids are common during pregnancy as a result of both constipation and changes in blood flow.

Crowding of the gastrointestinal tract FIGURE 11.5

During pregnancy, the uterus enlarges and pushes higher into the abdominal cavity, exerting pressure on the stomach and intestines.

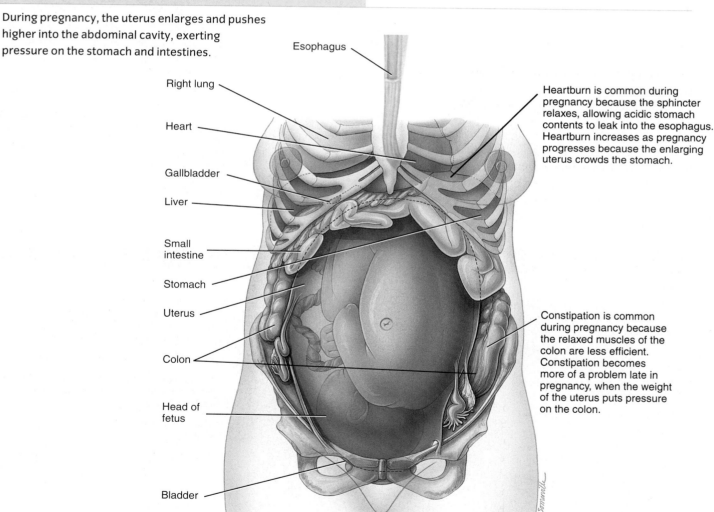

Esophagus

Right lung

Heart

Gallbladder

Liver

Small intestine

Stomach

Uterus

Colon

Head of fetus

Bladder

Heartburn is common during pregnancy because the sphincter relaxes, allowing acidic stomach contents to leak into the esophagus. Heartburn increases as pregnancy progresses because the enlarging uterus crowds the stomach.

Constipation is common during pregnancy because the relaxed muscles of the colon are less efficient. Constipation becomes more of a problem late in pregnancy, when the weight of the uterus puts pressure on the colon.

COMPLICATIONS OF PREGNANCY

Most of the 4.3 million women who give birth every year in the United States have healthy pregnancies. However, almost 13% of babies are born too soon, 9.7% have low or very low birth weights, and 6.8 out of 1000 of those born alive die in their first year of life.[9] In the United States, 13 out of every 100,000 women die as a result of childbirth.[10] If complications that occur during pregnancy are caught early, they can usually be managed, resulting in the delivery of a healthy baby.

High blood pressure

About 5 to 10% of pregnant women experience high blood pressure during pregnancy. **Hypertensive disorders of pregnancy**, also known as **pregnancy-induced hypertension**, refers to a spectrum of conditions involving elevated blood pressure during pregnancy. It accounts for nearly 16% of pregnancy-related maternal deaths in the United States.[11] It is especially common in mothers under 18 and over 35 years of age, low-income mothers, and mothers with chronic hypertension or kidney disease.

About one-third of the hypertensive disorders of pregnancy are due to chronic hypertension that was present before the pregnancy, but the remainder are related to the pregnancy. The least problematic of these is **gestational hypertension**, an abnormal rise in blood pressure that occurs after the 20th week of pregnancy. Gestational hypertension may signal the potential for a more serious condition called **preeclampsia**. Preeclampsia is characterized by high blood pressure along with fluid retention and excretion of protein in the urine; it can result in a weight gain of several pounds within a few days. It is dangerous to the baby because it reduces blood flow to the placenta, and it is dangerous to the mother because it can progress to a more severe form of pregnancy-induced hypertension called **eclampsia**, in which life-threatening seizures occur. Women with preeclampsia require bed rest and careful medical monitoring. The condition usually resolves after delivery.

> **preeclampsia**
> A condition characterized by elevated blood pressure, a rapid increase in body weight, protein in the urine, and edema. Also called *toxemia*.

> **eclampsia**
> Convulsions or seizures brought on by seriously high blood pressure during pregnancy (preeclampsia). Untreated, it can lead to coma or death.

The causes of pregnancy-induced hypertension are not fully understood. At one time, low-sodium diets were prescribed to prevent preeclampsia, but studies have not found such diets to be beneficial in lowering blood pressure or preventing this condition.[12] Calcium may play a role in preventing pregnancy-induced hypertension; calcium supplements have been found to reduce the risk of high blood pressure and preeclampsia.[13] Although calcium supplements are not routinely recommended for healthy pregnant women, pregnant teens, individuals with inadequate calcium intake, and women who are known to be at risk of developing pregnancy-induced hypertension may benefit from additional dietary calcium.[14]

Gestational diabetes

Diabetes that develops in a pregnant woman is known as **gestational diabetes**. It is more common in obese women and those with a family history of type 2 diabetes and occurs more frequently among African American, Hispanic/Latino American, and Native American women than among Caucasian women.[15] Gestational diabetes usually resolves after the birth, but the mother has a 20 to 50% chance of developing diabetes in the next 5 to 10 years.[16] A woman with gestational diabetes requires treatment to normalize maternal blood glucose levels. Because glucose in the mother's blood passes freely across the placenta, when the mother's blood glucose levels are high, the growing fetus receives extra glucose and hence extra calories. The baby grows rapidly and is at risk for being large for gestational age and consequently at increased risk for difficult delivery and abnormal blood glucose levels at birth. Babies born to mothers with gestational diabetes are at increased risk of developing diabetes as adults.[16]

> **gestational diabetes**
> A condition characterized by high blood glucose levels that develop during pregnancy.

CONCEPT CHECK STOP

HOW are nutrients and oxygen transferred from mother to fetus?

HOW does a mother's weight during pregnancy affect the birth weight of her child?

Why do heartburn and constipation tend to increase later in pregnancy?

HOW does gestational diabetes in a mother affect the baby?

Nutritional Needs During Pregnancy

During pregnancy, the mother's diet must provide all of her nutrients as well as those needed for the baby's growth and development. Because the increase in nutrient needs is greater than the increase in energy needs, a nutrient-dense diet is essential.

ENERGY AND MACRONUTRIENT NEEDS

Although pregnant women are eating for two, they don't need to eat twice as much as they normally do. During the first trimester, energy needs are not increased above nonpregnant levels. During the second and third trimesters, an additional 340 and 452 Calories/day, respectively, is recommended (**FIGURE 11.6**).[17]

Protein needs are increased during pregnancy because protein is needed for the synthesis of new blood cells, formation of the placenta, enlargement of the uterus and breasts, and growth of the baby (see Figure 11.6). An additional 25 g of protein above the RDA for nonpregnant women, or 1.1 g/kg/day, is recommended for the second and third trimesters of pregnancy.

To ensure sufficient glucose to fuel the fetal and maternal brains during pregnancy, the RDA for carbohydrate is increased by 45 g, to 175 g/day. If this carbohydrate comes from whole grains, fruits, and vegetables, it will also provide the additional 3 g of fiber/day recommended during pregnancy.

Although it is not necessary to increase total fat intake during pregnancy, additional amounts of the essential fatty acids linoleic and α-linolenic acid are recommended because these are incorporated into the placenta and fetal tissues. The long-chain polyunsaturated fatty acids DHA and arachidonic acid are important because they not only support maternal health but are essential for eye and nervous system development in the infant.[18]

Despite increases in the recommended intakes of protein, carbohydrate, and specific fatty acids during pregnancy, the distribution of calories from protein, carbohydrate, and fat should be about the same as that recommended for the general population.

Energy and macronutrient recommendations
FIGURE 11.6

This graph illustrates the percentage increase above nonpregnant levels in the recommended daily intake of energy, protein, carbohydrate, fiber, essential fatty acids, and water for a 25-year-old pregnant woman in her third trimester.

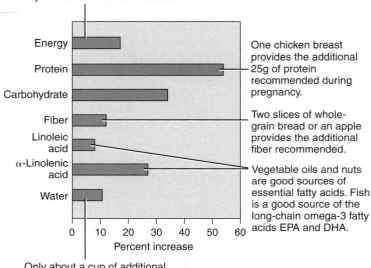

A snack of a sandwich, an apple, and a glass of milk will easily add the extra calories needed by a woman in her third trimester.

One chicken breast provides the additional 25g of protein recommended during pregnancy.

Two slices of whole-grain bread or an apple provides the additional fiber recommended.

Vegetable oils and nuts are good sources of essential fatty acids. Fish is a good source of the long-chain omega-3 fatty acids EPA and DHA.

Only about a cup of additional water is needed per day.

Micronutrient needs during pregnancy FIGURE 11.7

The graph illustrates the percentage increase in recommended micronutrient intakes for a 25-year-old woman during the third trimester of pregnancy.

The need for B vitamins increases as energy needs increase.

The need for folate, vitamin B$_{12}$, iron, and zinc increases to support the formation of new maternal and fetal cells.

The requirements for zinc and vitamin B$_6$ rise to meet the need for increased protein synthesis.

Calcium, phosphorus, magnesium, vitamin D, and vitamin C are needed to provide for the growth and development of bone and connective tissue.

Vitamin A is needed for cell differentiation and development. Low intake can cause low birth weight and premature birth, but too much can increase the risk of heart defects, cleft palate, and other developmental defects.

Iodine and selenium are needed for the synthesis of thyroid hormones. Iodine deficiency causes developmental disorders.

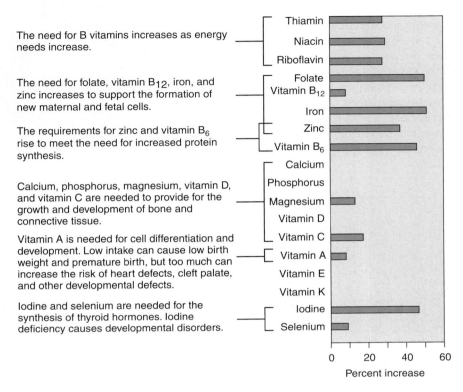

met with the extra food the mother consumes. For others, the increased need is met because their absorption is increased during pregnancy. For a few, including calcium, vitamin D, folate, vitamin B$_{12}$, iron, and zinc, there is a risk that the woman will not consume adequate amounts without supplementation.

Calcium and vitamin D

During gestation, the fetus accumulates about 30 g of calcium, mostly during the last trimester, when the bones are growing rapidly and the teeth are forming. However, the AI is not increased during pregnancy because calcium absorption doubles.[20] The AI for calcium can be met by consuming three to four servings of dairy products daily. Women who are lactose intolerant can meet their calcium needs with yogurt, cheese, reduced-lactose milk, calcium-rich vegetables, calcium-fortified foods, and calcium supplements. Many pregnant women fail to consume adequate amounts of calcium. Low calcium intake increases the risk that the mother will develop preeclampsia.[13]

Adequate vitamin D is essential to ensure efficient calcium absorption. Evidence is accumulating that the AI for vitamin D during pregnancy should be increased above current levels and that the amount typically contained in most prenatal supplements (10 µg/day) is insufficient.[21] Vitamin D deficiency is a particular risk for dark-skinned women living at latitudes greater than 40 degrees north or south—for example, farther north than New York City.[22]

Folate and vitamin B$_{12}$

Folate is needed for the synthesis of DNA and hence for cell division. Adequate folate intake before conception and during early pregnancy is crucial because rapid cell division occurs in the first days and weeks of pregnancy.

Low folate levels increase the risk of abnormalities in the formation of the *neural tube*, which forms the baby's brain and spinal cord (see Chapter 7, Figure 7.15). Neural tube closure, a critical step in neural tube development, occurs between 21 and 28 days after conception, often before a woman knows she is pregnant. Therefore, the recommended intake for all women capable of becoming pregnant is 400 µg daily of synthetic folic acid from fortified

FLUID AND ELECTROLYTE NEEDS

During pregnancy, a woman will accumulate 6 to 9 liters of water. Some of this water is intracellular, resulting from the growth of tissues, but most is due to increases in the volume of blood and the fluid between cells. The need for water increases from 2.7 L/day in nonpregnant women to 3 L/day during pregnancy.[19] Despite changes in the amount and distribution of body water during pregnancy, there is no evidence that the requirements for potassium, sodium, and chloride are different for pregnant women than for nonpregnant women.

VITAMIN AND MINERAL NEEDS

Many vitamins and minerals are needed for the growth of new tissues in both mother and child (FIGURE 11.7). For many of these nutrients, the increased need is easily

What a Scientist Sees

Folate Fortification and Neural Tube Defects

Consumers reading this label see that the pasta is made from a coarse flour called semolina, with added niacin, thiamin, riboflavin, iron, and folic acid. In 1998, the U.S. government began requiring the addition of folic acid to pasta and other enriched grain products in order to increase intake in women of childbearing age, with the goal of reducing the incidence of neural tube defects. Enriched grains were chosen for fortification because they are commonly consumed in regular amounts by this target population. Because high folic acid intake can mask the symptoms of vitamin B_{12} deficiency, the amount added to enriched grains was kept low enough to avoid this problem in any segment of the population but high enough to reduce the risk of neural tube defects. A scientist can see that this public health measure has succeeded. Since the initiation of folic acid fortification, the incidence of neural tube defects has been reduced by 25% in the United States and 50% in Canada.[25,26] Why has the incidence of neural tube defects not been cut to zero?

INGREDIENTS:
Durum semolina,
niacin,
ferrous
sulfate (iron),
thiamin mononitrate,
riboflavin,
folic acid

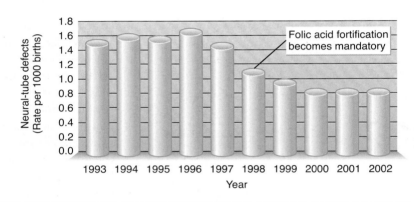

foods, supplements, or a combination of the two, in addition to a varied diet that is rich in natural sources of folate, such as leafy greens, legumes, and orange juice (see *What a Scientist Sees*).

Folate continues to be important even after the neural tube closes. Folate deficiency can cause megaloblastic (macrocytic) anemia in the mother, and inadequate folate intake is associated with premature and low-birth-weight infants and fetal growth retardation.[23] During pregnancy, the RDA is 600 µg of dietary folate equivalents per day.[24]

Vitamin B_{12} is essential for the regeneration of active forms of folate. A deficiency of vitamin B_{12} can therefore result in megaloblastic (macrocytic) anemia. Based on the amount of vitamin B_{12} transferred from mother to fetus during pregnancy and on the increased efficiency of vitamin B_{12} absorption during pregnancy, the RDA for pregnancy is set at 2.6 µg/day.[24] This recommendation is easily met by consuming a diet containing even small amounts of animal products. Pregnant women who consume vegan diets must include vitamin B_{12} supplements or foods fortified with vitamin B_{12} to meet their needs as well as those of the fetus.

Iron and zinc
Iron needs are high during pregnancy because iron is required for the synthesis of hemoglobin and other iron-containing proteins in both maternal and fetal tissues. The RDA for pregnant women is 27 mg/day, 50% higher than the recommended amount for non-pregnant women.[27] Many women start pregnancy with diminished iron stores and quickly become iron deficient. This occurs even though iron absorption is increased during pregnancy and iron losses decrease because menstruation ceases. Iron deficiency anemia during pregnancy has been associated with low birth weight and preterm delivery.[28] Because most of the transfer of iron from mother to fetus occurs during the last trimester, babies who are born prematurely may not have time to accumulate sufficient iron.

It takes a well-planned diet to meet iron needs during pregnancy. Red meat is a good source of the more absorbable heme iron, and leafy green vegetables and fortified cereals are good sources of nonheme iron. Consuming citrus fruits, which are high in vitamin C, or meat, which contains heme iron, along with foods that are good sources of nonheme iron, can enhance iron absorption. Iron supplements are typically recommended during the second and third trimesters, and iron is included in prenatal supplements.

Zinc is involved in the synthesis and function of DNA and RNA and the synthesis of proteins. It is therefore extremely important for growth and development. Zinc deficiency during pregnancy is associated with increased risks of fetal malformations, premature birth, and low birth weight.[29] Because zinc absorption is inhibited by high iron intake, iron supplements may compromise zinc status if the mother's diet is low in zinc. The RDA for zinc is 13 mg/day for pregnant women age 18 and younger and 11 mg/day for pregnant women age 19 and older.[27] As is the case with iron, the zinc in red meat is more absorbable than zinc from other sources.

MEETING NUTRIENT NEEDS WITH FOOD AND SUPPLEMENTS

The energy and nutrient needs of pregnancy can be met by following the recommendations of MyPyramid for Pregnancy and Breastfeeding (FIGURE 11.8).

MyPyramid for pregnancy and breastfeeding FIGURE 11.8

This MyPyramid Plan for Moms (www.mypyramid.gov) is for a 26-year-old woman who is 5 feet 4 inches tall, gets 30 to 60 minutes of exercise a day, and weighed 125 pounds before she became pregnant. Energy needs are not increased during the first trimester, so the recommended amounts from each group for the first trimester are the same as for a nonpregnant woman.

Based on the information you provided, these are your recommended amounts from each food group. For more information, go to MyPyramid.gov.

	GRAINS Make half your grains whole	VEGETABLES Vary your veggies	FRUITS Focus on fruits	MILK Get your calcium-rich foods	MEAT & BEANS Choose lean with protein
1st Trimester	7 ounces	3 cups	2 cups	3 cups	6 ounces
2nd Trimester	8 ounces	3 cups	2 cups	3 cups	6½ ounces
3rd Trimester	9 ounces	3½ cups	2 cups	3 cups	6½ ounces

*These are only estimates of your needs. Check with your health care provider to make sure you are gaining weight appropriately.

*The calories and amounts of food you need change with each trimester of pregnancy. Your plan may show different amounts of food for different months, to meet your changing nutritional needs. Changing the amount of calories you eat each trimester also helps you gain weight at the correct rate.

Know your limites on fats, sugars, and sodium		
	OILS Aim for this much	EXTRAS Limit excess solid fats and sugars to this much
1st Trimester	6 teaspoons	290 Calories
2nd Trimester	7 teaspoons	360 Calories
3rd Trimester	8 teaspoons	410 Calories

Even when a healthy diet based on MyPyramid for Pregnancy and Breastfeeding is consumed, it is difficult to meet all the vitamin and mineral needs of pregnancy. Therefore, a prenatal supplement is generally prescribed for all pregnant women. These supplements include the additional folic acid and iron discussed earlier.[1] A prenatal supplement, however, must be taken along with, not in place of, a carefully planned diet (FIGURE 11.9) (see the *Case Study*).

FOOD CRAVINGS AND AVERSIONS

Most women experience some food cravings and aversions during pregnancy. The foods most commonly craved are ice cream, sweets, candy, fruit, and fish (see *What Should I Eat?* on page 378). Common aversions include coffee, highly seasoned foods, and fried foods. It is not known why women have these cravings and aversions. It has been suggested that hormonal or physiological changes during pregnancy—in particular, changes in taste and smell—may be the cause, but psychological and behavioral factors are also involved.

Usually the foods that pregnant women crave are not harmful and can be safely included in the diet to meet not only nutritional needs but also emotional needs and individual preferences. However, **pica** during

pica An abnormal craving for and ingestion of nonfood substances that have little or no nutritional value.

Prenatal supplements FIGURE 11.9

Prenatal supplements such as this one typically do not provide enough calcium to meet the needs of a pregnant woman because to do so, the tablet would have to be very large. They also lack protein needed for tissue synthesis; complex carbohydrates needed for energy; essential fatty acids for brain and nerve tissue development; fiber and fluid, which help prevent constipation; and the phytochemicals found in a healthy diet.

Supplement Facts

Serving Size 1 Tablet
Servings Per Container 60

Amount Per 1 Tablet	% Daily Value
Vitamin A (as beta carotene) 5000 IU	63%
Vitamin C (as ascorbic acid) 85 mg	100%
Vitamin D (as cholecalciferol) 400 IU	200%
Vitamin E (as d-alpha tocopheryl) acetate (Covitol™) 22 IU	67%
Vitamin K 90 mcg	100%
Thiamin 1.4 mg	100%
Riboflavin 1.6 mg	100%
Niacin (as niacinamide) 17 mg	100%
Vitamin B6 (as pyridoxine HCl) 2.6 mg	137%
Folic acid 1000 mcg	167%
Vitamin B12 (as cyanocobalamin) 2.6 mg	100%
Pantothenic Acid (as as d-calcium pantothenate) 6 mg	100%
Iron (as iron fumarate) 27 mg	100%
Iodine (kelp) 220 mcg	100%
Zinc (as monomethionine & gluconate) 11mg	100%
Selenium (as sodium selenate) 60 mcg	100%
Copper (as copper sulfate) 1000 mcg	100%
Calcium (as calcium carbonate) 200 mg	20%

* **Daily Values based on RDAs for pregnant women ages 19-50**
Other ingredients: stearic acid, vegetable stearate, silicon dioxide, croscarmellose sodium, microcrystalline cellulose, natural coating (contains hydroxypropyl methylcellulose, titanium dioxide, riboflavin, polyethylene glycol and polysorbate)

NUTRIENT NEEDS FOR A SUCCESSFUL PREGNANCY

Tina is a sedentary 29-year-old at the end of her fourth month of pregnancy. She is 5′ 6″ tall and weighed 140 pounds at the start of her pregnancy. She is concerned about gaining too much weight because her sister gained 50 pounds during her pregnancy and has had difficulty losing the excess weight since her baby was born. Tina would like to keep her weight gain below 20 pounds.

Tina's typical diet provides enough energy for a non-pregnant woman, but during her second and third trimesters, she needs additional calories and nutrients. To decide what to add to her diet, she compares her typical intake to her MyPyramid Plan for Moms. Her current diet includes 8 oz of grains, 1.5 cups of vegetables, 1 cup of fruit, 2 cups of milk, and 6 oz of meat and beans.

How should the amounts of food from each food group be changed in order for Tina to meet her needs during the second trimester of her pregnancy?

▼

Your answer:

Based on the graph below, how much weight would you recommend that Tina gain? Why would gaining only 20 pounds or gaining 50 pounds put the baby at risk?

▼

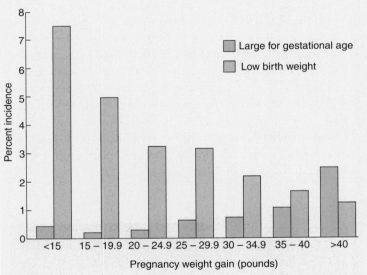

Tina is taking a prenatal supplement but is curious about whether her diet alone can meet her nutrient needs. She analyzes her diet and finds that she is meeting her needs for all nutrients except iron. Her current diet provides only 13.5 mg of iron—significantly less than the RDA of 27 mg for pregnant women.

Suggest some foods that Tina could include in her diet in order to obtain an additional 13.5 mg of iron.

▼

Your answer:

Your answer:

Do you think it is reasonable for Tina to consume 27 mg of iron each day from her diet alone? Why or why not?

▼

Your answer:

(Check your answers in Appendix K.)

WHAT SHOULD I EAT? | **During Pregnancy**

Use iProfile to plan a nutritious 300-Calorie snack for a pregnant woman.

Make nutrient-dense choices
- Have yogurt for a midmorning snack.
- Put some peanut butter on your banana to add some protein to your snack.
- Have a plate of pasta Florentine (with spinach)—it is both a natural and a fortified source of folate.

Drink plenty of fluids
- Have a glass of low-fat milk to boost fluid and calcium intake.
- Keep a bottle of water at your desk or in your car.
- Relax with a cup of tea.

Indulge your cravings, within reason
- Savor some ice cream—it adds calcium and protein.
- Enjoy your cookies with a glass of low-fat milk.

Pica FIGURE 11.10

This African American woman in Georgia is eating a white clay called kaolin, which some women crave during pregnancy. Eating kaolin is also a traditional remedy for morning sickness. This example of pica may be related to cultural beliefs and traditions, but pica is also believed to be triggered by nutrient deficiencies, stress, and anxiety. It is most common in African American women, women who live in rural areas, and those with a childhood or family history of pica.[30]

pregnancy can have serious health consequences. Women with pica commonly consume nonfoods such as clay, laundry starch, and ashes. Consuming large amounts of these substances can reduce intake of nutrient-dense foods, inhibit nutrient absorption, increase the risk of consuming toxins, and cause intestinal obstructions. Complications of pica include iron-deficiency anemia, lead poisoning, and parasitic infestations.[30] Anemia and high blood pressure are more common in those with pica than among other pregnant women, but it is not clear whether pica is a result of these conditions or a cause. In newborns, anemia and low birth weight are often related to pica in the mother (**FIGURE 11.10**).

CONCEPT CHECK STOP

Why is nutrient density so important during pregnancy?

How does calcium absorption change during pregnancy?

What nutrients are typically supplemented during pregnancy?

Factors That Increase the Risks Associated with Pregnancy

LEARNING OBJECTIVES

Define critical period in relation to fetal development.

Discuss how nutritional status can influence the outcome of pregnancy.

Explain how a pregnant woman's age and health status affect the risks associated with pregnancy.

Describe the effects of alcohol, mercury, and cocaine on the outcome of pregnancy.

nything that interferes with embryonic or fetal development can cause a baby to be born too soon or too small or result in birth defects. The embryo and fetus are particularly vulnerable to damage because their cells are dividing rapidly, differentiating, and moving to form organs and other structures. Developmental errors can be caused by deficiencies or excesses in the maternal diet and by harmful substances that are present in the environment, consumed in the diet, or taken as medications or recreational drugs. Any chemical, biological, or physical agent that causes a birth defect is called a **teratogen**. And because each organ system develops at a different time and rate, each has a **critical period** during which exposure to a teratogen is most likely to disrupt development and cause irreversible damage (FIGURE 11.11). Severe damage can result in miscarriage. Some women are at increased risk for complications during pregnancy because of their nutritional status, age, or preexisting health problems. Others are at risk due to exposure to harmful substances.

Critical periods of development FIGURE 11.11

The critical periods of development are different for different body systems. Because the majority of cell differentiation occurs during the embryonic period, this is the time when exposure to teratogens can do the most damage, but vital body organs can still be affected during the fetal period. One in every 33 babies born in the United States has a birth defect.[31]

During World War II, an embargo on food transport to the Netherlands in the winter of 1944–1945 caused the average intake per person per day to drop below 1000 Calories. Pregnant women gave birth to smaller babies. In adulthood, the affected babies were more likely than others to have diabetes, heart disease, obesity, and other chronic diseases.[34]

MATERNAL NUTRITIONAL STATUS

Before pregnancy, proper nutrition is important to allow conception and maximize the likelihood of a healthy pregnancy. Women with reduced body fat due to starvation diets, anorexia nervosa, or excessive exercise may have abnormal hormone levels. When hormone levels are too low, ovulation does not occur, and conception is not possible. Too much body fat can also reduce fertility by altering hormone levels. Deficiencies or excesses of specific nutrients can affect both fertility and the outcome of pregnancy.

During pregnancy, maternal malnutrition can cause fetal growth retardation, low birth weight, birth defects, premature birth, spontaneous abortion, or stillbirth. The effects of malnutrition vary, depending on when during the pregnancy it occurs.[32] As discussed earlier, inadequate folate intake in the first few weeks of pregnancy can affect neural tube development.[24] Too much vitamin A, particularly early in pregnancy, increases the risk of kidney problems and central nervous system abnormalities in the offspring.[27] To reduce the risk of excess vitamin A, supplements consumed during pregnancy should contain the vitamin A precursor, β-carotene, which is not damaging to the fetus.

Maternal malnutrition not only interferes with fetal growth and development but also causes changes that can affect the child's risk of developing chronic diseases later in life. Epidemiological studies suggest that compared to normal-weight newborns, individuals who are small or disproportionately thin at birth and during infancy have increased rates of heart disease, high blood pressure, stroke, high blood cholesterol, diabetes, obesity, and osteoporosis in adult life (FIGURE 11.12).[33]

One of the greatest risk factors for poor pregnancy outcome is poverty, which limits access to food, education, and health care.[35] Low-income women are unlikely to receive medical care until late in pregnancy and consequently have a high incidence of low-birth-weight and preterm infants. A federally funded program that addresses the nutritional needs of pregnant women is the **Special Supplemental Nutrition Program for Women, Infants, and Children (WIC)**. This program provides vouchers for the purchase of nutritious foods and referrals to health and other services for low-income women who are pregnant, postpartum, or breast feeding, and for infants and children up to age 5 who are at risk of malnutrition.

MATERNAL AGE AND HEALTH STATUS

Pregnancy places stresses on the body at any age, but the stresses have a greater impact on women in their teens and those age 35 or older. Pregnant teens are still growing, so their nutrient intake must meet their needs for growth as well as for pregnancy. Pregnant teenagers are at increased risk of pregnancy-induced hypertension and are more likely to deliver preterm and low-birth-weight babies. Even teenagers who deliver normal-birth-weight infants may stop growing themselves.[36] To produce a healthy baby, a pregnant teenager needs early medical intervention and nutrition counseling (FIGURE 11.13). Although the rate of teenage pregnancy has decreased over the past decade, from 62 babies/1000 teens in 1991 to 42/1000 in 2006, it remains a major public health problem.[37]

Nutrient needs of pregnant teens
FIGURE 11.13

Because the nutrient needs of pregnant teens are different from those of pregnant adults, the DRIs include a special set of nutrient recommendations for this age group. The percentage increase in micronutrient needs above nonpregnant levels is shown here are for 14- to 18-year-old girls during the second and third trimesters of pregnancy.

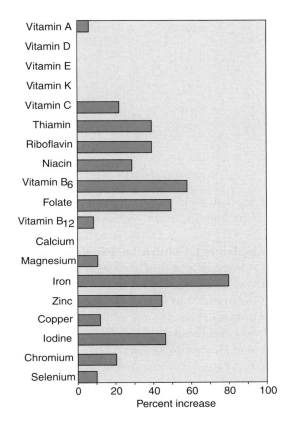

The nutritional requirements for older women during pregnancy are no different from those for women in their 20s, but pregnancy after age 35 carries additional risks. Older women are more likely to already have one or more medical conditions, such as cardiovascular disease, kidney disorders, obesity, or diabetes. These preexisting conditions increase the risks associated with pregnancy. For example, a woman who has preexisting high blood pressure is at increased risk for having a low-birth-weight baby, and a woman who has diabetes is more likely to have a baby who is large for gestational age. Older women are also more likely to develop gestational diabetes, pregnancy-induced hypertension, and other complications. They have a higher incidence of low-birth-weight infants. In addition, their infants are more likely to have chromosomal abnormalities, especially **Down syndrome** (FIGURE 11.14). The frequency of twins and triplets is higher among older mothers in part because of their greater use of fertility treatments. Multiple pregnancies increase nutrient needs and the risk of preterm delivery.

Women with a history of miscarriage or birth defects are also at increased risk. For example, a woman who has had a number of miscarriages is more likely to have another, and a woman who has had one child with a birth defect has an increased risk for defects in subsequent pregnancies. Another factor that increases risks is frequent pregnancies. An interval of less than 18 months between pregnancies increases the risk of delivering a small-for-gestational age infant. An interval of only 3 months increases the risk of a preterm infant as well as the risk of neonatal death.[39] One reason for these increased risks is that the mother may not have replenished the nutrient stores depleted in the first pregnancy before becoming pregnant again.

Incidence of Down syndrome FIGURE 11.14

Down syndrome is caused by a defect during egg or sperm formation that results in extra genetic material in the baby. It causes distinctive facial characteristics, developmental delays and other health problems. The incidence of Down syndrome rises significantly with maternal age of 35 years or more. However, while older mothers are more likely to carry a Down syndrome baby, 80% of Down syndrome births are to mothers under age 35, as younger women have more babies overall.[38]

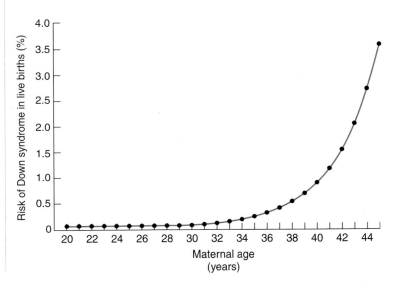

Sources of caffeine TABLE 11.2

Food or medication	Amount	Caffeine (mg)
Coffee, regular brewed	1 cup (240 ml)	100–200
Coffee, decaffeinated	1 cup	3–12
Black tea, brewed	1 cup	40–120
Green tea, brewed	1 cup	8–30
Pepsi	20 oz	63
Mountain Dew	20 oz	118
Energy drink	8.5 oz	50–300
Hot chocolate	1 cup	7
Brownie	1	14
Chocolate bar	1 oz	15
NoDoz	1 tablet	100
Excedrin	1 tablet	65
Empirin, Anacin	1 tablet	32

EXPOSURE TO TOXIC SUBSTANCES

A pregnant woman's exposure to toxins in food, water, and the environment can affect the developing fetus. Even substances that seem innocuous can be dangerous. For example, herbal remedies, including herbal teas, should be avoided unless their consumption during pregnancy has been determined to be safe.[4]

Caffeine When consumed in excess, coffee and other caffeine-containing beverages have been associated with increased risks of miscarriage or low birth weight.[40] It is recommended that pregnant women avoid consuming more than 200 mg of caffeine per day (TABLE 11.2).

Mercury in fish Fish has both benefits and risks for pregnant women. It is a source of lean protein for tissue growth and of omega-3 fatty acids and iodine needed for brain development, but if it is contaminated with mercury, consumption during pregnancy can cause developmental delays and brain damage. Rather than avoid fish, pregnant women should be informed consumers. Exposure to mercury can be controlled by avoiding varieties of fish that are highest in mercury and limiting intake of fish that contain lower amounts mercury (TABLE 11.3).

Food safety during pregnancy[41] TABLE 11.3

Don't eat swordfish, shark, king mackerel, or tilefish, which can be high in mercury.

Eat up to 1 serving (6 oz) per week of canned albacore or chunk white tuna and up to 12 oz per week of fish and shellfish that are lower in mercury, such as salmon, shrimp, canned light tuna, pollock, catfish, and cod.

Check local advisories about the safety of fish caught in local waters. If no advice is available, eat up to 6 oz per week but don't consume any other fish during that week.

Don't drink raw (unpasteurized) milk or consume products made with unpasteurized milk, such as certain Mexican-style soft cheeses.

Don't eat refrigerated smoked fish, cold deli salads, or refrigerated pâtés or meat spreads.

Don't eat hot dogs unless they have been reheated to steaming hot.

Don't eat raw or undercooked meat, poultry, fish, shellfish, or eggs.

Don't eat unwashed fruits and vegetables, raw sprouts, or unpasteurized juice.

Dangers of alcohol use during pregnancy FIGURE 11.15

The facial characteristics associated with fetal alcohol syndrome (FAS), which include a low nasal bridge, short nose, distinct eyelids, and thin upper lip, can be seen in this 3-year-old girl. Newborns with FAS may be shaky and irritable, with poor muscle tone. Other problems associated with FAS include heart and urinary tract defects, impaired vision and hearing, and delayed language development. Below-average intellectual function is the most common and most serious effect.

Food-borne illness

The immune system is weakened during pregnancy, increasing susceptibility to and the severity of certain food-borne illnesses. *Listeria* infections are about 20 times more likely during pregnancy and are especially dangerous for pregnant women, often resulting in miscarriage, premature delivery, stillbirth, or infection of the fetus.[42] About one-quarter of babies born with *Listeria* infections do not survive. The bacteria are commonly found in unpasteurized milk, soft cheeses, and uncooked hot dogs and lunch meats (see Table 11.3).

Toxoplasmosis is an infection caused by a parasite. If a pregnant woman becomes infected, there is about a 40% chance that she will pass the infection to her unborn baby.[43] Some infected babies develop vision and hearing loss, intellectual disability, and/or seizures. The toxoplasmosis parasite is found in cat feces, soil, and undercooked infected meat (see Table 11.3). Pregnant women should follow the safe food-handling recommendations discussed in Chapter 13.

Alcohol

Alcohol consumption during pregnancy is one of the leading causes of preventable birth defects. Alcohol is a teratogen that is particularly damaging to the developing nervous system.[44] It also indirectly affects fetal growth and development because it is a toxin that reduces blood flow to the placenta, thereby decreasing the delivery of oxygen and nutrients to the fetus. Use of alcohol can also impair maternal nutritional status, further increasing the risks to the fetus.

Prenatal exposure to alcohol can cause a spectrum of disorders, depending on the amount, timing, and duration of the exposure. One of the most severe outcomes of alcohol use during pregnancy is delivery of a baby with **fetal alcohol syndrome (FAS)**

> **fetal alcohol syndrome (FAS)**
> A characteristic group of physical and mental abnormalities in an infant resulting from maternal alcohol consumption during pregnancy.

(FIGURE 11.15). Not all babies who are exposed to alcohol while in the uterus have FAS, but many have some alcohol-related problems. **Alcohol-related neurodevelopmental disorders (ARND)** are functional or mental impairments linked to prenatal alcohol exposure, and **alcohol-related birth defects (ARBD)** are malformations in the skeleton or major organ systems. These conditions are less severe than FAS but occur about three times more often. Because alcohol consumption in each trimester has been associated with fetal abnormalities and there is no level of alcohol consumption that is known to be safe, complete abstinence from alcohol is recommended during pregnancy.

Cigarette smoke

If a woman smokes cigarettes during pregnancy, her baby will be affected before birth and throughout life. The carbon monoxide in cigarette smoke binds to hemoglobin in maternal and fetal blood, reducing the amount of oxygen delivered to fetal tissues. The nicotine absorbed from cigarette smoke is a teratogen that can affect brain development.[45] It also constricts arteries and limits blood flow, reducing the amounts of oxygen and nutrients delivered to the fetus.[46] Cigarette smoking during pregnancy reduces birth weight and increases the risks of stillbirth, preterm delivery, neurobehavioral problems, and early infant death.[4,45] In women who don't smoke, environmental exposure to cigarette smoke has been found to increase the risk of having a low-birth-weight baby. The risks of **sudden infant death syndrome (SIDS, or crib death)** and respiratory problems are also increased in children exposed to cigarette smoke both in the uterus and after birth. The effects of maternal smoking follow children throughout life; these children are more likely to have frequent colds and develop lung problems later in life.[47]

> **sudden infant death syndrome (SIDS, or crib death)**
> The unexplained death of an infant, usually during sleep.

Drug use Certain drugs—whether over-the-counter, prescribed, or illegal—can affect both fertility and fetal development. For example, the acne medications Accutane and Retin-A are derivatives of vitamin A that can cause birth defects if used during pregnancy. A woman who is considering becoming pregnant should discuss her plans with her physician in order to determine the risks associated with any medication she is taking.

Substance abuse during pregnancy is a national health issue. It is estimated that from 1 to 11% of babies born each year have been exposed to drugs during the prenatal period. These percentages include only the use of illegal drugs; they would be much higher if alcohol and nicotine were included.[48]

Marijuana and cocaine can cross the placenta and enter the fetal blood. There is little evidence that marijuana affects fetal development, but cocaine use creates problems for both the mother and the infant before, during, and after delivery.[49] Cocaine is a central nervous system stimulant, but many of its effects during pregnancy occur because it constricts blood vessels, thereby reducing the delivery of oxygen and nutrients to the fetus. Cocaine use during pregnancy is also associated with an increased risk of miscarriage, fetal growth retardation, premature labor and delivery, low birth weight, and birth defects.[50] Exposure to cocaine and other illegal drugs before birth has also been shown to affect infant behavior and influence learning and attention span during childhood.[51]

CONCEPT CHECK STOP

Why does the effect of a given teratogen vary, depending on when a pregnant woman is exposed to it?

How does malnutrition during pregnancy affect the health of the child later in life?

Why are the requirements for some nutrients different in pregnant teenage girls than in pregnant adult women?

How much alcohol can be safely consumed during pregnancy?

Lactation

The need for many nutrients is even greater during lactation than during pregnancy. The milk produced by a breast-feeding mother must meet all the nutrient needs of her baby, who is bigger and more active that he or she was in the womb. To meet these needs, a lactating woman must choose a varied, nutrient-dense diet that follows the MyPyramid recommendations for breast-feeding women.

MILK PRODUCTION AND LET-DOWN

Lactation involves both the synthesis of milk components—proteins, lactose, and lipids—and the movement of these components through the milk ducts to the nipple (**FIGURE 11.16**). Milk production and

Anatomy of milk production FIGURE 11.16

Throughout pregnancy, hormones prepare the breasts for lactation by stimulating the enlargement and development of the milk ducts and milk-producing glands, called *alveoli* (singular *alveolus*). During lactation, milk travels from the alveoli through the ducts to the milk storage sinuses and then to the nipple.

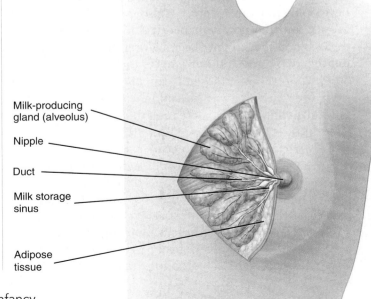

Milk-producing gland (alveolus)

Nipple

Duct

Milk storage sinus

Adipose tissue

This graph illustrates the percentage increase in energy and macronutrient recommendations for a 25-year-old woman during the third trimester of pregnancy and the first 6 months of lactation.

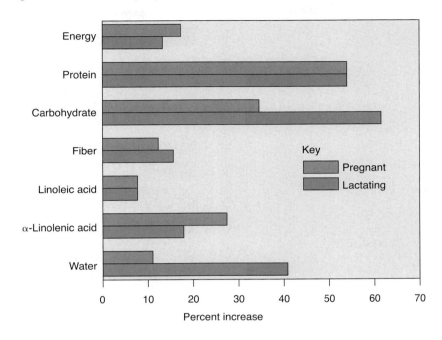

let-down are triggered by hormones that are released in response to an infant's suckling. The pituitary hormone **prolactin** stimulates milk production; the more the infant suckles, the more milk is produced. Let-down is caused by **oxytocin**, another pituitary hormone. Oxytocin release is also stimulated by suckling, but as nursing becomes more automatic, oxytocin release and let-down may occur in response to just the sight or sound of an infant. Let-down can be inhibited by nervous tension, fatigue, or embarrassment. Because let-down is essential for breast feeding and makes suckling easier for the child, slow let-down can make feeding difficult.

let-down
The release of milk from the milk-producing glands and its movement through the ducts and storage sinuses.

ENERGY AND NUTRIENT NEEDS DURING LACTATION

Human milk contains about 70 Calories/100 milliliters (160 Calories/cup). During the first 6 months of lactation, an average infant consumes 600 to 900 mL (about 2.5 to 4 cups)/day, so approximately 500 Calories are required from the mother each day. Much of this energy must come from the diet, but some can come from maternal fat stores. Because some of the energy for milk production comes from fat stores, the increase in recommended energy intake is lower during lactation than during pregnancy, even though total energy demands are greater (FIGURE 11.17). An additional 330 Calories/day above nonpregnant, nonlactating needs are recommended during the first 6 months of lactation, and an additional 400 Calories are recommended for the second 6 months. Beginning 1 month after birth, most lactating women lose 0.5 to 1 kg (1 to 2 lbs)/month for 6 months. Rapid weight loss is not recommended during lactation because it can decrease milk production.

To ensure adequate protein for milk production, the RDA for lactation is increased by 25 g/day. The recommended intakes of total carbohydrate, fiber, and the essential fatty acids linoleic and α-linolenic acid are also higher during lactation (see Figure 11.17).[17]

To avoid dehydration and ensure adequate milk production, lactating women need to consume about 1 L of additional water per day.[19] Consuming an extra glass of milk, juice, or water at each meal and whenever the infant nurses can help ensure adequate fluid intake. The recommended intakes for several vitamins

Micronutrient needs during lactation FIGURE 11.18

This graph illustrates the percentage increase in vitamin and mineral recommendations for a 25-year-old woman during the third trimester of pregnancy and the first 6 months of lactation.

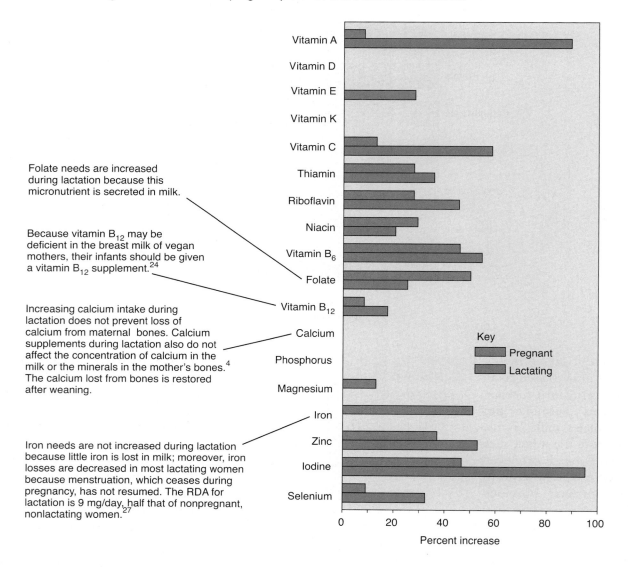

Folate needs are increased during lactation because this micronutrient is secreted in milk.

Because vitamin B_{12} may be deficient in the breast milk of vegan mothers, their infants should be given a vitamin B_{12} supplement.[24]

Increasing calcium intake during lactation does not prevent loss of calcium from maternal bones. Calcium supplements during lactation also do not affect the concentration of calcium in the milk or the minerals in the mother's bones.[4] The calcium lost from bones is restored after weaning.

Iron needs are not increased during lactation because little iron is lost in milk; moreover, iron losses are decreased in most lactating women because menstruation, which ceases during pregnancy, has not resumed. The RDA for lactation is 9 mg/day, half that of nonpregnant, nonlactating women.[27]

and minerals are increased during lactation to meet the needs for synthesizing milk and to replace the nutrients secreted in the milk (FIGURE 11.18). Maternal intake of vitamins C, B_6, B_{12}, A, and D can affect the composition of milk. For other nutrients, including calcium and folate, levels in the milk are maintained at the expense of maternal stores.

CONCEPT CHECK STOP

What causes milk let-down?

Where does the energy for milk production come from?

Why is the recommended calcium intake for a new mother not increased while she is lactating?

Nutrition for Infants

LEARNING OBJECTIVES

Explain how growth charts are used to monitor the nutritional well-being of infants.

Discuss the importance of choosing foods that are appropriate for a child's developmental stage.

Compare the benefits of breast feeding and formula feeding.

List three foods that should not be fed to infants and explain why.

A fter the umbilical cord is cut, a newborn must actively obtain nutrients rather than being passively fed through the placenta. The energy and nutrients an infant consumes must support his or her continuing growth and development, as well as his or her increasing activity level.

INFANT GROWTH AND DEVELOPMENT

During **infancy**—the first year of life—growth is extremely rapid. Healthy infants follow standard patterns of growth—that is, whether a newborn weighs 6 pounds or 8 pounds at birth, the rate of growth should be approximately the same: rapid initially and slowing slightly as the infant approaches his or her first birthday. A rule of thumb is that an infant's birth weight should double by 4 months of age and triple by 1 year of age. In the first year of life, most infants increase their length by 50%. Growth is the best indicator of adequate nutrition in an infant.

Growth charts Growth charts can be used to compare an infant's growth with that of other infants of the same age (**FIGURE 11.19**).[53] The resulting ranking,

Growth charts FIGURE 11.19

This weight-for-age growth chart for boys from birth to 36 months of age can be used to compare a boy's weight at a particular age to standards for the general population. Growth charts for this age group are also available to monitor length for age and head circumference for age in boys and girls.

CDC Growth Charts: United States

Weight-for-age percentiles: Boys, birth to 36 months

This infant's birth weight was at the 40th percentile, and he remained at this percentile into childhood.

SOURCE: Developed by the National Center for Health Statistics in collaboration with the Nation Center for Chronic Disease Prevention and Health Promotion (2000).

Age	Birth to 4 months	4 to 6 months	6 to 9 months	9 to 12 months
Developmental milestone	The infant takes milk by means of a licking motion of the tongue called *suckling*, which strokes or milks the liquid from the nipple. Solid food placed in the mouth at an early age is usually pushed out as the tongue thrusts forward.	The tongue is held farther back in the mouth, allowing solid food to be accepted without being expelled. The infant can hold his or her head up and is able to sit, with or without support.	The infant can sit without support, chew, hold food, and easily move hand to mouth.	The infant can drink from a cup and feed him/herself.
Foods	Breast milk or iron-fortified infant formula	Breast milk or formula, iron-fortified infant cereal. Rice cereal is usually the first solid food introduced because it is easily digested and less likely than other grains to cause allergies. After cereals, puréed vegetables and fruits can be introduced.	Breast milk or formula, iron-fortified infant cereal, puréed or strained vegetables, fruits, meats and beans, limited finger foods.	Breast milk or formula, iron-fortified infant cereal, chopped vegetables, soft fruits, meats and beans, fruit juice, nonchoking finger foods such as dry cereal, cooked pasta, and cut well-cooked vegetables.

NATIONAL GEOGRAPHIC

or percentile, indicates where the infant's growth falls in relation to population standards. For example, if a newborn boy is at the 20th percentile for weight, 19% of newborn boys weigh less and 80% weigh more. Children usually remain at the same percentile as they grow. For instance, a child who is at the 50th percentile for height and the 25th percentile for weight generally remains close to these percentiles throughout childhood. Small and premature infants often follow a pattern that is parallel to but below the growth curve for a period of time and then experience catch-up growth that brings them into the same range as children of the same age.

Slight variations in growth rate are normal, but a consistent pattern of not following the established growth curve or a sudden change in growth pattern is cause for concern and could indicate overnutrition or undernutrition. For example, a rapid increase in weight without an increase in height may indicate that the infant is being overfed. Because overweight children are more likely to be overweight as adults, this pattern of weight increase should be addressed early in life.

Growth that is slower than the predicted pattern indicates **failure to thrive**, a catchall term for any type of growth failure

failure to thrive Inability of a child's growth to keep up with normal growth curves.

in a young child. The cause may be a congenital condition, disease, poor nutrition, neglect, abuse, or psychosocial problems. The treatment is usually an individualized plan that includes adequate nutrition and careful monitoring by physicians, dietitians, and other health-care professionals. Just as there are critical periods in prenatal life, there are critical periods during infancy when undernutrition can have permanent effects on growth and development. Malnutrition during infancy has a great impact on learning and behavior because the first year of life is a critical period for brain development.

Developmental milestones
In addition to getting bigger, infants develop physically, intellectually, and socially. Adequate nutrition is essential for achieving these developmental milestones, and they in turn affect how the infant obtains nourishment. Although most of an infant's nutritional needs are met by breast milk or infant formula, solid and semi-solid foods can be gradually introduced into the diet starting at 4 to 6 months of life. By this time, the infant's feeding abilities and gastrointestinal tract are mature enough to handle solid foods (FIGURE 11.20).

ENERGY AND NUTRIENT NEEDS OF INFANTS

The rapid growth and high metabolic rate of infants increase their need for energy, protein, and vitamins and minerals that are important for growth. Human milk and commercially produced formula are designed to meet infants' nutrient needs. Nevertheless, infants may still be at risk for iron, vitamin D, and vitamin K deficiencies and for suboptimal levels of fluoride.

Energy and macronutrients

Infants require more calories and protein per kilogram of body weight than do individuals at any other time of life (**FIGURE 11.21A**).[17] As infants grow older, their rate of growth slows, but they become more mobile, so the amount of energy they need for activity increases. Because infants change so much during the first year, energy recommendations are made for three age groups—0 to 3 months, 4 to 6 months, and 7 to 12 months—and nutrient recommendations for two age groups—0 to 6 months and 7 to 12 months (see inside cover).

The combination of high energy demands and a small stomach means that infants require an energy-dense diet.

Healthy infants consume about 55% of their energy as fat during the first 6 months of life and 40% during the second 6 months. These percentages are far higher than the 20 to 35% of energy from fat recommended in the adult diet (**FIGURE 11.21B**). This energy-dense diet allows the small volume of food that fits in an infant's stomach to provide enough energy to meet the infant's needs.

Fluid needs

Infants have a higher proportion of body water than do adults, and they lose proportionately more water in urine and through evaporation. Urine losses are high because the kidneys are not fully developed and hence are unable to reabsorb as much water as adult kidneys. Water losses through evaporation are proportionately higher in infants than in adults because they have a larger surface area relative to body weight. As a result, they need to consume more water per unit of body weight than do adults. Nevertheless, healthy infants who are exclusively breast fed do not require additional water.[19] In older infants, some water is obtained from food and from beverages other than milk. When water losses are increased by diarrhea or vomiting, additional fluids may be needed.

Energy and macronutrient needs FIGURE 11.21

A The total amount of energy required by a newborn is less than the amount needed by an adult. When this amount is expressed as Calories/kg of body weight, however, infants require about three times more energy than an adult male. ▼

B Comparing the distribution of calories from carbohydrate, fat, ▶ and protein in human milk with that recommended for an adult illustrates proportionally how much more fat infants need. As an infant grows and solid foods are introduced into the diet, the percentage of calories from carbohydrate in the diet increases, and the percentage from fat decreases.

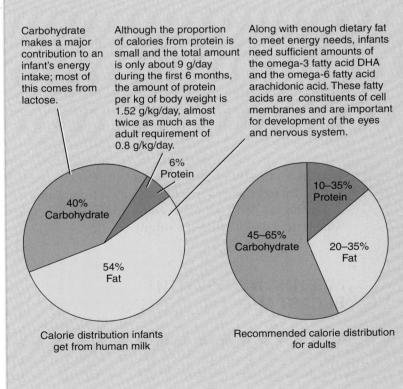

Carbohydrate makes a major contribution to an infant's energy intake; most of this comes from lactose.

Although the proportion of calories from protein is small and the total amount is only about 9 g/day during the first 6 months, the amount of protein per kg of body weight is 1.52 g/kg/day, almost twice as much as the adult requirement of 0.8 g/kg/day.

Along with enough dietary fat to meet energy needs, infants need sufficient amounts of the omega-3 fatty acid DHA and the omega-6 fatty acid arachidonic acid. These fatty acids are constituents of cell membranes and are important for development of the eyes and nervous system.

Calorie distribution infants get from human milk

Recommended calorie distribution for adults

Micronutrients at risk Iron is the nutrient that is most commonly deficient in infants who are consuming adequate energy and protein. Iron deficiency usually is not a problem during the first 6 months of life because infants have iron stores at birth and the iron in human milk, though not abundant, is very well absorbed. The AI for iron from birth to 6 months is 0.27 mg/day. After 4 to 6 months, iron stores are depleted, but iron needs remain high. The RDA for infants 7 to 12 months old increases to 11 mg/day.[27] By this age, the diet of breast-fed infants should contain other sources of iron. Formula-fed infants should be fed iron-fortified formula.

Breast milk is low in vitamin D. Therefore, it is recommended that breast-fed infants receive 5 µg/day of vitamin D as drops beginning at 2 months of age and continuing until they are consuming about 500 mL (2 cups) of vitamin D-fortified formula or milk daily.[54] Infant formulas contain 10 µg of vitamin D (twice the AI) per liter of formula. Light-skinned infants can synthesize enough vitamin D if their faces are exposed to the sun for 15 minutes per day; a longer time is required for darker-skinned babies.

Infants are at risk for vitamin K deficiency because little vitamin K crosses the placenta, and the infant's gut is sterile, so there are no bacteria to synthesize this vitamin. Because lack of vitamin K can cause bleeding, it is recommended that all newborns receive an intramuscular injection containing 0.5 to 1.0 mg of vitamin K,[55] which provides enough of the vitamin to last until the intestines have been colonized with bacteria that synthesize it.

Fluoride is important for tooth development, even before the teeth erupt. Breast milk is low in fluoride, and formula manufacturers use unfluoridated water in preparing liquid formula. Therefore, breast-fed infants, infants who are fed premixed formula, and those who are fed formula mixed with low-fluoride water at home are often given fluoride supplements beginning at 6 months of age. In areas where drinking water is fluoridated, infants who are fed formula reconstituted with tap water should not be given fluoride supplements.

MEETING NEEDS WITH BREAST MILK OR FORMULA

Because of its health and nutritional benefits, breast feeding is the recommended choice for the newborn of a healthy, well-nourished mother. Health professionals in the United States recommend exclusive

Breast feeding vs. formula feeding FIGURE 11.22

A After the first year, breast feeding is not necessary to meet the infant's nutrient needs, but in developing nations, where other foods offered to young children are nutrient poor, breast feeding after the first year helps prevent malnutrition. The World Health Organization recommends breast feeding for 2 years or more.[58] In both developed and developing nations, breast feeding after the first year continues to provide nutrition, comfort, and an emotional bond between mother and child.

breast feeding for the first 6 months of life and breast feeding with complementary foods for at least the first year and as long thereafter as mutually desired (FIGURE 11.22).[56,57] As infants begin consuming other foods, their demand for milk is reduced, and milk production decreases, but lactation can continue as long as suckling is maintained.

Whether they are breast fed or formula fed, young infants should be fed frequently, on demand. For breast-fed infants, a feeding should last approximately 10 to 15 minutes at each breast. Bottle-fed newborns may consume only a few ounces at each feeding; as the infant grows, the amount consumed will increase to 4 to 8 ounces. A well-fed newborn, whether breast fed or bottle fed, should urinate enough to soak six to eight diapers a day and gain about 0.15 to 0.23 kg (0.33 to 0.5 lb)/week.

Nutrients in breast milk and formula

Human milk is tailored to meet the needs of human infants. The composition of milk changes continuously to suit the needs of a growing infant. The first milk, called **colostrum**, which is produced by the breast for up to a week after delivery, has beneficial effects on the gastrointestinal tract, acting as a laxative that helps the baby excrete the thick, mucusy stool produced during

colostrum
The first milk, produced by the breast late in pregnancy and for up to a week after delivery. Compared to mature milk, it contains more water, protein, immune factors, minerals, and vitamins and less fat.

B During bottle feeding, the infant's head should be higher than its stomach, and the bottle should be tilted so that there is no air in the nipple. Just as breast-fed infants alternate breasts, bottle-fed infants should be held alternately on the left and right sides to promote equal development of the head and neck muscles.

C Infants should never be put to bed with a bottle because saliva flow decreases during sleep, and the formula remains in contact with the teeth for many hours. This causes **nursing bottle syndrome**, rapid and serious decay of the upper teeth. Usually the lower teeth are protected by the tongue.

life in the womb. Colostrum looks watery, but the nutrients it supplies meet the infant's needs until mature milk production begins. Mature breast milk contains an appropriate balance of nutrients in forms that are easily digested and absorbed. Infant formulas try to replicate human milk as closely as possible in order to match the growth, nutrient absorption, and other benefits associated with breast feeding (**TABLE 11.4**).

Nutritional composition of breast milk and infant formula TABLE 11.4

Nutrient	Amount in breast milk	Amount in formula	Comparisons
Protein (g/100 mL)	1.8	1.4	The relatively low protein content of human milk and formula protects the immature kidneys from a too-high load of nitrogen wastes. Alpha-lactalbumin, the predominant protein in human milk, forms a soft, easily digested curd in the infant's stomach. Most formula is made from cow's milk, modified to mimic the protein concentration and amino acid composition of human milk.
Fat (g/100 mL)	4	4.8	The fat in human milk is easily digested. Human milk is high in cholesterol and the essential fatty acids linoleic acid and α-linolenic acid, as well as their long-chain derivatives arachidonic acid and DHA, which are essential for normal brain development, eyesight, and growth. The fat in formula is derived from vegetable oils and provides linoleic and α-linolenic acid. Some formulas are also supplemented with arachiconic acid and DHA.
Carbohydrate (g/100 mL)	7	7.3	Lactose, the primary carbohydrate in human milk and most formula, enhances calcium absorption. Because it is digested slowly, it stimulates the growth of beneficial acid-producing bacteria.
Sodium (mg/100 mL)	1.3	0.7	Because breast milk and formula are both low in sodium, the fluid needs of breast-fed and formula-fed infants can be met without an excessive load on the kidneys.
Calcium (mg/100 mL)	22	53	The 2:1 ratio of calcium to phosphorus in breast milk and formula enhances calcium absorption.
Phosphorus (mg/100 mL)	14	38	
Iron (mg/100 mL)	0.03	0.1	Iron and zinc are present in limited amounts in breast milk but are readily absorbed.[56] Most infant formulas are fortified with iron and zinc because the forms present are less absorbable than those in breast milk.
Zinc (mg/100 mL)	3.2	5.1	
Vitamin D (IU/100 mL)	4	41	Formulas are fortified with vitamin D, which is present at low levels in breast milk.

Health benefits of breast feeding Despite a nutritional profile that is similar, infant formula can never exactly duplicate the composition of human milk. Antibody proteins and immune-system cells pass from the mother to her child in the breast milk, providing immune protection for the infant.[59] A number of enzymes and other proteins in breast milk prevent the growth of harmful microorganisms, and several of the carbohydrates in breast milk protect against viruses that cause diarrhea. One substance favors the growth of the beneficial bacterium *Lactobacillus bifidus* in the infant's colon; this bacterium inhibits the growth of disease-causing organisms. Growth factors and hormones present in human milk promote maturation of the infant's gut and immune defenses and enhance digestion.

Breast-fed babies have fewer allergies, ear infections, respiratory illnesses, and urinary tract infections than do formula-fed babies, and they are less likely to suffer from constipation and diarrhea. There is also evidence that breast feeding reduces the risk of SIDS and may also reduce the risk that a child will develop asthma, chronic digestive diseases, obesity, type 1 and 2 diabetes, and childhood leukemia.[60] In addition, the strong suckling required for breast feeding aids in the development of the facial muscles, thus contributing to speech development and correct formation of the teeth. Also, breast-fed babies are unlikely to be overfed because the amount of milk consumed cannot be monitored visually. Caregivers often mistakenly encourage infants to finish every bottle rather than respond to cues that the infant is full. This tendency can result in overfeeding and excess weight gain in bottle-fed infants.

For the mother, breast feeding can be a relaxing, emotionally enjoyable interaction that strengthens the bond between her and the infant. It is less expensive than formula feeding and more convenient because it involves less equipment and preparation. In addition, breast feeding causes uterine contractions that help the uterus return to its normal size more quickly after delivery. Although the effect of breast feeding on maternal weight loss is unclear, there is evidence that women who breast feed may have a lower risk of developing type 2 diabetes and breast and ovarian cancers.[60] Breast feeding also inhibits ovulation, lengthening the time between pregnancies; however, because it does not always prevent ovulation, breast feeding cannot be relied on for birth control.

When is formula feeding better? Despite the benefits of breast milk, formula feeding may be the best option in some cases. Common illnesses such as colds and skin infections are not passed to the infant in breast milk, but tuberculosis, cytomegalovirus, and HIV infection are.[59,61] Some drugs can also pass from the mother to the baby in breast milk, which means that women who are taking medications should check with their physician about whether it is safe to breast feed. Because alcohol and drugs such as cocaine and marijuana can be passed to a baby in breast milk, alcoholic and drug-addicted mothers are counseled not to breast feed. Nicotine from cigarette smoke is also rapidly transferred from maternal blood to milk, and heavy smoking may decrease the supply of milk.

Although alcoholic mothers are counseled not to breast feed, occasional limited alcohol consumption while breast feeding is probably not harmful if alcohol intake is timed so as to minimize the amount present in milk when the infant is fed. Alcohol is most concentrated an hour after consumption and is cleared from the milk at about the same rate at which it disappears from the bloodstream.

Feeding an infant with formula requires more preparation and washing than breast feeding, but it can give the mother a break because other family members can share the responsibility. For preterm infants and those with genetic abnormalities, formula may be the best option because there are special formulas to meet these infants' unique needs. If an infant is too small or weak to take a bottle, pumped breast milk or formula can be fed through a tube.

SAFE FEEDING FOR THE FIRST YEAR

Whether infants are breast fed or formula fed, care must be taken to ensure that their needs are met and their food is safe. If proper measurements are not used in preparing formula, the infant can receive an excess or a deficiency of nutrients and an improper ratio of nutrients to fluid (FIGURE 11.23A). If the water and equipment used in preparing formula are not clean or if the prepared formula is left unrefrigerated, food-borne illness may result. Because sanitation is often lacking in developing nations, infections that lead to diarrhea and dehydration occur more frequently in formula-fed infants than in breast-fed infants. Bacterial contamination is not a concern when a baby is breast fed, but care must be taken to avoid contamination when milk is pumped from the breast and stored for later feedings (FIGURE 11.23B).

A concern that is unique to feeding breast milk is that substances in the maternal diet may pass into the milk and cause adverse reactions in the infant. For example, caffeine in the mother's diet can make the infant jittery and excitable, so a mother should avoid consuming large amounts of caffeine while breast feeding. Most of these reactions seem to be unique to a particular mother and child, so as long as a food does not affect the infant's health or response to feeding, it can be included in the mother's diet.

Food allergies

Food allergies are common in infants because their digestive tracts are immature and therefore allow the absorption of incompletely digested proteins, which trigger a response from the immune system (see Chapters 3 and 6). After about 3 months of age, the risk of developing food allergies is reduced because incompletely digested proteins are less likely to be absorbed. Many children who develop food allergies before age 3 years eventually outgrow them. Allergies that appear after 3 years of age are more likely to be a problem throughout the individual's life.

Exclusive breast feeding for the first 4 to 6 months reduces an infant's risk of developing a food allergy.[62] If a formula-fed baby becomes allergic to the milk proteins used in the formula, soy formulas should be used. For infants who cannot tolerate soy protein, formulas made from predigested proteins are an option.

Appropriate introduction of solid and semisolid foods can reduce the risk of an infant developing food allergies. The most commonly recommended first food is iron-fortified infant rice cereal mixed with formula or breast milk because this cereal is easily digested and rarely causes allergic reactions. After rice has been successfully included in the diet, other grains can be introduced, with wheat cereal given last because it is most likely to cause an allergic reaction. Each new food should be offered for a few days without the addition of any other new foods. If an allergic reaction occurs, it is then easier to determine that the newly introduced food caused it. Foods that cause symptoms such as rashes, digestive upsets, or respiratory problems should be discontinued, and the symptoms should no longer be present before any other new foods are added.

Safe infant feeding FIGURE 11.23

A To avoid bacterial contamination, wash hands before preparing formula. Clean bottles and nipples by washing them in a dishwasher or placing them in boiling water for 5 minutes. Boil water for 1 to 2 minutes and cool it before using it to mix powdered formula or dilute concentrates. Cover and refrigerate opened cans of ready-to-feed and liquid concentrate formula and use the formula within the period indicated on the can. Prepare formula immediately before a feeding and discard any excess. ▼

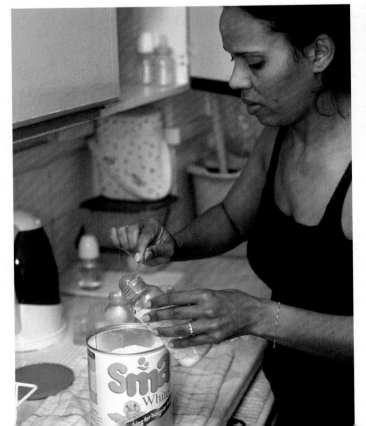

B When breast feeding isn't possible milk can be pumped from ▲ the breast and fed from a bottle. To ensure the safety of pumped milk, wash hands, breast pumps, bottles, and nipples. Breast milk that is not immediately fed to the baby can be kept refrigerated for 24 to 48 hours. Warming breast milk in a microwave is not recommended because microwaving destroys some of its immune properties and may result in dangerously hot milk. The best way to warm milk is by running warm water over the bottle.

Nutrition for Infants   393

Developmentally appropriate foods

Foods that are offered to infants should be appropriate for their digestive and developmental abilities (see Figure 11.20). Cow's milk should never be fed to infants because it is too high in protein and too low in iron.[63] At 1 year of age, whole cow's milk can be offered; it can be used until 2 years of age, after which reduced-fat or low-fat milk can be used. As a child becomes familiar with more variety, food choices should be made from each of the food groups. To avoid choking, foods that can easily lodge in the throat, such as carrots, grapes, and hot dogs, should not be offered to infants or toddlers.

Fruit juice can be fed from a cup when an infant is 9 to 10 months old, but excess quantities of apple and pear juice should be avoided because they contain sorbitol, a poorly absorbed sugar alcohol that can cause diarrhea. The American Academy of Pediatrics recommends that infants not be given juice at bedtime or offered juice from bottles or covered cups that allow them to consume juice easily throughout the day.[64] Added sugars should be offered in moderation to ensure a nutrient-dense diet. Honey should not be fed to children less than 1 year old because it may contain spores of *Clostridium botulinum*, the bacterium that causes botulism poisoning (discussed in Chapter 13). Older children and adults are not at risk from botulism spores because the environment in a mature gastrointestinal tract prevents the bacteria from growing.

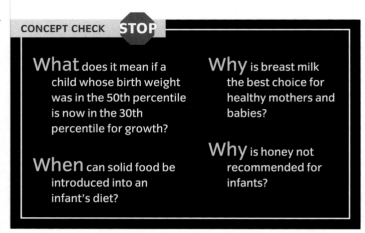

CONCEPT CHECK STOP

What does it mean if a child whose birth weight was in the 50th percentile is now in the 30th percentile for growth?

When can solid food be introduced into an infant's diet?

Why is breast milk the best choice for healthy mothers and babies?

Why is honey not recommended for infants?

SUMMARY

1 Changes in the Body During Pregnancy

1. During the first 8 weeks of development, all the organ systems necessary for life are formed in the **embryo**. Over the remaining weeks of pregnancy, the **fetus** grows, and organs develop and mature. The **placenta** transfers nutrients and oxygen from maternal blood to fetal blood and removes wastes from the fetus. At birth, a healthy baby weighs 3 to 4 kg (6.5 to 9 lbs). **Low-birth-weight** infants and infants who are **large for gestational age** are at increased risk of health problems.

2. During pregnancy, the mother's body undergoes many changes to support the pregnancy and prepare for **lactation**. Recommended weight gain during pregnancy is 11 to 16 kg (25 to 35 lbs) for normal-weight women. Too little or too much weight gain can place both mother and baby at risk, but weight loss should never be attempted during pregnancy. Normal-weight, underweight, overweight, and obese mothers should gain weight at a steady rate during pregnancy, but the total amount of weight gain recommended is different depending on prepregnancy weight.

3. During healthy pregnancies, moderate-intensity exercise that does not increase the risk of abdominal trauma, falls, or joint stress can be beneficial and safe.

4. The hormones that direct changes in maternal physiology and fetal growth and development sometimes cause unwanted side effects, including **edema**, **morning sickness**, heartburn, constipation, and hemorrhoids.

5. **Hypertensive disorders of pregnancy** increase risk for the mother and baby. **Gestational hypertension** involves an increase in blood pressure during pregnancy. **Preeclampsia** is a more severe condition, characterized by edema, weight gain, and protein in the urine and can progress to life-threatening **eclampsia**. High blood glucose in the mother, called **gestational diabetes**, results in babies who are large for gestational age because extra glucose crosses the placenta from mother to baby.

2 Nutritional Needs During Pregnancy

1. During pregnancy, the requirements for energy, protein, carbohydrate, essential fatty acids, water, and many vitamins and minerals increase above nonpregnant levels.

2. The AI for calcium is not increased because the increased need during pregnancy is met by an increase in absorption. Vitamin D deficiency is a concern, particularly for darker-skinned women. Adequate folic acid early in pregnancy reduces the risk of neural tube defects. Iron needs are high, and deficiency is common during pregnancy.

3. MyPyramid for Pregnancy and Breastfeeding can help pregnant women select foods to meet their nutritional needs. A prenatal supplement containing iron and folic acid and other vitamins and minerals is generally prescribed for all pregnant women.

4. Food cravings are common during pregnancy. Most are harmless, but **pica** can reduce the intake of nutrient-dense foods, inhibit nutrient absorption, increase the risk of consuming toxins and infectious organisms, and cause intestinal obstructions.

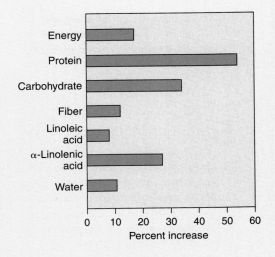

3 Factors That Increase the Risks Associated with Pregnancy

1. The rapidly developing embryo and fetus are susceptible to damage from poor nutrition and physical, chemical, or other environmental **teratogens**. Malnutrition during pregnancy can cause fetal growth retardation, low infant birth weight, birth defects, premature birth, spontaneous abortion, and stillbirth.

2. Pregnant teenagers are at increased risk because they are still growing themselves. Women over age 35 are at increased risk because they are more likely to have preexisting health conditions and to develop gestational diabetes, pregnancy-induced hypertension, or other complications during pregnancy.

3. Excessive caffeine intake can increase the risk of miscarriage. Following guidelines on fish consumption can minimize exposure to mercury, which can cause brain damage in a fetus.

Pregnant women are particularly susceptible to food-borne illness and should follow safe food handling recommendations. Alcohol consumption during pregnancy is a leading cause of brain damage and other birth defects. Exposure to cigarette smoke causes low birth weight and increases the risk of stillbirth, preterm delivery, and behavioral problems in the baby. The use of illegal drugs such as cocaine also increases the risk of low birth weight and birth defects.

4 Lactation

1. Milk production and **let-down** are triggered by hormones released in response to the suckling of an infant.

2. Lactation requires energy and nutrients from the mother to produce adequate milk. The energy for milk production comes from the diet and maternal fat stores. Maternal needs for protein, fluid, and many vitamins and minerals are even greater during lactation than during pregnancy.

5 Nutrition for Infants

1. Growth is the best indicator of adequate nutrition in an infant. Healthy infants follow standard patterns of growth. Growth charts can be used to compare an infant's growth with the growth of infants of the same age. Slow growth indicates **failure to thrive**, whereas excess weight gain may predispose to obesity. Adequate nutrition is essential for achieving developmental milestones, and they in turn affect how an infant can obtain nourishment.

2. Infants require more calories and protein per kilogram of body weight than do individuals at any other time of life. Fat and fluid needs are also proportionately higher than in adults. Infants are at risk for deficiencies of iron, vitamin D, and vitamin K, as well as low fluoride intake.

3. Breast milk is the ideal food for infants. It meets nutrient needs; it is always available; it requires no special equipment, mixing, or sterilization; and it provides immune protection. There are many infant formulas on the market that are patterned after human milk and provide adequate nutrition to a baby. Formula is the best option when the mother is ill or is taking prescription or illicit drugs, or when the infant has special nutritional needs.

4. Introducing solid foods between 4 and 6 months of age adds iron and other nutrients to the diet. Newly introduced foods should be appropriate to the child's stage of development and offered one at a time in order to monitor for food allergies.

KEY TERMS

1. Keep a 3-day diet record. Use iProfile to analyze the nutrient composition of your diet. Would your diet meet the energy, protein, and micronutrient needs of a 25-year-old pregnant woman who is 65 inches tall, weighed 130 lbs at the start of her pregnancy, and is now in her second trimester? If not, what foods or supplements would need to be added to meet these needs?

2. Many people object to infant formula manufacturers advertising their products in developing nations. Do you feel it is appropriate to promote the use of formula in developing nations? Why or why not?

3. HIV, the virus that causes AIDS, passes via breast feeding to one out of seven infants born to HIV-infected mothers, yet in developing countries, some HIV-positive women are advised to breast feed. Explain why this might be, considering what you know about the benefits of breast feeding.

4. If an infant is born weighing 6 lbs, what should the baby weigh at 4 months of age and at 12 months? Why?

5. Chelsea, a vegan woman, has just found out she is pregnant. What nutrient deficiencies are common for vegans? for pregnant women? What supplements would you recommend Chelsea take during her pregnancy?

6. Marina, a 16-year-old, is 4 months pregnant. She is 5 ft 4 inches tall and weighed 110 pounds before she became pregnant. Her typical diet, which provided 1800 Calories, 60 g of protein, and 15 mg of iron, met her needs before she became pregnant. What changes in the amounts of energy, protein, and iron would you recommend now that Marina is in her second trimester?

What is happening in this picture ?

Supplemental nursing systems such as this one allow pumped breast milk to be fed to an infant via a tube attached near the mother's nipple. The infant suckles but does not have to work as hard to get adequate milk.

Why might an infant need to be fed in this manner?

What benefits does it offer the mother?

What benefits does it offer the infant?

(Check your answers in Appendix L.)

1. Which process is indicated by the number 5?

   a. fertilization
   b. implantation
   c. lactation
   d. ovulation

2. The function of the _____ is to transfer nutrients and oxygen from the maternal blood to the fetal blood.

   a. amniotic sac
   b. placenta
   c. uterus
   d. oviduct

3. An infant born at term, weighing 4.5 pounds at birth, is considered _____.

   a. large for gestational age
   b. premature
   c. very low birth weight
   d. low birth weight

4. Newborn infants receive an injection of _____ to prevent the possibility of hemorrhage.

   a. iron
   b. folate
   c. vitamin D
   d. vitamin K

5. Use the figure to determine how much of the weight gained during pregnancy is due to an increase in body fluids.

   a. about 4 pounds
   b. about 2 pounds
   c. as much as 10 pounds
   d. less than 4 pounds

Total	25-35 lbs
Fetus	7-8 lbs
Amniotic fluid	2 lbs
Placenta	1-2 lbs
Uterus	2 lbs
Maternal blood	3-4 lbs
Breast tissue	2 lbs
Extracellular fluids	4 lbs
Maternal fat	4-11 lbs

6. A woman who enters pregnancy with excess weight (BMI > 30) should _____.

   a. lose about 5 to 10 lbs during her pregnancy
   b. gain about 11 to 20 lbs during her pregnancy
   c. not gain any additional weight during her pregnancy
   d. limit her intake to 1200 Calories per day

7. Which of the following is not associated with preeclampsia?

   a. high blood glucose
   b. a rise in blood pressure
   c. edema
   d. protein in the urine

8. The recommended intake for which of the following is not increased during pregnancy?

a. calcium
b. iron
c. protein
d. zinc

9. During which weeks of development is exposure to a teratogen most likely to result in a heart defect in the embryo or fetus?

a. first 3 week
b. about 3 to 7 weeks
c. 7 to 8 weeks
d. any time after 9 weeks

Fertilization to implantation	Embryonic development		Fetal development

Embryonic or fetal age (weeks)   3   8   9   38

Neural tube defects affect about 1 in 1000 pregnancies. — Central nervous system

Heart defects are the most common birth defect, affecting about 1 in every 100 to 200 babies. — Heart

Extremities

Eyes

Ears

■ Indicates when damage from teratogens is likely to be greatest   Teeth

■ Indicates when damage from teratogens may be less severe   External genitalia

10. The hormone responsible for the let-down of milk is

_____.

a. estrogen
b. prolactin
c. progesterone
d. oxytocin

11. When should solid food be introduced into an infant's diet?

a. within 2 weeks of birth
b. around 4 to 6 months of age
c. at 9 months of age
d. after 1 year

12. The leading cause of preventable birth defects and intellectual disability is _____ during pregnancy.

a. coffee consumption
b. tobacco use
c. alcohol consumption
d. cocaine use

13. According to this growth chart, a 16-month-old infant who weighs 21 pounds is at about the _____ percentile for weight.

a. 5th   c. 25th
b. 10th   d. 50th

CDC Growth Charts: United States

Weight-for-age percentiles: Boys, birth to 36 months

97th 95th 90th 75th 50th 25th 10th 5th 3rd

Age (months)   Birth 3 6 9 12 15 18 21 24 27 30 33 36

SOURCE: Developed by the National Center for Health Statistics in collaboration with the Nation Center for Chronic Disease Prevention and Health Promotion (2000).

CDC
CENTER FOR DISEASE CONTROL AND PREVENTION

14. Colostrum is _____.

a. a type of infant formula that is fortified with omega-3 fatty acids
b. the first stool passed by the infant after delivery
c. the first fluid produced by the breast after delivery
d. the mature milk produced in the later part of a feeding

15. Which of the following statements about breast milk is false?

a. It contains immune factors that protect the baby from infections.
b. It provides about 50% of calories from fat.
c. It contains a high concentration of iron.
d. The proteins it contains are easily digested.

Nutrition from 1 to 100

In *As You Like It*, Shakespeare allotted a human life seven acts to be played upon the world's stage, beginning with "the infant, mewling and puking in the nurse's arms" and ending in "second childishness . . . sans teeth, sans eyes, sans taste." While our senses and abilities do diminish as we age, with proper nutrition and health maintenance, we may not quite reach the state of helplessness described by the Bard before the final curtain falls.

For "the whining schoolboy"—and girl— "with . . . shining morning face," nutrition and healthy development go hand in hand. As the adolescent becomes "the lover," then "the soldier" of young adulthood, we may think we've stopped growing, but good nutrition is still necessary to maintain health and build a solid foundation of well-being for the mature "justice, in fair round belly with good capon lin'd", Shakespeare's archetype of middle age.

Just as there are unique nutritional concerns in infancy, childhood, adolescence, and adulthood, there are nutritional issues that arise in the closing years of life, symbolized by Shakespeare in "the lean and slipper'd pantaloon . . . a world too wide for his shrunk shank." Even in Elizabethan England, poets recognized the muscle-withering aspects of old age. As one ages, physical, social, and mental changes present a new set of challenges to maintaining a healthy nutrition regimen.

Good nutrition habits adopted in our early years will serve us well through the seven acts of our own "strange eventful history."

NATIONAL GEOGRAPHIC

Nutrition for Children

N utrient intake during childhood affects health in adulthood. The foods offered to a child must supply the energy and nutrients needed for growth and development as well as for maintenance and activity. They must also be appropriate for the child's stage of physical development and suit his or her developing tastes. A nutritious, well-balanced eating pattern and an active lifestyle allow children to grow to their potential and can prevent or delay the onset of the chronic diseases that plague adults. Therefore, teaching healthy eating and exercise habits will benefit not only today's children but also tomorrow's adults.

ENERGY AND NUTRIENT NEEDS OF CHILDREN

As children grow and become more active, their requirements for energy and most nutrients increase. The average 2-year-old needs about 1000 Calories and 13 grams of protein/day. By age 6, that child needs about 1600 Calories and 19 g of protein/day.[1] The total amount of protein and energy needed continue to increase as children grow into adults; however, the amounts needed per kilogram of body weight decrease (**FIGURE 12.1**).

The recommended range of carbohydrate intake for children is the same as for adults: 45 to 65% of total energy intake. To provide enough energy to support rapid growth and development, the recommended range of fat intake is higher for children than for adults: 30 to 40% of total energy intake for 1- to 3-year-olds and 25 to 35% for 4- to 18-year-olds. As children grow, the recommended proportion of calories from fat decreases to avoid increasing the risk of developing chronic diseases.

Infants have high fluid needs, but by 1 year of age, their evaporative losses have decreased and their kidneys have matured, decreasing the loss of fluid in urine. Therefore, as with adults, in most situations children can meet their fluid needs by drinking enough to satisfy thirst.[2] Fluid needs increase with illness, when the environmental temperature is high, and when activity increases sweat losses.

Because children are smaller than adolescents and adults, the recommended amounts of most micronutrients are also smaller (see inside cover). Recommended intakes do not differ for boys and girls until about age 9, at which time sexual maturation causes differences in nutrient requirements. Like adults, children who consume a varied, nutrient-dense diet can meet all their vitamin and mineral requirements with food. However, in the United States today, diets that frequently include fast-food meals and high-sugar and high-fat snacks put many children at risk for inadequate vitamin and mineral intake.[3] Deficiencies of calcium, vitamin D, and iron are of particular concern.

Calcium, vitamin D, and bone health

Calcium intake in school-age children has been declining, primarily due to a decrease in the consumption of dairy products. Adequate calcium intake during childhood is essential for achieving maximum peak bone mass, which is important for preventing osteoporosis later in life (see Chapter 8). The AI for calcium is 500 milligrams/day for toddlers (ages 1 to 3) and 800 mg/day for young children (ages 4 to 8).[4]

Vitamin D, which is needed for calcium absorption, is also essential for bone health. Low intakes of milk combined with limited sun exposure may put many children at risk for vitamin D deficiency.[5] The AI is 5 µg/day for children, adolescents, and young adults.

Energy needs FIGURE 12.1

As children grow, their larger body size causes the total amount of energy they need to increase, but as growth slows, energy needs/kilogram of body weight decline.

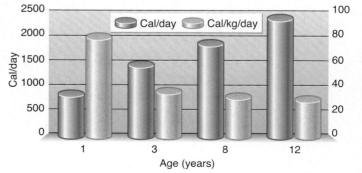

Iron and anemia Children's iron needs are high because iron is required for growth. The RDA is 7 mg/day for toddlers and 10 mg/day for young children; the latter recommendation is higher than the RDA for adult men. The high needs and finicky eating habits of young children often lead to iron deficiency anemia, a condition that can impair learning ability, intellectual performance, and stamina, as well as affect mood.[6,7] If anemia is diagnosed, iron supplements are usually prescribed until the child's iron stores have been replenished. These supplements should be kept out of the reach of children to prevent iron toxicity from supplement overdoses (see Chapter 8).

DEVELOPING HEALTHY EATING HABITS

Much of what we choose to eat as adults depends on what we learned to eat as children. Caregivers are responsible for deciding what foods should be offered to a child and when, and where they should be eaten. The child must then decide whether to eat, what foods to eat, and how much to consume.[8] As children grow older, their choices are increasingly affected by social activities, what they see at school, and what their friends are eating.

What to offer?
Children should be offered a balanced and varied diet that is adequate in energy and essential nutrients and is appropriate to their developmental needs. A healthy meal plan is based on whole grains, vegetables, and fruits; includes adequate milk and other high-protein foods; and contains moderate amounts of fat and sodium. MyPyramid for Kids can be used as a guide for meeting these dietary goals (Figure 12.2).

MyPyramid for kids Figure 12.2

MyPyramid for kids uses child-friendly graphics to recommend amounts of food from each group. The recommendations shown here are for a 3-year-old and an 8-year-old who engage in more than 60 minutes of activity daily. Food choices to meet these amounts should be spread throughout the meals and snacks served each day.

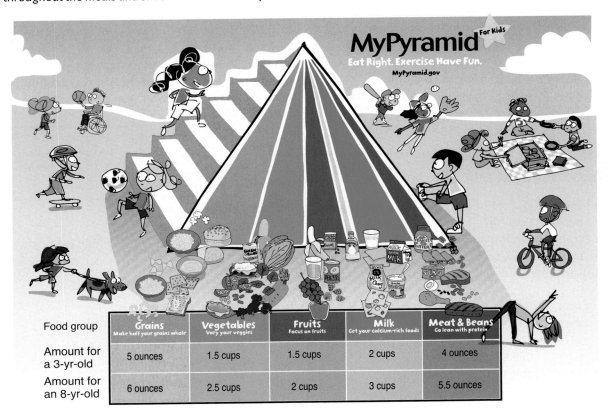

Food group	Grains Make half your grains whole	Vegetables Vary your veggies	Fruits Focus on fruits	Milk Get your calcium-rich foods	Meat & Beans Go lean with protein
Amount for a 3-yr-old	5 ounces	1.5 cups	1.5 cups	2 cups	4 ounces
Amount for an 8-yr-old	6 ounces	2.5 cups	2 cups	3 cups	5.5 ounces

Limiting juice consumption
FIGURE 12.3

Because of the sweet taste of juice, overconsumption is a concern. Drinking too much juice, even if it is 100% juice, can cause diarrhea, over- or undernutrition, and dental caries. It is recommended that juice not be offered to children in containers that can be carried around, encouraging continuous sipping.[9]

It isn't always easy to persuade a child to eat a variety of foods from all the food groups, as recommended by MyPyramid. To increase variety, new foods should be introduced into a child's diet regularly. Children's food preferences are learned through repeated exposure to foods; a new food may need to be offered 8 or 10 times before the child will accept it. Children are also more likely to eat a new food if it is introduced at the beginning of a meal, when the child is hungry, and if the child sees his or her parents or peers eating it. Incorporating healthy foods into familiar dishes can also increase the variety of the diet. Vegetables can be added to soups and casseroles, for example, and lean meats can be added to spaghetti sauce, stews, or pizza. Getting children to consume the recommended amount of fruit is usually not difficult, but most

servings should come from fruit, with limited amounts from 100% juice, not fruit drinks or cocktails. The American Academy of Pediatrics recommends limiting juice to 4 to 6 ounces/day for children ages 1 to 6 and 8 to 12 oz for children age 7 and older (**FIGURE 12.3**).[9]

No matter how erratic children's food intake may be, caregivers should continue to offer a variety of healthy foods at each meal and let children select what and how much they will eat. Children, like adults, tend to eat greater quantities when larger portions are provided.[10] When children are allowed to serve themselves, they eat more appropriate portions than they do when a large portion is put in front of them.

The best indicator that a child is receiving adequate nourishment, neither too little nor too much, is a normal growth pattern. Growth is most rapid in the first year of life, when an infant's length increases by 50%, or about 10 inches. In the second year of life, children generally grow about 5 inches; in the third year, 4 inches; and thereafter, about 2 to 3 inches/year. Although growth often occurs in spurts, growth patterns are predictable and can be monitored by comparing a child's growth pattern with standard patterns shown on growth charts (Appendix B).[11] The stature a child will eventually attain is affected by genetic, environmental, and lifestyle factors. A child whose parents are 5 feet tall may not have the genetic potential to grow to 6 feet.

When a child does not get enough to eat, weight gain slows, and if the deficiency continues, growth in height slows. If food intake is excessive, a child is at risk for becoming obese and developing the chronic diseases that are increasingly common in American adults (see *What Should I Eat?*).

WHAT SHOULD I EAT?   **Childhood**

Use iProfile to find snacks that are high in iron.

Serve children frequent nutritious meals and snacks
- Smear peanut butter on a banana or an apple.
- Offer some carrots with yogurt dip.
- Try to have at least four colors in every meal.
- Cut and arrange foods in interesting shapes.

Sneak in more fruits and vegetables
- Bake bananas and berries into breads and muffins.
- Add vegetables to soups, tacos, and casseroles.
- Blend fruit into shakes and smoothies.
- Mix extra vegetables into spaghetti sauce.

Include calcium where you can
- Have macaroni and cheese.
- Make oatmeal with milk rather than water.
- Make cream soup by adding milk.
- Serve pudding and custard.

Add iron
- Make your spaghetti sauce with meat.
- Cook your stew in an iron pot.
- Beef up your tacos and burritos.
- Serve iron-fortified breakfast cereal.

Breakfast and School Performance

This breakfast looks appealing, but regardless of what's on the table, many children and teens do not make time for breakfast; they are more likely to skip breakfast than to skip any other meal.[12] What a scientist sees is the impact breakfast has on nutritional status and school performance. Skipping breakfast may result in a span of 15 or more hours without food. Because breakfast provides energy and nutrients to the brain, children who skip it are more likely to have academic, emotional, and behavioral problems than those who eat breakfast.[13] Studies have found that compared with nonbreakfast eaters, children who participate in school breakfast programs have better nutrient intakes, and these improvements in nutrient intakes are associated with improvements in academic performance, reductions in hyperactivity, better psycho-social behaviors, and less absence and tardiness (see graph).[14] In addition to enhancing learning by fueling the brain after the overnight fast, in what other ways might breakfast contribute to better school performance?

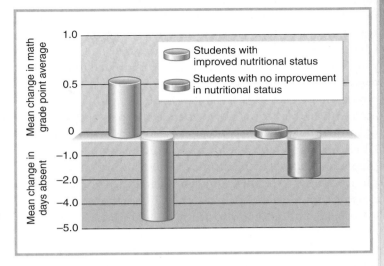

Implementation of a free school breakfast program in the Boston Public Schools improved the nutritional status of many students. Those whose nutritional status improved showed greater improvements in math grades and fewer school absences than students whose nutritional status was not improved.[14]

When and where to offer meals and snacks Because children have small stomachs and high nutrient needs, they need to consume small, nutrient-dense meals and snacks, ideally every two to three hours throughout the day. Establishing a consistent meal pattern is important because children thrive on routine and feel secure when they know what to expect. Starting the day with a good breakfast is particularly important; children who eat breakfast are more likely to meet their daily nutrient needs and do better in school (see *What a Scientist Sees*).[12] Snacks should be as nutritious as meals to ensure that nutrient needs are met (TABLE 12.1).

Typical meal and snack patterns for 3- and 8-year-old children TABLE 12.1

Food	Amount		Food	Amount	
	3-Year-Old	**8-Year-Old**		**3-Year-Old**	**8-Year-Old**
Breakfast			**Snack**		
Cereal	1/2 cup	1 cup	Yogurt	1/2 cup	1 cup
Milk, 2%	1/2 cup	1 cup	Berries	3/8 cup	3/4 cup
Banana	1/2 medium	1 medium			
			Dinner		
Snack			Rice	1/2 cup	1 cup
Peanut butter	2 Tbsp	2 Tbsp	Chicken drumsticks	1	2
Wheat crackers	5	5	Broccoli	4 florets	6 florets
			Milk, 2%	1/2 cup	1 cup
Lunch			Ice cream	1/2 cup	1/2 cup
Vegetable soup	1/2 cup	1 cup			
Grilled tuna sandwich	half	1	**Snack**		
Tomato	1/4 medium	1/2 medium	Graham crackers	1	2
Orange	1/2 medium	1 medium	Milk	1/2 cup	1/2 cup
Milk, 2%	1/2 cup	1 cup			

The setting in which a meal is consumed is also important. Children who eat dinner with their families have a higher-quality diet than those who don't.[15] Children learn by example; therefore, the eating patterns, attitudes, and feeding styles of their caregivers influence what they learn to eat. When meals are shared and caregivers make healthy food choices, children are likely to follow their example. Eating meals together also helps children connect with family and culture and is associated with better school performance and decreased risk of unhealthy weight loss practices and substance abuse. Children need companionship, conversation, and a pleasant location at mealtimes. They should be given plenty of time to finish eating. Slow eaters are unlikely to finish eating if they are abandoned by siblings who run off to play and adults who leave to wash dishes. Moreover, if mealtime is to be a nutritious, educational, and enjoyable experience, it should not be a battle zone. Food is not a reward or a punishment: It is simply nutrition.

Meals at day care or school

It is not easy to ensure that meals eaten away from home are nutritious because there is no guarantee that what is served at school or brought from home will be eaten. A packed lunch should contain foods that the child likes and that do not require refrigeration. For children who do not bring meals from home, federal school breakfast and lunch programs provide free or low-cost meals containing age-appropriate foods.

The goals of the **National School Lunch Program** are to improve the dietary intake and nutritional health of children in the United States and to promote nutrition education by teaching children to make appropriate food choices.[16] Each meal includes servings of milk, high-protein foods, vegetables, fruit, and grains and must provide one-third of the RDA for protein, vitamin A, vitamin C, iron, calcium, and energy and contain no more than 30% of energy from fat and 10% from saturated fat. In addition to lunches, federal guidelines regulate foods sold at snack bars and in vending machines that compete with school lunch programs. These must provide at least 5% of the RDA for one or more of the following: protein, vitamin A, vitamin C, niacin, riboflavin, calcium, and iron. An analysis of the foods students choose to eat from the meal offered found that students who participated in the school lunch program consumed more vegetables, milk and milk products, and meat and meat substitutes, and fewer soft drinks and/or fruit drinks than did nonparticipants.[17]

NUTRITION AND HEALTH CONCERNS IN CHILDREN

The diets of U.S. children today are not as healthy as they could be, and as a result children are not as healthy as they could be (**FIGURE 12.4**). Some of the nutrition and health concerns regarding children in the United States are related to their dietary and exercise patterns. The high-calorie, high-salt, high-saturated-fat diet and low-activity lifestyle that contribute to obesity and chronic disease in adults are having the same effects in children. Other nutrition-related health concerns in children include dental caries and lead poisoning.

The rising rate of childhood obesity

It is estimated that more than 16% of U.S. children and adolescents ages 2 through 19 are obese.[18] Along with obesity come a number of other chronic conditions, including type 2 diabetes, high blood pressure, and elevated blood cholesterol, as well as social and psychological challenges (**FIGURE 12.5**).[19,20]

How good are children's diets? FIGURE 12.4

Only a small percentage of children in the United States have "good" diets, based on how well they meet the recommendations of MyPyramid. Most American children consume too few fruits and vegetables and whole grains and too much fat, salt, and sugar. As children grow older, their diets worsen.

Body mass index-for-age percentiles: Boys, 2 to 20 years percentile

A 10-year old boy with a BMI of 23 would be in the obese category (95th percentile or greater).

A 10-year old boy with a BMI of 21 would be in the overweight category (85th to less than 95th percentile).

A 10-year old boy with a BMI of 18 would be in the healthy weight category (5th percentile to less than 85th percentile).

A 10-year old boy with a BMI of 13 would be in the underweight category (less than 5th percentile).

95th percentile
85th percentile
5th percentile

Age (years)

◀ A child's weight is assessed by determining his or her BMI and plotting it on a gender-specific BMI-for-age growth chart to determine his or her percentile (see Chapter 11). The BMI percentile is then used to classify the child as obese, overweight, healthy weight, or underweight.[21]

1988–1994
1999–2002
2003–2006

▲ Results from the National Health and Nutrition Examination Surveys illustrate the increase in the percentage of children who are obese over the past 20 years.[18,22,23]

▲ Obese children are frequently ridiculed and teased; this may result in a poor self-image, low self-esteem, and social isolation. Social isolation, in turn, results in boredom, depression, inactivity, and withdrawal—all of which can increase eating and decrease activity, worsening the problem.

◀ Obese children are at risk for type 2 diabetes, high blood cholesterol levels, and elevated blood pressure.

Type 2 diabetes is a progressive disease that increases in severity over time. The longer an individual has diabetes, the greater the risk of complications that can lead to blindness, kidney failure, heart disease, or amputations (see Chapter 4).[19]

Elevated blood cholesterol levels during childhood and adolescence (170 mg/100 milliliters or greater) are associated with higher blood cholesterol and higher mortality rates from cardiovascular disease in adulthood. The American Academy of Pediatrics recommends blood cholesterol monitoring for children and teenagers with a family history of heart disease or high blood cholesterol.[24]

Children who have blood pressure at the high end of normal are more likely to develop high blood pressure as adults. As with adults, blood pressure can be affected by the amount of body fat, the total pattern of dietary intake, including sodium intake, and activity level.

Addressing the issue of excess weight in children requires changes in both eating and activity patterns. Because children are still growing, weight loss is rarely recommended. Rather, overweight children should be encouraged to slow their weight gain while they continue to grow taller. This allows them to "grow into" their weight. A child who is at the 85th percentile for BMI at age 7 and gains only a few pounds a year can be at the 75th percentile by age 9.

It can be difficult to modify a child's food consumption patterns. Denying food may promote further overeating by making the child feel that he or she will not obtain enough to satisfy hunger. Thus, restrictions on food intake should be relatively mild, and the focus instead should be on offering nutrient-dense foods. As with adults, the Dietary Guidelines and the DRIs recommend that children be physically active for at least an hour per day. This may be difficult for overweight children, who are often embarrassed by their bodies and shy away from group activities.

Increases in physical activity need to be gradual in order to make exercise a positive experience. A good way to start is to limit time spent watching television and playing video and computer games and encourage active games, walks after dinner, bike rides, hikes, swimming, volleyball, and other activities that the whole family can enjoy together. Learning to enjoy sports and exercise in childhood will set the stage for an active lifestyle in adulthood.

Watching television has a major influence on children's energy balance because it affects both food intake and activity level (**FIGURE 12.6** and the *Case Study*). Sitting in front of the television encourages snacking and reduces activity. Television also affects the quality of the diet because commercials introduce children to foods to which they might otherwise not be exposed. Children who view food ads choose those food products more often than children who are not exposed to the ads.[25]

Keeping teeth healthy: Preventing dental caries
A diet that is high in sugary foods promotes the formation of dental caries (see Chapter 4). Because the primary teeth guide the growth of the permanent teeth, maintaining healthy primary teeth is just as important as preserving the permanent ones. Much of the added sugar in children's diets comes from soft drinks and other sweetened beverages; when these are sipped slowly between meals, the duration of the contact between sugar and bacteria on the surface of the teeth is prolonged, increasing the risk of tooth decay.

Hyperactivity
Hyperactivity is a problem in 5 to 10% of school-age children, occurring more frequently in boys than in girls. Hyperactivity involves extreme physical activity, excitability, impulsiveness, distractibility, short attention span, and low tolerance for frustration. Hyperactive children have more difficulty learning but usually are of normal or above-average intelligence.

Television affects food intake and activity level FIGURE 12.6

A Hours spent watching television are hours when physical activity is at a minimum. Children who watch four or more hours of TV per day are 40% more likely to be overweight than those who watch an hour or less a day.[26] ▼

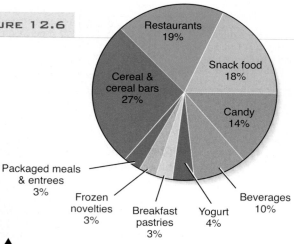

Restaurants 19%
Snack food 18%
Cereal & cereal bars 27%
Candy 14%
Packaged meals & entrees 3%
Frozen novelties 3%
Breakfast pastries 3%
Yogurt 4%
Beverages 10%

▲
B During children's television programming, food is the most frequently advertised product category. This pie chart, which illustrates the types of food advertised on Saturday morning children's television programming, shows that almost half of the commercials advertise candy, snack foods, beverages, and pastries.[27]

UNDER- AND OVERNUTRITION

Sam is 8 years old and has gained 5 pounds in the past three months. His parents are worried because all Sam wants to do is watch TV. Because Sam's parents are both overweight, they are concerned that he will also have a weight problem, so they take him to see their pediatrician.

Based on this growth chart, how has Sam's BMI percentile changed over the past year?

▼

CDC Growth Charts: United States

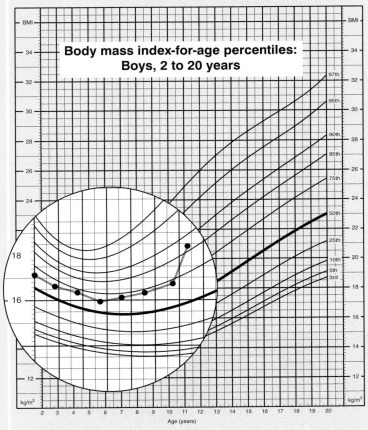

Body mass index-for-age percentiles:
Boys, 2 to 20 years

Your answer:

Reviewing Sam's diet and exercise patterns, the doctor learns that Sam has been watching TV or playing video games for about six hours a day. A recall of his intake shows that he eats doughnuts and milk for breakfast, gets lunch from the school lunch program, and then snacks so much on chips and candy when he gets home from school that he doesn't really eat dinner. He likes fruit, refuses to eat vegetables, and drinks 5 to 6 cups of whole milk daily.

What nutrients are likely to be excessive or deficient in this dietary pattern?

▼

Your answer:

A blood test reveals that Sam has iron deficiency anemia. The pediatrician prescribes an iron supplement and refers Sam and his parents to a dietitian. She recommends that the family switch to 1% milk to reduce Sam's energy and saturated fat intake and to a fortified cereal for breakfast to increase his iron intake, and that they limit Sam's after-school snacking to fruit so he can eat a better evening meal.

Why might excessive consumption of dairy products contribute to Sam's anemia?

▼

Your answer:

How might Sam's iron deficiency have contributed to his weight gain?

▼

Your answer:

(Check your answers in Appendix K.)

Hyperactivity is now considered part of a larger syndrome known as **attention-deficit/ hyperactivity disorder (ADHD)**.

A popular misconception is that hyperactivity is caused by eating sugar, but research on sugar intake and behavior has failed to support this hypothesis.[28,29] The hyperactive behavior observed after sugar consumption is more likely the result of situational factors. For example, the excitement of a birthday party rather than the sugar in the cake is most likely the cause of hyperactive behavior.

Other possible causes of hyperactivity include caffeine consumption, lack of sleep, overstimulation, desire for more attention, or lack of physical activity. Specific foods and food additives have also been implicated as causes of hyperactivity. Numerous studies have failed to provide sufficient evidence for the efficacy of any dietary treatment for ADHD. However, some children are sensitive to specific additives and may benefit from a diet that eliminates them.[29]

Lead toxicity

Lead is an environmental contaminant that can be toxic, especially in children under age 6. Children can be exposed to lead in air pollution, old house paint, lead plumbing, and certain ceramics. Children are at particular risk for lead toxicity because they absorb lead much more efficiently than do adults.[30] Once it has been absorbed from the gastrointestinal tract, lead circulates in the bloodstream and then accumulates in the bones and, to a lesser extent, the brain, teeth, and kidneys. Lead disrupts the functioning of neurotransmitters and thus interferes with the functioning of the nervous system.

In young children, lead poisoning can cause learning disabilities and behavior problems.[31,32] There is evidence that even blood lead levels below 10 microgram/ 100 ml, which were once thought to be safe, may impair IQ in young children.[32] Higher levels of lead can contribute to iron deficiency anemia, changes in kidney function, nervous system changes, and even seizures, coma, and death.

Because of the risks of lead toxicity from environmental contamination, lead is no longer used in house paint, gasoline, or solder. As a result, the number of children ages 1 to 5 with elevated blood lead levels decreased from 77.8% in 1976–1980 to only 1.6% in 1999–2002.[31]

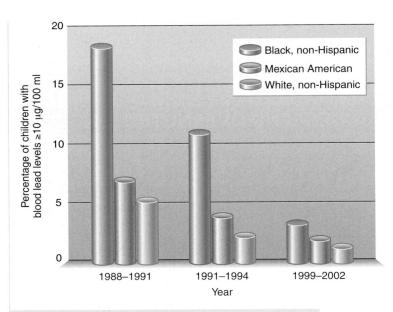

Percentage of children with elevated levels of lead in the blood FIGURE 12.7

Minority children are at higher risk for lead toxicity than others, partly due to differences in socioeconomic status.[31] Low-income children often live in older buildings that still have lead paint and plumbing. They are more likely to be malnourished, which increases their risk because lead is absorbed better from an empty stomach and when other minerals, such as calcium, zinc, and iron, are deficient.

Despite these gains, certain ethnic groups remain at higher risk of elevated blood lead levels than others (FIGURE 12.7). The effects of lead poisoning are permanent, but if high levels are detected early, the lead can be removed with medical treatment. Most children in the United States are at sufficient risk of lead exposure that they should have their blood lead concentration measured at least once.[33]

CONCEPT CHECK STOP

How do children's energy and protein requirements change as they age?

What factors affect children's food choices?

How does television viewing affect eating and exercise patterns?

Why is lead toxicity more common in low-income children than in others?

Nutrition for Adolescents

LEARNING OBJECTIVES

Describe how growth and body composition are affected by puberty.

Compare the energy needs of adolescents with those of children and adults.

Explain why iron and calcium are of particular concern during the teen years.

Use MyPyramid to plan a day's diet that would appeal to a teenager.

A dolescents are a unique population in many ways, and they have unique nutritional needs. The physical, emotional, mental, and social changes of adolescence transform a child into an adult. Organ systems develop and grow, **puberty** occurs, body

> **puberty** A period of rapid growth and physical changes that ends in the attainment of sexual maturity.

composition changes, and the growth rates and nutritional requirements of boys and girls diverge (**FIGURE 12.8**). The physiological changes associated with sexual maturation affect nutrient requirements, and social and psychological changes that occur during adolescence influence nutrient intakes.

Visualizing

Adolescent growth FIGURE 12.8

The **adolescent growth spurt** is an 18- to 24-month period of peak growth velocity that begins at about ages 10 to 13 in girls and 12 to 15 in boys. During a 1-year growth spurt, girls can gain 3.5 in. in height and boys 4 in.

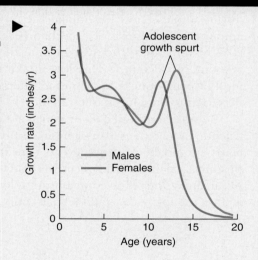

During the adolescent growth spurt, boys gain some fat but add so much lean mass as muscle and bone that their percentage of body fat actually decreases. Girls gain proportionately more body fat and less lean tissue. By age 20, females have about twice as much adipose tissue as males and only about two-thirds as much lean tissue. ▼

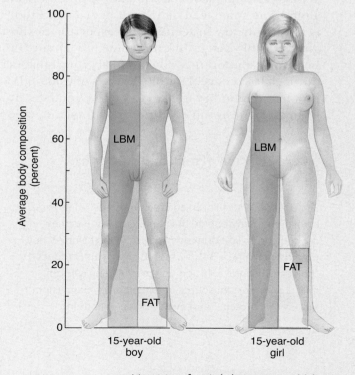

◀ At age 13, some boys are physically still children, while others have matured sexually. Because there are large individual variations in the age at which these growth and developmental changes occur, the stage of maturation is often a better indicator of nutritional requirements than is chronological age.

ENERGY AND NUTRIENT NEEDS OF ADOLESCENTS

The DRIs provide recommendations for adolescents in two age groups: 9 through 13 and 14 through 18. Separate recommendations are made for boys and girls because their needs begin to differ during the adolescent years.

Energy and energy-yielding nutrients

The proportions of calories from carbohydrate, fat, and protein recommended for adolescents are similar to those for adults, but the total amount of energy needed by teenagers usually exceeds adult needs. Boys require more energy than girls because they have more muscle and their bodies are larger. Protein requirements per kilogram of body weight are the same for boys and girls, but because boys are generally heavier, they require more total protein than do girls.

Vitamins

The need for most of the vitamins rises to adult levels during adolescence. The requirement for B vitamins, which are involved in energy metabolism, is much higher in adolescence than in childhood because of higher energy needs. The rapid growth of adolescence further increases the need for vitamin B_6, which is important for protein synthesis, and for folate and vitamin B_{12}, which are essential for cell division. The high calorie intakes of teens help them meet most of their vitamin needs, but inadequate intakes of riboflavin and vitamin D put some teens at risk for deficiency. Riboflavin is frequently low in teens' diets, especially in those of girls, possibly due to low milk intake. Vitamin D is important to support the rapid skeletal growth that occurs during adolescence. Low blood levels of vitamin D are a problem due to low intakes as well as limited synthesis from sunlight in those with dark skin pigmentation or inadequate exposure to sunlight during the winter months (see Chapter 7).[34]

Iron

The need for iron rises between childhood and adolescence. Iron is needed to synthesize hemoglobin for the expansion of blood volume and myoglobin for the increase in muscle mass. Because blood volume expands at a faster rate in boys than in girls, boys require more iron for tissue synthesis than do girls. However, in girls the onset of menstruation increases iron losses, making total iron needs greater in young women. The RDA is set at 11 mg/day for boys and 15 mg/day for girls ages 14 to 18. Girls are more likely than boys to consume less than the recommended amount because they require more iron, tend to eat fewer iron-rich foods, and consume fewer overall calories. As a result, iron deficiency is common in adolescent females, affecting about 9% of girls ages 12 to 15 and 16% of young women ages 16 to 19.[35]

Calcium

The adolescent growth spurt increases both the length and mass of bones. Adequate calcium is essential for forming healthy bone. The AI for calcium rises from 800 mg/day in children ages 4 to 8 to 1300 mg/day during adolescence, but intake is typically below these amounts in both sexes.[4] Fewer than 10% of girls and only 25% of boys ages 9 to 13 consume the recommended amount of calcium.[36] This low intake may reduce the level of peak bone mass achieved, increasing the risk of developing osteoporosis later in life.

Because milk and cheese, which are major sources of calcium in teen diets, can be high in saturated fat, adolescents should be encouraged to consume low-fat dairy products, calcium-fortified cereals, and vegetable sources of calcium. One of the contributors to low calcium intake is the use of soda, rather than milk, as a beverage (**Figure 12.9**).

Consumption of milk and soft drinks
Figure 12.9

Since the 1970s, children and teens (ages 2 to 18 years) have more than doubled the number of calories they consume from soft drinks while cutting the calories they obtain from milk by 34%.[37] This has significantly reduced their calcium intake. In addition to providing calcium, milk is an important source of phosphorus, magnesium, potassium, protein, riboflavin, vitamin A, and zinc.

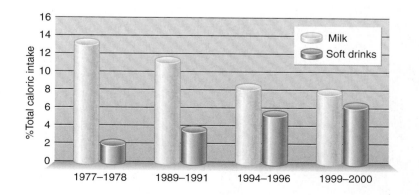

MyPyramid recommendations for teens
FIGURE 12.10

The recommendations shown here are for 11- and 16-year-old boys and girls who engage in more than 60 minutes of activity daily. The 10 oz of grains recommended for an active 16-year-old boy may seem like a huge amount. But when spread over the course of a day (in the form of, say, a large bowl of cereal and toast for breakfast, two tacos for lunch, and a dinner that includes spaghetti and garlic bread), it is an amount that is easily consumed by a teenage boy.

Food group	GRAINS	VEGETABLES	FRUITS	MILK	MEAT & BEANS
Amount for an 11-yr-old male	7 ounces	3 cups	2 cups	3 cups	6 ounces
Amount for an 11-yr-old female	6 ounces	2.5 cups	2 cups	3 cups	5.5 ounces
Amount for an 18-yr-old male	10 ounces	4 cups	2.5 cups	3 cups	7 ounces
Amount for an 18-yr-old female	8 ounces	3 cups	2 cups	3 cups	6.5 ounces

MEETING TEENS' NUTRITIONAL NEEDS

During adolescence, physiological changes dictate nutritional needs, but peer pressure may dictate food choices. Parents often have little control over what adolescents eat, and skipped meals and meals away from home are common. A food is more likely to be selected because it tastes good, it is easy to grab, or friends are eating it than because it is a healthy choice. No matter when foods are consumed throughout the day, an adolescent's diet should follow the recommendations of MyPyramid for the appropriate age, gender, and activity level (see FIGURE 12.10 and *What Should I Eat?*). The best indicators of adequate intake are satiety and a growth pattern that follows the curve of the growth charts.

Use iProfile to calculate the calcium content of your favorite fast-food meal.

WHAT SHOULD I EAT?   Adolescence

Balance unhealthy choices with healthy ones
- Have milk with your burger and fries.
- Eat an extra vegetable with dinner.
- Put peppers on your pizza.
- Try fresh fruit for dessert.

Eat breakfast
- Grab some toast with peanut butter.
- Stick a cereal bar or muffin in your backpack.
- Have a yogurt on the go.

Snack well
- Reach for an apple, a pear, or an orange before the cookies and chips.
- Dip your chips in salsa, guacamole, or hummus.
- Nibble on nuts and seeds.
- Crunch some baby carrots.

Count up your calcium
- Drink milk—low-fat milk has fewer calories than soda.
- Put extra milk on your cereal.
- Make a shake by mixing yogurt and fruit in the blender.
- Have cheese with crackers, on pizza, or in tacos.

Make fast food fit There is nothing wrong with an occasional fast-food meal, but a steady diet of burgers, fries, and tacos will likely contribute to an overall unhealthy diet. Fast food is typically high in fat and sodium and low in fruits and vegetables.[38] Most teens in the United States consume more than the recommended amounts of fat and sodium and fewer fruits and vegetables than recommended. The lettuce and tomatoes that garnish a burger or taco are not enough to meet the serving recommendations for vegetables. French fries, which are high in fat and salt, are the most frequently consumed vegetable. To fit fast food into a healthy diet, make more nutrient-dense fast-food choices and make sure other meals and snacks eaten throughout the day supply the nutrients that are not obtained from fast food. Many fast-food franchises now offer fruit, salads, yogurt, and milk. And some of the old standbys are not bad choices. A plain, single-patty hamburger provides a lot less fat and energy than one with two patties and a high-fat sauce. A chicken sandwich can be a healthy choice if it is grilled or barbecued, not breaded and fried (TABLE 12.2).

Keep vegetarian choices healthy It is not uncommon for a teen to decide to consume a vegetarian diet even if the rest of the family does not. Some give up meat for health reasons or to lose weight, while others give up meat because they are concerned about animals and the environment. A vegetarian diet can be a healthy choice when it is carefully planned to meet nutrient needs, not just to eliminate meat. A poorly planned vegetarian diet will be no healthier than any other poorly planned diet. Adequate protein is generally not a problem, but meatless diets can be low in iron and zinc. Teenage vegans, who consume no animal products, may also be at risk for a vitamin B_{12} deficiency and inadequate calcium and vitamin D intake. We generally think of vegetarian diets as being low in fat, but one that relies on high-fat dairy products can be high in total fat, saturated fat, and cholesterol (FIGURE 12.11).

SPECIAL CONCERNS FOR TEENS

Peer pressure to fit in and concern about physical appearance probably have a greater impact on behavior during adolescence than at any other time in life. Many girls want to lose weight even if they are not overweight, and boys want to gain weight in order to achieve a strong, muscular appearance.

Eating disorders As discussed in Chapter 9, the excessive concern about weight, low self-esteem, and poor body image that are common during the teenage years contribute to the development of eating disorders. These disorders can be fatal, but even in less severe cases, the nutritional consequences of an eating disorder can affect growth and development during adolescence and have a lifelong impact on bone health.

The impact of athletics Participation in competitive sports may affect adolescent nutrient needs and eating patterns. Like adult athletes, teen athletes have increased nutrient needs; they require more water, energy, protein, carbohydrate, and micronutrients than do their less active peers. Individuals involved in sports such as football that require the athlete to be large and heavy usually do not have trouble eating enough to meet these additional needs, but they may compromise their health by experimenting with anabolic steroids or other ergogenic supplements in an effort to "bulk up." As discussed in Chapter 10, steroids can stunt growth in adolescence as

Make healthier fast-food choices TABLE 12.2	
Instead of . . .	**Choose . . .**
Double-patty hamburger with cheese, mayonnaise, special sauce, and bacon	Regular single-patty hamburger without mayonnaise, special sauce, and bacon
Breaded and fried chicken sandwich	Grilled chicken sandwich
Chicken nuggets or tenders	Grilled chicken strips
Large French fries	Baked potato, side salad, or small order of fries
Fried chicken wings	Broiled skinless wings
Crispy-shell chicken taco with extra cheese and sour cream	Grilled-chicken soft taco without sour cream
Nachos with cheese sauce	Tortilla chips with bean dip
12-in. meatball sub	6-in. turkey breast sub with lots of vegetables
Thick-crust pizza with extra cheese and meat toppings	Thin-crust pizza with extra veggies
Doughnut	Cinnamon and raisin bagel with low-fat cream cheese

Healthy vegetarian choices FIGURE 12.11

Cheese pizza and ice cream are high-saturated fat, high-cholesterol vegetarian choices. In contrast, whole-grain pita bread stuffed with chickpeas, corn, spinach, and tomatoes served with

reduced-fat milk, is low in saturated fat and cholesterol, high in complex carbohydrate and fiber, and a good source of calcium and iron.

well as lead to sexual and reproductive disorders, heart disease, liver damage, acne, and aggressive, violent behavior. Teens participating in gymnastics and wrestling may restrict their food intake in order to stay light and lean. Weight restriction at this stage of life may affect nutritional status and maturation and increase the risk of developing an eating disorder.[39] In female athletes, the combination of hard training and weight restriction can lead to the *female athlete triad* (see Chapter 10).[40]

Tobacco use Approximately 20% of high school students in the United States smoke cigarettes.[41] Smoking increases the risk of cardiovascular disease and lung cancer. Smoking can limit appetite, and many teens start smoking in order to control their weight and are afraid to quit because they fear that they will gain weight if they do.[42] Smoking may also have an impact nutrient intake; a study of smokers found that they eat more saturated fat and fewer fruits and vegetables than do nonsmokers.[43] This dietary pattern increases the risk of developing heart disease and cancer.

Alcohol use Although it is illegal to sell alcohol to adolescents, alcoholic beverages are commonly available at teen social gatherings, and peer pressure to consume them is strong. Surveys of American youth suggest that about 44.7% of students in 9th through 12th grade have had at least one drink during the previous month and 26% have engaged in **binge drinking**.[44] It is estimated that about 40% of college students "binge" on alcohol at least once during a two-week period.[45] Alcohol is a drug that has short-term effects that occur soon after ingestion and long-term health consequences that are associated with overuse. It provides 7 Calories/gram but no nutrients, and often alcohol is consumed instead of foods that are nutritious. Once it has been ingested, alcohol alters nutrient absorption and metabolism and affects overall health. These effects are discussed in greater depth in the last section of the chapter.

> **binge drinking**
> The consumption of five or more drinks in a row for males or four or more for females.

CONCEPT CHECK STOP

How does puberty affect body composition in males and females?

How do the energy needs of teens compare with those of adults?

What factors contribute to low calcium intake in teens?

What could a teen choose at a fast-food restaurant to boost vegetable intake?

Nutrition for the Adult Years

he benefits of a healthy diet do not stop when you stop growing. Good nutrition throughout your adult years can keep you healthy and active into your 80s and beyond. In the United States, **life expectancy** is 77.8 years.[46] However, **healthy life expectancy** is only about 69 years.[47] This means that, on average, the last 9 years of life are restricted by disease and disability.

The goal of successful aging is to increase not only life expectancy but healthy life expectancy. Achieving this goal is particularly important because we live in a nation with an aging population (**FIGURE 12.12A**). Keeping older adults healthy will benefit not only the aging individuals themselves but also the family members who must find the time and resources to care for them and the public health programs that attempt to meet their needs. Although nutrition is not the key to immortality, a healthy diet can prevent malnutrition and delay the onset of chronic diseases that typically begin in middle age and reduce the quality of life in older adults (**FIGURE 12.12B**).

> **life expectancy**
> The average length of life for a particular population of individuals.

The number of older adults is rising FIGURE 12.12

A About 12% of the U.S. population is 65 years of age or over; by 2030 this percentage is expected to reach 20%.[48] The **oldest old** (≥ 85 years), one of the fastest-growing age groups, have more activity limitations and chronic conditions and require more public health dollars and services than do younger adults.[49]

B Chronological age is not always the best indicator of a person's health. A person who is 75 may have the vigor and health of someone who is 55, or vice versa. Some older adults are healthy, independent, and active, while others are chronically ill, dependent, and at high risk for malnutrition.

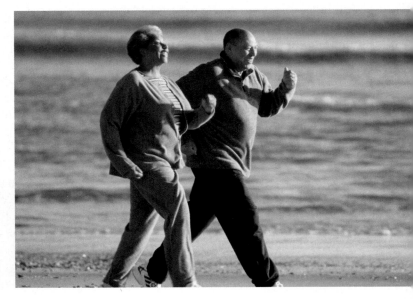

Genes determine the efficiency with which cells are maintained and repaired and also determine our susceptibility to age-related diseases, such as cardiovascular disease and cancer, but lifestyle and environment also affect how fast we age.

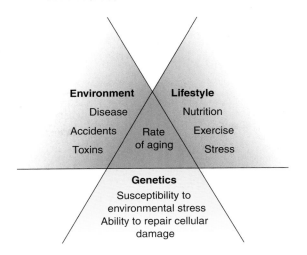

WHAT IS AGING?

aging The inevitable accumulation of changes associated with and responsible for an ever-increasing susceptibility to disease and death.

Aging is universal to all living things, but it is a process that we still don't fully understand. We know that as organisms grow older, the number of cells in their bodies decreases and the functioning of the remaining cells declines. This loss of cells and cell function occurs throughout life, but the effects are not felt for many years because organisms start out life with more cells and cell function than they need. This reserve capacity allows an organism to continue functioning normally despite a decrease in the number and function of cells. In young adults, the reserve capacity of organs is 4 to 10 times that required to sustain life. As a person ages and reserve capacity decreases, the effects of aging become evident in all body systems. With this loss of function comes a reduction in the ability to repair damage and resist infection, so older people may die from diseases from which they could easily have recovered when they were younger.

life span

The maximum age to which members of a species can live.

The human **life span** is about 120 years, but how long individuals live and the rate at which they age are determined by the genes they inherit, their lifestyle, and the extent to which they are able to avoid accidents, disease, and environmental toxins (FIGURE 12.13). A person with a family history of heart disease who eats a healthy diet and exercises regularly may never develop heart disease. In contrast, someone with no family history of heart disease who is inactive, smokes, and eats a poor diet may develop heart problems.

NUTRITION AND HEALTH CONCERNS THROUGHOUT ADULTHOOD

The physiological and health changes that accompany aging affect energy and nutrient requirements, how some nutrient requirements must be met, and the risk of malnutrition. In order to best recommend nutrient intakes for adults of all ages, the DRIs include four adult age categories: young adulthood (ages 19–30), middle age (ages 31–50), adulthood (ages 51–70), and older adulthood (over age 70). These recommendations are designed to meet the needs of the majority of healthy individuals in each age group. Although the incidence of chronic diseases and disabilities increases with advancing age, these increases are not considered when making general nutrient intake recommendations.

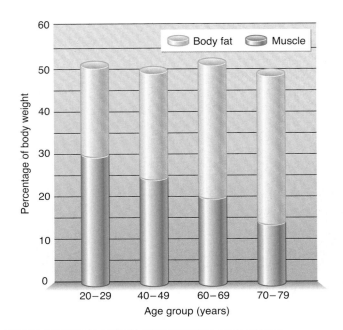

Body composition and energy needs[50]

FIGURE 12.14

Some of the decline in energy needs in older adults is due to a decrease in lean body mass;[50] the less lean tissue a person has, the lower his or her BMR. The EER for an 80-year-old man is almost 600 Calories less than for a 20-year-old man of the same size and activity level. For women, the difference in EER between an 80- and a 20-year-old of the same height, weight, and physical activity level is about 400 Calories/day.

Energy and energy-yielding nutrient recommendations

Adult energy needs typically decline with age, due primarily to a decreases in BMR and activity level (**FIGURE 12.14**). The need for most nutrients does not change, however, so in order to meet nutrient needs without exceeding energy needs, older adults must consume a nutrient-dense diet. For example, adult protein requirements do not change with age; therefore, older adults must consume a diet that is higher in protein relative to calories than that of younger adults.

The proportions of carbohydrate and fat recommended in the diet also remain the same in older adults as in younger adults. In order to ensure adequate vitamin, mineral, and fiber intake, most dietary carbohydrate should come from unrefined sources. Adequate fiber, when consumed with adequate fluid, helps prevent constipation, hemorrhoids, and diverticulosis—

conditions that are common in older adults. High-fiber diets may also be beneficial in the prevention and management of diabetes, cardiovascular disease, and obesity.

Sources of dietary fat should also be chosen with nutrient density in mind. A diet with 20 to 35% of energy from fat that contains adequate amounts of the essential fatty acids and limits saturated fat, *trans* fat, and cholesterol is recommended.

Meeting the water needs of older adults

The recommended water intake for older adults is the same as for younger adults; but meeting these needs may be more challenging in older adults. With age there is a reduction in the sense of thirst, which can decrease fluid intake. In addition older adults are likely to have mobility limitations that limit their access to beverages. The risk of dehydration is further increased in older adults by greater water losses. The kidneys are no longer as efficient at conserving water and many older adults take medications that increase water loss.

Risk of vitamin and mineral deficiencies in older adults

The physiological changes of aging and the decrease in calorie needs put older adults at risk for deficiency of several vitamins and minerals. For some of these, recommended intakes are increased or special recommendations are made about how needs should be met (**FIGURE 12.15**).

The RDA for vitamin B_{12} is not increased in individuals over age 50, but it is recommended that these people meet their RDA for vitamin B_{12} by consuming foods that are fortified with this vitamin or by taking a supplement containing vitamin B_{12}. This is because food-bound vitamin B_{12} is not absorbed efficiently in many older adults due to *atrophic gastritis*, an inflammation of the stomach lining that causes a reduction in stomach acid (see Chapter 7).[52,53] Reduced secretion of stomach acid also allows microbial overgrowth in the stomach and small intestine, and the greater number of microbes compete for available vitamin B_{12}, further reducing vitamin B_{12} absorption. It is estimated that 10 to 30% of American adults over age 50, and 40% of those in their 80s, have atrophic gastritis. The vitamin B_{12} in fortified foods and supplements is not bound to proteins, so it is absorbed even when stomach acid levels are low. Atrophic gastritis may also reduce the absorption of iron, folate, calcium, and vitamin K.

Calcium status is a problem in the elderly because calcium intake is low and intestinal absorption decreases with age. Without sufficient calcium, bone mass decreases, and the risk of bone fractures due to osteoporosis increases. The reduction in estrogen that occurs with menopause also increases the risk of osteoporosis in women by increasing the rate of bone breakdown and decreasing the absorption of calcium from the intestine. The AI for adults over age 51 is 1200 mg, 200 mg greater than the AI for younger adults.

Vitamin D, which is necessary for adequate calcium absorption, is also a concern in the elderly. Intake is often low, and synthesis in the skin is reduced due to limited exposure to sunlight and because the capacity to synthesize vitamin D in the skin decreases with age. The AI for men and women ages 51 to 70 has been set at 10 µg/day. For individuals over age 70, this is further increased to 15 µg/day. As discussed in Chapter 7, many experts now believe that in the absence of adequate exposure to sunlight, 20 to 25 µg of vitamin D is needed per day in all adults and children.[54]

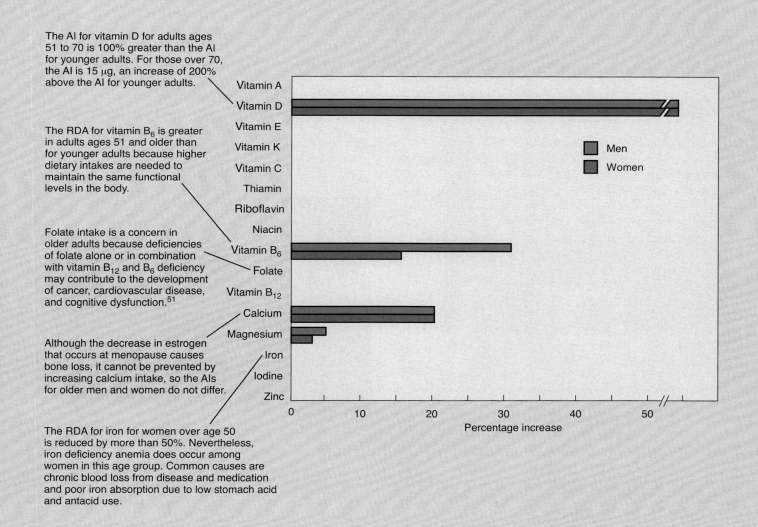

Vitamin and mineral needs of older adults FIGURE 12.15

This graph illustrates the percentage increase in micronutrient recommendations for adults age 51 and older compared with those of young adults ages 19 to 30.

The AI for vitamin D for adults ages 51 to 70 is 100% greater than the AI for younger adults. For those over 70, the AI is 15 µg, an increase of 200% above the AI for younger adults.

The RDA for vitamin B_6 is greater in adults ages 51 and older than for younger adults because higher dietary intakes are needed to maintain the same functional levels in the body.

Folate intake is a concern in older adults because deficiencies of folate alone or in combination with vitamin B_{12} and B_6 deficiency may contribute to the development of cancer, cardiovascular disease, and cognitive dysfunction.[51]

Although the decrease in estrogen that occurs at menopause causes bone loss, it cannot be prevented by increasing calcium intake, so the AIs for older men and women do not differ.

The RDA for iron for women over age 50 is reduced by more than 50%. Nevertheless, iron deficiency anemia does occur among women in this age group. Common causes are chronic blood loss from disease and medication and poor iron absorption due to low stomach acid and antacid use.

A Many of the physiological changes associated with age can affect nutritional status. This illustration shows how the decreases in muscle mass and immune function that occur with age contribute to malnutrition and how, in turn, malnutrition makes these problems worse. ▶

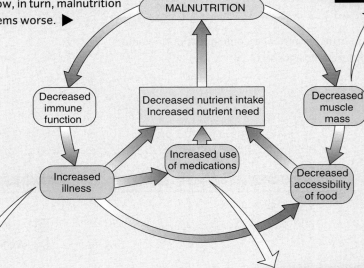

B The thighs of this 25-year-old (left) and 65-year-old (right) are of similar size, but in the older man a significant amount of muscle has been replaced by fat (shown in white). In a malnourished individual, the loss of muscle mass and strength would be even greater. Loss of muscle can limit the ability to shop for and prepare food, and decreased intake contributes to further muscle loss.

**Diagram labels:**
- MALNUTRITION
- Decreased immune function
- Decreased nutrient intake / Increased nutrient need
- Decreased muscle mass
- Increased illness
- Increased use of medications
- Decreased accessibility of food

▲

C The incidence of cancer increases with age.[55] One reason for the higher incidence is that the immune system's ability to destroy cancer cells declines. Reduced immune function also increases the frequency of infectious diseases and reduces the ability to recover from these diseases.

Bar graph — Y-axis: Percentage of U.S. adults who have had cancer (0, 5, 10, 15, 20, 25, 30); X-axis: Age (18–44, 45–64, 65–74, 75+)

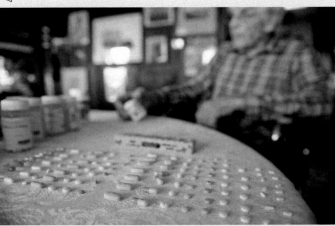

▲

D It is common for older adults to take multiple medications. Shown here are the pills this 73-year-old man takes each week. Medications can affect nutritional status by interfering with taste, chewing, and swallowing; by causing loss of appetite, gastrointestinal upset, constipation, or nausea; and by increasing nutrient losses or decreasing nutrient absorption.

FACTORS THAT INCREASE THE RISK OF MALNUTRITION IN OLDER ADULTS

The aging process itself usually does not cause malnutrition in healthy, active adults, but nutritional health can be compromised by the physical changes that occur with age, the presence of disease, and economic, psychological, and social circumstances.[56] These factors can increase the risk of malnutrition by altering nutrient needs and decreasing the motivation to eat and the ability to acquire and enjoy food. Malnutrition then exacerbates some of these factors, contributing to a downward health spiral from which it is difficult to recover (FIGURE 12.16A).

Physiological changes

With age comes a decline in muscle size and strength (see FIGURE 12.16B). This decline affects both the skeletal muscles needed to move the body and the heart and respiratory muscles needed to deliver oxygen to the tissues. Some of this change is due to changes in hormone levels and muscle protein synthesis, but lack of exercise is also an important contributor.[57] The changes in muscle strength contribute not only to **physical frailty**, which is characterized by general weakness, impaired mobility and balance, and poor endurance, but also to the risk of falls and fractures. In the oldest old, those age 85 years and older, loss of muscle strength is the limiting factor determining whether they can continue to live independently.

The immune system's ability to fight disease declines with age. With this decline, the incidence of infections, cancers, and autoimmune diseases increases, and the effectiveness of immunizations declines (see FIGURE 12.16C).

In turn, increases in infections and chronic disease can lead to increased use of medications that affect nutritional status (see FIGURE 12.16D). Malnutrition exacerbates the decrease in immune function.[58]

Acute and chronic illness

More than 75% of the older population suffers from some form of illness or disability, and the incidence increases with advancing age.[59] These conditions affect the ability to maintain good nutritional health because they can change nutrient requirements, decrease the appeal of food, and impair the ability to obtain and prepare an adequate diet.

Some illnesses change the type of diet that is recommended. For instance, kidney failure reduces the ability to excrete protein waste products, so the diet must be lower in protein. Blood pressure is affected by sodium intake, so a low-sodium diet is recommended for individuals with high blood pressure. Dietary restrictions like these limit food choices and can affect the palatability of the diet and thereby contribute to malnutrition in the elderly.

Physical disabilities can limit a person's ability to obtain and prepare food. The most common reason for physical disability among older adults is **arthritis**, a condition that causes pain in joints when they are moved (FIGURE 12.17). Arthritis affects more than 45 million Americans.[60] Half of all individuals age 70 and older with arthritis need help with the activities of daily living, including preparing and eating meals.[3]

> **arthritis** A disease characterized by inflammation of the joints, pain, and sometimes changes in structure.

Osteoarthritis FIGURE 12.17

Osteoarthritis, the most common form of arthritis, occurs when the cartilage that cushions the joints degenerates, allowing the bones to rub together and cause pain. Anti-inflammatory medications help reduce the pain. Supplements of glucosamine and chondroitin have also been found to improve symptoms, as well as slow the progression of the disease in some patients.[61]

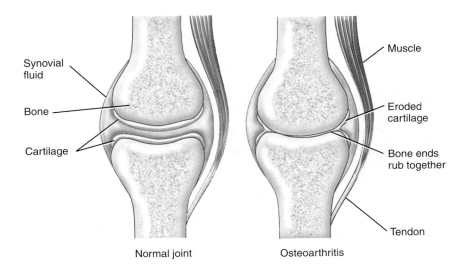

Synovial fluid

Bone

Cartilage

Muscle

Eroded cartilage

Bone ends rub together

Tendon

Normal joint   Osteoarthritis

Cataracts FIGURE 12.18

Cataracts cause the lens of the eye to become cloudy and impair vision. When cataracts obscure vision, the affected lens can be removed and replaced with an artificial plastic lens.

Visual disorders are also more common with age. **Macular degeneration** is the most common cause of blindness in older Americans. The **macula** is a small area of the retina of the eye that distinguishes fine detail. If the number of viable cells in the macula is reduced, visual acuity declines, ultimately resulting in blindness. **Cataracts** is another common cause of declining vision. Among people who live to age 85, half will develop cataracts that impair vision (**FIGURE 12.18**).[62] Oxidative damage is believed to cause both macular degeneration and cataracts. Therefore, a diet that is high in foods containing antioxidant nutrients and phytochemicals might slow or prevent these eye disorders.

Changes in mental status can affect nutrition by interfering with the response to hunger and the ability to eat and to obtain and prepare food. The incidence of **dementia** increases with age. Dementia involves impairment in memory, thinking, or judgment that is se-

macular degeneration Degeneration of a portion of the retina that results in loss of visual detail and eventually in blindness.

cataracts A disease of the eye that results in cloudy spots on the lens (and sometimes the cornea), which obscure vision.

dementia A deterioration of mental state that results in impaired memory, thinking, and/or judgment.

vere enough to cause personality changes and affect daily activities and relationships with others. Causes of dementia include multiple strokes, alcoholism, dehydration, side effects of medication, vitamin B_{12} deficiency, and **Alzheimer's disease**. Regardless of the cause, these neurological problems can affect the ability to consume a healthy diet.

Another cause of altered mental status in the elderly is depression. Social, psychological, and physical factors all contribute to depression in the elderly. Retirement and the death and relocation of friends and family can cause social isolation, which contributes to depression. Physical disability causes loss of independence. The inability to engage in normal daily activities, easily visit with friends and family, and provide for personal needs contributes to depression. Depression can make meals less appetizing and decrease the quantity and quality of foods consumed, thereby increasing the risk of malnutrition.

Alzheimer's disease A disease that results in a relentless and irreversible loss of mental function.

Use of medications

The higher frequency of acute and chronic illnesses in the elderly makes it likely that they will be taking multiple medications (see Figure 12.16D).[63] Medications can affect nutritional status, and nutritional status can alter the effectiveness of medications. The more medications are taken, the greater the chance of side effects that affect nutritional status, such as decreased appetite, changes in taste, and nausea. Diet can also change the effectiveness of medications. For example, vitamin K hinders the action of anticoagulants, which are taken to reduce the risk of blood clots. On the other hand, omega-3 fatty acids, such as those in fish oils, inhibit blood clotting and may intensify the effect of an anticoagulant drug and cause bleeding.

Economic and social issues

Approximately 3.4 million older adults live below the poverty level, and many must live on a fixed income, making it difficult to afford health care, especially medications, and a healthy diet.[64] Food costs and limited food preparation facilities can reduce the types of foods available. In 2007, 7.3 million elderly Americans experienced **food insecurity**,[65] which occurs when the availability of nutritionally adequate, safe food or the ability to acquire food in socially acceptable ways is limited. This in turn increases the risk of malnutrition.

KEEPING HEALTHY THROUGHOUT THE ADULT YEARS

There is no secret dietary factor that will bestow immortality, but good nutrition and an active lifestyle are major determinants of successful aging (see *What a Scientist Sees*). A well-planned, nutritionally adequate diet can extend an individual's years of healthy life by preventing malnutrition and delaying the onset of chronic diseases. Regular exercise can help maintain muscle mass, bone strength, and cardiorespiratory function, helping to prolong independent living. For those with economic, social, or physical limitations, food assistance programs or assisted living can help prevent food insecurity.

The Secrets of Longevity

This woman is over 100 years old. She lives in Okinawa, a series of islands lying between mainland Japan and Taiwan. Okinawans enjoy not only the longest life expectancy in the world (81.2 years) but also the longest *healthy* life expectancy. A scientist sees that genes play a role, but an active lifestyle and a low-calorie, nutrient-dense diet are also important reasons for Okinawans' long, healthy lives. Most Okinawans are farmers, an occupation with a high energy demand. And most consume a nutrient-dense diet of vegetables and fish and typically eat only until they are 80% full. The high energy expenditure and low calorie intake result in periods of caloric restriction.[66] *Caloric restriction* refers to a diet that limits calories but provides enough of all the essential nutrients. Insects, worms, mice, and other rodents that are fed a calorie-restricted diet live longer—as much as 50% longer—than animals that eat more calories. Calorie-restricted animals have a lower incidence of age-related chronic diseases, better immune function, lower blood glucose, and better overall organ function than do animals whose diets are not calorie restricted. The people of Okinawa provide evidence that caloric restriction can also extend human life.[66] They maintain a low BMI, and the incidence of the chronic diseases of aging is much lower among Okinawans than among people living in the United States or on mainland Japan (see graph).

It is estimated that during one period of caloric restriction Okinawans consumed 11% fewer calories than they expended.[66] This would mean that someone who needs 2000 Calories/day would consume only 1780 Calories/day. Could you eliminate 220 Calories from your diet every day and still meet all your nutrient needs?

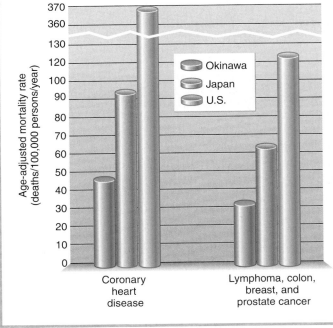

DETERMINE: A checklist of the warning signs of malnutrition TABLE 12.3

Disease	Any disease, illness, or condition that causes changes in eating can predispose a person to malnutrition. Memory loss and depression can also interfere with nutrition if they affect food intake.
Eating poorly	Eating either too little or too much can lead to poor health.
Tooth loss/ mouth pain	Poor health of the mouth, teeth, and gums interferes with the ability to eat.
Economic hardship	Having to, or choosing to, spend less than $25 to $30 per person per week on food interferes with nutrient intake.
Reduced social support	Not having contact with people on a daily basis has a negative effect on morale, well-being, and eating.
Multiple medicines	The more medicines a person takes, the greater the chances of side effects such as weakness, drowsiness, diarrhea, changes in taste and appetite, nausea, and constipation.
Involuntary weight loss or gain	Unintentionally losing or gaining weight is a warning sign that should not be ignored. Being overweight or underweight also increases the risk of malnutrition.
Needs assistance in self-care	Difficulty walking, shopping, and cooking increases the risk of malnutrition.
Elder above age 80	The risks of frailty and health problems increase with increasing age.

Identifying older adults at risk

To address concerns about the nutritional health of elderly individuals, the federal Nutrition Screening Initiative promotes screening for and intervention with nutrition-related problems in older adults. This program is working to increase awareness of nutritional problems among the elderly by involving practitioners and community organizations as well as relatives, friends, and others caring for the elderly in evaluating the nutritional status of the aging population. This program developed the DETERMINE checklist (TABLE 12.3), based on an acronym for the physiological, medical, and socioeconomic situations that increase the risk of malnutrition among the elderly. The elderly themselves, as well as family members and caregivers, can use this tool to determine when malnutrition is a potential problem.

Meeting nutrient needs

Meeting the nutrient needs of older adults can be challenging (see *What Should I Eat?*). Because energy needs are reduced while most micronutrient needs remain the same or increase, food choices must be nutrient dense. In addition, the medical, social, and economic challenges that often accompany aging make it more difficult to meet these needs. Many older adults need supplements of vitamin D, vitamin B_{12}, and calcium to meet their nutrient needs. However, supplements should not take the place of a balanced, nutrient-dense diet that is high in whole grains, fruits, and vegetables (FIGURE 12.19). In addition to essential nutrients, these foods contain phytochemicals and other substances that may protect against disease.

WHAT SHOULD I EAT? Advancing Age

Use iProfile to find foods that are fortified with vitamin B_{12}.

Consume plenty of fluids and fiber
- Drink a beverage with every meal.
- Keep a bottle of water handy and sip on it.
- Use whole-wheat bread.
- Bake bran muffins.

Pay attention to vitamin B_{12}, calcium, and vitamin D
- Make sure your cereal is fortified with vitamin B_{12}.
- Drink milk; it gives you both calcium and vitamin D.
- Sit in the sun to get some vitamin D with no calories at all.
- Add some canned salmon to a salad for lunch.

Antioxidize
- Have a bowl of strawberries or blueberries.
- Choose colorful vegetables to boost carotenoids.
- Use vegetable oils in cooking to supply vitamin E.
- Eat some nuts, but not too many—they are high in calories.

Work on your meals for one
- Ask the grocer to break up larger packages of eggs and meats.
- Buy in bulk and share with a friend.
- Make a whole pot but freeze it in meal-size portions.
- Top a baked potato with leftover vegetables or sauces.

MyPyramid amounts for older adults
FIGURE 12.19

The MyPyramid recommendations shown here are for sedentary 50- and 70-year-old men and women. The MyPyramid plan for sedentary 70-year-old women allows only 150 discretionary Calories/day. To meet this allowance, food choices must be nutrient dense. High-fiber foods are important because fiber is often low in the diets of older adults. Sufficient beverage consumption is important to ensure that water needs are met.

MyPyramid
STEPS TO A HEALTHER YOU
MyPyramid.gov

Food group	GRAINS	VEGETABLES	FRUITS	MILK	MEAT & BEANS
Amount for a 50-yr-old male	7 ounces	3 cups	2 cups	3 cups	6 ounces
Amount for a 50-yr-old female	6 ounces	2.5 cups	1.5 cups	3 cups	5 ounces
Amount for a 70-yr-old male	6 ounces	2.5 cups	2 cups	3 cups	5.5 ounces
Amount for a 70-yr-old female	5 ounces	2 cups	1.5 cups	3 cups	5 ounces

Older adults who have physical limitations need to choose foods that they can easily prepare and consume. For those who have difficulty preparing foods, pre-cooked foods, frozen dinners, and canned soup or dry soup mixes can provide a meal with almost no preparation. Medical nutritional products, such as Ensure or Boost, can also be used to supplement intake.

Physical activity for older adults
Regular physical activity can extend years of active, independent life, reduce the risk of disability, and improve the quality of life for older adults. Exercise also allows an increase in food intake without weight gain, so micronutrient needs are met more easily. A physical activity program for older adults should improve endurance, strength, flexibility, and balance.[67] Endurance activities such as walking, biking, and swimming provide protection against chronic disease (FIGURE 12.20). Strengthening exercises increase strength and lean body mass and slow the rate of bone loss. Lifting small weights or stretching elastic bands at an intensity that requires some physical effort can provide resistance training. Flexibility makes the

Physical activity for older adults FIGURE 12.20

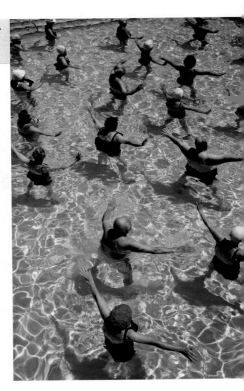

Exercise classes and other group-based activities can be a good way for older adults to start an exercise program. Water activities such as water aerobics and swimming do not stress the joints and hence can be used to improve endurance in individuals with arthritis or other bone and joint disorders. Some weight-bearing exercise, such as walking, is encouraged to promote bone health.

tasks of everyday life easier and reduces the risk of injuries. Flexibility exercises should include those that move the muscle through a full range of motion, such as arm circles, as well as those that stretch a muscle its full length. Improvements in strength, endurance, and flexibility all enhance balance, which reduces the risk of falls. Specific balance exercise such as those practiced in tai chi and yoga can further improve balance.

Overcoming economic and social issues

Overcoming economic limitations may involve providing education about economics and food preparation or providing assistance with shopping and food preparation. Options for people with limited incomes include reduced-cost meals at senior centers, federal food assistance programs (discussed in Chapter 14), food banks, and soup kitchens.

Another problem that contributes to poor nutrient intake in older adults is loneliness. Living, cooking, and eating alone can decrease interest in food. Programs that provide nutritious meals in communal settings promote social interaction and can improve nutrient intake. For those who are unable to attend communal meals, home-delivered meals are available. Studies have shown that compared to others, individuals who receive these meals have better-quality diets.[68]

Overcoming physical limitations: Assisted living

The physical and psychological declines associated with aging eventually cause many people to require assistance in everyday living. Assisted living facilities allow individuals to live in their own apartments but provide help as needed with activities such as eating, bathing, dressing, housekeeping, and taking medications. These facilities provide an interim level of care for those who cannot live safely on their own but do not require the total care provided in a nursing home. Eventually many older adults will need to live in a nursing home. Even though nursing homes provide access to food and medical care, their residents are at increased risk for malnutrition because they are more likely to have medical conditions that increase nutrient needs or interfere with food intake or nutrient absorption, and because they are dependent on others to provide for their care. Even when adequate meals are provided, many nursing home residents require assistance in eating and frequently do not consume all the food served, thus increasing their likelihood of developing deficits of energy, water, and other nutrients.[69]

CONCEPT CHECK STOP

What is the goal of successful aging?

What nutrients have higher recommended intakes for older adults than for younger adults?

Why are older adults at risk for malnutrition?

Where can older adults get assistance in meeting their nutrient needs?

The Impact of Alcohol Throughout Life

LEARNING OBJECTIVES

Define moderate alcohol consumption.

Explain how alcohol is absorbed and metabolized.

Describe the short- and long-term problems of excess alcohol consumption.

Discuss the potential benefits of moderate alcohol consumption.

Since the dawn of civilization, almost every human culture has produced and consumed some type of alcoholic beverage. Depending on the times and the culture, alcohol use has been touted, casually accepted, denounced, and even outlawed.

Whether alcohol consumption represents a risk to health or provides some benefits depends on who is drinking and how much is consumed. When consumed by a pregnant woman, alcohol can cause birth defects in the developing child. When consumed during childhood and adolescence, when the brain is still developing

Alcoholic beverages consist primarily of water, ethanol, and sugars, with few other nutrients. A drink, defined as about 5 oz of wine, 12 oz of beer, or 1.5 oz of distilled spirits, contains 12 to 14 g of alcohol, providing about 90 Calories (7 Calories/g). The remaining calories come from sugars.

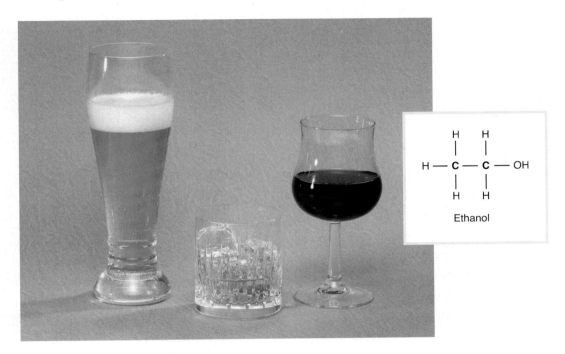

Ethanol

and changing, alcohol can cause permanent reductions in learning and memory.[70]

When consumed in excess by anyone, alcohol has medical and social consequences that negatively affect drinkers and those around them. It can reduce nutrient intake and affect the storage, mobilization, activation, and metabolism of nutrients. Its breakdown produces toxic compounds that damage tissues, particularly the liver.

When consumed in moderation by healthy adults, however, alcohol consumption provides some health advantages. The Dietary Guidelines define moderate alcohol consumption as no more than one drink per day for women and two drinks per day for men (FIGURE 12.21).

ALCOHOL ABSORPTION, TRANSPORT, AND EXCRETION

Chemically, any molecule that contains an —OH group is an **alcohol**, but we usually use the term to refer to **ethanol** and often to any beverage that contains ethanol (see Figure 12.21). Ethanol is a small molecule that is rapidly and almost completely absorbed in the upper gastrointestinal tract. Because some alcohol is absorbed directly from the stomach, its effects are almost immediate, especially when consumed on an empty stomach. If there is food in the stomach, absorption is slowed because food dilutes the alcohol in the stomach and slows the rate of stomach emptying.

Once it has been absorbed, alcohol enters the bloodstream and is rapidly distributed throughout all body water. Peak blood alcohol concentrations are attained approximately one hour after ingestion. Many variables affect blood alcohol level, including the kind and quantity of alcoholic beverage consumed, the speed at which the beverage is consumed, the food consumed with it, the weight and gender of the consumer, and the

ethanol The alcohol in alcoholic beverages; it is produced by yeast fermentation of sugar.

A Blood alcohol levels are higher in women than in men after consuming the same amount of alcohol. This may be due to lower levels of the enzymes that break down alcohol or to the fact that women have less body water than men, so the alcohol they consume is distributed in a smaller amount of body water.

B In the lungs, some alcohol diffuses out of the blood, into the air, and is exhaled. The amount of alcohol lost through the lungs is reliable enough to estimate blood alcohol level by using a Breathalyzer test.

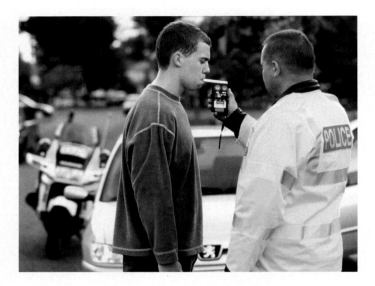

activity of alcohol-metabolizing enzymes in the body (FIGURE 12.22A).

Because alcohol is a toxin and cannot be stored in the body, it must be eliminated quickly. Absorbed alcohol travels to the liver, where it is given metabolic priority and is therefore broken down before other molecules. About 90% of the alcohol is metabolized by the liver. The remainder is excreted through the urine or eliminated via the lungs during exhalation (FIGURE 12.22B). The alcohol that reaches the kidney acts as a diuretic, increasing fluid excretion. Therefore, excessive alcohol intake can contribute to dehydration.

ALCOHOL METABOLISM

In people who occasionally consume moderate amounts of alcohol, most of the alcohol is broken down in the liver by the enzyme alcohol dehydrogenase (ADH) (FIGURE 12.23). This enzyme has also been found in all parts of the gastrointestinal tract.[71] When greater amounts of alcohol are consumed, a second pathway in the liver, called the microsomal ethanol-oxidizing system (MEOS), also metabolizes alcohol.[72] The rate at which ADH breaks down alcohol is fairly constant, but MEOS activity increases when more alcohol is consumed. MEOS also metabolizes other drugs, so as activity increases in response to high alcohol intake, it can alter the metabolism of other drugs.

ADVERSE EFFECTS OF ALCOHOL

The consumption of alcohol has short-term effects that interfere with organ function for several hours after ingestion. Chronic alcohol consumption has long-term effects that cause disease both because the alcohol interferes with nutritional status and because alcohol metabolism produces toxic compounds.

Short-term effects When alcohol intake exceeds the liver's ability to break it down, the excess accumulates in the bloodstream. The circulating alcohol acts as a depressant, impairing mental and physical abilities. First, alcohol affects reasoning; if drinking continues, the brain's vision and speech centers are affected. Next, large-muscle control becomes impaired, causing lack of coordination. Finally, if alcohol consumption continues, it can result in **alcohol poisoning**, a serious condition that can slow breathing, heart rate, and the gag reflex, leading to loss of consciousness, choking, coma, and even death. This most frequently occurs in cases of *binge drinking*. Even if an individual does not experience a loss of consciousness, excess drinking may still cause memory loss. Drinking enough alcohol to cause amnesia is called **blackout drinking**. Blackout drinking puts people at risk because they have no memory of events that occurred during the blackout. During alcohol-related memory blackouts, people may engage in risky behaviors such as having unprotected sexual intercourse, vandalizing property, or driving a car—and have no memory of it afterward.

The effects of alcohol on the central nervous system are what make driving while under the influence of alcohol so dangerous. Alcohol affects reaction time, eye–hand coordination, accuracy, and balance. Not only does alcohol impair one's ability to operate a motor vehicle, but it also impairs one's judgment in making the deci-

sion to drive. Abuse of alcohol also contributes to domestic violence and is a factor in more than 100,000 deaths per year, including almost 40% of all traffic fatalities.[73]

Alcoholism
One risk associated with regular alcohol consumption is the possibility of alcohol addiction, or **alcoholism**. The risk of alcoholism is increased in individuals who begin drinking at a younger age. Alcoholism, like any other drug addiction, is a physiological condition that needs treatment. It is believed to have a genetic component that makes some people more likely to become addicted, but environmental factors also play a significant role.[74] Thus, someone with a genetic predisposition toward alcoholism whose family and peers do not consume alcohol is much less likely to become addicted than someone with the same genes who drinks regularly with friends.

Alcohol metabolism FIGURE 12.23

The alcohol dehydrogenase (ADH) pathway predominates when small amounts of alcohol are consumed. The microsomal ethanol-oxidizing system (MEOS) becomes important when larger amounts are consumed. The MEOS reaction requires oxygen and the input of energy to break down alcohol. It also generates reactive oxygen molecules that can contribute to liver disease.

HOW IT WORKS
View in your WileyPLUS course

1. ADH breaks down alcohol to produce acetaldehyde.

2. Acetaldehyde is toxic and is degraded to produce acetyl-CoA.

3. The breakdown of alcohol and acetaldehyde releases electrons that can be used to produce ATP and also results in changes that inhibit the circular pathway, limiting breakdown of acetyl-CoA.

4. Acetyl-CoA that cannot enter the circular pathway is used to synthesize fatty acids, which accumulate in the liver.

5. When larger amounts of alcohol are consumed, MEOS also converts alcohol into acetaldehyde, which is then broken down to form acetyl-CoA.

Process Diagram

The Impact of Alcohol Throughout Life   429

Alcoholic cirrhosis Figure 12.24

The liver on the left is normal. The one on the right has cirrhosis. This is an irreversible condition in which fibrous deposits scar the liver and interfere with its functioning. Because the liver is the primary site of many metabolic reactions, cirrhosis is often fatal.

Alcoholic liver disease

The most significant physiological effects of chronic alcohol consumption occur in the liver. The metabolism of alcohol by ADH promotes fat synthesis (see Figure 12.23), which leads to the accumulation of fat in the liver. Metabolism by MEOS generates reactive oxygen molecules, which cause oxidation of lipids, membrane damage, and altered enzyme activities. Whether alcohol is broken down by ADH or MEOS, toxic acetaldehyde is formed. Acetaldehyde binds to proteins and inhibits chemical reactions and mitochondrial function, allowing more acetaldehyde to accumulate and causing further liver damage.

Chronic alcohol consumption leads to three types of alcoholic liver disease. **Fatty liver** is the accumulation of fat in liver cells. It occurs in almost all people who drink heavily due to increased synthesis and deposition of fat. If drinking continues, this condition may progress to **alcoholic hepatitis**. Both of these conditions are reversible if alcohol consumption is stopped and good nutritional and health practices are followed. If alcohol consumption continues, **cirrhosis** may develop (Figure 12.24).

alcoholic hepatitis Inflammation of the liver caused by alcohol consumption.

cirrhosis Chronic and irreversible liver disease characterized by loss of functioning liver cells and accumulation of fibrous connective tissue.

Alcohol, malnutrition, and other health problems

Malnutrition is one of the complications of long-term excessive alcohol consumption. Alcohol contributes energy—7 Calories/gram—but few nutrients; it may replace more nutrient-dense energy sources in the diet. In addition to decreasing nutrient intake, alcohol interferes with nutrient absorption. Alcohol causes inflammation of the stomach, pancreas, and intestine, which impairs digestion of food and absorption of nutrients into the blood. Deficiency of the B vitamin thiamin is a particular concern with chronic alcohol consumption. Alcohol also contributes to malnutrition by altering the storage, metabolism, and excretion of other vitamins and some minerals.

In addition to causing liver disease and malnutrition, heavy drinking is associated with cancer of the oral cavity, pharynx, esophagus, larynx, breast, liver, colon, rectum, and stomach.[75,76] Even moderate alcohol consumption has been found to increase the risk of certain cancers in women.[77] Alcohol use also increases the risk of hypertension, heart disease, and stroke.[78] Some of this effect is related to the fact that calories consumed as alcohol are more likely to be deposited as fat in the abdominal region, and excess abdominal fat increases the risk of high blood pressure, heart disease, and diabetes.

BENEFITS OF ALCOHOL CONSUMPTION

For some adults, moderate alcohol consumption may be beneficial. Consuming alcoholic beverages can stimulate appetite, improve mood, and enhance social interactions. Light to moderate drinking can also reduce the risk of heart disease and stroke. The primary mechanisms by which alcohol lowers cardiovascular risk are by raising blood levels of HDL cholesterol and by inhibiting the formation of blood clots. The phytochemicals in red wine are thought to make it more cardioprotective than other alcoholic beverages.[79]

Whether or not the benefits of alcohol consumption outweigh the risks, drinking is a personal decision that must take into account medical and social considerations. But anyone who chooses to drink should do so in moderation. Alcohol should be consumed slowly; no more than one drink every 1.5 hours. Sipping, not gulping, allows the liver time to break down what has already been consumed. Alternating nonalcoholic and alcoholic drinks will also slow down the rate of alcohol intake and prevent dehydration. Alcohol absorption is most rapid on an empty stomach. Consuming alcohol with meals slows its absorption and may also enhance its protective effects on the cardiovascular system.

CONCEPT CHECK **STOP**

HOW much beer per day constitutes moderate drinking for a man?

HOW can alcohol metabolism lead to fatty liver?

What are the symptoms of alcohol toxicity?

HOW does moderate alcohol intake reduce the risk of cardiovascular disease?

SUMMARY

1 Nutrition for Children

1. A child's diet should meet the needs for growth, development, and activity as well as reduce the risk of chronic disease later in life. Energy and protein needs per kilogram of body weight decrease as children grow, but total needs increase. The acceptable range of fat intake is higher for young children than for adults. Calcium and iron intakes are often low in children's diets, putting them at risk for low bone density and anemia.

2. In order to meet the nutrient needs of children and develop nutritious habits, caregivers should offer a variety of healthy foods at meals and snacks throughout the day. Children can then choose what and how much they consume. The **National School Lunch Program** provides low-cost school lunches designed to meet nutrient needs and promote healthy diets.

3. The typical diet of U.S. children contributes to their rising obesity rates as well as an increasing incidence of diabetes, high blood cholesterol, and high blood pressure. Watching television contributes to childhood obesity by promoting the intake of foods that are high in calories, fat, and sugar and by reducing the amount of exercise children get. A diet high in sugary foods can increase the risk of dental caries. Children are at particular risk for lead toxicity. Reductions in the use of lead in paint and gasoline have decreased the incidence of high blood lead levels.

2 Nutrition for Adolescents

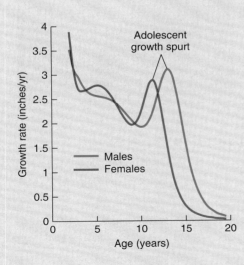

1. During adolescence, the changes associated with **puberty** have an impact on nutrient requirements. Body composition and the nutritional requirements of boys and girls diverge. Energy and protein requirements are higher than in adulthood, and vitamin requirements increase to meet the needs of rapid growth. Calcium intake is often low in the adolescent diet, particularly if soda replaces milk. Iron deficiency anemia is common in adolescent girls due to low intake and iron losses through menstruation.

2. The food choices of adolescents are usually determined more by social activities, peer pressure, and participation in athletics than by nutrient needs. Teens can improve their diets by making healthier fast-food choices. Poorly planned vegetarian diets can be low in iron, zinc, calcium, vitamin D, and vitamin B_{12} and high in saturated fat and cholesterol.

3. Psychological and social changes occurring during the adolescent years make eating disorders more common than at any other time. Adolescent nutritional status may also be affected by weight loss diets and supplements to enhance athletic performance and the use of cigarettes or alcohol.

3 Nutrition for the Adult Years

1. As a population, Americans are living longer but not necessarily healthier lives. Increasing the number of healthy years is an important public health goal. The genes people inherit, as well as their diet, lifestyle, and other environmental factors, determine how long they live.

2. Energy needs decrease with age, but the needs for protein, water, fiber, and most micronutrients remain the same. Decreases in nutrient intake and absorption and changes in the metabolism or absorption of certain micronutrients, including vitamin B_{12}, vitamin D, and calcium, put older adults at risk for deficiency. Iron requirements decrease in women after menopause, but many older adults are at risk for iron deficiency due to poor absorption or blood loss from disease or medications.

3. Older adults are at risk for malnutrition due to the physiological changes that accompany aging, such as the decline in muscle mass and immune function. Acute and chronic illnesses, which are more common in the elderly, may change nutrient requirements, decrease the appeal of food, and impair the ability to obtain and prepare an adequate diet. Medications to treat these diseases may also affect nutritional status. Physical disabilities such as **arthritis** and **macular degeneration**, and changes in mental status caused by **dementia** or depression, and social and economic factors increase the risk of **food insecurity**.

4. A nutrient-dense diet and regular exercise can prevent malnutrition, delay the chronic diseases associated with aging, and increase independence in older adults. The DETERMINE checklist helps identify older adults who are at risk for malnutrition. Economic or physical assistance may be required to meet nutritional needs.

4 The Impact of Alcohol Throughout Life

1. Alcohol, which refers to **ethanol**, is absorbed rapidly, causing the blood alcohol level to rise and its effects to be felt almost immediately. Absorption is slowed when there is food in the stomach. Alcohol is metabolized primarily in the liver. Some is excreted in urine and exhaled in expired air.

2. Moderate amounts of alcohol are broken down by the enzyme alcohol dehydrogenase (ADH). When greater amounts of alcohol are consumed, a second pathway in the liver, called the microsomal ethanol-oxidizing system (MEOS), also metabolizes alcohol. Alcohol metabolism increases fat synthesis in the liver and generates reactive oxygen molecules that can contribute to liver disease.

3. In the short term, excess alcohol consumption causes **alcohol poisoning**, which interferes with brain function. Chronic alcohol consumption can lead to **alcoholism** and can damage the liver, resulting in **fatty liver**, **alcoholic hepatitis**, and eventually **cirrhosis**. Excess alcohol consumption also increases the risks of malnutrition and of developing hypertension, heart disease, and stroke, as well as certain types of cancer.

4. Moderate alcohol consumption can decrease the risk of heart disease by increasing HDL cholesterol and reducing blood clot formation.

KEY TERMS

CRITICAL AND CREATIVE THINKING QUESTIONS

1. Plot these height and weight measurements that were recorded for a girl from age 6 to age 9 on a growth chart and discuss any problems this pattern suggests.

Age	Height (in.)	Weight (lb)
6	45	44
7	48	53
8	50	77
9	52	97

2. Use MyPyramid to design a day's menu for a 15-year-old boy who spends two hours a day playing soccer.

3. Use MyPyramid to design a day's menu for a sedentary 70-year-old woman who must limit her sodium intake.

4. Use iProfile to look up the nutrient composition of your favorite fast-food meal. What is the percentage of calories from carbohydrate, protein, and fat in the meal? Compare the percentage of calories from carbohydrate, fat, and protein in the meal with the percentages recommended for a 10-year-old boy. Assuming that he exercises for 30 to 60 minutes a day, would he be able to eat this meal and still keep his day's intake within the recommended percentages? Why or why not?

5. With age, there is a loss of smell and taste sensation. How might you design meals for a senior center to compensate for this?

6. Jared is 8 years old. He refuses to eat breakfast before leaving for school. What can Jared's parents do to ensure that he has a nutritious meal before school starts?

7. Angela is 55 years old and has a family history of heart disease. She eats a healthy diet that is high in whole grains, fruits, and vegetables, and she does not smoke or consume alcohol. She recently heard that moderate alcohol consumption can help reduce her risk of heart disease. Should she start consuming alcohol? Why or why not?

What is happening in this picture ?

Dara Torres is shown after receiving one of the three silver medals she won in swimming events at the 2008 Olympic Games. At age 41, what we consider middle age, she is twice the age of many of her competitors and the oldest Olympic swimmer ever.

■ How does her physiological age compare with her chronological age?

■ How do you think her lean body mass compares with that of the average 41-year-old woman?

SELF-TEST

(Check your answers in Appendix L.)

1. Which of the following statements is not supported by the graph?

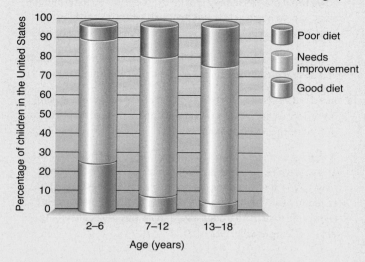

a. Fewer than 25% of children and teens consume a good diet.
b. Diet quality gets worse as children get older.
c. The majority of children and teens consume a diet that needs improvement.
d. More teenagers ages 13 to 18 eat a good diet than eat a poor diet.

2. Which of the following statements about lead exposure in children is false?

a. The incidence of high blood lead levels is greater among low-income children than among high-income children.
b. Malnutrition decreases lead absorption.
c. High lead levels cause learning disabilities in children.
d. The number of children with high blood levels in the United States has declined since 1990.

3. Television affects the nutritional status of children in all except which of the following ways?

a. helping them recognize the importance of fresh fruits and vegetables
b. exposing them to new snack foods
c. providing an environment that encourages snacking
d. reducing the time spent engaged in activity

4. Nutrients most likely to be deficient in an adolescent's diet are _____.

a. sodium and selenium
b. iodine and vitamin A
c. iron and calcium
d. protein and zinc

5. Which of the following statements about energy requirements is true?

a. Total energy needs are higher in childhood than at any other time of life.
b. Energy needs per kilogram of body weight increase as children grow.
c. Energy needs are the same for adolescent boys and girls.
d. Energy needs are lower in older adults than in younger adults.

6. Which of the following statements about iron is false?

a. Iron deficiency is a risk in children, adolescents, and older adults.
b. The RDA is higher in a 60-year-old women than in a 20-year-old woman.
c. Iron needs increase in adolescent males due to increases in muscle mass.
d. Iron needs increase in adolescent females due to menstrual losses.

7. Which of the following could contribute to low calcium status in children and teens?

a. spending too little time outdoors
b. replacing milk with soda
c. having lactose intolerance
d. eating a vegan diet
e. all of the above

8. The graph shows changes in body composition that occur from _____.

a. infancy to childhood
b. childhood to adolescence
c. young adulthood to older adulthood
d. moderate to excessive alcohol consumption

9. Life expectancy refers to _____.

a. the average age to which people in a population live
b. how long an individual will live
c. the longest any person can live
d. how long an individual remains healthy

10. Which of the following statements about vitamin B_{12} is false?

a. Absorption from food is reduced in individuals with atrophic gastritis.
b. Older adults are not at risk for vitamin B_{12} deficiency.
c. It is recommended that older adults meet vitamin B_{12} needs with supplements and/or fortified foods.
d. Vegan diets must include supplements or foods fortified with vitamin B_{12} to meet needs.

11. The DETERMINE checklist is used to _____.

a. qualify recipients for federal food assistance programs
b. check for adverse reactions between food and prescription medications
c. assess the risk of malnutrition in older adults
d. decide whether an older adult needs assisted living

12. For which of the following nutrients is the recommended intake greater in older adults than in younger adults?

a. vitamin D
b. protein
c. vitamin A
d. vitamin C

13. _____ is a type of alcoholic liver disease that results in irreversible scaring.

a. Fatty liver
b. Alcohol poisoning
c. Cirrhosis
d. Alcoholic hepatitis

14. Which of the following statements about the U.S. population is illustrated by this graph?

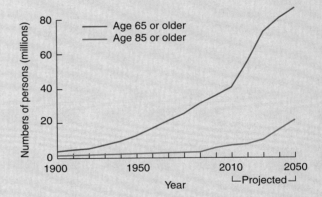

a. The number of people who are over age 65 is expected to more than double between 2010 and 2050.
b. By 2050, 20% of the population will be over 85.
c. The life expectancy of the population is expected to increase between 2010 and 2050.
d. The average healthy life expectancy is expected to increase between 2010 and 2050.

15. Which of the following statements about alcohol is true?

a. It is absorbed faster on a full stomach than on an empty stomach.
b. It can contribute to malnutrition.
c. Moderate alcohol consumption lowers HDL cholesterol levels.
d. It can reduce the risk of cancer.

How Safe Is Our Food Supply?

In the spring of 2008, the FDA warned consumers to avoid eating certain types of tomatoes because they had been linked to outbreaks of illness caused by *Salmonella* bacteria. Restaurants removed tomatoes from their menus, and supermarkets discarded suspect varieties and sold only those that authorities had certified as safe. Tomato producers suffered greatly. That summer, however, jalapeno peppers grown in Mexico were identified as the actual culprit. Tomatoes were exonerated and returned to hamburgers and salads, but the industry continued to reel from the economic impact of the embargo.

Also in 2008, residents of the Colorado town of Alamosa were forced to subsist on bottled and trucked-in water for weeks when *Salmonella* was found to have contaminated the town's water supply. In 2006, when spinach was found to be unsafe to eat due to contamination with the bacterium *E. coli*, the ensuing ban had a severe impact on California's Salinas Valley growers, even after the source was found to be a pig farm outside the spinach-growing region. Almost annually in recent years, huge lots of ground beef have been recalled because they have been found to be contaminated with *E. coli*.

Despite these frightening incidents, however, most foods arrive in our homes safe and fit to eat, and they remain that way if we handle them properly. The modern food-supply chain is perhaps the safest in human history, but danger still lurks, principally in the huge volume of food processed for consumers, as well as inadequate sanitation practices at home.

Keeping Food Safe

LEARNING OBJECTIVES

Name the primary cause of food-borne illness.

Explain why a contaminated food does not cause illness in everyone who eats it.

Discuss the roles of the federal agencies responsible for the safety of the U.S. food supply.

Explain how a HACCP system helps prevent food-borne illness.

Have you ever had food poisoning? Whether you know it or not, you probably have. Oftentimes what we call the 24-hour flu is actually food poisoning, also called **food-borne illness**. Most food-borne illness is caused by consuming food that has been contaminated by **microbes**; occasionally it is caused by toxic chemicals or other contaminants that find their way into food.

Whether or not you get sick from eating a contaminated food depends on how potent the contaminant is, how much of it you consume, and how often you consume it, as well as on your age, size, and health. Some food contaminants cause harm even when minute amounts are consumed, and almost any substance can be toxic if a large enough amount of it is consumed. How well a substance is absorbed and how it is metabolized by the body affect toxicity. Dietary factors and nutritional status can affect absorption. For example, mercury, which is extremely toxic, is not absorbed well if the diet is high in selenium, and lead absorption is decreased by the presence of iron and calcium in the diet. Contaminants that are stored in the body after being absorbed are more likely to be toxic because they accumulate over time, eventually causing symptoms of toxicity. Contaminants that are easily excreted from the body are less likely to cause toxicity.

An individual's size, overall health and nutritional status, and immune function affect his or her risk of food-borne illness. Infants and children are at greater risk than adults because their immune systems are immature and

> **food-borne illness** An illness caused by consumption of contaminated food.

> **microbes** Microscopic organisms, or microorganisms, including bacteria, viruses, and fungi.

their small size means that a given amount of contaminant represents a greater amount per unit of body weight than it would in an adult. Elderly people, people with AIDS, and those receiving chemotherapy or other immunosuppressant drugs are at increased risk because their immune

Agencies that monitor the food supply
TABLE 13.1

INTERNATIONAL ORGANIZATIONS

Food and Agriculture Organization of the United Nations (FAO): Specializes in promoting and sharing knowledge in all aspects of food quality and safety and in all stages of food production: harvest, post-harvest handling, storage, transport, processing, and distribution.

World Health Organization (WHO): Develops international food safety policies, food inspection programs, and standards for hygienic food preparation; promotes technologies that improve food safety and consumer education about safe food practices. Works closely with the FAO.

FEDERAL ORGANIZATIONS

U.S. Food and Drug Administration (FDA): Ensures the safety and quality of all foods sold across state lines with the exception of red meat, poultry, and egg products; inspects food processing plants; inspects imported foods with the exception of red meat, poultry, and egg products; sets standards for food composition; oversees use of drugs and feed in food-producing animals; enforces regulations for food labeling, food and color additives, and food sanitation.

U.S. Department of Agriculture (USDA) Food Safety and Inspection Service (FSIS): Enforces standards for the wholesomeness and quality of red meat, poultry, and egg products produced in the United States or imported from other countries. If a food is suspect, it can be tested for contamination and denied entry into the country.

U.S. Environmental Protection Agency (EPA): Regulates pesticide levels and must approve all pesticides before they can be sold in the United States; establishes water quality standards.

National Marine Fisheries Service: Oversees the management of fisheries and fish harvesting; operates a voluntary program of inspection and grading of fish products.

National Oceanic and Atmospheric Administration (NOAA): Oversees fish and seafood products. Its Seafood Inspection Program inspects and certifies fishing vessels, seafood processing plants, and retail facilities for compliance with federal sanitation standards.

Centers for Disease Control and Prevention (CDC): Monitors and investigates the incidence and causes of food-borne diseases.

STATE AND LOCAL GOVERNMENTS

Oversee all food within their jurisdiction; inspect restaurants, grocery stores, and other retail food establishments, as well as dairy farms and milk processing plants, grain mills, and food manufacturing plants within local jurisdictions.

systems may be compromised. Pregnancy weakens the immune system, putting pregnant women and their unborn babies at risk. Poor nutritional status and chronic conditions such as diabetes and kidney disease may decrease the body's ability to detoxify harmful substances.

THE ROLE OF GOVERNMENT

The safety of the food supply is monitored by agencies at international, federal, state, and local levels (TABLE 13.1). Federal agencies set standards and establish regulations for the safe handling of food and water and for the information included on food labels. They regulate the use of additives, packaging materials, and agricultural chemicals; inspect food processing and storage facilities; monitor domestic and imported foods for contamination; and investigate outbreaks of food-borne illness.

Each year, 76 million people in the United States experience a food-borne illness.[1] Media coverage of outbreaks of food-borne illness on cruise ships, of deaths from *E. coli* infection, and of cows infected with mad cow disease have heightened public concern and led to the development of the National Food Safety Initiative. The goal of this initiative is to reduce the incidence of food-borne illness by improving food safety practices and policies throughout the United States. Because food can be contaminated anywhere in the supply chain—from where it is grown to when it is served in your home—the program targets food safety from farm to table (FIGURE 13.1).

Keeping food safe from farm to table FIGURE 13.1

Keeping food safe involves identifying possible points of contamination along a food's journey from the farm to the dinner table and implementing controls to prevent or contain contamination.

1 **Farm** Crops can be contaminated with bacteria before they are even harvested. Good agricultural practices help minimize contamination during growing, harvesting, sorting, packing, and storage.

2 **Processing** Contamination of processing equipment can transfer microbes to food. To prevent contamination, processors must follow guidelines concerning cleanliness and training of workers, as well as a protocol that anticipates how biological, chemical, or physical hazards are most likely to occur and establish appropriate measures to prevent them from occurring.

3 **Transportation** During transport, poor sanitation and inadequate refrigeration can contaminate food and allow microbes to grow. Clean containers and vehicles, plus refrigeration can prevent the growth of food-borne bacteria.

5 **Table** Even a safe food can be contaminated in the home. Consumers can prevent food-borne illness at their table by learning to handle, store, and prepare food safely.

4 **Retail** Food can become contaminated during handling or storage in grocery stores or during preparation in restaurants. The FDA's Food Code provides recommendations for the handling and service of food in an effort to help owners and employees at retail establishments prevent food-borne illness. Local health inspections ensure cleanliness and proper procedures.

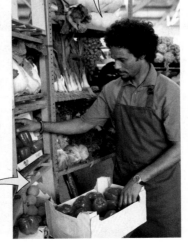

Process Diagram

THE ROLE OF FOOD MANUFACTURERS AND RETAILERS

The responsibility for providing safe food to the marketplace falls on the shoulders of food manufacturers, processors, and distributors. To meet this responsibility, they must establish and implement a **Hazard Analysis Critical Control Point (HACCP)** system. A HACCP system analyzes food production, processing, and transport, with the goal of identifying potential sources of contamination and points where measures can be taken to control contamination. Then, by monitoring these **critical control points**, contamination can be prevented or eliminated (**FIGURE 13.2**). Unlike traditional methods of protecting the food supply, which use visual spot checks and random testing to catch contamination after it occurs, HACCP systems are designed to *prevent* contamination.

> **Hazard Analysis Critical Control Point (HACCP)**
>
> A food safety system that focuses on identifying and preventing hazards that could cause food-borne illness.

THE ROLE OF THE CONSUMER

Although government agencies, manufacturers, and retailers are involved in creating a safe food supply, consumers also need to assume responsibility for their food. Even a food that has been manufactured, packaged, and transported with great care can cause food-borne illness if it is not handled carefully at home. In fact, most cases of food-borne illness are caused by foods prepared at home.[2] Consumers can prevent most food-borne illness through careful food handling, storage, and preparation (discussed in depth later in the chapter). They can also protect themselves and others by reporting incidents involving unsanitary, unsafe, deceptive, or mislabeled food to the appropriate agencies (**TABLE 13.2**).

Process Diagram

HACCP in liquid egg production FIGURE 13.2

The scrambled eggs served in your cafeteria at school or work most likely came out of a carton rather than a shell. To produce this product, eggs are shelled, mixed together in large vats, heated to kill microbial contaminants, packaged, and either refrigerated or frozen. A contaminated batch could sicken hundreds of people. This example shows how a HACCP system might be used to prevent contaminated eggs from reaching the consumer.

1 **Conduct a hazard analysis** The manufacturer analyzes its processing steps for potential hazards and determines what preventive measures can be taken. In the case of eggs, there is a large potential for contamination with the bacterium *Salmonella*. Adequate heating is a preventive measure that can eliminate this hazard.

2 **Identify the critical control points** Critical control points are the steps in a food's processing at which the hazard can be eliminated. In the case of egg processing, the critical control point is heating the shelled egg mixture in a large chamber.

3 **Establish critical limits** Critical limits are the parameters that will prevent the hazard. In the case of these eggs, the critical limits are sufficient heating time and temperature to ensure that *Salmonella* bacteria are killed.

How to report food-related issues TABLE 13.2

Before reporting a food-related problem, get all the facts. Determine whether you have used the product as intended and according to the manufacturer's instruction. Check to see if the item is past its expiration date. After these steps have been taken, report the incident to the appropriate agency:

• **Problems related to any food except meat and poultry, including adverse reactions:** Report emergencies to the FDA's main emergency number, which is staffed 24 hours a day: 301-443-1240. Nonemergencies can be reported to the FDA consumer complaint coordinator in your area, which you can find at www.fda.gov/safety/reportaproblem.

• **Issues related to meat and poultry:** Report first to your state department of agriculture and then to the USDA Meat and Poultry Hotline (1-888-MPHotline or mphotline.fsis@usda.gov).

• **Restaurant food and sanitation problems:** Report directly to your local or state health department.

• **Issues related to alcoholic beverages:** Report to the U.S. Department of the Treasury's Bureau of Alcohol, Tobacco, Firearms, and Explosives.

• **Pesticide, air, and water pollution:** Report first to your state environmental protection department and then to the U.S. EPA.

• **Products purchased at the grocery store:** Return to the store. Grocery stores are concerned with the safety of the foods they sell, and they will take responsibility for tracking down and correcting the problem. They will either refund your money or replace the product.

CONCEPT CHECK STOP

What causes food-borne illness?

Why might the same food make one person sick and not another person?

Who is responsible for the safety of the food you eat?

How does HACCP differ from traditional visual food inspection?

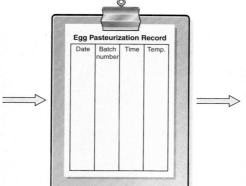

Egg Pasteurization Record

Date	Batch number	Time	Temp.

4 Establish monitoring procedures Procedures need to be in place to continually monitor the critical control points. With egg processing, each batch is tested for the presence of *Salmonella*. If the temperature is not hot enough or the heating is not continued long enough, *Salmonella* can survive, as shown here by the growing bacterial colonies.

5 Establish corrective action If a critical limit is not met, corrective action is necessary. Batches of eggs that are contaminated with *Salmonella* are discarded, and the temperature of the heat chamber is adjusted to ensure that *Salmonella* in the next batch will be killed.

6 Record keeping Extensive records are kept, documenting the monitoring of critical control points, verification activities, and corrective actions taken. This enables the manufacturer to trace the source of the problem in the event of an outbreak of food-borne illness.

7 Verification procedures Review of plans and records helps ensure that the HACCP plan is working and only safe eggs are reaching the consumer.

Pathogens in Food

LEARNING OBJECTIVES

Distinguish food-borne infection from food-borne intoxication.

Discuss three types of bacteria that commonly cause food-borne illness.

Explain how viruses, molds, and parasites can make us sick.

Describe how careful food handling can prevent food-borne illness.

Most cases of food-borne illness in the United States are caused by food that has been contaminated with **pathogens**. The pathogens that most commonly affect the food supply include bacteria, viruses, molds, and parasites. A typical case of food-borne illness causes a short bout of flulike symptoms, including abdominal pain, nausea, diarrhea, and vomiting. However, more severe symptoms, such as kidney failure, arthritis, paralysis, miscarriage, and even death, sometimes occur.

pathogen
A biological agent that causes disease.

Any food-borne illness caused by pathogens that multiply in the human body is called a **food-borne infection**. Contracting a food-borne infection usually involves consumption of a large number of pathogens that infect the body or produce toxins within the body. Any food-borne illness caused by consuming a food that contains toxins produced by pathogens is referred to as **food-borne intoxication**. Even food that contains only a few pathogens can cause food-borne intoxication if the pathogens have produced enough toxin. Avoiding food-borne illness—both infection and intoxication—requires knowing how to handle and store food in ways that will prevent contamination and prevent or minimize the growth of pathogens that may already be present in the food. Even a food that is contaminated with pathogens can be safe if it is prepared in a manner that destroys any pathogens or toxins that are present.

BACTERIA IN FOOD

Bacteria are present in the soil, on our skin, on most surfaces in our homes, and in the food we eat. Most are harmless, some are beneficial, and a few are pathogenic, causing food-borne infection or intoxication.[3]

Visualizing

How bacteria contaminate our food FIGURE 13.3

A Because poultry farms house large numbers of chickens in close proximity, one infected chicken can infect thousands of others. *Salmonella* can infect the ovaries of hens and contaminate the eggs before the shells are formed, so that the bacteria are present inside the shell when the eggs are laid. Therefore, eggs should never be eaten raw. ▼

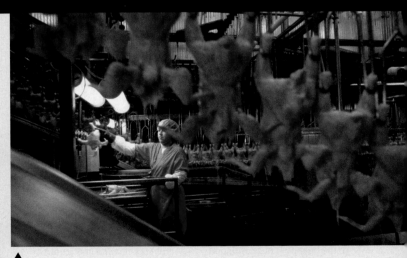

▲

B In processing plants, *Salmonella* and *Campylobacter* from infected birds can be transferred to the meat of healthy birds. Consumers should always handle raw chicken as if it contains pathogens.

NATIONAL GEOGRAPHIC

Bacterial food-borne infection

It is estimated that about 2 million to 4 million people become infected with the bacterium *Salmonella* each year in the United States.[3] Contaminated meat, dairy products, seafood, fresh produce, and cereal have caused outbreaks, but poultry and eggs are the foods most commonly contaminated with the bacterium (**FIGURE 13.3A** and **B**). Because *Salmonella* is killed by heat, foods that are likely to be contaminated should be cooked thoroughly.

Campylobacter jejuni is the leading cause of acute bacterial diarrhea in developed countries.[4] Common sources are undercooked chicken, unpasteurized milk, and untreated water (**FIGURE 13.3B** and **C**). This organism grows slowly in cold temperatures and is killed by heat, so thorough cooking and careful storage help prevent infection.

Escherichia coli, commonly called *E. coli*, is a bacterium that inhabits the gastrointestinal tracts of humans and other animals. It comes into contact with food through fecal contamination of water or unsanitary handling of food. Some strains of *E. coli* are harmless, but others can cause serious food-borne infection. One strain of *E. coli*, found in water contaminated by human or animal feces, is the cause of "travelers' diarrhea." Another strain, *E. coli* O157:H7, produces a toxin in the body that causes abdominal pain, bloody diarrhea, and in severe cases a form of kidney failure called **hemolytic-uremic syndrome**, which can be fatal.[5]

E. coli O157:H7 entered the public spotlight in 1993, when it led to the deaths of several children who had consumed undercooked, contaminated hamburgers from a fast-food restaurant (**FIGURE 13.3D**). Thorough cooking of the hamburgers would have killed the bacteria that caused these deaths. *E. coli* can also contaminate produce such as lettuce, spinach, and green onions and cause illness if the produce is eaten raw.

Each year in the United States, an estimated 2,500 persons become seriously ill due to infection with *Listeria monocytogenes*, and of these, 500 die.[6] In most people *Listeria* infection just causes flulike symptoms, but in high-risk groups, such as children, pregnant women, and the elderly, it can cause meningitis and serious blood infections. *Listeria* is ubiquitous in the environment and can survive and grow at refrigerator temperatures. Because it can grow at cool temperatures, this bacterium can infect ready-to-eat foods such as hot dogs and lunchmeats, even if they have been kept properly refrigerated. To prevent infection, ready-to-eat meats should be heated to the steaming point, and unpasteurized dairy products should be avoided.

The food-borne infection caused by the bacterium *Vibrio vulnificus* usually causes gastrointestinal upset but can be deadly in people with compromised immune systems. The most common way in which people become

D *E. coli* O157:H7 can live in the intestines of healthy cattle and contaminate the meat after slaughter. Ground beef contaminated with *E. coli* O157:H7 is a particular concern because the pathogens are mixed throughout during grinding rather than remaining on the surface, as they do on steaks and chops. The *E. coli* on the outside of the meat are quickly killed during cooking, but those in the interior survive if the meat is not cooked thoroughly. *E. coli*–contaminated meat that comes into contact with a grinder may contaminate hundreds of pounds of ground beef.

C *Campylobacter* are often carried by healthy cattle and by flies on farms. As a result, the bacteria are commonly present in unpasteurized (raw) milk. Unpasteurized milk is also a common source of *Listeria*. During pasteurization, milk is heated to a temperature that is high enough to kill both *Campylobacter* and *Listeria*. ▼

infected is by eating raw or undercooked shellfish, particularly oysters. *Vibrio* bacteria grow in warm seawater. The incidence of *Vibrio* infection is higher during the summer months, when warm water favors growth.

Bacterial food-borne intoxication

Staphylococcus aureus is a common cause of bacterial food-borne intoxication. These bacteria live in human nasal passages and can be transferred to food through coughing or sneezing. They can then grow on the food, producing a toxin that causes vomiting soon after ingestion.

Another cause of food-borne intoxication is the bacterium *Clostridium perfringens*. It is often called the *cafeteria germ* because it grows in foods that are stored in large containers like those used in cafeterias. Little oxygen gets to the food at the center of a large container, thus providing an excellent growth environment for bacteria such as these, which thrive in low-oxygen environments. *C. perfringens* are difficult to kill because they form heat-resistant **spores**. Spores are a stage of bacterial life that remains dormant until environmental conditions favor their growth. *C. perfringens* may cause illness through both infection and intoxication.

The deadliest of all bacterial food toxins is produced by *Clostridium botulinum*. Heat-resistant spores of *C. botulinum* are found in soil, water, and the intestinal tracts of animals. The toxin is produced when the spores begin to grow and develop. When consumed, the toxin blocks nerve function, resulting in vomiting, abdominal pain, double vision, and paralysis that leads to respiratory failure. If untreated, **botulism** is often fatal, but modern detection methods and rapid administration of antitoxin have reduced mortality rates. *C. botulinum* grows in low-oxygen, low-acid conditions, so improperly canned foods and foods such as potatoes or stew that are held in large containers where there is little exposure to oxygen pro-

vide optimal conditions for botulism spores to germinate (**FIGURE 13.4**).

Infant botulism is a type of botulism that is seen only in infants. Though rare, it occurs worldwide and is the most common form of botulism in the United States.[7] It is caused by ingestion of botulism spores. When ingested, the spores germinate in the infant's gastrointestinal tract, producing toxin. Some of the toxin is absorbed into the bloodstream, causing weakness, paralysis, and respiratory problems. In the absence of complications, infants generally recover. Only infants are affected, because in adults, competing intestinal microflora prevent spores from germinating. Because honey can be contaminated with botulism spores, it should never be fed to infants under 1 year of age.

VIRUSES IN FOOD

Unlike bacteria, the viruses that cause human diseases cannot grow and reproduce in foods. Human viruses can reproduce only inside human cells. They make us sick by turning our cells into virus-producing factories (**FIGURE 13.5**).

Noroviruses are a group of viruses that cause gastroenteritis, or what we commonly call "stomach flu." These viruses are believed to be responsible for about 50% of all food-borne gastroenteritis outbreaks in the United States.[8] Norovirus illness is contracted either by eating food that is contaminated with the virus or by touching a contaminated surface and then putting your fingers in your mouth. Shellfish can be contaminated with norovirus if the water in which they live is polluted with human or animal feces. Cooking destroys noroviruses, so uncooked foods and water are the most common cause of norovirus food-borne illness. Norovirus infection can be spread from one

Canned foods and botulism FIGURE 13.4

Because acid prevents the germination of *Clostridium botulinum* spores, foods that are low in acid, such as green beans, corn, peppers, asparagus, and mushrooms, are more likely to cause botulism than are acidic foods. To avoid botulism, discard bulging cans, as the bulge could indicate the presence of gas produced by the bacteria as they grow. Once it has formed, botulism toxin can be destroyed by boiling for at least 10 minutes, but if the safety of a food is in question, it should be thrown away; even a taste of a food contaminated with botulism toxin can be deadly.

infected person to another, so it spreads swiftly where many people congregate in a small area. You may have heard of it as a cause of food-borne illness aboard cruise ships. These outbreaks make headlines, but norovirus outbreaks are just as likely in nursing homes, restaurants, hotels, and dormitories as they are aboard cruise ships.

Hepatitis A is another viral infection that can be contracted from food or water that is contaminated with fecal matter. Hepatitis A infection causes liver inflammation, jaundice, fever, nausea, fatigue, and abdominal pain. The infection can require a recovery period of several months, but it does not require treatment and does not cause permanent liver damage. Hepatitis in drinking water is destroyed by chlorination. Cooking destroys the virus in food, and good sanitation can prevent its spread. A vaccine that protects against hepatitis A infection is available.

How viruses make us sick FIGURE 13.5

Viruses make us sick by reproducing inside our cells. Viruses that cause food-borne illness enter the body through the gastrointestinal (GI) tract. Other types of viruses may enter the body through open cuts, the respiratory tract, or the genital tract.

HOW IT WORKS
View in your WileyPLUS course

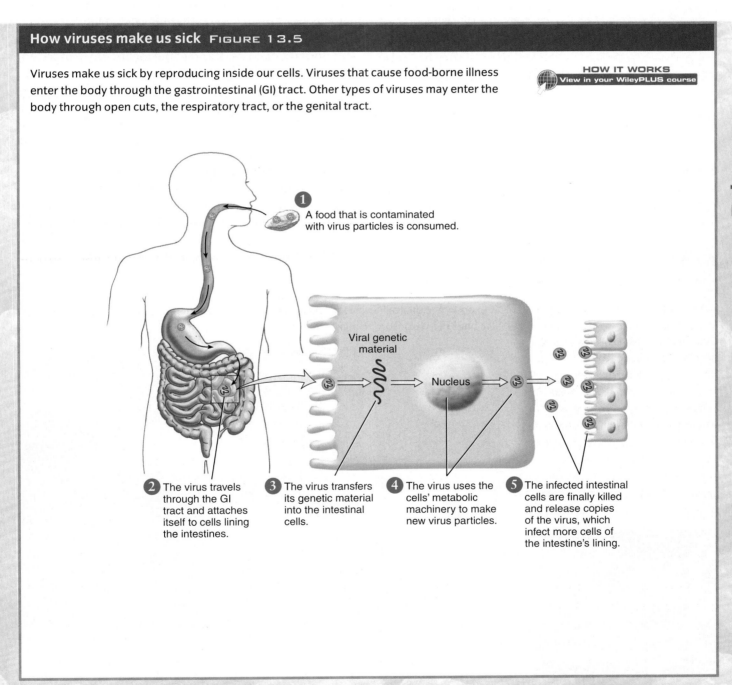

1 A food that is contaminated with virus particles is consumed.

Viral genetic material

Nucleus

2 The virus travels through the GI tract and attaches itself to cells lining the intestines.

3 The virus transfers its genetic material into the intestinal cells.

4 The virus uses the cells' metabolic machinery to make new virus particles.

5 The infected intestinal cells are finally killed and release copies of the virus, which infect more cells of the intestine's lining.

Process Diagram

MOLDY FOODS

Many types of **mold** grow on foods such as bread, cheese, and fruit. Under certain conditions, these molds produce toxins (**FIGURE 13.6**). More than 250 different mold toxins have been identified. Cooking and freezing stop mold growth but do not destroy toxins that have already been produced. If a food is moldy, it should be discarded, the area where it was stored should be cleaned, and neighboring foods should be checked to see if they have also become contaminated.

> **mold**
> Multicellular fungi that form filamentous branching growths.

PARASITES IN FOOD

> **parasites**
> Organisms that live at the expense of others.

Some **parasites** are microscopic single-celled animals, while others are worms large enough to be seen with the naked eye. Parasites that can be transmitted through consumption of contaminated food and water cause food-borne illness. *Giardia lamblia* is a single-celled parasite that is often contracted by hikers who drink untreated water from streams contaminated with animal feces. *Giardia* infection is also becoming a problem in day-care centers where diapers are changed and hands and surfaces are not thoroughly washed.[3] *Cryptosporidium parvum* is another single-celled parasite that is commonly spread by contaminated water, but cases have also been reported in patients who have eaten contaminated raw fruits and vegetables.[10]

Trichinella spiralis is a parasite that is found in raw and undercooked pork and game meats. Once ingested, these small, wormlike organisms find their way to the muscles, where they grow, causing flulike symptoms. Fish are another common source of parasitic infections because they carry the larvae of parasites such as roundworms, flatworms, flukes, and tapeworms (**FIGURE 13.7**). As the popularity of eating raw fish has increased, so has the incidence of parasitic infections from fish. Parasites, including those in fish, are killed by thorough cooking. If raw fish is consumed, parasitic infections can be avoided by eating fish that has been frozen.

Mold toxin and liver cancer FIGURE 13.6

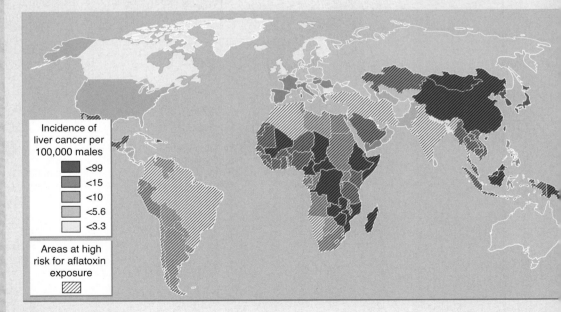

A The filamentous growths seen in this electron micrograph belong to the mold *Aspergillus flavus*. It produces *aflatoxin*, which is among the most potent carcinogens and mutagens known. This mold commonly grows on corn, rice, wheat, peanuts, almonds, walnuts, sunflower seeds, and spices such as black pepper and coriander. The level of aflatoxin that may be present in foods in the United States is regulated to prevent toxicity. ▼

B Exposure to aflatoxin can lead to liver cancer. Many regions with high rates of liver cancer also have high exposure to aflatoxin.[9]

Incidence of liver cancer per 100,000 males
- <99
- <15
- <10
- <5.6
- <3.3

Areas at high risk for aflatoxin exposure

Herring worm FIGURE 13.7

The body cavity of this herring contains the larval form of the small roundworm *Anisakis* simplex, also called herring worm. When consumed in raw fish, these parasites invade the stomach and intestinal tract, causing *Anisakis* disease, which is characterized by severe abdominal pain. The fresher the fish is when it is eviscerated, the less likely it is to cause this disease because the larvae move from the fish's stomach to its flesh only after the fish dies.

PRIONS IN FOOD

The strangest, scariest, yet rarest food-borne illness is caused not by a microbe but by a protein, called a **prion**, that has folded improperly. Abnormal prions are believed to be the cause of mad cow disease, or **bovine spongiform encephalopathy (BSE)**, a deadly degenerative neurological disease that affects cattle. The human form of this disease is **variant Creutzfeldt-Jakob Disease (vCJD)**. People are believed to contract it by eating tissue from a cow infected with BSE (**FIGURE 13.8**).[11] Symptoms of vCJD begin as mood swings and numbness and within about 14 months progress to dementia and death.

vCJD is believed to be transmitted by consumption of the brain and nervous tissue, intestines, eyes, or tonsils of contaminated animals, but thus far meat (if free of central nervous system tissue) and milk have not been found to transmit either BSE or vCJD.[3] Even though cooking does not destroy prions, the risk of acquiring vCJD is extremely small. Safeguards are in place to prevent cattle in the United States from contracting BSE. These include restrictions on the import of animals and animal products from countries where BSE has occurred, restrictions on what can be included in cattle feed, and testing for BSE before meat is released into the food supply.[12] Several cows with BSE have been identified in the United States, but meat from these animals did not enter the food supply. Thus far there has been no known instance of U.S. beef causing a case of vCJD.

> **prion** A pathogenic protein that is the cause of degenerative brain diseases called spongiform encephalopathies. *Prion* is short for *proteinaceous infectious particle*.

How prions multiply FIGURE 13.8

The abnormal prions that cause BSE differ from normal proteins in the way they are folded—that is, in their three-dimensional structure. When the improperly folded form of a prion is introduced into the brain after a person has eaten contaminated tissue, it can reproduce by corrupting neighboring proteins, essentially changing their shape so that they, too, become abnormal prions. Because the abnormal prions are not degraded normally, they accumulate and form clumps called plaques. These plaques cause deadly nervous tissue damage.

1. Normal prion proteins are present in the brain.

2. Abnormal prion proteins arise spontaneously or enter from the diet.

3. Normal and abnormal prion proteins come into contact with each other.

4. Normal prions are converted into abnormal prions.

5. Abnormal prion proteins accumulate in the brain, leading to the formation of plaques that damage brain tissue.

Process Diagram

Summary of bacterial, viral, and parasitic food-borne illnesses TABLE 13.3

Microbe	Sources	Symptoms	Onset (time after consumption)	Duration
Bacteria				
Salmonella	Fecal contamination, raw or undercooked eggs and meat, especially poultry	Nausea, abdominal pain, diarrhea, headache, fever	6–48 hours	1–2 days
Campylobacter jejuni	Unpasteurized milk, untreated water, undercooked meat and poultry	Fever, headache, diarrhea, abdominal pain	2–5 days	1–2 weeks
Listeria monocytogenes	Raw milk products, soft ripened cheeses, deli meats and cold cuts, raw and undercooked poultry and meats, raw and smoked fish, raw vegetables	Fever, headache, stiff neck, chills, nausea, vomiting. May cause spontaneous abortion or stillbirth in pregnant women.	Days to weeks	Days to weeks
Vibrio vulnificus	Raw seafood from contaminated water	Cramps, abdominal pain, weakness, watery diarrhea, fever, chills	15–24 hours	2–4 days
Staphylococcus aureus	Human contamination from coughs and sneezes; eggs, meat, potato and macaroni salads	Severe nausea, vomiting, diarrhea	2–8 hours	2–3 days
Escherichia coli O157:H7	Fecal contamination, undercooked ground beef	Abdominal pain, bloody diarrhea, kidney failure	5–48 hours	3 days–2 weeks or longer
Clostridium perfringens	Fecal contamination, deep-dish casseroles	Nausea, diarrhea, abdominal pain	8–22 hours	6–24 hours
Clostridium botulinum	Improperly canned foods, deep casseroles, honey	Lassitude, weakness, vertigo, respiratory failure, paralysis	18–36 hours	10 days or longer (must administer antitoxin)
Shigella	Fecal contamination of water or foods, especially salads such as chicken, tuna, shrimp, and potato salads	Diarrhea, abdominal pain, fever, vomiting	12–50 hours	5–6 days
Yersinia enterocolitica	Pork, dairy products, and produce	Diarrhea, vomiting, fever, abdominal pain; often mistaken for appendicitis	24–48 hours	Weeks
Viruses				
Norovirus	Fecal contamination of water or foods, especially shellfish and salad ingredients	Diarrhea, nausea, vomiting	1–2 days	2–6 days
Hepatitis A	Human fecal contamination of food or water, raw shellfish	Jaundice, liver inflammation, fatigue, fever, nausea, anorexia, abdominal discomfort	10–50 days	1–2 weeks to several months
Parasites				
Giardia lamblia	Fecal contamination of water and uncooked foods	Diarrhea, abdominal pain, gas, anorexia, nausea, vomiting	5–25 days	1–2 weeks, but may be chronic
Cryptosporidium parvum	Fecal contamination of food or water	Severe watery diarrhea	Hours	2–4 days, but sometimes weeks
Trichinella spiralis	Undercooked pork, game meat	Muscle weakness, flulike symptoms	Weeks	Months
Anisakis simplex	Raw fish	Severe abdominal pain	1 hour–2 weeks	3 weeks
Toxoplasma gondii	Meat, primarily pork	Toxoplasmosis (can cause central nervous system disorders, flulike symptoms, and birth defects in the offspring of women exposed during pregnancy, see Chapter 11)	10–23 days	May become chronic

WHAT BUG HAS YOU DOWN?

There are certainly a wide variety of food-borne pathogens that can make you sick (TABLE 13.3 on the previous page). Recent improvements in governmental outbreak surveillance, attentiveness by healthcare professionals, and testing frequency and accuracy have made it possible to identify even more cases of food-borne illness than was possible a few years ago. Given this and the extensive media coverage of outbreaks of food-borne illness and recalls of contaminated foods, one would expect that the incidence of food-borne illness has been rising. In fact, there has been no increase over the past 4 years.[13] Public awareness of the problem and education on how to handle food safely should make food-borne illness even less frequent in the future.

PREVENTING MICROBIAL FOOD-BORNE ILLNESS

Microbes in food multiply when they are presented with the right conditions for growth. The first step in preventing microbial food-borne illness is to minimize the presence of microbes by choosing food carefully (TABLE 13.4). Preparing food in a clean kitchen reduces **cross-contamination**. Storing food at refrigerator or freezer temperatures either limits or stops microbial growth. Heating foods to the recommended temperature kills microbes and destroys toxins (see FIGURE 13.9 on the next page). Foods that are served cold should be kept cold until they are served. Frozen foods should be kept frozen and then thawed in the refrigerator or microwave before cooking, not thawed at room temperature, which favors microbial growth. Cooked food should be handled with care and kept hot until it is served. When in doubt about the safety of a food, throw it out.

Cross-contamination can occur when uncooked foods containing live microbes come into contact with foods that have already been cooked. Therefore, cooked meat should never be returned to the same dish that held the raw meat, and sauces used to marinate uncooked foods should never be used as a sauce on cooked food. Cooked food should be refrigerated as soon as possible after it has been served. The temperature range that is most favorable for microbial growth is the range at which food usually sits between service and storage. Large portions of food should be divided before refrigeration so they will cool quickly. Most leftovers should be kept for only a few days.

> **cross-contamination**
> The transfer of contaminants from one food or object to another.

Safe grocery choices TABLE 13.4

- Purchase food from reputable venders.
- Make sure jars are closed and seals are unbroken and that safety "buttons" on jar lids have not popped.
- Reject cans that are rusted, dented, or bulging.
- Make sure food packaging is secure.
- Select frozen foods from below the frost line in the freezer.
- Make sure frozen foods are solidly frozen and do not contain frost or ice crystals.
- Check voluntary freshness dates and avoid foods with expired dates:

  o **Sell-by or pull-by date:** Used by manufacturers to tell grocers when to remove their product from the shelves. You should buy the product before this date, but if the food has been handled and stored properly, it is usually still safe for consumption after it. For example, milk is usually still good at least a week beyond its sell-by date if it has been properly refrigerated.

  o **Best if used by, use-by, quality assurance, or freshness date:** Used to specify the last date on which the product will retain maximum freshness, flavor, and texture. Beyond this date, the product's quality may diminish, but the food may still be safe if it has been handled and stored properly.

  o **Expiration date:** Used to specify the last day on which a product should be eaten. State governments regulate these dates for perishable items, such as milk and eggs. The FDA regulates only the expiration dates of infant formula.

Fight Bac! is an educational campaign conducted by the Partnership for Food Safety Education. It is designed to teach food-handling practices that will keep food safe from bacteria and prevent food-borne illness. Fight Bac! recommends that consumers follow four steps—clean, separate, cook, and chill—to prevent food-borne illness. (www.fightbac.org) ▶

Meats and casseroles should be cooked, and leftovers reheated, until they reach the internal temperatures shown here, which will ensure that microbes have been killed. Use a food thermometer to make sure that the food is cooked to a safe internal temperature; color is not a good indicator of safety. ▼

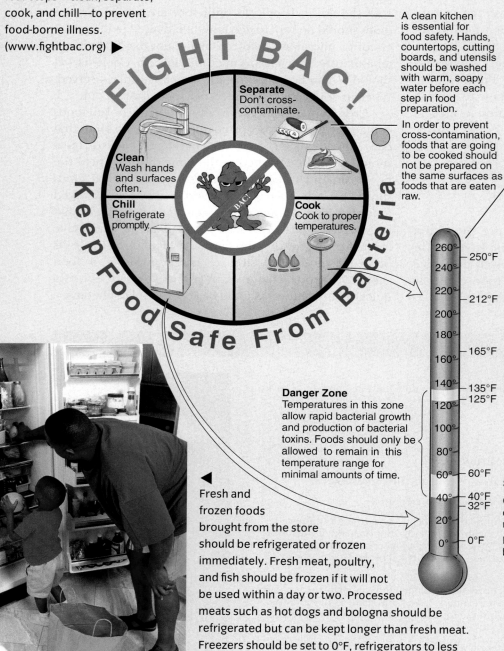

A clean kitchen is essential for food safety. Hands, countertops, cutting boards, and utensils should be washed with warm, soapy water before each step in food preparation.

In order to prevent cross-contamination, foods that are going to be cooked should not be prepared on the same surfaces as foods that are eaten raw.

FIGHT BAC!

Keep Food Safe From Bacteria

Separate Don't cross-contaminate.

Clean Wash hands and surfaces often.

Chill Refrigerate promptly.

Cook Cook to proper temperatures.

Safe Cooking Temperatures[14]	
Food item	**Internal temperature (°F) or description**
Beef roasts and steaks	145 medium rare 160 medium 170 well done
Ground meat	160
Pork	160 medium 170 well done
Poultry	165
Fish	145 or until the flesh is opaque and separates easily with a fork
Eggs	Until the yolk and white are firm, not runny (egg dishes 160)
Leftovers and casseroles	165

260°
250°F — Canning temperature for low-acid foods in pressure cooker

240°
220°
212°F — Range of cooking temperatures to kill most bacteria. The amount of time needed decreases as the temperature increases.

200°
180°
165°F — Minimum temperature for reheating foods. Warming temperatures control growth but allow survival of some bacteria.

160°
140°
135°F
125°F — Some growth may occur: Many bacteria survive.

Danger Zone Temperatures in this zone allow rapid bacterial growth and production of bacterial toxins. Foods should only be allowed to remain in this temperature range for minimal amounts of time.

120°
100°
80°
60°
60°F — Some bacterial growth may occur in this zone.

40°
40°F
32°F — Cold temperatures allow slow growth for a few cold-tolerant organisms but stop the growth of most.

20°
0°
0°F — Freezing temperatures prevent bacterial growth but some bacteria are able to survive.

◀ Fresh and frozen foods brought from the store should be refrigerated or frozen immediately. Fresh meat, poultry, and fish should be frozen if it will not be used within a day or two. Processed meats such as hot dogs and bologna should be refrigerated but can be kept longer than fresh meat. Freezers should be set to 0°F, refrigerators to less than 40°F.

▲ Temperature is one of the best weapons consumers have for preventing food-borne illness. Low temperatures slow or stop microbial growth, and high temperatures kill microorganisms.

NATIONAL GEOGRAPHIC

Although most food-borne illness in the United States is caused by food prepared in homes, an outbreak in a commercial or institutional establishment usually involves more people and is more likely to be reported (see the *Case Study*). Food in retail establishments has many opportunities to be contaminated because of the large volume of food handled and the large number of people involved in its preparation. Consumers should choose restaurants with safety in mind. Restaurants should be clean, and cooked foods should be served hot. Cafeteria steam tables should be kept hot enough that the water is steaming and food is kept above 135°F. Cold foods, such as salad bar items, should be kept either refrigerated or on ice to keep the food at 41°F or colder.

CASE STUDY

FOOD DETECTIVES

On Friday, over half of the 200 children enrolled at the local elementary school were either absent or went home sick sometime during the school day. Symptoms included nausea and vomiting, diarrhea, abdominal pain, and fever. Food-borne illness was suspected, and the local health department was notified. Inspectors were able to trace the source of the outbreak to the Spring Celebration held at the school on Thursday. For this event, the first-graders made cupcakes, the second-graders cookies, the third-graders fruit salad, and the fourth-graders frozen custard. All the children were interviewed about which of these foods they had eaten that day, and the information was used to compile the following graph:

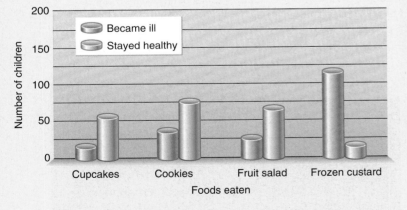

Based on the graph, which food is the most likely cause of the illness? Why?

Your answer:

Physicians saw many of the sick children, and the bacterium *Salmonella enteritidis* was isolated from their stool samples. The health inspectors determined that the fourth-graders had used six grade-A raw eggs to make the frozen custard.

How can eggs become contaminated with *Salmonella*?

Your answer:

The cookie and cupcake recipes also called for eggs. Why are these unlikely to be the cause of the problem?

Your answer:

Suggest a reason why 20 children who consumed the frozen custard did not get ill.

Your answer:

What could the fourth-graders have done to avoid the risk of *Salmonella* in their frozen custard?

Your answer:

(Check your answers in Appendix K.)

A Picnic for Bacteria

Looks great—lots of food and people together on a warm, sunny day. Most people see lunch, but those concerned with food-borne illness see trouble. If a food is contaminated with pathogenic bacteria, it won't take long before enough bacteria are present to cause food-borne illness. The number of bacterial cells doubles each time the cells divide, resulting in an exponential growth curve like the one shown here. If 10 bacterial cells contaminate the egg salad during preparation and then it sits in the warm sun for 4 hours, during which time the cells divide every 20 minutes, there will be 40,960 bacterial cells in the salad when you scoop a portion of it onto your plate.

Limiting bacterial growth is a consideration any time food must be carried out of the home. Any food that is transported should be kept cold. Lunches should be transported to and from work or school in a cooler or an insulated bag and refrigerated upon arrival. Perishable foods that are brought home from work or school uneaten should be thrown out and not saved for another day. What foods would be the safest to include in lunch boxes and serve at picnics? Why?

Picnics, potluck suppers, and other large events where food is served provide a prime opportunity for bacteria to flourish because food is often left at room temperature or in the sun for long periods before it is consumed. When diners serve themselves, cross-contamination from dirty hands or used plates and utensils is possible. Unlike the food in salad bars at restaurants, the food at a family picnic is not placed under a sneeze guard to prevent contamination from coughs and sneezes. All food that is served outdoors at a family picnic or county fair should be approached with food safety in mind (see *What a Scientist Sees*).

CONCEPT CHECK **STOP**

How does *Clostridium botulinum* cause food-borne illness?

What pathogenic bacteria commonly contaminate chicken and eggs?

How do viruses make us sick?

How does refrigeration help prevent food-borne illness?

Agricultural and Industrial Chemicals in Food

Chemicals used in agricultural production and industrial wastes contaminate the environment and can find their way into the food supply. How harmful these chemicals are depends on how long they remain in the environment and whether they are stored in the organisms that consume them or can be broken down and excreted by these organisms. Some contaminants are eliminated from the environment quickly because they are broken down by microorganisms or chemical reactions. Others remain in the environment for very long periods, and when taken up by plants and small animals, they are not metabolized or excreted. When these plants or small animals are consumed by larger animals that are in turn eaten by still larger animals, the contaminants accumulate, reaching higher concentrations at each level of the food chain (**FIGURE 13.10**). This process is called **bioaccumulation**. Because the toxins are not eliminated from the body, the greater the amount consumed, the greater the amount present in the body.

bioaccumulation
The process by which compounds accumulate or build up in an organism faster than they can be broken down or excreted.

Contamination throughout the food chain FIGURE 13.10

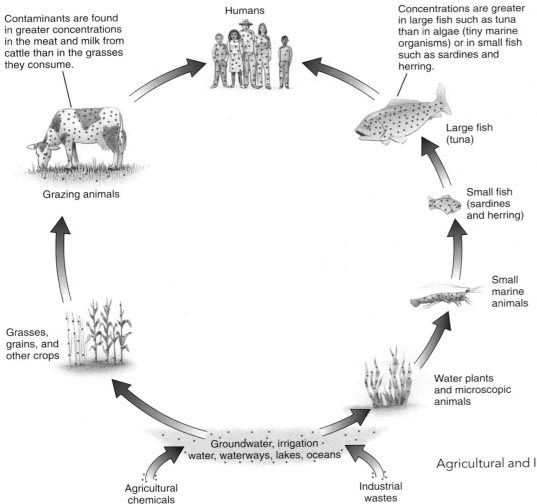

Contaminants are found in greater concentrations in the meat and milk from cattle than in the grasses they consume.

Grazing animals

Grasses, grains, and other crops

Agricultural chemicals

Groundwater, irrigation water, waterways, lakes, oceans

Industrial wastes

Water plants and microscopic animals

Small marine animals

Small fish (sardines and herring)

Large fish (tuna)

Humans

Concentrations are greater in large fish such as tuna than in algae (tiny marine organisms) or in small fish such as sardines and herring.

Industrial pollutants and agricultural chemicals that contaminate the water supply enter the food chain and accumulate as they are passed through the chain. Fat-soluble contaminants concentrate in body fat and cannot be excreted. An animal that occupies a higher level in the food chain has higher concentrations of these contaminants because it consumes all the contaminants that have been eaten by organisms at lower feeding levels.

PESTICIDES: RISKS AND BENEFITS

Pesticides are used to prevent plant diseases and insect infestations. They are applied both to crops in the fields and to harvested produce in order to prevent spoilage and extend shelf life. Crops that are grown using pesticides generally produce higher yields and look more appealing because they have less insect damage. Once they have been applied, however, pesticides can travel into water supplies, soil, and other parts of the environment. Because pesticides enter the environment, pesticide residues are found not only on the treated plants but also in meat, poultry, fish, and dairy products (see Figure 13.10).

The potential risks of pesticides to consumers depend on the size, age, and health of the person who consumes the pesticides and on the type and amount consumed.[15] To protect public health and the environment, the types of pesticides that may be used on food crops, how often they may be used, and the amount of residue that may remain when foods reach consumers are regulated. The EPA approves and registers pesticides that are used in food production and establishes allowable limits, or **tolerances**, for both children and adults.[16] To establish tolerances for pesticides, the risk of toxicity is weighed against the benefit that the pesticide provides. The risks are based on the known incidence of toxicity and the amount of the pesticide to which consumers are likely to be exposed. Tolerance levels are then set at the minimum amount of the pesticide needed to be effective; these levels are often several hundred times lower than the level that has been found to cause reactions in test animals.

The FDA and EPA monitor pesticide residues in foods. In general, pesticide residue levels in both domestic and imported foods have been found to be well below federally permitted limits (**FIGURE 13.11**).[17] Although repeated consumption of large doses of any one pesticide could be harmful, such a situation is unlikely because most people consume a variety of foods that have been produced in many different locations.

Integrated pest management

One way to limit pesticide use is through **integrated pest management (IPM)**. IPM is a method of agricultural pest control that combines chemical and nonchemical

> **integrated pest management (IPM)** A method of agricultural pest control that integrates nonchemical and chemical techniques.

> **organic food** Food that is produced, processed, and handled in accordance with the standards of the USDA National Organic Program.

Legend:
- No residue found
- Residue found but levels are below tolerance levels
- Residue found that exceeds tolerance or for which no tolerance has been established in the sampled food.

Domestic samples: 0.8%, 33.7%, 65.5%
Imported samples: 4.3%, 25.3%, 70.4%

Pesticide tolerances FIGURE 13.11

An analysis of samples of domestically produced food and imported food from 100 countries found no pesticide residues in 65.5% of domestic and 70.4% of imported samples.[18] To further reduce pesticide risks and exposure in the United States, more effective, less toxic chemical pesticides are being developed; the use of older, more toxic products is decreasing; and production methods that result in low-pesticide and pesticide-free produce are being implemented.

methods and emphasizes the use of natural toxins and more effective pesticide application. For example, increasing the use of naturally pest-resistant crop varieties that thrive without the use of pesticides can reduce costs and do less environmental damage. IPM programs use information about the life cycles of pests and their interaction with the environment to manage pest damage economically and with the least possible hazard to people, property, and the environment.

Organic food production

Organic food production methods emphasize the recycling of resources and the conservation of soil and water to protect the environment. Organic food is produced without using most conventional pesticides, fertilizers made with synthetic ingredients, sewage sludge, genetically modified ingredients, irradiation, antibiotics, or growth hormones (**FIGURE 13.12**). Organic farming techniques reduce farm workers' exposure to pesticides and decrease the quantity of pesticides introduced into the food supply and the environment. However, organic foods are not risk free. Manure is often used for fertilizer. If the manure is not treated properly, it can increase the risks of microbial food-borne illness, and runoff can pollute lakes and streams. Irrigation water, rain, and a variety of other sources can introduce traces of synthetic pesticides and other agricultural chemicals that are not approved for organic use into organically grown foods. The threshold for pesticide residues in organic foods is set at 5% of the EPA's pesticide-residue tolerance.[19]

INDUSTRIAL CONTAMINANTS

Industrial chemicals that contaminate the environment find their way into the food supply. Fish accumulate substances from the water in which they live and feed. Shellfish accumulate contaminants because they feed by passing large volumes of water through their bodies. Pollutants in the water can also contaminate crops and move through the food chain into meat and milk (see Figure 13.10).

One group of carcinogenic compounds that pollutes the environment is **polychlorinated biphenyls (PCBs)**. Prior to the 1970s, these chemicals were used in the manufacture of electrical capacitors and transformers, plasticizers, waxes, and paper. PCBs in runoff from manufacturing plants contaminated water, particularly near the Great Lakes. PCBs are no longer produced, but because they do not degrade, they are still in the environment and accumulate in fish caught in contaminated waters. PCBs are a particular problem for pregnant and lactating women because prenatal exposure to PCBs and consumption of contaminated breast milk can damage the fetal and infant nervous system and cause learning deficits. Pregnant and breast-feeding women should check with their local health department for recommendations regarding fish consumption.

Other contaminants from manufacturing, such as chlordane (used to control termites), radioactive substances such as strontium-90, and toxic metals such as cadmium, lead, arsenic, and mercury, have found their way into fish and shellfish. Cadmium and lead can interfere with the absorption of other minerals. Cadmium can

Labeling organic foods FIGURE 13.12

The USDA sets standards regarding substances that are approved for and prohibited from use in organic food production. Before a food can be labeled "organic," the USDA must certify the farming and processing operations that produce and handle the food. Products that meet the definition of "100% organic" or "organic" may display the USDA "organic" seal shown here.

Labeling term	Meaning
100% organic	Contains 100% organically produced raw or processed ingredients.
Organic	Contains at least 95% organically produced raw or processed ingredients.
Made with organic ingredients	Contains at least 70% organically produced ingredients.

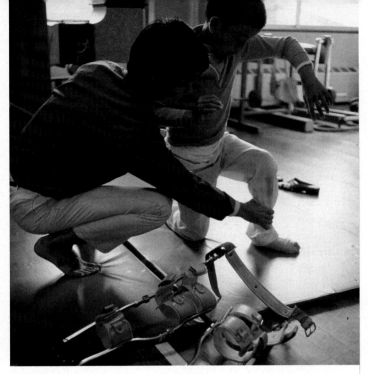

Mercury poisoning FIGURE 13.13

This Japanese boy has Minamata disease, a neurological syndrome caused by mercury poisoning. The disease first appeared in Minamata, Japan, in 1956 and was caused by the release of mercury into the water by a local chemical factory. The mercury accumulated in the fat of fish and shellfish that were eaten by the local population.

cause kidney damage, and lead can impair brain development. Arsenic is believed to increase the risk of cancer. Mercury, which has been found in large fish, particularly swordfish, king mackerel, tilefish, and shark, damages nerve cells (FIGURE 13.13).[20] Because mercury is more damaging during prenatal development, pregnant women are advised to avoid certain types of fish and limit their consumption of others (see Chapter 11).

ANTIBIOTICS AND HORMONES

Antibiotics and hormones are administered to animals to improve health, increase growth, or otherwise enhance food production. To prevent these chemicals from being passed on to consumers, both the types of drugs used and when they can be administered are regulated, and animal tissues are monitored for drug residues.[21]

Animals are treated with antibiotics when they are sick, and some animals are also given antibiotics to prevent disease and promote growth. This treatment increases the amount of meat produced and reduces costs, but if it is used improperly, antibiotic residues can remain in the meat. Another concern is the creation of antibiotic-resistant bacteria. When exposed to an antibiotic, bacteria that are resistant to it survive and produce offspring that are also resistant. If these antibiotic-resistant bacteria infect humans, the resulting illness cannot be treated with that antibiotic. Because nearly half the antibiotics produced in the United States are used to prevent disease in animals, this use is suspected of being a major contributor to the development of antibiotic-resistant strains of bacteria.[22]

Hormones are used to increase weight gain in sheep and cattle and milk production in dairy cows. Some hormones, such as estrogen and testosterone, occur naturally. Generally these are administered in slow-release form, and their levels are no higher in treated animals than in untreated animals. Before a synthetic hormone can be used, it must be demonstrated that hormone residues in meat from treated animals are within safe limits.

A synthetic hormone that has created public concern is genetically engineered **bovine somatotropin (bST)**. bST is produced naturally by cows and stimulates milk production. Genetically engineered bST is produced by bacteria and injected into cows to further increase milk production (FIGURE 13.14). Milk from cows that have been treated with genetically engineered bST is indistinguishable from other milk.

Bovine somatotropin FIGURE 13.14

Consumer groups are concerned that the injection of cows with bST may cause health problems for humans who consume the milk. The FDA has concluded that bST causes no serious long-term health effects,[23] and it does not require milk from bST-treated cows to be specially labeled. Some dairies voluntarily label their products as bST free.

A Pesticide residues on fruits and vegetables can be removed or reduced by peeling or washing with tap water and scrubbing with a brush, if appropriate. In the case of leafy vegetables such as lettuce and cabbage, the outer leaves can be removed and discarded. Washing apples, cucumbers, eggplant, squash, and tomatoes may not remove all the pesticides because these fruits and vegetables are coated with wax in order to maintain freshness by sealing in moisture, but wax also seals in pesticides. The wax and pesticides can be removed by peeling, but removing the peel also eliminates fiber and some micronutrients.

B Exposure to chemical contaminants can be minimized by choosing saltwater fish caught well offshore, away from polluted coastal waters. Fish that live near the shore or spend part of their life cycle in freshwater are more likely to contain contaminants. Smaller species of fish are safer because they are earlier in the food chain, and smaller fish within a species are safer because they are younger and hence have had less time to accumulate contaminants (see Figure 13.10).

CHOOSING WISELY TO MINIMIZE AGRICULTURAL AND INDUSTRIAL CONTAMINANTS

Even though individual consumers cannot detect chemical contaminants in food, care in selection and preparation can reduce the amounts consumed. One of the easiest ways to reduce risk is to choose a wide variety of foods, thus avoiding excessive consumption of contaminants that may be present in any one food. To reduce exposure to pesticide residues in fruits and vegetables, consumers can choose organic foods or locally grown produce. Locally grown produce contains fewer pesticides because the pesticides used to prevent spoilage and extend the shelf life of shipped produce are not needed. Exposure to pesticide residues on conventionally grown produce can be minimized by washing and in some cases peeling (**FIGURE 13.15A**). Pesticides and other toxins that are ingested by animals concentrate in fat, so intake can be reduced by trimming all fat from meat and removing the skin from poultry.

Intake of pesticides and other chemical pollutants from fish and seafood products can also be minimized by choosing wisely and consuming a variety of fish (**FIGURE 13.15B**). To minimize consumption of contaminants, remove the skin, fatty material, and dark meat

Avoid ingesting pathogenic microbes
- Make sure your burger is well done.
- Skip the runny eggs and have them scrambled.
- Pass on the dough! Treat yourself to chocolate chip cookies only after they come out of the oven.
- Slice up some melon, but make sure the knife, the cutting board, and the skin of the melon are clean before you slice it.

Reduce pesticides and pollutants in your food
- Buy locally grown produce.
- Look for the organic symbol.
- Try the small fish in the pond.
- Make a salad after you have washed the lettuce or peeled off the outer leaves.
- Trim the fat and don't eat the skin of poultry and fish.

from fish. Use cooking methods such as broiling, poaching, boiling, and baking, which allow contaminants from the fatty portions of fish to drain out. Do not eat the "tomale" in lobster. The tomale, a green paste inside the abdominal cavity of a cooked lobster, serves as the liver and pancreas and is the organ in which toxins accumulate. The analogous organ in blue crabs, called the "mustard" because of its yellow color, should also be avoided (see *What Should I Eat?*).

CONCEPT CHECK STOP

How can a pesticide used on broccoli plants end up in milk?

What can you do to minimize PCBs in your diet?

How can organic food cause food-borne illness?

Technology for Keeping Food Safe

LEARNING OBJECTIVES

Describe how temperature is used to prevent food spoilage.

Discuss how irradiation preserves food.

Explain how packaging protects food.

Discuss the risks and benefits of food additives.

Food spoils when its taste, texture, or nutritional value is changed either by enzymes that are naturally present in the food or by microbes that grow on the food. For thousands of years, humans have treated food in order to prevent spoilage. Techniques that preserve food work by destroying enzymes present in the food, by killing microbes, or by slowing microbial growth (**TABLE 13.5**).

Most of the oldest methods of food preservation—heating, cooling, drying, smoking, and adding substances such as sugar or salt—are still used today. In addition, newer methods, such as irradiation and specialized packaging, have been developed. While all these technologies offer benefits, they can also create risks. Some risk arises when substances find their way into food, either accidentally or as a normal part of the production process. The FDA considers any substance that can be expected to become part of a food a **food additive** and regulates the types and amounts of food additives that may be present in a particular food. Unexpected substances that enter food are considered **accidental contaminants** and are not regulated.

food additive
A substance that is intentionally added to or can reasonably be expected to become a component of a food during processing.

accidental contaminants
Substances not regulated by the FDA that unexpectedly enter the food supply.

HIGH AND LOW TEMPERATURE

Cooking food is one of the oldest methods of ensuring that food is safe. Cooking kills disease-causing organisms and destroys most toxins. Other preservation techniques that rely on high temperature to kill microbes include

FAT TOM TABLE 13.5

The acronym FAT TOM reminds us of the factors that affect microbial growth. Most food preservation techniques modify one or more of these factors to stop or slow microbial growth.

Food	This is where the bacteria grow.	
Acidity	Most bacteria grow best at a pH near neutral. Some food additives, such as citric acid and ascorbic acid (vitamin C), are acids, which prevent microbial growth by lowering the pH of food.	
Time	The longer a food sits at an optimum growth temperature, the more bacteria it will contain. Preservation methods such as canning and pasteurization kill microbes by heating food to an appropriate temperature for the right amount of time.	
Temperature	The high temperatures of canning, cooking, and pasteurization kill microbes, and the low temperatures of freezing and refrigeration slow or stop microbial growth.	
Oxygen	In order to grow, most bacteria need oxygen, so packaging that eliminates oxygen prevents their growth.	
Moisture	Bacteria need water to grow, so preservation methods such as drying or use of high concentrations of salt or sugar, which draw water away by osmosis, prevent bacteria from growing.	

pasteurization The process of heating food products in order to kill disease-causing organisms.

aseptic processing The placement of sterilized food in a sterilized package using a sterile process.

pasteurization, sterilization, and **aseptic processing** (FIGURE 13.16). Lowering the temperature of food by means of refrigeration or freezing does not kill microbes but preserves the food and protects consumers because it slows or stops microbial growth.

Preservation techniques that rely on temperature benefit consumers by providing appealing, safe foods, but these foods are not risk free, particularly if they are handled incorrectly. If foods are not heated long enough or to a high enough temperature, or if they are not kept cold enough, they could pose a risk of food-borne illness. In addition, some types of cooking can generate hazardous chemicals. Carcinogenic chemicals produced during the cooking of meats include **polycyclic aromatic hydrocarbons (PAHs)** and **heterocyclic amines (HCAs)**. PAHs are formed when fat drips on a grill and burns. They rise with the smoke and are deposited on the surface of the food. PAH formation can be minimized by selecting lower-fat meat and using a layer of aluminum foil to prevent fat from dripping on the coals. HCAs are produced by the burning of amino acids and other substances in meats and are formed during any type of high-temperature cooking. HCA formation can be reduced by precooking meat, marinating meat before cooking, cooking at lower temperatures, and reducing cooking time by using smaller pieces of meat and avoiding overcooking. The cooking temperatures recommended by the FDA are designed to prevent microbial food-borne illness and minimize the production of PAHs and HCAs. Because PAHs and HCAs are considered accidental contaminants, their amounts in food are not regulated by the FDA.

Another contaminant formed during food preparation is **acrylamide**. It is formed as a result of chemical reactions that occur during high-temperature baking or frying, particularly in carbohydrate-rich foods. The highest levels of acrylamide are found in French fries and snack chips. Smaller amounts are found in coffee and in foods made from grains, such as breakfast cereal and cookies. High doses can cause cancer and reproductive problems in experimental animals and act as a neurotoxin in humans. Thus far, dietary exposure to acrylamide has not been associated with cancer in humans, and more research is needed to determine whether long-term, low-level exposure has any cumulative effects.[24] Methods for reducing the amounts and potential toxicity of acrylamide in foods are being investigated.[25]

Aseptic processing FIGURE 13.16

The juice boxes that fit so conveniently into school lunch bags are produced by aseptic processing. This technique heats foods to temperatures that result in sterilization. The sterilized foods are then placed in sterilized packages, using sterilized packaging equipment. If the package remains unopened, juice or milk packaged aseptically can remain free of microbial growth at room temperature for years.

Irradiated foods FIGURE 13.17

A Irradiated foods must be labeled with the radura symbol shown here and the statement "treated with radiation" or "treated by irradiation." This symbol is not required on the labels of foods that contain irradiated spices or other irradiated ingredients. ▼

TREATED BY IRRADIATION

NON - IRRADIATED -   IRRADIATED - (0.2 M RAD)

▲

B Irradiation increases the safety and shelf life of foods and does not compromise nutritional quality or noticeably change food texture, taste, or appearance, as long as it is properly applied to a suitable product. After two weeks in cold storage, the strawberries on the right, which were treated by irradiation, remain free of mold, whereas the untreated strawberries on the left, which were picked at the same time, are covered with mold.

FOOD IRRADIATION

irradiation
A process that exposes foods to radiation in order to kill contaminating organisms and retard the ripening and spoilage of fruits and vegetables.

Food **irradiation**, also called cold pasteurization, is used in more than 40 countries to treat everything from frog legs to rice. Irradiation exposes food to high doses of X-rays, gamma radiation, or high-energy electrons in order to kill microbes and insects and inactivate enzymes that cause germination and ripening of fruits and vegetables (**FIGURE 13.17**).[26]

Because irradiation produces compounds that are not present in the original foods, it is treated as a food additive, and the level of radiation that may be used is regulated. At the allowed levels of radiation, the amounts of these compounds produced are almost negligible and have not been found to be a risk to consumers.[27]

Food irradiation is used relatively infrequently in the United States because of a lack of irradiation facilities and because of public suspicion of the technology. The word *irradiation* fosters the belief that the food becomes radioactive. Opponents to food irradiation claim that it introduces carcinogens, depletes the nutritional value of food, and is used to allow the sale of previously contaminated foods. In fact, irradiated food is not radioactive, and scientific studies conducted over the past 50 years have found that the benefits of irradiation outweigh the potential risks.[28] Irradiation can decrease the amounts of certain nutrients in foods, but these nutrient losses are similar to those that occur with canning or refrigerated storage.[27]

Because irradiation can be used in place of chemical treatments, it reduces consumers' exposure to chemical pesticides and preservatives. It is one of the technologies promoted by the National Food Safety Initiative because of its potential for improving the safety of food and reducing the incidence of food-borne illness.

FOOD PACKAGING

Packaging plays an important role in food preservation; it keeps molds and bacteria out, keeps moisture in, and protects food from physical damage. An open package of refrigerated cheddar cheese will be moldy in a few days, but an unopened package will stay fresh for weeks.

Food packaging is continually being improved. In the past two decades, for instance, consumer demand for fresh and easy-to-prepare foods has led manufacturers to offer partially cooked pasta, vegetables, seafood, fresh and cured meats, and dry products such as whole-bean and ground coffee in packaging that, if unopened, will keep perishable food fresh much longer than will conventional packaging. **Modified atmosphere packaging (MAP)** uses plastics or other packaging materials that are impermeable to oxygen. The air inside the package is vacuumed out in order to remove the oxygen. The product can then remain packaged in a vacuum, or the package can be infused with another gas, such as carbon dioxide or nitrogen. The lack of oxygen prevents the growth of aerobic bacteria, slows the ripening of fruits and vegetables, and slows down oxidation reactions,

> **modified atmosphere packaging (MAP)**
> A preservation technique used to prolong the shelf life of processed or fresh food by changing the gases surrounding the food in the package.

which cause discoloration in fruits and vegetables and rancidity in fats.

MAP is often used to package cooked entrees such as pasta primavera or beef teriyaki. The raw ingredients are sealed in a plastic pouch, the air is vacuumed out, and the pouch and its contents are partially precooked and immediately refrigerated. This processing eliminates the need for the extreme cold of freezing or the extreme heat of canning, so flavor and nutrients are better preserved. Because these products are not heated to temperatures high enough to kill all bacteria and are not stored at temperatures low enough to prevent all bacteria from growing, they could pose a food safety risk. To ensure safety, fresh refrigerated foods should be purchased only from reputable vendors, used before the expiration date printed on the package, refrigerated until use, and heated according to the time and temperature directions on the package.

Packaging can protect food from spoilage, but even the best packaging can introduce risk if it becomes part of the food. A variety of substances found in paper and plastic containers and packaging, and even dishes, can leach into food (**FIGURE 13.18**). Substances that are known to contaminate food are regulated by the EPA and the FDA. However, these regulations apply only to the intended use of the product. When a product is used improperly, substances from its packaging can migrate into food. For instance, some plastics migrate into food when heated in a microwave oven. Thus, only containers designed for microwave cooking should be used when microwaving food.

Bisphenol A from plastics FIGURE 13.18

The transfer of bisphenol A, a chemical found in polycarbonate plastic used to manufacture hard, transparent water bottles, baby bottles, and food containers as well as the coating inside cans, is a concern for pregnant women and infants. A review by the U.S. National Toxicology Program found that although there is negligible risk of adverse effects in most adults, exposure of pregnant women to bisphenol A could affect fetal brain development, and exposure of infants and children to the chemical could affect the nervous system and accelerate puberty.[29] Eating fewer canned foods and drinking from glass or aluminum, rather than plastic, containers can minimize exposure.

FOOD ADDITIVES

direct food additives
Substances intentionally added to foods. They are regulated by the FDA.

indirect food additives
Substances that are expected to unintentionally enter foods during manufacturing or from packaging. They are regulated by the FDA.

What keeps bread from molding, gives margarine its yellow color, and keeps Parmesan cheese from clumping in the shaker? The answer to all these questions is food additives. Substances that are intentionally added to foods are called **direct food additives**. Other substances that get into food unintentionally—such as the oil used to lubricate food processing machinery—are referred to as **indirect food additives**. The FDA regulates the amounts and types of direct and indirect food additives in food.

turer that wants to use a new food additive must submit to the FDA a petition that describes the chemical composition of the additive, how it is manufactured, and how it is detected in food. The manufacturer must prove that the additive will be effective for its intended purpose at the proposed levels, that it is safe for its intended use, and that its use is necessary. Additives may not be used to disguise inferior products or deceive consumers. They cannot be used if they significantly destroy nutrients or if the same effect can be achieved through sound manufacturing processes.

More than 600 chemicals defined as food additives were already in common use when legislation regulating food additives was passed. To accommodate substances that the FDA or the USDA had already determined to be safe, they were designated as **prior-sanctioned substances** and are exempt from regulation. The nitrates and nitrites used to retard the growth of *Clostridium botulinum* in cured meats are prior-sanctioned substances, for instance. However, their use has been controversial because they form carcinogenic **nitrosamines** in the digestive tract. They are still allowed in foods, however, because they prevent botulism, and there is little evidence that they pose a serious risk in the amounts consumed in the human diet (**FIGURE 13.19**).[30]

Regulating food additives Food additives improve food quality and help protect us from disease, but if the wrong additive is used or the wrong amount is added, it could do more harm than good. Any manufac-

Reducing nitrosamine risk FIGURE 13.19

To minimize any risk posed by nitrosamines without increasing the risk of bacterial food-borne illness, the FDA limits the amount of nitrate and nitrite that can be added to food and requires the addition of antioxidants such as vitamin C, which reduce nitrosamine formation, to foods that contain these additives. Consumers can reduce nitrosamine exposure by limiting their consumption of cured meat to 3 to 4 ounces per week and maintaining adequate intakes of the antioxidant vitamins C and E.

INGREDIENTS: MECHANICALLY SEPARATED CHICKEN, WATER, PORK, MODIFIED CORN STARCH, DEXTROSE, SALT, BEEF, CONTAINS 2% OR LESS OF THE FOLLOWING CORN SYRUP, FLAVORINGS, SODIUM PHOSPHATES, POTASSIUM LACTATE, SODIUM DIACETATE, SODIUM ASCORBATE (VITAMIN C), OLEO RESIN OF PAPRIKA, SODIUM NITRITE

A second category that is not subject to food additive regulation consists of substances **generally recognized as safe (GRAS)**, based either on their history of use in food before 1958 or on published scientific evidence. However, just because a substance is on the GRAS or prior-sanctioned list doesn't mean that it is safe or that it will stay on these lists. If new evidence emerges which suggests that a substance in either category is unsafe, the FDA may take action to require that the substance be removed from food products.

Substances that are toxic at some level of consumption may be harmless at a lower level. To ensure that additives are safe, most of those that are allowed in foods can be added only at levels 100 times below the highest level that has been shown to have no harmful effects. This is a greater margin of safety than exists for many vitamins and other naturally occurring substances.

The regulations for substances that cause cancer are far more rigid because of the **Delaney Clause**, part of the 1958 Food Additives Amendment. It states that a substance that induces cancer in either an animal species or humans, at any dosage, may not be added to food. Debate continues regarding whether the Delaney Clause should be liberalized to allow the use of substances that are added at a level so low that they would not represent a significant health risk.

Identifying food additives Food additives are used to make food safer; maintain palatability and wholesomeness; improve color, flavor, or texture; aid in processing; and enhance nutritional value (see TABLE 13.6 on the next page). Their use ensures the availability of wholesome, appetizing, and affordable foods that meet consumer demands throughout the year. The FDA's database "Everything Added to Food in the United States" lists more than 3000 additives.[31] Many of these, such as sugar and spices, are used in homes every day. Other additives may sound like a chemical soup: calcium propionate in bread, disodium EDTA in kidney beans, and BHA in potato chips. Understanding what these chemicals are used for can help make the ingredient list a source of information rather than a cause for concern.

Sensitivities to additives Some individuals are allergic or sensitive to certain food additives. For example, the flavor enhancer monosodium glutamate (MSG), commonly used in Chinese food, can cause adverse reactions known as *MSG symptom complex* or *Chinese restaurant syndrome* in sensitive individuals (see Chapter 6). Sulfites can cause symptoms ranging from stomachache and hives to severe asthma. Sulfites are used as preservatives in baked goods, canned foods, condiments, and dried fruits. Sensitive individuals can identify foods that contain sulfites by checking food labels. The forms of sulfites allowed in packaged foods include sulfur dioxide, sodium sulfite, sodium and potassium bisulfite, and sodium and potassium metabisulfite. Foods served in restaurants may also contain sulfites. For example, a potato dish served in a restaurant may be prepared using potatoes that were peeled and soaked in a sulfite solution before cooking.

Color additives can also cause adverse reactions. FD&C yellow no. 5, for instance, listed as tartrazine on medicine labels, may cause itching and hives in sensitive people. It is found in beverages, desserts, and processed vegetables. Color additives are listed in the ingredient list along with other food additives. Colors in foods are classified as certified or exempt. Certified colors are human-made, meet strict specifications for purity, and must be listed by name in the ingredient list. Colors that are exempt from certification include pigments from natural sources such as dehydrated beets and carotenoids; these may be listed collectively in the ingredient list as "artificial color."

CONCEPT CHECK ⬡**STOP**

What is pasteurization?

How does irradiation help extend the shelf life of food?

How does modified atmosphere packaging prevent food spoilage?

Why are food additives regulated?

Common food additives[32] TABLE 13.6

Type of additive	What's on the label	What they do	Where they are used
Preservatives	Ascorbic acid, citric acid, sodium benzoate, calcium propionate, sodium erythorbate, sodium nitrite, calcium sorbate, potassium sorbate, BHA, BHT, EDTA, tocopherols	Maintain freshness; prevent spoilage caused by bacteria, molds, fungi, or yeast; slow or prevent changes in color, flavor, or texture; and delay rancidity	Jellies, beverages, baked goods, cured meats, oils and margarines, cereals, dressings, snack foods, fruits and vegetables
Sweeteners	Sucrose, glucose, fructose, sorbitol, mannitol, corn syrup, high-fructose corn syrup, saccharin, aspartame, sucralose, acesulfame potassium (acesulfame-K), neotame	Add sweetness with or without extra calories	Beverages, baked goods, table-top sweeteners, many processed foods
Color additives	FD&C blue nos. 1 and 2, FD&C green no. 3, FD&C red nos. 3 and 40, FD&C yellow nos. 5 and 6, orange B, citrus red no. 2, annatto extract, beta-carotene, grapeskin extract, cochineal extract or carmine, paprika oleoresin, caramel color, fruit and vegetable juices, saffron, colorings or color added	Prevent color loss due to exposure to light, air, temperature extremes, and moisture; enhance colors; give color to colorless and "fun" foods	Processed foods, candies, snack foods, margarine, cheese, soft drinks, jellies, puddings and pie fillings
Flavors, spices, and flavor enhancers	Natural flavoring, artificial flavor, spices, monosodium glutamate (MSG), hydrolyzed soy protein, autolyzed yeast extract, disodium guanylate or inosinate	Add specific flavors or enhance flavors already present in foods	Many processed foods, puddings and pie fillings, gelatin mixes, cake mixes, salad dressings, candies, soft drinks, ice cream, BBQ sauce
Nutrients	Thiamine hydrochloride, riboflavin (vitamin B_2), niacin, niacinamide, folate or folic acid, beta-carotene, potassium iodide, iron or ferrous sulfate, alpha-tocopherols, ascorbic acid, vitamin D, amino acids (L-tryptophan, L-lysine, L-leucine, L-methionine)	Replace vitamins and minerals lost in processing; add nutrients that may be lacking in the diet	Flour, breads, cereals, rice, pasta, margarine, salt, milk, fruit beverages, energy bars, breakfast drinks
Emulsifiers	Soy lecithin, mono- and diglycerides, egg yolks, polysorbates, sorbitan monostearate	Allow smooth mixing and prevent separation; reduce stickiness; control crystallization; keep ingredients dispersed	Salad dressings, peanut butter, chocolate, margarine, frozen desserts
Stabilizers and thickeners, binders, and texturizers	Gelatin, pectin, guar gum, carrageenan, xanthan gum, whey	Produce uniform texture, improve "mouth-feel"	Frozen desserts, dairy products, cakes, pudding and gelatin mixes, dressings, jams and jellies, sauces
pH control agents and acidulants	Lactic acid, citric acid, ammonium hydroxide, sodium carbonate	Control acidity and alkalinity, prevent spoilage	Beverages, frozen desserts, chocolate, low-acid canned foods, baking powder
Leavening agents	Baking soda, monocalcium phosphate, calcium carbonate	Promote rising of baked goods	Breads and other baked goods
Anti-caking agents	Calcium silicate, iron ammonium citrate, silicon dioxide	Keep powdered foods free-flowing, prevent moisture absorption	Salt, baking powder, confectioners' sugar
Humectants	Glycerin, sorbitol	Retain moisture	Shredded coconut, marshmallows, soft candies, confections

Biotechnology

Biotechnology alters the characteristics of organisms by making selective changes in their DNA. The concept is not new. For centuries, farmers have selected seeds from plants with the most desirable characteristics to plant for the next year's crop, bred the animals that grew fastest or produced the most milk to improve the productivity of the next generation of animals, and cross-bred plant varieties to combine the desired traits of each. However, these traditional methods may require many generations to produce the desired results. Biotechnology uses **genetic engineering** to select genes for specific traits. Genetic engineering has significantly sped up the process of modifying the traits of organisms. Like all other new technologies, however, it may introduce new risks.

> **biotechnology**
> The process of manipulating life forms via genetic engineering in order to provide desirable products for human use.

> **genetic engineering**
> A set of techniques used to manipulate DNA for the purpose of changing the characteristics of an organism or creating a new product.

HOW BIOTECHNOLOGY WORKS

Genetically modified (GM) crops are created through genetic engineering: A piece of DNA containing the gene for a desired characteristic is taken from plant, animal, or bacterial cells and transferred to plant cells (**FIGURE 13.20**).

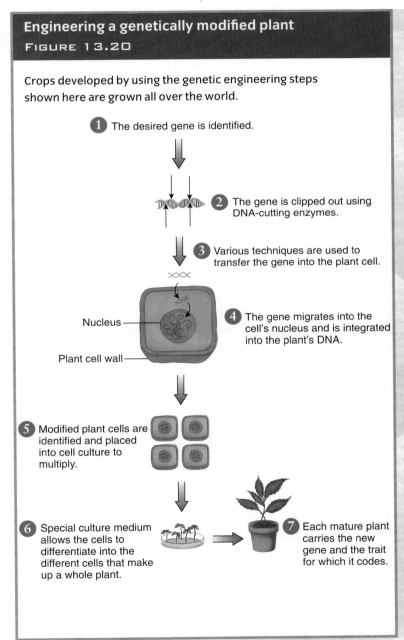

Process Diagram

Engineering a genetically modified plant
FIGURE 13.20

Crops developed by using the genetic engineering steps shown here are grown all over the world.

1. The desired gene is identified.

2. The gene is clipped out using DNA-cutting enzymes.

3. Various techniques are used to transfer the gene into the plant cell.

4. The gene migrates into the cell's nucleus and is integrated into the plant's DNA.

Nucleus

Plant cell wall

5. Modified plant cells are identified and placed into cell culture to multiply.

6. Special culture medium allows the cells to differentiate into the different cells that make up a whole plant.

7. Each mature plant carries the new gene and the trait for which it codes.

recombinant DNA DNA that has been formed by joining DNA from different sources.

transgenic An organism with a gene or group of genes intentionally transferred from another species or breed.

The DNA is then referred to as **recombinant DNA** because the new DNA is a combination of the DNA from two organisms. The modified cells are then allowed to divide into more and more cells and eventually differentiate into the various types of cells that make up a whole plant. The new plant is a **transgenic** organism. Each cell in the new plant contains the transferred gene for the desired trait. This technique is used to introduce characteristics such as disease and drought resistance into plants. Genetic engineering is more difficult in animals because animal cells do not take up genes as easily as plant cells do, and making copies of these cells (clones) is also more difficult. However, these techniques have been used to produce cows that yield more milk, cattle and pigs with more meat on them, and sheep that grow more wool.[33]

APPLICATIONS OF BIOTECHNOLOGY

The techniques of biotechnology can be used in a variety of ways in food production to alter quantity, quality, cost, safety, and shelf life. By making plants resistant to herbicides, insects, and various plant diseases, this technology has increased crop yields and reduced damage from insects and plant diseases (**FIGURE 13.21A** and **B**). By altering enzyme activity and other traits, biotechnology is being used to increase the shelf life of fresh fruits and vegetables and create products that have greater consumer appeal, such as seedless grapes and watermelons.

Biotechnology is also used in food processing. Rennet, an enzyme used in cheese production; enzymes used in the production of high-fructose corn syrup; and the enzyme lactase, used to reduce the lactose content of milk, are now all produced by GM microbes.

Biotechnology also has great potential for addressing the problem of world hunger and malnutrition. Although world hunger is rooted in political, economic, and cultural issues that cannot be resolved by agricultural technology alone, GM crops that target some of the major nutritional deficiencies worldwide are being developed. To address protein deficiency, varieties of corn, soybeans, and sweet potatoes with enhanced levels of essential amino acids are being developed. To address iron deficiency, rice has been engineered to contain more iron.[37] To address vitamin A deficiency, genes that code for the production of enzymes needed for the synthesis of the vitamin A precursor β-carotene have been inserted into rice (**FIGURE 13.21C**).[38]

RISKS AND REGULATION OF BIOTECHNOLOGY

The rapid advancement of biotechnology during the past decade has created the potential for health problems and environmental damage. Regulations are in place to control the use of genetic engineering and GM products. The National Academy of Sciences has concluded that the risks posed by biotechnology are the same as those posed by crops produced by traditional plant breeding.[39] Nevertheless, many consumers and scientists believe that these conclusions are premature and that the potential impact of this booming technology has not yet become apparent. They urge that this technology be used with caution to avoid health or environmental impacts that outweigh the benefits.

Consumer concerns Consumer safety concerns related to GM foods include the possibility that the nutrient content of a food may have been negatively affected or that an allergen or a toxin may have inadvertently been introduced into a food that was previously safe. For example, if DNA from fish or nuts—foods that commonly cause allergic reactions—were introduced into soybeans or corn, these foods would then be dangerous to individuals allergic to fish or nuts. To prevent this kind of situation from occurring unintentionally, biotechnology companies have established systems for monitoring the allergenic potential of proteins used for plant genetic engineering.[40] In 1996, allergy testing successfully prevented soybeans containing a gene from a Brazil nut from entering the market.[41]

Environmental concerns An environmental concern about GM crops is that they will be used to the exclusion of other varieties, thereby reducing biodiversity. The ability of populations of organisms to adapt to new conditions, diseases, or other hazards depends on the presence of many different species and varieties that provide a diversity of genes. If farmers plant only GM insect-resistant, high-yielding crops, other species and varieties may eventually become extinct, and the genes for the traits they possess may be lost forever.

Another environmental issue is the possibility that GM crops will create "superweeds." This might occur, for example, if a trait such as increased rate of growth introduced into a domesticated plant species were passed on to a related wild species. This could produce a fast-growing weed, or superweed, that would compete with the domesticated species. As a safeguard, plant developers are avoiding introducing genes for traits that could increase a plant's competitiveness or other undesirable properties in weedy relatives.

There is also concern that crops that have been engineered to produce pesticides will promote the evolution of pesticide-resistant insects. An illustration is the case of insects that feed on plants modified to produce the Bt toxin (see Figure 13.21A). As more and more of the insects' food supply consists of plants that produce this pesticide, only insects that carry genes that make them resistant to Bt toxin survive and reproduce. This increases the number of Bt-resistant insects and therefore reduces the effectiveness of Bt toxin as a method of pest control. Although an important concern when growing GM crops, pesticide-resistant insects may also evolve when pesticides are sprayed on crops.

Visualizing

The potential of biotechnology FIGURE 13.21

A Insect-resistant corn is created by inserting a gene from the bacterium *Basillus thuringiensis* (or Bt). The gene produces a protein called Bt toxin that is toxic to certain insects, such as this European corn borer, but safe for humans and other animals. The presence of the new gene improves the crop yield and also reduces the amounts of chemical pesticides that need to be applied.

B In the 1990s the papaya crop in Hawaii was severely diminished by the papaya ring-spot virus (PRSV). In response, researchers developed papaya that is genetically enhanced to resist PRSV. The seeds were released for commercialization in 1998, allowing Hawaiian papaya production to rebound.[34] This was the first genetically enhanced fruit crop on the market. Genes for resistance to various viruses have also been used to create virus-resistant strains of potatoes, squash, cucumbers, and watermelons.[35]

C Half the world's population depends on rice as a dietary staple, but rice is a poor source of vitamin A. Genetically modified rice, called golden rice (seen here compared with white rice) for the color imparted by the β-carotene pigment, has the potential to significantly increase vitamin A intake. One variety contains enough provitamin A in 1/2 cup of dry rice to provide more than 50% of the RDA for a child.[36]

Biotechnology 467

Despite concerns about the impact of GM crops, the number of acres planted with them worldwide has risen steadily. The most common GM crops are soybeans, corn, cotton, and rapeseed (or canola). Therefore, foods produced in the United States that contain corn or high-fructose corn syrup, such as many breakfast cereals, snack foods, and soft drinks; foods made with soybeans; and foods made with cottonseed and canola oils, are likely to contain GM ingredients.

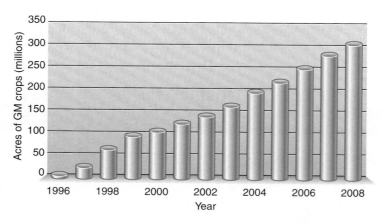

Regulation of GM food products

Experts estimate that 70 to 75% of all processed foods on U.S. grocery shelves contain GM ingredients (FIGURE 13.22).[42] You don't recognize these foods as genetically modified because they appear no different from other foods, and food manufacturers are not required to provide special labeling unless the food is known to pose a potential risk.

To ensure that GM plants and foods cause no harm to consumers or to the environment, the FDA, the USDA, and the EPA are all involved in overseeing plant biotechnology. Safety and environmental issues are monitored at all stages of the process. The FDA regulates the safety and labeling of foods containing GM ingredients. Labeling of foods containing GM ingredients is required only if the nutritional composition of the food has been altered; if it contains potentially harmful allergens, toxins, pesticides, or herbicides; if it contains ingredients that are new to the food supply; or if it has been changed significantly enough so that its traditional name no longer applies. Premarket approval is required when the new food contains a substance that is not commonly found in foods or when it contains a substance that does not have a history of safe use in foods. To prevent material from a new plant variety intended for food use from inadvertently entering the food supply before its safety has been established, the FDA has asked developers to provide them with information about the safety of the new plants at a relatively early stage of development.[43]

The USDA regulates agricultural products and research concerning the development of new plant varieties, including those developed through genetic engineering. The EPA regulates any pesticides that may be present in foods and sets tolerance levels for these pesticides. This includes GM plants containing proteins that protect them from insects or disease.

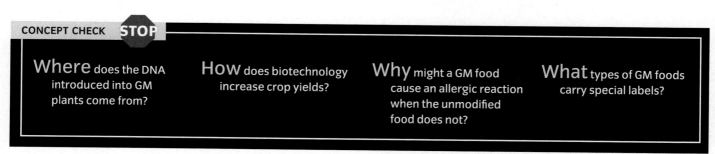

CONCEPT CHECK STOP

Where does the DNA introduced into GM plants come from?

How does biotechnology increase crop yields?

Why might a GM food cause an allergic reaction when the unmodified food does not?

What types of GM foods carry special labels?

SUMMARY

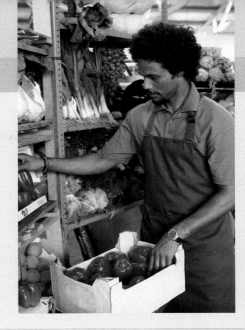

1 Keeping Food Safe

1. Most **food-borne illness** is caused by food contaminated with disease-causing **microbes**; occasionally it can be caused by chemical contaminants in food. The harm caused by contaminants in the food supply depends on the type of toxin, dose, length of time over which the contaminant is consumed, how it is metabolized and excreted, and the size, age, and health of the consumer.

2. The food supply is monitored for safety by food manufacturers and regulatory agencies at the international, federal, state, and local levels. Federal programs promote the use of **Hazard Analysis Critical Control Point (HACCP)** systems to prevent and eliminate food contamination rather than catch it after it occurs. Consumers can prevent most cases of food-borne illness by following safe food-handling and preparation guidelines.

2 Pathogens in Food

1. The **pathogens** that affect the food supply include bacteria, viruses, molds, parasites, and prions. Some bacteria cause **food-borne infection** because they are able to grow in the gastrointestinal tract when ingested. Others produce toxins in food, and consumption of the toxin causes **food-borne intoxication**.

2. Viruses do not grow on food, but when consumed in food, they can reproduce in human cells and cause food-borne illness.

3. **Molds** that grow on foods produce toxins that can harm consumers.

4. **Parasites** include microscopic single-celled animals, as well as worms that

can be seen with the naked eye. They are consumed in contaminated water or food.

5. Improperly folded **prion** proteins cause **bovine spongiform encephalopathy (BSE)** in cattle. The risk of acquiring the human form of this deadly degenerative neurological disease is extremely low.

6. The risk of food-borne illness can be decreased through proper food selection, preparation, and storage to kill pathogens or minimize their growth.

3 Agricultural and Industrial Chemicals in Food

1. Contaminants in the environment can find their way into the food supply. Those that deposit in the fatty tissue of animals are not eliminated, leading to

bioaccumulation as they pass through the food chain.

2. Pesticides help increase crop yields and the quality of produce. To decrease the risk of pesticide toxicity, **tolerances** are established, and foods are monitored for pesticide residues. Safer pesticides are being developed, and U.S. farmers are reducing the amounts applied by using **integrated pest management (IPM)** and **organic food** production methods.

3. Industrial pollutants such as PCBs have contaminated some waterways and the fish and shellfish that live in them. Larger, longer-lived fish and those that

live in contaminated waters have the highest concentrations.

4. Antibiotics and hormones are used in animal food production. The amounts entering the food supply pose little risk, but the use of antibiotics contributes to the development of antibiotic-resistant strains of bacteria.

5. Consumers can reduce the amounts of pesticides and other environmental contaminants in food through carefully selecting and handling produce, selecting low-fat saltwater varieties of fish caught far offshore in unpolluted waters, and trimming fat from meat, poultry, and fish before cooking.

4 Technology for Keeping Food Safe

1. Heating foods to high temperatures, cooling them to low temperatures, and altering levels of acidity, moisture, and oxygen prevent food spoilage and lengthen shelf life by killing microbes or slowing their growth.

2. **Irradiation** preserves food by exposing it to radiation. This process kills microbes, destroys insects, and slows the germination and ripening of fruits and vegetables.

3. Packaging keeps molds and bacteria out of foods, keeps moisture in, and protects food from physical damage. **Modified atmosphere packaging** reduces the oxygen available for microbial growth. The safety of packaging materials must be considered because components of packaging can leach into food.

4. **Direct food additives** are used to preserve or enhance the appeal of food. **Indirect food additives** are substances known to find their way into food during cooking, processing, and packaging. Both are FDA regulated. **Accidental contaminants**, which enter food when it is handled or prepared incorrectly, are not regulated by the FDA.

Nucleus

Plant cell wall

5 Biotechnology

1. **Biotechnology** produces **genetically modified (GM)** crops by transferring a gene for a desired characteristic from one organism to another. The result is a **transgenic** organism.

2. Biotechnology has the potential to improve the volume, safety, and quality of the food supply, but it also has the potential to introduce allergens or toxins into foods or to negatively affect nutrient content. Environmental concerns with the use of GM crops include reduction of biologic diversity, creation of "super weeds," and evolution of pesticide-resistant insects. Regulations are in place to control the use of genetic engineering and GM products.

KEY TERMS

CRITICAL AND CREATIVE THINKING QUESTIONS

1. After 67 people became ill from consuming food at a company picnic, investigators determined that the tossed green salad, the egg salad, and the turkey slices were all contaminated with *Campylobacter*. Invent a scenario that would explain how all three became contaminated.

2. A restaurant decides not to replace an old dishwasher, even though it no longer heats the water to above 135°F. What are the potential risks associated with this decision? How else could the restaurant sanitize the dishes?

3. The chicken Amy brings home from the store is contaminated with *Salmonella*. She prepares a meal by grilling the chicken and making a salad. List the steps in the preparation of this meal that might result in cross-contamination and increase the likelihood of *Salmonella* infection. What steps could Amy take to prevent food-borne illness?

4. A town's voters decide that they can improve their own health and protect the environment by banning the production and sale of all but organically produced foods. What are the risks and benefits of this decision?

5. Fermentation, a process that uses microbes to convert carbohydrates into alcohols or acids, is used to produce alcoholic beverages, and yogurt. Explain how fermentation converts milk into yogurt and why yogurt will keep longer than milk.

6. A train crash spills a load of industrial waste into a river that feeds into a local reservoir. Bottled water is provided to the residents of the community. How might this spill impact other segments of the food supply?

7. *Brassica* is a genus of plants that includes cabbage and broccoli, as well as a number of weeds. What risks might be associated with the use of a new genetically engineered variety of *Brassica* that grows faster and produces more seeds than traditional varieties?

What is happening in this picture ?

These rye plants are infected with a fungus. When the grain is consumed, the fungal toxins cause a syndrome called ergotism. The symptoms include prickling skin sensations, facial distortions, incomprehensible speech, paralysis, hallucinations, convulsions, and dementia. Ergotism may have caused some of the symptoms exhibited by individuals who were supposedly cursed by the "witches" of 17th-century Salem, Massachusetts.[44]

How could ergotism cause individuals to appear "bewitched"?

Why might moldy rye have been more of a problem in the 17th century than it is today?

Why doesn't baking prevent this ailment?

(Check your answers in Appendix L.)

1. What is the major cause of food-borne illness in the United States today?

   a. pesticides
   b. microbes
   c. environmental toxins
   d. antibiotics

2. Which factor does not affect the likelihood that a contaminant will cause food-borne illness in an individual?

   a. body size
   b. immune status
   c. age
   d. dose of toxin
   e. time of year

3. Foods on the GRAS list _____.

   a. are definitely safe
   b. have been used for years without ill effect
   c. are green
   d. do not need to be listed in an ingredient list

4. Which of the following is not true of a HACCP system?

   a. It relies on visual food inspections.
   b. It identifies steps in food production where contamination can occur or be prevented.
   c. Designing and implementing a HACCP system is the responsibility of a food manufacturer.
   d. It requires extensive record keeping.
   e. It monitors critical points in food production and takes corrective action if criteria are not met.

5. The foods that most frequently cause *Salmonella* infection are _____.

   a. beef and pork
   b. dairy products
   c. eggs and poultry
   d. shellfish

6. Pathogenic bacteria are killed by _____.

   a. freezing
   b. cooking
   c. refrigeration
   d. marinating

7. Below what temperature should food be refrigerated to reduce bacterial growth?

   a. A
   b. B
   c. C
   d. D

8. Which organism can cause food-borne intoxication and can be present in honey and home-canned foods?

   a. *Escherichia coli*
   b. *Clostridium perfringens*
   c. *Clostridium botulinum*
   d. *Salmonella*

9. Which of the following is most likely to be a concern in hamburger that is cooked to well done on a grill?

   a. polycyclic aromatic hydrocarbons (PAHs)
   b. *Escherichia coli*
   c. *Giardia*
   d. prions

10. Raw hamburger patties are taken to the grill on a platter. After being cooked, they are returned to the unwashed platter and served. This is an example of _____.

   a. efficient use of kitchen equipment
   b. food intoxication
   c. cross-contamination
   d. a HACCP system

11. Glass that enters food from a broken jar is _____.

   a. regulated as an indirect food additive
   b. not regulated
   c. safe because it is sterilized
   d. regulated as an accidental contaminant

12. Which organism is most likely to contain the highest concentration of industrial contaminants?

   a. A
   b. B
   c. C
   d. D

Groundwater, irrigation water, waterways, lakes, oceans

Agricultural chemicals

Industrial wastes

13. At what step in this process is recombinant DNA formed?

   a. 1
   b. 3
   c. 4
   d. 6
   e. 7

14. The potential benefits of biotechnology include all of the following except _____.

   a. increased biodiversity
   b. enhanced disease resistance
   c. improved crop yields
   d. reduced pesticide use

15. This insignia means the food _____.

   a. is not safe to eat
   b. has been irradiated
   c. is radioactive
   d. can safely be stored without refrigeration

Feeding the World 14

Works of fantasy and literature are filled with speculation about the impact of a growing population on a world of limited food supplies. In Harry Harrison's 1966 novel *Make Room! Make Room!*, the 35 million people populating New York City in 1999 subsist on seaweed, oatmeal, rationed water, and soy biscuits, with meat a rare, expensive commodity illegally procured from "meatleggers." In the 1999 film *The Matrix*, a character betrays his comrades for a *virtual* steak dinner—not even the real thing.

Of course, 1999 has come and gone, along with the rest of the 20th century, and one may argue that we are not quite in the dire straits anticipated by these and many other fantasists. Even though disaster has been averted thus far, however, the production, distribution, safety, consumption, and sustainability of the world's food and water resources remain matters of great concern to governments and individuals. Although a large part of the world's population faces undernutrition and starvation on a daily basis, leading to a plethora of public health issues, another portion faces problems caused by too rich a diet, which can lead to overnutrition, obesity, and a different—but equally dangerous and costly—set of public health issues.

Throughout history, governments have concerned themselves with adequate food production and distribution for burgeoning populations, but individual self-interest has often defeated more altruistic—and sensible—nutrition objectives. Global and national economic and political interests may either alleviate or exacerbate world nutrition conditions.

The Two Faces of Malnutrition

LEARNING OBJECTIVES

Compare the problems of under- and overnutrition in the world today.

Discuss the impact of undernutrition throughout the life cycle.

Explain how nutrition transition affects the incidence of obesity.

For most of us, the image that comes to mind when we think of malnutrition around the world is one of undernutrition: **hunger** and **starvation**. This image is certainly valid because about 923 million people around the world are chronically undernourished and more than a third of all deaths in children under age 5 are due to undernutrition, which kills nearly 6 million children each year.[1–4] At the same time that health organizations are struggling with issues of undernutrition, however, rates of illness related to overnutrition are soaring. The overweight and the undernourished both suffer from malnutrition and experi-

hunger Recurrent involuntary lack of food that over time may lead to malnutrition.

starvation A severe reduction in nutrient and energy intake that impairs health and eventually causes death. It is the most extreme form of malnutrition.

ence high levels of sickness and disability, shorter life expectancies, and lower levels of productivity. These two faces of malnutrition complicate the goal of solving the problem of malnutrition worldwide.

THE IMPACT OF UNDERNUTRITION

In populations where hunger is a chronic problem, there is a **cycle of malnutrition** (FIGURE 14.1A). The cycle begins when women consume a nutrient-deficient diet during pregnancy. These women are more likely than others to give birth to low-birth-weight infants who are susceptible to illness and early death.

Visualizing

The cycle of malnutrition FIGURE 14.1

▲ A Malnutrition affects the health and productivity of individuals at every stage of life. It often begins in the womb, continues through infancy and childhood, and extends into adolescence and adulthood. Interruption of this cycle of malnutrition at any point can benefit both the individuals affected and their society. Healthy children can then grow into healthy adults who produce healthy offspring and can contribute fully to society.

▲ B Low-birth-weight infants are at increased risk for complications, illness, and early death. Survivors often suffer lifelong physical and cognitive disabilities. A higher number of low-birth-weight infants means a higher infant mortality rate. Every year, more than 20 million low-birth-weight babies are born, 96% of them in developing countries.[6]

The **infant mortality rate** and the number of low-birth-weight births are indicators of a population's health and nutritional status (FIGURE 14.1B). In most industrialized countries the infant mortality rate is less than 7 per 1000 live births; in developing countries, the rate is often over 100 per 1000 live births.[5] Low-birth-weight infants who do survive require extra nutrients, which usually are not available. Malnutrition in infancy and childhood has a profound effect on growth and development as well as on susceptibility to infectious disease. Infectious diseases are more common in undernourished children, and undernourished children may die of infectious diseases that would not be life threatening in well-nourished children (FIGURE 14.1C).

Malnutrition in children causes **stunting** (FIGURE 14.1D), which is used as an indicator of undernutrition in a population's children. Stunting in childhood produces smaller adults who have a reduced work capacity and are unable to contribute optimally to their society's economic and social development. Stunted, malnourished women

are more likely than others to give birth to low-birth-weight babies. In addition, abdominal obesity in adulthood is more common in those who have experienced lower birth weight and early-childhood stunting.[8] Abdominal obesity increases the risk of morbidity from cardiovascular disease, hypertension, and diabetes.

OVERNUTRITION: A WORLD ISSUE

For the first time in history, with over 1 billion overweight or obese adults worldwide, the number of over-nourished people exceeds the number who are undernourished.[9,10] If recent trends continue, by 2030 up to 57.8% of the world's adult population could be either overweight or obese.[11] Because obesity increases the risk of cardiovascular disease, hypertension, stroke, type 2 diabetes, certain cancers, and arthritis, among other conditions, it is a major contributor to the global burden of chronic disease and disability.

The prevalence of overweight and obesity is also growing among children worldwide.[12] According to the latest estimates about 22 million children under age 5 are overweight, and at least 155 million school-age children are overweight or obese.[13] In some countries, a high prevalence of overweight children now exists alongside a high prevalence of undernourished children.[14]

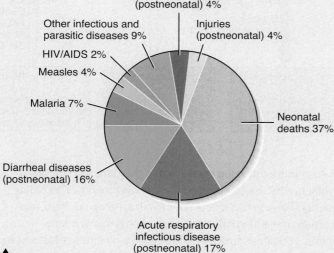

Causes of death in neonates and children under 5 in the world

- Noncommunicable disease (postneonatal) 4%
- Injuries (postneonatal) 4%
- Other infectious and parasitic diseases 9%
- HIV/AIDS 2%
- Measles 4%
- Malaria 7%
- Neonatal deaths 37%
- Diarrheal diseases (postneonatal) 16%
- Acute respiratory infectious disease (postneonatal) 17%

▲ **C** Well over half of all deaths in children under 5 years are due to infectious disease.[4] Mortality from infections is increased among malnourished children. It is estimated that 35% of deaths in children under age 5 occurs due to the presence of undernutrition. Immunizations against infectious disease are less effective in malnourished children because their immune systems cannot respond normally.

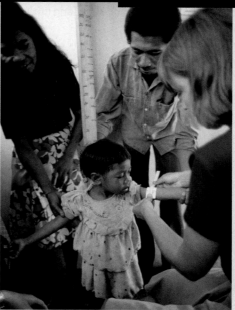

▲ **D** In developing countries, more than 30% of children less than 5 years of age suffer from stunting.[7] Deficiencies of energy, protein, vitamin A, iodine, iron, and zinc, as well as prolonged infections, have been implicated as causes.

WHY DO UNDERNUTRITION AND OVERNUTRITION EXIST SIDE BY SIDE?

We see the problems of undernutrition and overnutrition existing side by side because diets and lifestyles change as economic conditions improve. Traditional diets in developing countries are based on a limited number of foods—primarily starchy root vegetables. As incomes increase and food availability improves, the diet becomes more varied and includes more energy-dense foods such as meat, milk, fat, and sugar. Along with these dietary changes, there is a decrease in activity due to occupations that are less physically demanding, greater access to transportation, more labor-saving technology, and more passive leisure time (**FIGURE 14.2A**).

Some of the effects of this **nutrition transition** are positive: Life expectancy increases, and the frequencies of low birth weight, infectious diseases, and nutrient deficiencies decrease. However, at the same time, rates of heart disease, cancer, diabetes, obesity, and childhood obesity increase (**FIGURE 14.2B**).[19,20] Increased reliance on animal proteins and refined and processed foods increases the amounts of energy and natural resources needed to produce the food, and in the long term, these higher rates of consumption may damage the environment and deplete nonrenewable resources.

nutrition transition A series of changes in diet, physical activity, health, and nutrition that occurs as poor countries become more prosperous.

CONCEPT CHECK STOP

HOW prevalent are undernutrition and overnutrition around the world?

What does a high incidence of stunting indicate?

HOW does nutrition transition affect a population's health?

Nutrition transition FIGURE 14.2

A This schematic represents the dietary changes that occur with nutrition transition and the health consequences associated with these changes.[15] A diet that falls somewhere between the traditional rural diet, which may be inadequate in energy, protein, or micronutrients, and the affluent Western diet, which meets nutrient needs but is high in fat and sugar and low in fiber, is optimal for health.

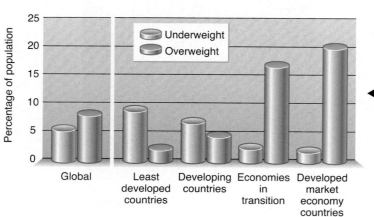

B As countries develop economically, they face many of the problems that are common in industrialized countries, including obesity.[10] In Argentina, Colombia, Mexico, Paraguay, Peru, and Uruguay, more than half of the population is overweight or obese.[16] Countries such as China and India, which have historically been plagued by undernutrition, must now also contend with overnutrition.[17,18] And in parts of Africa, obesity is now considered a major disease, along with AIDS and malnutrition.

Causes of Hunger Around the World

The specific reasons for hunger and **food insecurity** vary with time and location, but the underlying cause is that whatever food is available is not distributed equitably. This inequitable distribution results in either a shortage of food or the wrong combination of foods to meet nutrient needs. This situation, in turn, results in protein-energy malnutrition and individual nutrient deficiencies.

> **food insecurity**
> A situation in which people lack adequate physical, social, or economic access to sufficient, safe, nutritious food that meets their dietary needs and food preferences for an active and healthy life.

> **famine**
> A widespread lack of access to food due to a disaster that causes a collapse in the food production and marketing systems.

FOOD SHORTAGES

The most obvious example of a food shortage is **famine**. Drought, floods, earthquakes, and crop destruction by diseases or pests are natural causes of famines. Human causes include wars and civil conflicts (**FIGURE 14.3**).

Food shortages due to famine are very visible because they cause many deaths in an area during a short period, but chronic food shortages take a greater toll. Chronic shortages occur when economic inequities result in lack of money, health care, and education for individuals or populations; when the population outgrows the food supply; when cultural and religious practices limit food choices; or when environmental damage limits the amount of food that can be produced.

Poverty Almost 1.4 billion people around the world live below the international poverty line, earning less than $1.25 per day.[21] Poverty is central to the problem of hunger and undernutrition (**FIGURE 14.4** on the next page). In addition to creating food insecurity, poverty reduces access to health care, increasing the prevalence of disease and disability. When diseases go untreated, nutrient needs are increased, a situation that further limits the ability to obtain an adequate diet and contributes to malnutrition. Those who are poor also have less access to education, and this lack of access contributes to undernutrition and disease and reduces opportunities to escape poverty.

Famine FIGURE 14.3

This girl awaits relief food in a nation beset by famine. Regions that produce barely enough food for survival under normal conditions are vulnerable to the disaster of famine. This situation is analogous to a man standing in water up to his nostrils: If all is calm, he can breathe, but if there is a ripple, he will drown. When a ripple such as a natural or civil disaster occurs, it reduces the margin of survival and creates famine.

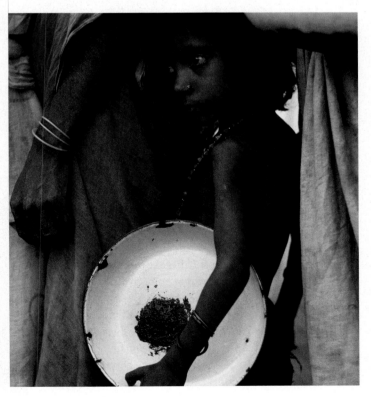

Visualizing

Nearly all (96%) of the world's undernourished people live in the developing world, where poverty is most prevalent. [22] In wealthy countries, social safety nets, such as soup kitchens, government food assistance programs, and job training programs, help the hungry obtain food or money to buy food, but in poor countries a family that cannot grow enough food or earn enough money to buy food may have nowhere to turn for help.[23]

Clinics such as this one in Nicaragua are not accessible to many people in the developing world. Lack of immunizations and treatment for infections and other illnesses results in increased incidence and morbidity from infectious disease and a decrease in survival rates from chronic diseases such as cancer. Lack of health care also increases infant mortality and the incidence of low-birth-weight births.

NATIONAL GEOGRAPHIC

When young children must work in the fields with their parents, it is difficult for them to attend school. Lack of education contributes to undernutrition and disease because it leads to inadequate care for infants, children, and pregnant women. Lack of education about food preparation and storage can affect food safety and the health of the household: Unsanitary food preparation increases the incidence of gastrointestinal diseases, which contribute to malnutrition.

NATIONAL GEOGRAPHIC

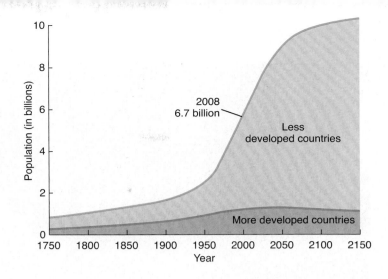

World population growth FIGURE 14.5

About 90% of the world's population growth is occurring in less-developed countries. Developing countries cannot escape poverty because their economies cannot keep pace with such rapid population growth. Efforts to produce enough food can damage the soil and deplete environmental resources, further reducing the capacity to produce food in the future.

Overpopulation

Overpopulation exists when a region has more people than its natural resources can support. A fertile river valley can support more people per acre than can a desert environment. But even in fertile regions of the world, if the number of people increases excessively, resources are overwhelmed, and food shortages occur. At present, enough food is produced throughout the world to prevent hunger if that food is distributed equitably, but demand is rising. The human population is currently growing at a rate of more than 82 million persons per year (FIGURE 14.5).[24] This rate of growth could eventually outstrip the planet's ability to produce enough food to feed the world's population.

In addition, the demand for grain is increasing as a result of increased consumption of more grain-intensive livestock products and the recent sharp acceleration in the use of grain to produce ethanol to fuel cars.[25] The increased demand has contributed to dramatic increases in food prices, which have made it even more challenging for low- and middle-income families worldwide to obtain enough food. The rising price of grain and fuel oil has also reduced the amount of food aid, widening the gap between the amount of food available and the amount needed to meet nutritional needs.[26]

Cultural practices

In some cultures, access to food may be limited for certain individuals in households. For example, because they are viewed as less important, women and girls may receive less food than men and boys. How much food is available to an individual within a household depends on gender, control of income, education, age, birth order, and genetic endowments.

The cultural acceptability or unacceptability of foods also contributes to food shortages and malnutrition. If available foods are culturally unacceptable, a food shortage exists unless the population can be educated to accept the new food. For example, insects are eaten in some cultures and are an excellent source of protein, but in other cultures they are unacceptable as food.

Limited environmental resources

The land and other resources available to produce food are limited. Some resources, such as minerals and fossil fuels, are present in finite amounts and are nonrenewable—that is, once they have been used, they cannot be replaced within a reasonable amount of time. Others, such as soil and water, are **renewable resources** because they will be available indefinitely if they used at a rate at which Earth can restore them. For example, when agricultural land is used wisely—when crops are rotated, erosion is prevented, and contamination is limited—it can be reused almost endlessly. However, if land is not used carefully, damage caused by soil erosion, nutrient depletion, and accumulation of pollutants may reduce the amount of usable land over the long term.

> **renewable resources** Resources that are restored and replaced by natural processes and can therefore be used forever.

Modern mechanized agricultural methods that have increased food production use more energy and resources and cause more environmental damage than does more traditional labor-intensive farming. In industrialized nations, about 17% of the energy used is employed in food production.[27]

In general, the environmental cost of producing plant-based foods is lower than that of producing animal products, but it may still be substantial. Modern large-scale farming can erode the soil and deplete its nutrients. Fertilizers and pesticides can contaminate groundwater and eventually pollute waterways. And if a plant product is shipped over long distances, requires refrigeration or

Overfishing has severely reduced the numbers of many marine species. Pollution also threatens the world's fishing grounds. Oil spills and deliberate dumping occur offshore, and sewage, pesticides, organic pollutants, and sediments from erosion wash into coastal waters, where most fish spend at least part of their lives. Even aquaculture, designed to increase fish production, produces wastes that can pollute ocean water and harm other marine organisms.

freezing, or needs other types of processing, the environmental costs are increased even more.

Modern methods of raising cattle create both air and water pollution. The animals themselves produce methane, a greenhouse gas, in their gastrointestinal tracts. More methane is produced when animal sewage is stored in ponds and heaps. In fact, livestock is responsible for 18% of greenhouse gas emissions, a larger share than that of all the cars in the world combined. Livestock production also accounts for over 8% of global human water use and releases nutrients, pathogens, and other pollutants into waterways.[28]

As more countries undergo nutrition transition, the demand for meat-based diets will increase, as will the use of natural resources and energy. It is not only the resources of the land that are at risk. Population growth has increased the demand for fish to the point that the Earth's oceans are being depleted (FIGURE 14.6).

POOR-QUALITY DIETS

Even when there is enough food, malnutrition can occur if the quality of the diet is poor. The typical diet in developing countries is based on high-fiber grain products and has little variety. Adults who are able to consume a relatively large amount of this diet may be able to meet their nutrient needs. But individuals with high nutrient needs because they are ill or pregnant and those with limited capacity to consume this bulky grain diet such as children and elderly individuals are at risk for nutrient deficiencies. Deficiencies of protein, iron, iodine, and vitamin A are common with poor-quality diets. The images in FIGURE 14.7 will help you recall the information about these deficiencies discussed in earlier chapters.

Several other vitamin and mineral deficiencies have recently emerged or reemerged as problems throughout the world. Beriberi, pellagra, and scurvy—diseases caused by deficiencies of thiamin, niacin, and vitamin C, respectively—are rare in the developed world but still occur among extremely poor and underprivileged people and in large refugee populations. In many parts of the world, folate deficiency causes megaloblastic anemia during pregnancy and often compounds existing iron deficiency anemia. Deficiencies of the minerals zinc, selenium, and calcium are also of concern.[32] Zinc deficiency affects about one-third of the world's population and is believed to cause as many deaths as vitamin A deficiency or iron deficiency.[33] Selenium deficiency has been identified in population groups in China, New Zealand, and the Russian Federation. Inadequate calcium intake is a worldwide concern due to its association with osteoporosis.

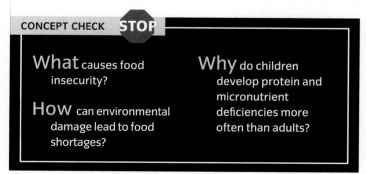

CONCEPT CHECK STOP

What causes food insecurity?

How can environmental damage lead to food shortages?

Why do children develop protein and micronutrient deficiencies more often than adults?

Protein and micronutrient deficiencies FIGURE 14.7

Protein-energy malnutrition is most common in children. When there is a general lack of food, the wasting associated with *marasmus* results, and when the diet is limited to starchy grains and vegetables, *kwashiorkor*, characterized by a bloated belly, can predominate. Other factors, such as metabolic changes caused by infection, may also play a role in the development of kwashiorkor. ▶

Marasmus

Kwashiorkor

Normal red blood cells

Iron deficiency anemia

◀ More than 2 billion people worldwide suffer from iron deficiency anemia, which is characterized by small, pale red blood cells. The lack of iron reduces the amount of hemoglobin produced, and the lack of hemoglobin lowers the blood's oxygen-carrying capacity.[29] In developing countries, intestinal parasites, which cause gastrointestinal blood loss, and acute and chronic infections, such as malaria, aggravate dietary iron deficiency. Iron deficiency can have a major impact on the health and productivity of a population.

Although goiter, seen here, is a more visible manifestation of iodine deficiency, the more subtle effects of deficiency on mental performance and work capacity may have a greater impact on the population as a whole. Iodine-deficient children have lower IQs and impaired school performance.[30] Iodine deficiency in children and adults is associated with apathy and decreased initiative and decision-making capabilities. ▼

▲

It is estimated that more than 150 million preschool children worldwide suffer from vitamin A deficiency.[31] Vitamin A deficiency leads to *xerophthalmia*, shown here. Vitamin A deficiency is the leading cause of preventable blindness among children. It also depresses immune function, thus increasing the risk of illness and death from infections, particularly measles and diarrheal disease.

Causes of Hunger in the United States

Most of the nutritional problems in the United States are related to overnutrition.[34] However, although news stories often focus on obesity, about 11% of households in the United States experience food insecurity (**FIGURE 14.8**).[35] This situation is caused not by a general food shortage but by an inequitable distribution of food and money. The incidence of hunger and food insecurity is higher among women, infants, children, elderly individuals, and those who are poor, homeless, ill, or disabled. However, a sudden decrease in income or increase in living expenses can put anyone at risk for food insecurity.

POVERTY AND FOOD INSECURITY

In the United States, as elsewhere in the world, poverty is the main cause of food insecurity. Poverty reduces access to food, education, and health care. About 12.5% of Americans (37.3 million people) live at or below the poverty level.[36] These individuals have less money to spend on food and often have less access to affordable food. Limited income also reduces the chances that healthier foods will be consumed. Choosing leaner meats and dairy products and whole grains costs more—about 35 to 40% of low-income consumers' food budgets.[37]

Poverty reduces access to food. The high price of real estate in cities has driven supermarkets into the suburbs, and because many low-income city families do not own cars, they must shop at small, expensive corner stores or pay cab fares if they wish to take advantage of lower prices at more distant, larger stores. The rural poor may have limited access to food because they live far from grocery stores. High poverty and unemployment rates among Native Americans and Alaska Natives contribute to food insecurity.[38] Migrant workers also have limited access to food because labor camps are in remote locations, and transportation is often unavailable. Low incomes and difficult working and living conditions among migrant workers further limit their ability to purchase food and prepare adequate meals.

Poverty also limits access to health care, leading to poorer health status. Iron deficiency is more than twice as frequent in low-income children than in children in higher-income families, and the incidence of heart disease, cancer, hypertension, and obesity increases with decreasing income.[39] As in developing nations, poverty is reflected in infant mortality rates. The average infant mortality in the U.S. population is about 6.7 per 1000 live births.[40] However, there are groups within the population that have infant mortality rates as high as those in impoverished nations. Among African Americans, the infant mortality rate is 13.6 per 1000 live births—more than twice that of the general population.[40] This difference mirrors the higher poverty rate in this group.

Food insecurity in the United States FIGURE 14.8

In 2007, approximately 89% of U.S. households were food secure and about 11%, or 13 million households, experienced food insecurity.[35]

88.9%

7.0%

4.1%

Food secure households

Households with low food security

Households with very low food security

Low food security means that families were able to avoid substantially disrupting their eating patterns or reducing food intake by using coping strategies, such as eating a less varied diet, participating in federal food assistance programs, or getting emergency food from community food pantries.

Very low food security means that the normal eating patterns of one or more household members was disrupted and food intake was reduced at times during the year because families had insufficient money or other resources to use for obtaining food. In 2007, about 4.7 million households, including 323,000 households with children, had very low food security.

Education and poverty FIGURE 14.9

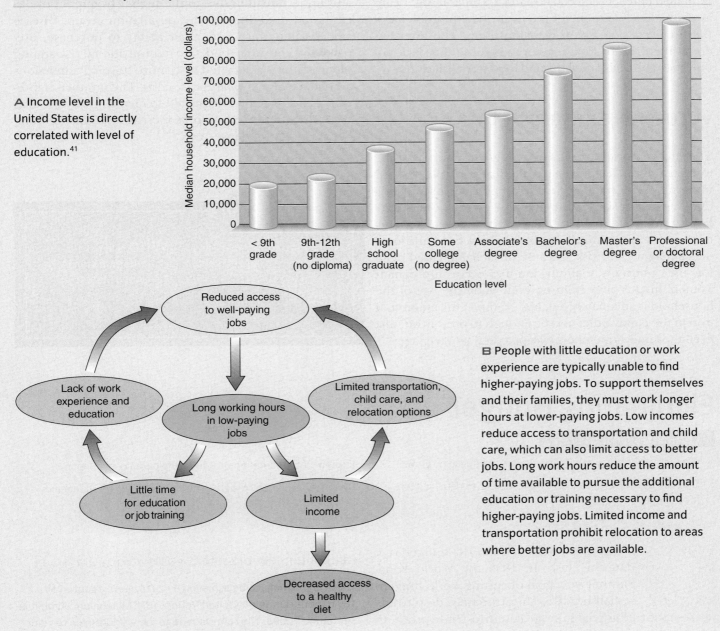

A Income level in the United States is directly correlated with level of education.[41]

Median household income level (dollars) — Education level:
< 9th grade / 9th-12th grade (no diploma) / High school graduate / Some college (no degree) / Associate's degree / Bachelor's degree / Master's degree / Professional or doctoral degree

Reduced access to well-paying jobs

Lack of work experience and education

Long working hours in low-paying jobs

Limited transportation, child care, and relocation options

Little time for education or job training

Limited income

Decreased access to a healthy diet

B People with little education or work experience are typically unable to find higher-paying jobs. To support themselves and their families, they must work longer hours at lower-paying jobs. Low incomes reduce access to transportation and child care, which can also limit access to better jobs. Long work hours reduce the amount of time available to pursue the additional education or training necessary to find higher-paying jobs. Limited income and transportation prohibit relocation to areas where better jobs are available.

Lack of education, which is both a cause and a consequence of poverty, also contributes to food insecurity (FIGURE 14.9). For people at or below the poverty level, educational opportunities are fewer and lower in quality than those for people with higher incomes. In the short term, lack of knowledge about food selection, food safety, and home economics can contribute to malnutrition. Too little food may cause the diet to be deficient in energy or particular nutrients, but poor food choices also allow food insecurity to coexist with obesity. Lack of education about food safety can also increase the incidence of food-borne illness. In the long term, lack of education prevents people from getting the higher-paying jobs that could allow them to escape poverty.

Poor families must use most of their income to pay for shelter, a situation that seriously reduces the chances that they will be adequately fed. The high cost of housing not only limits food budgets but also contributes to the growing problem of homelessness in the United States. It is estimated that between 600,000 and 2.5 million Americans are homeless,[42] and one of the major health problems of the homeless population is malnutrition. The homeless are at high risk of food insecurity because they lack not only money but also cooking and food storage facilities.

VULNERABLE STAGES OF LIFE

The high nutrient needs of pregnant and lactating women and small children put them at particular risk for undernutrition. Almost one-third of households with children headed by single women live below the poverty line. Poverty and food insecurity place these women and children at risk for malnutrition, and their special nutritional needs magnify this risk. Because of their increased need for some nutrients, malnutrition may occur in pregnant women, infants, and children even when the rest of the household is adequately fed. For example, the amount of iron in the family's diet may be enough to prevent anemia in all the family's members except a pregnant teenager.

Elderly individuals are vulnerable to food insecurity and undernutrition due to the higher frequency of diseases and disabilities in this population group. Disease and disability may limit their ability to purchase, prepare, and consume food. Greater nutritional risk among older adults is associated with more hospital admissions and hence higher health-care costs. The number of individuals over age 85 is expected to quadruple by 2050; as the number of elderly people increases, so will the number at risk for food insecurity.[43]

CONCEPT CHECK STOP

Why are some Americans hungry in a land of plenty?

Who is at risk for undernutrition in the United States?

How are education and poverty related?

Eliminating Hunger

LEARNING OBJECTIVES

Discuss two strategies that can help reduce population growth.

Discuss the role of sustainable agriculture in maintaining the food supply.

Explain how international trade can help eliminate hunger.

Describe five federal programs designed to alleviate hunger in the United States.

Solving the problem of world hunger is a daunting task. In 1996 the World Food Summit set a goal of cutting world hunger in half by 2015. Unfortunately, despite advances toward this goal in some countries, little progress has been made worldwide. Current estimates put the number of undernourished people in the world at 923 million, 80 million more than there were in the early 1990s.[1]

Solutions to world hunger need to address population growth, ensure that the nutrient needs of a large and diverse population are met with culturally acceptable foods, and increase food production while maintaining the global ecosystem (**FIGURE 14.10**). Meeting these goals will require input from politicians, nutrition scientists, economists, and the food industry.

Millennium development goals FIGURE 14.10

These eight goals, to be achieved by 2015, were adopted by 189 nations during the United Nations (UN) Millennium Summit in September, 2000. They correspond to the world's main development challenges. In order to achieve the first goal, stamping out hunger, most of the others must also be addressed.[44]

Emergency food relief FIGURE 14.11

Many organizations are working to combat world hunger. The American Red Cross and High Commissioner for Refugees of the UN concentrate on famine relief. The Food and Agriculture Organization (FAO) works to improve the production, intake, and distribution of food worldwide. The World Health Organization (WHO) focuses on international health and emphasizes the prevention of nutrition problems, and the UN Children's Fund (UNICEF) targets education and vaccination and responds to crisis situations to improve the lives of children.

Economic policies, technical advances, education, and legislative measures must put programs and policies in place to provide food in the short term, and in the long term they must establish sustainable programs to allow the continued production and distribution of acceptable foods.

PROVIDING SHORT-TERM FOOD AID

When people are starving, short-term food and medical aid must be provided right away. The standard approach has been to bring food into stricken areas (FIGURE 14.11). This food generally consists of agricultural surpluses from other countries and often is not well planned in terms of its nutrient content. Although this type of relief is necessary for a population to survive an immediate crisis such as famine, it does little to prevent future hunger.

CONTROLLING POPULATION GROWTH

In the long term, solving the problem of world hunger requires balancing the number of people and the amount of food that can be produced. The world's population has increased dramatically since the middle of the 20th century, but population growth has recently begun to slow. The birth rate worldwide has declined—from 5 children per woman in 1950 to 2.6 in 2009.[45,46] This downward trend in population growth must continue to ensure that food production and natural resources can support the population. Changes in cultural and economic factors as well as family planning and government policies can be used to influence the birth rate.

Economic and cultural factors that affect birth rate In many cultures, a large family is expected. A major reason for this expectation is high infant and child mortality rates. When infant mortality rates are high, people choose to have many children in order to ensure that some will survive. Higher birth rates in some developing countries are also due to the economic and societal roles of children. They are needed to work the farms, support the elders, and otherwise contribute to the economic survival of the family. Programs that foster economic development and ensure access to food, shelter, and medical care have been shown to cause a decline in birth rates because people feel secure having fewer children. Economic development also reduces the need for children as workers.

Education and Birth Rate

The large number of children in this impoverished Cambodian family is indicative of the uneven burden of population growth in the developing world. A scientist sees that one of the reasons for the many children in this family is lack of education for women. Education builds job skills that allow women to join the workforce, marry later in life, and have fewer children. Education increases the likelihood that women will have control over their fertility and gives them knowledge that can be used to improve the family's health and economic situation. The graph shows that higher literacy among women is associated with lower birth rates.[48] Women who are better educated have options other than having numerous children. What do you think a graph showing years of education versus birth rate in the United States would look like?

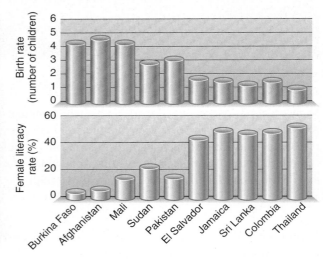

Another cultural factor that influences birth rate is gender inequality. Girls are often kept at home to work rather than being sent to school. In most developing countries, the literacy rate is lower for women than men, and fewer women attend primary and secondary school. This lack of education leaves women few options other than remaining home and having children. Providing education for girls has been shown to reduce birth rates (see *What a Scientist Sees*).[47]

Family planning and government policies

Changes in cultural and economic factors may reduce the desire for large families, but achieving this goal requires the availability of health and family planning services. To be successful, family-planning efforts must be acceptable to the population and compatible with cultural and religious beliefs. Governments around the world have used a number of approaches, such as provision of contraceptives, education, and economic incentives, to decrease population growth (FIGURE 14.12).

Access to birth control FIGURE 14.12

A birth control vendor explains condoms to women at a market in the Ivory Coast. The birth rate in this West African country declined from nearly 7 children per woman in 1988 to 4.1 in 2009, due in part to increased use of modern methods of birth control. Increased knowledge and availability of contraceptives is linked to a decrease in birth rate.[46]

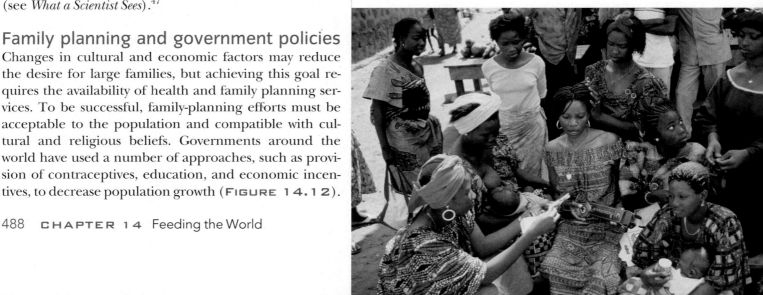

INCREASING FOOD PRODUCTION WHILE PROTECTING THE ENVIRONMENT

Advances in agricultural technology have allowed food production to keep pace with population growth. However, the use of energy-intensive modern agricultural techniques has contributed to serious environmental problems. Commercial inorganic fertilizers and pesticides and modern farm machinery increase food production but at the same time pollute the air and water. Overuse of land causes deterioration of soil quality, a condition that will limit food production in the future. For food production to continue to meet the needs of future generations, we must figure out how to continue to increase food yields and availability while conserving the world's natural resources (see the *Case Study*).

Sustainable agriculture uses food production methods that prevent damage to the environment and allow the land to restore itself so that food can be produced indefinitely. For example, contour plowing and terracing help prevent erosion, keeping the soil available for future crops. Rotating the crops grown in a field prevents the depletion of nutrients in

> **sustainable agriculture**
> Agricultural methods that maintain soil productivity and a healthy ecological balance while having minimal long-term impacts.

WHAT CAN YOU DO?

Keesha is concerned about the problems of hunger and malnutrition and the impact her choices have on the environment. Although she is a college student who cannot afford to make monetary contributions to relief organizations, she would like her everyday choices to have a minimal impact on the environment.

What are the advantages and disadvantages of these salad options in terms of convenience, food safety, and environmental impact?

▼

Your answer:

The following are some inexpensive changes Keesha can make to reduce her impact on the environment. What are the advantages and disadvantages of each?

Action	Advantages	Disadvantages
	Your answer:	*Your answer:*
Bike instead of drive on short trips around town.		
Buy a canvas bag to carry groceries.		
Bring juice in a thermos instead of buying a non-recyclable bottle.		
Compost vegetable scraps.		
Buy locally grown produce.		
Buy organically grown produce.		

(Check your answers in Appendix K.)

A sustainable farm FIGURE 14.13

A sustainable farm consists of a total agricultural ecosystem rather than a single crop. It may include field crops, fruit- and nut-bearing trees, herds of livestock, and forests.

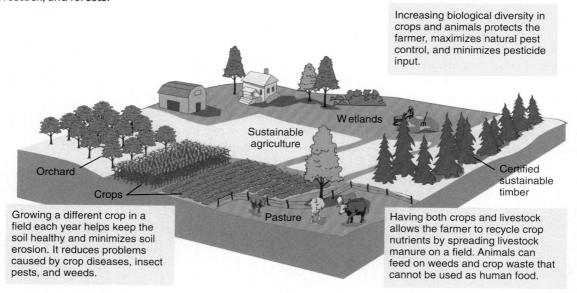

Increasing biological diversity in crops and animals protects the farmer, maximizes natural pest control, and minimizes pesticide input.

Wetlands

Sustainable agriculture

Orchard

Crops

Pasture

Certified sustainable timber

Growing a different crop in a field each year helps keep the soil healthy and minimizes soil erosion. It reduces problems caused by crop diseases, insect pests, and weeds.

Having both crops and livestock allows the farmer to recycle crop nutrients by spreading livestock manure on a field. Animals can feed on weeds and crop waste that cannot be used as human food.

the soil, reducing the need for fertilizers. Sustainable agriculture uses environmentally friendly chemicals that degrade quickly and do not persist as residues in the environment. It also relies on diversification. This approach to farming maximizes natural methods of pest control and fertilization and protects farmers from changes in the marketplace (FIGURE 14.13).

Sustainable agriculture is not a single program but involves choosing options that mesh well with the local soil, climate, and farming techniques. In some cases, organic farming, which does not use synthetic pesticides, herbicides, and fertilizers (see Chapter 13), may be the more sustainable option. Organic techniques have a smaller environmental impact because they reduce the use of agricultural chemicals and the release of pollutants into the environment. Organic farming is also advantageous in terms of soil quality and biodiversity, but it is a disadvantage when it comes to land use because crop yields are lower. A combination of organic and conventional techniques, as is used with integrated pest management (see Chapter 13), might improve land use and protect the environment.

Other sustainable programs include agroforestry, in which techniques from forestry and agriculture are used together to restore degraded areas; natural systems agri-

culture, which attempts to develop agricultural systems that include many types of plants and therefore function like natural ecosystems; and the technique of reducing fertilizer use by matching nutrient resources with the demands of the particular crop being grown. One modern technology that may be integrated with sustainable systems is genetic engineering. As we saw in Chapter 13, genetic engineering can increase crop yields by inserting genes that improve the efficiency with which plants convert sunlight into food or those that make plants resistant to herbicides, insects, and plant diseases.

INCREASING FOOD AVAILABILITY THROUGH ECONOMIC DEVELOPMENT AND TRADE

Hunger will exist as long as there is poverty. Even when food is plentiful, the poor do not have access to enough of the right foods to maintain their nutritional health. Economic development that leads to safe and sanitary housing, access to health care and education, and the resources to acquire enough food are essential if hunger is to be eliminated. Government policies can help reduce poverty and improve food security by increasing the population's income, lowering food prices, or funding food programs for those who are poor.

Economic development in the form of industrialization can also help provide food for a county's population by increasing access to international trade. The newly industrialized countries of Asia, such as South Korea, rely on imported food to decrease the number of hungry people in their populations. In general, countries around the world are becoming more dependent on food imports and on exports of food and other goods to pay for the food they import. This trade can increase the availability of food for the world's population as a whole.

Whether a country's agricultural emphasis is on producing **subsistence crops** or **cash crops** influences the availability of food for its people. Shifting to cash crops improves the country's cash flow but uses local resources to produce crops for export and limits the ability of its people to produce enough food to feed their families. For example, if a large portion of the arable land in a country is used to grow cash crops such as coffee and tea, little agricultural land remains for growing grains and vegetables that nourish the local population. If, however, the cash from the crop is used to purchase nutritious foods from other countries, this decision may help alleviate undernutrition.

> ■ **subsistence crops** Crops that are grown as food for the local population.

> ■ **cash crops** Crops that are grown to be sold for monetary return rather than as food for the local population.

ENSURING A NUTRITIOUS FOOD SUPPLY

To ensure the nutritional health of a population, the foods that are grown or imported must supply both sufficient energy and adequate amounts of all essential nutrients. If the diet does not provide enough of all the essential nutrients, either the dietary pattern must be changed, commonly consumed foods must be fortified, or supplements containing deficient nutrients must be provided. To make these changes effectively, consumers have to know how to choose foods that provide the needed nutrients and how to handle them safely.

Nutrition education
Education can help improve nutrient intake by teaching consumers what foods to grow, which foods to choose, and how to prepare them safely.

Education is particularly important when introducing a new crop. No matter how nutritious it may be, a new plant variety is not beneficial unless local farmers know how to grow it and the population accepts it as a food source and knows how to prepare it for consumption. For instance, white yams are common in some regions but are a poor source of β-carotene, which the body can use to make vitamin A. If the yellow yam, which is rich in β-carotene, became an acceptable choice, the amount of vitamin A available to the population would increase.

Food safety is also a concern when changing traditional dietary practices. For example, introducing papaya to the diet as a source of vitamin A will not improve nutritional status if it is washed in unsanitary water and causes dysentery among the people it is meant to nourish.

Education to encourage breast feeding can also improve nutritional status and health (FIGURE 14.14). To achieve optimal growth, development, and health, WHO recommends that infants be exclusively breast fed for the first six months of life. After that, other foods should be offered, while breast feeding continues for up to two years of age or beyond.[49]

Nutritional and health benefits of breast feeding FIGURE 14.14

Breast milk provides infants with optimal nutrition and immune factors that reduce the risk of infectious diseases. In developing nations, where infant mortality from infectious disease is high, mothers are advised to breast feed even if they are HIV positive because the risk of the baby dying of malnutrition and other infections outweighs the risk of transmitting the virus in the milk.[50] When infants are not breast fed, education about nutritious substitutes for breast milk and safe preparation of formulas is essential.

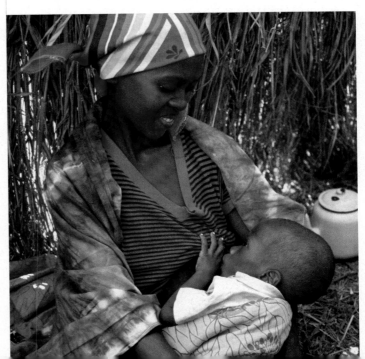

Fortifying the food supply

Although food fortification will not provide energy for a hungry population, it can increase the protein quality of the diet and eliminate micronutrient deficiencies. In order to solve a nutritional problem in a population, fortification must be implemented wisely. Fortification works only if vulnerable groups consume centrally processed foods. The foods selected for fortification should be among those that are consistently consumed by the majority of the population so that extensive promotion and reeducation are not needed to encourage their consumption. The nutrient should be added uniformly and in a form that optimizes its utilization.

Fortification has been used successfully in preventing health problems in the United States: Fortification of cow's milk to increase vitamin D intake was a major factor in the elimination of infantile rickets, and enrichment of grains with niacin helped eliminate pellagra. Fortification of salt with iodine has been used successfully to eliminate iodine deficiency diseases in countries around the world (**Figure 14.15**).

Providing supplements

Supplementing specific nutrients for at-risk segments of the population can help reduce the prevalence of malnutrition. Of countries where vitamin A deficiency is a public health problem, about three quarters have policies supporting regular vitamin A supplementation in children. Many have also adopted WHO's recommendation to provide all breast-feeding women with a high-dose supplement of vitamin A within eight weeks of delivery. This improves maternal vitamin A status and raises the amount of vitamin A that is present in breast milk and is therefore passed to the infant.

Many countries have adopted programs to supplement children older than 6 months with iron and pregnant women with iron and folate.

ELIMINATING FOOD INSECURITY IN THE UNITED STATES

As with world hunger, eliminating hunger in the United States involves improving economic security, keeping food affordable, providing food aid to the hungry, and offering education about healthy diets that will meet nutrient needs and reduce diseases related to overconsumption.

The nutrition safety net

Federal programs that provide access to affordable food and promote healthy eating have been referred to as a nutrition safety net for the American population (**Table 14.1**). The nutrition assistance programs include a combination of general nutrition assistance with specialized programs targeted to groups with particular nutritional risks: children, seniors, infants, women during and after pregnancy, Native Americans living on reservations, people with disabilities, and homeless people.[51] One of every 5 Americans receives some kind of food assistance, at a total cost of about $54 billion per year.[52]

Iodized salt FIGURE 14.15

This logo is used around the world as an indicator of iodized salt. Over the past decade, the number of countries with salt iodization programs has increased dramatically. It is estimated that 66% of households worldwide now have access to iodized salt.[30] As a result, the number of countries where iodine deficiency disorders are a public health problem has been cut in half.

Programs to prevent undernutrition in the United States TABLE 14.1

Program	Target population	Goals and methods
Supplemental Nutrition Assistance Program (SNAP)	Low-income individuals	Increases access to food by providing coupons or debit cards that can be used to purchase food at a grocery store
Commodity Supplemental Food Assistance Program	Low-income pregnant women, breast-feeding and non-breast-feeding postpartum women, infants and children under age 6, and elderly people	Provides food by distributing USDA commodity foods
Special Supplemental Nutrition Program for Women, Infants, and Children (WIC)	Low-income pregnant women, breast-feeding and non-breast-feeding postpartum women, and infants and children under age 5	Provides vouchers for the purchase of foods (including infant formula and infant cereal) high in nutrients that are typically lacking in the program's target population; provides nutrition education and referrals for health care
WIC Farmers' Market Nutrition Program	WIC participants	Increases access to fresh produce by providing vouchers that can be used to purchase produce at authorized local farmers' markets.
National School Breakfast Program	Low-income children	Provides free or low-cost breakfasts at school to improve the nutritional status of children
National School Lunch Program	Low-income children	Provides free or low-cost lunches at school to improve the nutritional status of children
Special Milk Program	Low-income children	Provides milk for children in schools, camps, and child-care institutions with no federally supported meal program
Summer Food Service Program	Low-income children	Provides free meals and snacks for children when school is not in session
Child and Adult Care Food Program	Children up to age 12 and elderly and disabled adults	Provides nutritious meals to children and adults in day-care settings
Team Nutrition	School-age children	Provides nutrition education, training and technical assistance, and resources to participating schools with the goal of improving children's lifelong eating and physical activity habits
Head Start	Low-income preschool children and their families	Provides education, including nutrition education
Nutrition Program for the Elderly	Individuals age 60 and over and their spouses	Provides free congregate meals in churches, schools, senior centers, or other facilities and delivers food to homebound people
Senior Farmers' Market Program	Low-income seniors	Provides coupons that can be exchanged for eligible foods at farmers' markets, roadside stands, and community-supported agricultural programs
Homeless Children Nutrition Program	Preschoolers living in shelters	Reimburses providers for meals served
Emergency Food Assistance Program	Low-income people	Provides commodities to soup kitchens, food banks, and individuals for home use
Healthy People 2010	U.S. population	Sets national health promotion objectives to improve the health of the U.S. population through health-care system and industry involvement, as well as individual actions
Expanded Food and Nutrition Education Program (EFNEP)	Low-income families	Provides education in all aspects of food preparation and nutrition
Temporary Assistance for Needy Families (TANF)	Low-income households	Provides assistance and work opportunities to needy families by granting states federal funds to implement welfare programs
Food Distribution Program on Indian Reservations	Low-income households living on reservations and Native Americans living near reservations	Provides food by distributing USDA commodity foods

The largest USDA program designed to make sure that all people have access to an adequate diet is the Supplemental Nutrition Assistance Program (SNAP) (previously known as the Food Stamp Program). SNAP provides monthly benefits in the form of coupons or debit cards that can be used to purchase food, thereby supplementing the food budgets of low-income individuals. Together with SNAP, four other programs that target high-risk populations—the National School Lunch Program, the Special Supplemental Nutrition Program for Women, Infants, and Children (WIC), the Child and Adult Care Food Program, and the National School Breakfast Program—account for 95% of the USDA's expenditure for food assistance.

In addition to federal nutrition assistance programs, church, community, and charitable emergency food shelters provide for the basic nutritional needs of many Americans. In the United States, about 150,000 non-profit food distribution programs help direct food to those in need.[53] The leading hunger-relief charity in the United States is Feeding America, which provides food assistance to over 25 million low-income people per year. It includes a network of food banks across the country and supports thousands of local charitable organizations, such as food pantries and soup kitchens, that distribute food directly to hungry Americans.

Virtually all these food distribution programs use food obtained through **food recovery**, which involves collecting food that is wasted in fields, commercial kitchens, restaurants, and grocery stores and distributing it to those in need (**FIGURE 14.16**). It is estimated that over 25% of America's food—enough to feed 49 million people—goes to waste each year.[54]

Nutrition education People who have more nutrition information and greater awareness of the relationship between diet and health consume healthier diets. Healthy diets not only improve current health by optimizing growth, productivity, and well-being but are essential for preventing chronic diseases. Increasing knowledge about nutrition can reduce medical costs and improve the quality of life.

Education can help individuals with lower incomes stretch their limited food dollars by making wise choices at the store and reducing food waste at home. It can promote community gardens to increase the availability of seasonal vegetables. It can teach people how to prepare foods received from commodity distribution programs and food banks. It can explain safe food handling and preparation methods. Knowing which foods to choose and how to handle them safely is as important in preventing malnutrition as having the money to buy enough food. In addition to the programs described in Table 14.1, the *Dietary Guidelines for Americans*, MyPyramid, and food labels educate the general public about making wise food choices (see *What Should I Eat?*).

WHAT SHOULD I EAT? | Environmental Impact

Use iProfile to compare the nutrients in a vegetarian versus a meat-based meal.

Make your meals green

- Reduce the amount of meat in your meal.
- Eat vegetarian at least some of the time.
- Buy in bulk in order to cut down on packaging.
- Use reusable bags to take your groceries home.
- Choose locally grown or organically produced foods.
- Eat lower on the food chain—more plant foods and small fish.
- Cook from scratch—use fewer processed foods.
- Grow and eat some of your own vegetables.

CONCEPT CHECK STOP

How does educating women help control population growth?

What impact does sustainable agriculture have on the world's food supply?

How can growing cash crops improve a nation's food supply?

What is the nutrition safety net?

SUMMARY

1 The Two Faces of Malnutrition

1. In poorly nourished populations, a **cycle of malnutrition** exists in which poorly nourished women give birth to low-birth-weight infants at risk for disease and early death. If these children survive, they grow into adults who are physically unable to fully contribute to society. In populations where malnutrition is prevalent, low birth weight, a high **infant mortality rate**, **stunting**, and infections are more common.

2. Overnutrition coexists with **hunger** and **starvation** in both developed and developing nations around the world. As economic conditions improve, **nutrition transition** to more Western diet and lifestyle patterns contribute to the growing problem of overnutrition.

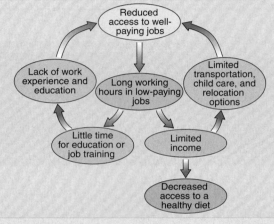

2 Causes of Hunger Around the World

1. The underlying cause of hunger and **food insecurity** is that the food available in the world is not distributed equitably. **Famine** results from natural and human-caused disasters that temporarily disrupt food production and distribution. Chronic food shortage occurs when economic inequities result in lack of money, health care, and education; when overpopulation and limited natural resources create a situation in which there are more people than food; when cultural practices limit food choices; and when **renewable resources** are misused, limiting the ability to continue to produce food.

2. Deficiencies of protein, iron, iodine, and vitamin A are common worldwide when the quality of the diet is poor. Pregnant women, children, elderly individuals, and those who are ill may not be able to meet their nutrient needs with the available diet.

3 Causes of Hunger in the United States

1. Both undernutrition and overnutrition are problems in the United States. As in developing nations, undernutrition and food insecurity are associated with poverty, which limits education and access to health care and adequate housing.

2. High nutrient needs increase the risk of malnutrition in women and children, and disease and disability increase risk in elderly individuals.

4 Eliminating Hunger

1. Short-term solutions to hunger provide food through relief at the local, national, and international levels.

2. Eliminating world hunger in the long term requires controlling population growth. This can be addressed by improving economic conditions, providing education, particularly for women, and ensuring access to family planning services.

3. **Sustainable agriculture** helps eliminate hunger by allowing food to be produced without damaging the environment.

4. Economic development helps prevent hunger by eliminating poverty and ensuring access to health care and education. It also increases access to international trade, which can be used to import food or to export **cash crops** to bring more money into the country.

5. Food fortification and dietary supplementation can be used to increase protein quality and eliminate micronutrient deficiencies, improving the overall quality of the diet.

6. Nutrition programs in the United States focus on maintaining a nutrition safety net that provides access to affordable food and education to promote healthy eating.

KEY TERMS

CRITICAL AND CREATIVE THINKING QUESTIONS

1. Describe the living conditions of people and regions of the world most likely to be affected by undernutrition and the living conditions of people and regions of the world most likely to be affected by overnutrition.

2. The percentage of the U.S. corn crop that is used to make ethanol biofuel has increased over the past decade. How might this impact food insecurity in the United States and around the world?

3. Discuss which food assistance programs listed in Table 14.1 would benefit homeless people and which would not.

4. Keep a record of how much money you spend on food in a day and use this information to estimate your monthly food costs. Would you be able to meet the recommendations of MyPyramid on a budget of $3 a day? Which food groups contain the most expensive choices?

5. Compare the cost of a single-serving bottle of orange juice with the same size serving poured from a half-gallon container. Compare the cost of these two products from a large super-market and from a small corner convenience store. Explain why someone might be forced to pay the higher prices for orange juice.

6. The diet in a developing country is deficient in iodine. To solve the problem, the government imports iodized salt, but iodine deficiency continues to be a problem. Why might this be the case?

7. Research one area of the world where hunger and undernutrition are a major problem. What is the cause of undernutrition in this area? What solutions are in place or proposed to solve these problems?

What is happening in this picture ?

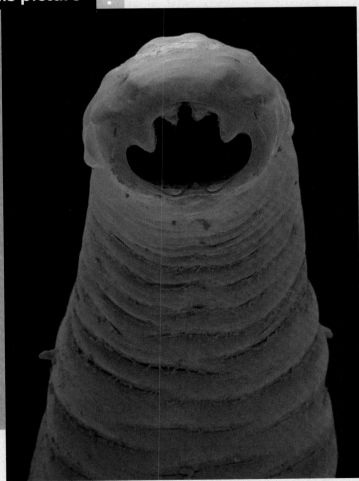

This 250 fold magnification shows the mouth of a hookworm, which it uses to attach to the lining of the small intestine and feed on blood. Hookworm larvae penetrate the skin, infecting people when they walk barefoot in contaminated soil. Hookworm infection affects 740 million people in tropical developing countries.[55]

Why do you think the infection is more common in poor tropical and subtropical regions than elsewhere?

How does hookworm infection affect iron status?

How would hookworm infection affect a population's productivity?

(Check your answers in Appendix L.)

1. The cycle of malnutrition can be broken by _____.

    a. better health care for children
    b. increasing the availability of nutritious foods for adults
    c. better health care and nutrition for women during pregnancy
    d. any of the above

2. Which of the following statements about overweight and underweight is not supported by the graph?

    a. Underweight is less of a problem in developed than in developing countries.
    b. Overweight occurs in developing as well as developed countries.
    c. In developed countries underweight is only a problem among children.
    d. As a country develops economically the incidence of overweight increases.

3. Which of the following statements is true of stunting?

    a. It is an indicator of the health and well-being of populations of children.
    b. It is an indicator of the health and well-being of adults.
    c. It is measured with body mass index.
    d. It is highest in well-nourished populations.

4. Which of the following dietary changes is not associated with nutrition transition?

    a. consumption of a wider variety of foods
    b. an increase in the fat and sugar content of the diet
    c. an increase in the consumption of animal products
    d. an increase in the fiber content of the diet

5. What proportion of the world's undernourished people live in the developing world?

    a. half
    b. one third
    c. over 90%
    d. less than a quarter

6. The yellow section of this graph of population growth most likely represents population growth in _____.

    a. developed countries
    b. the entire world
    c. less-developed countries
    d. North America

7. Which of the following statements is true of population growth?

   a. Population growth parallels economic growth.
   b. Education and economic growth slow population growth.
   c. Education increases population growth.
   d. Economic growth and education do not affect population growth.

8. Deficiencies of which three micronutrients are major world health problems?

   a. vitamins A, K, and D
   b. iodine, vitamin A, and iron
   c. iodine, iron, and chromium
   d. iron, biotin, and vitamin E

9. Crops that are grown and consumed locally are _____.

   a. sustainable crops
   b. cash crops
   c. subsistence crops
   d. renewable crops

10. Which product is not made from a renewable resource?

    a. paper towels
    b. plastic bags
    c. bread
    d. wooden crates

11. Fortifying _____ will be most likely to eliminate a nutrient deficiency in a country's population.

    a. commonly eaten foods
    b. locally grown foods
    c. foods eaten seasonally
    d. expensive foods

12. Which of the following statements is not supported by the information in the pie chart?

    a. In 4.1% of households, food intake was reduced at times during the year.
    b. Food insecurity is highest among women and children.
    c. Food insecurity is a problem for more than 10% of U.S. households.
    d. Most U.S. households are food secure.

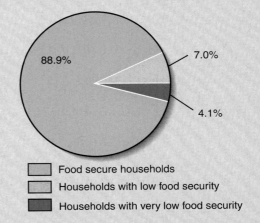

88.9%   7.0%   4.1%

▢ Food secure households
▢ Households with low food security
▢ Households with very low food security

13. Which group in the U.S. population is at risk for undernutrition?

    a. homeless people
    b. children
    c. women
    d. all of the above

14. What is the largest federal program designed to make sure that all Americans have access to an adequate diet?

    a. Special Supplemental Nutrition Program for Women, Infants, and Children (WIC)
    b. National School Lunch Program
    c. National School Breakfast Program
    d. Supplemental Nutrition Assistance Program (SNAP)

15. Which of the following statements about breast feeding is true?

    a. It decreases risk of malnutrition in infants.
    b. It is important only for the first 6 months of life.
    c. It is not recommended in poor countries.
    d. Is never recommended for women who are HIV positive.

Appendices

Appendix A
Additional DRI Tables

DRI tables for Vitamins and for Minerals are on the front and back covers of this text.

Acceptable Macronutrient Distribution Ranges (AMDR) for Healthy Diets as a Percent of Energy

Age	Carbohydrate	Added Sugars	Total Fat	Linoleic Acid	α- Linoleic Acid	Protein
1–3 y	45–65	≤25	30–40	5–10	0.6–1.2	5–20
4–18 y	45–65	≤25	25–35	5–10	0.6–1.2	10–30
≥19 y	45–65	≤25	20–35	5–10	0.6–1.2	10–35

Source: Institute of Medicine, Food and Nutrition Board. "Dietary Reference Intakes for Energy, Carbohydrates, Fiber, Fat, Protein, and Amino Acids." Washington, D.C.: National Academies Press, 2002.

Dietary Reference Intakes: Recommended Intakes for Individuals: Carbohydrates, Fiber, Fat, Fatty Acids, Protein, and Water

Life Stage Group	Carbohydrate (g/day)	Fiber (g/day)	Fat (g/day)	Linoleic Acid (g/day)	α-Linoleic Acid (g/day)	Protein (g/kg/day)	Protein (g/day)	Water (liters)
Infants								
0–6 mo	60*	ND	31*	4.4*†	0.5*‡	1.52*	9.1*	0.7*
7–12 mo	95*	ND	30*	4.6*†	0.5*‡	1.5	13.5	0.8*
Children								
1–3 y	130	19*	ND	7*	0.7*	1.10	13	1.3*
4–8 y	130	25*	ND	10*	0.9*	0.95	19	1.7*
Males								
9–13 y	130	31*	ND	12*	1.2*	0.95	34	2.4*
14–18 y	130	38*	ND	16*	1.6*	0.85	52	3.3*
19–30 y	130	38*	ND	17*	1.6*	0.80	56	3.7*
31–50 y	130	38*	ND	17*	1.6*	0.80	56	3.7*
51–70 y	130	30*	ND	14*	1.6*	0.80	56	3.7*
>70 y	130	30*	ND	14*	1.6*	0.80	56	3.7*
Females								
9–13 y	130	26*	ND	10*	1.0*	0.95	34	
14–18 y	130	26*	ND	11*	1.1*	0.85	46	2.1*
19–30 y	130	25*	ND	12*	1.1*	0.80	46	2.3*
31–50 y	130	25*	ND	12*	1.1*	0.80	46	2.7*
51–70 y	130	21*	ND	11*	1.1*	0.80	46	2.7*
>70 y	130	21*	ND	11*	1.1*	0.80	46	2.7*
Pregnancy	175	28*	ND	13*	1.4*	1.1	RDA + 25g	3.0*
Lactation	210	29*	ND	13*	1.3*	1.1	RDA + 25g	3.8*

ND = not determined. *Values are AI (Adequate Intakes), † Refers to all ω-6 polyunsaturated fatty acids, ‡Refers to all ω-3 polyunsaturated fatty acids.

Source: Institute of Medicine, Food and Nutrition Board. "Dietary Reference Intakes for Energy, Carbohydrates, Fiber, Fat, Fatty Acids, and Protein." Washington, D.C.: National Academies Press, 2002.

Dietary Reference Intake Values for Energy: Estimated Energy Requirement (EER) Equations and Values for Active Individuals by Life Stage Group

Life Stage Group	EER Prediction Equation	EER for Active Physical Activity Level (kCal\day)[a]	
		Male	Female
0–3 mo	EER = (89 × weight of infant in kg − 100) + 175	538	493 (2 mo)[c]
4–6 mo	EER = (89 × weight of infant in kg − 100) + 56	606	543 (5 mo)[c]
7–12 mo	EER = (89 × weight of infant in kg − 100) + 22	743	676 (9 mo)[c]
1–2 y	EER = (89 × weight of infant in kg − 100) + 20	1046	992 (2 y)[c]
3–8 y			
Male	EER = 88.5 − (61.9 × Age in yrs) + PA[b][(26.7 × Weight in kg) + (903 × Height in m)] + 20	1742 (6 y)[c]	
Female	EER = 135.3 − (30.8 × Age in yrs) + PA[b][(10.0 × Weight in kg) + (934 × Height in m)] + 20		1642 (6 y)[c]
9–13 y			
Male	EER = 88.5 − (61.9 × Age in yrs) + PA[b][(26.7 × Weight in kg) + (903 × Height in m)] + 25	2279 (11 y)[c]	
Female	EER = 135.3 − (30.8 × Age in yrs) + PA[b][(10.0 × Weight in kg) + (934 × Height in m)] + 25		2071 (11 y)[c]
14–18 y			
Male	EER = 88.5 − (61.9 − Age in yrs) + PA[b][(26.7 × Weight in kg) + (903 × Height in m)] + 25	3152 (16 y)[c]	
Female	EER = 135.3 − (30.8 × Age in yrs) + PA[b][(10.0 × Weight in kg) + (934 × Height in m)] + 25		2368 (16 y)[c]
19 and older			
Males	EER = 662 − (9.53 × Age in yrs) + PA[b][(15.91 × Weight in kg) + (539.6 × Height in m)]	3067 (19 y)[c]	
Females	EER = 354 − (6.91 × Age in yrs) + PA[b][(9.36 × Weight in kg) + (726 × Height in m)]		2403 (19 y)[c]
Pregnancy			
14–18 y			
1st trimester	Adolescent EER + 0		2368 (16 y)[c]
2nd trimester	Adolescent EER + 340 Cal		2708 (16 y)[c]
3rd trimester	Adolescent EER + 452 Cal		2820 (16 y)[c]
19–50 y			
1st trimester	Adult EER + 0		2403 (19 y)[c]
2nd trimester	Adult EER + 340 Cal		2743 (19 y)[c]
3rd trimester	Adult EER + 452 Cal		2855 (19 y)[c]
Lactation			
14–18 y			
1st 6 mo	Adolescent EER + 330 Cal		2698 (16 y)[c]
2nd 6 mo	Adolescent EER + 400 Cal		2768 (16 y)[c]
19–50 y			
1st 6 mo	Adult EER + 330 Cal		2733 (19 y)[c]
2nd 6 mo	Adult EER + 400 Cal		2803 (19 y)[c]

[a] The intake that meets the average energy expenditure of active individuals at a reference height, weight, and age.

[b] See table entitle "Physical Activity Coefficients (PA Values) for Use in EER Equations" to determine the PA value for various ages, genders, and activity levels.

[c] Value is calculated for an individual at the age in parentheses.

Physical Activity Coefficients (PA Values) for Use in EER Equations

Age and Gender	Sedentary	Low Active	Active	Very Active
3 to 18 y				
Boys	1.00	1.13	1.26	1.42
Girls	1.00	1.16	1.31	1.56
≥19 y				
Men	1.00	1.11	1.25	1.48
Women	1.00	1.12	1.27	1.45

Source: Institute of Medicine, Food and Nutrition Board."Dietary Reference Intakes for Energy, Carbohydrates, Fiber, Fat, Protein, and Amino Acids." Washington, D.C.: National Academies Press, 2002.

Dietary Reference Intakes: Tolerable Upper Intake Levels (UL[a]): Vitamins

Life Stage Group	Vitamin A (µg/day)[b]	Vitamin C (mg/day)	Vitamin D (µg/day)	Vitamin E (mg/day)[c,d]	Vitamin K	Thiamin	Riboflavin	Niacin (mg/day)[d]	Vitamin B6 (mg/day)	Folate (µg/day)[d]	Vitamin B12	Pantothenic Acid	Biotin	Choline (mg/day)	Carotenoids[e]
Infants															
0–6 mo	600	ND[f]	25	ND	ND	ND	ND	ND	ND	ND	ND	ND	ND	ND	ND
7–12 mo	600	ND	25	ND	ND	ND	ND	ND	ND	ND	ND	ND	ND	ND	ND
Children															
1–3 y	600	400	50	200	ND	ND	ND	10	30	300	ND	ND	ND	1.0	ND
4–8 y	900	650	50	300	ND	ND	ND	15	40	400	ND	ND	ND	1.0	ND
Males, Females															
9–13 y	1,700	1,200	50	600	ND	ND	ND	20	60	600	ND	ND	ND	2.0	ND
14–18 y	2,800	1,800	50	800	ND	ND	ND	30	80	800	ND	ND	ND	3.0	ND
19–70 y	3,000	2,000	50	1,000	ND	ND	ND	35	100	1,000	ND	ND	ND	3.5	ND
>70 y	3,000	2,000	50	1,000	ND	ND	ND	35	100	1,000	ND	ND	ND	3.5	ND
Pregnancy															
≤18 y	2,800	1,800	50	800	ND	ND	ND	30	80	800	ND	ND	ND	3.0	ND
19–50 y	3,000	2,000	50	1,000	ND	ND	ND	35	100	1,000	ND	ND	ND	3.5	ND
Lactation															
≤18 y	2,800	1,800	50	800	ND	ND	ND	30	80	800	ND	ND	ND	3.0	ND
19–50 y	3,000	2,000	50	1,000	ND	ND	ND	35	100	1,000	ND	ND	ND	3.5	ND

[a] UL = The maximum level of daily nutrient intake that is likely to pose no risk of adverse effects. Unless otherwise specified, the UL represents total intake from food, water, and supplements. Due to lack of suitable data, ULs could not be established for vitamin K, thiamin, riboflavin, vitamin B12, pantothenic acid, biotin, or carotenoids. In the absence of ULs, extra caution may be warranted in consuming levels above recommended intakes.

[b] As preformed vitamin A only.

[c] As α-tocopherol; applies to any form of supplemental α-tocopherol.

[d] The ULs for vitamin E, niacin, and folate apply to synthetic forms obtained from supplements, fortified foods, or a combination of the two.

[e] β-Carotene supplements are advised only to serve as a provitamin A source for individuals at risk of vitamin A deficiency.

[f] ND = Not determinable due to lack of data of adverse effects in this age group and concern with regard to lack of ability to handle excess amounts. Source of intakes should be from food only to prevent high levels of intake.

Source: Dietary Reference Intake Tables: The Complete Set. Institute of Medicine, National Academy of Sciences. Available online at www.nap.edu. Reprinted with permission from *Dietary Reference Intakes: The Essential Guide to Nutrient Requirements*, 2006, by the National Academy of Sciences, Washington, D.C.

Dietary Reference Intakes: Tolerable Upper Intake Levels (UL^a): Minerals

Life Stage Group	Arsenic^b (mg/day)	Boron (mg/day)	Calcium (g/day)	Chromium	Copper (µg/day)	Fluoride (mg/day)	Iodine (µg/day)	Iron (mg/day)	Magnesium^c (mg/day)	Manganese (mg/day)	Molybdenum (µg/day)	Nickel (mg/day)	Phosphorus (g/day)	Selenium (µg/day)	Silicon^d	Vanadium^e (mg/day)	Zinc (mg/day)	Sodium (g/day)	Chloride (g/day)	Potassium
Infants																				
0–6 mo	ND^f	ND	ND	ND	ND	0.7	ND	40	ND	ND	ND	ND	ND	45	ND	ND	4	ND	ND	ND
7–12 mo	ND	ND	ND	ND	ND	0.9	ND	40	ND	ND	ND	ND	ND	60	ND	ND	5	ND	ND	ND
Children																				
1–3 y	ND	3	2.5	ND	1,000	1.3	200	40	65	2	300	0.2	3	90	ND	ND	7	1.5	2.3	ND
4–8 y	ND	6	2.5	ND	3,000	2.2	300	40	110	3	600	0.3	3	150	ND	ND	12	1.9	2.9	ND
Males, Females																				
9–13 y	ND	11	2.5	ND	5,000	10	600	40	350	6	1,100	0.6	4	280	ND	ND	23	2.2	3.4	ND
14–18 y	ND	17	2.5	ND	8,000	10	900	45	350	9	1,700	1.0	4	400	ND	ND	34	2.3	3.6	ND
19–70 y	ND	20	2.5	ND	10,000	10	1,100	45	350	11	2,000	1.0	4	400	ND	1.8	40	2.3	3.6	ND
>70 y	ND	20	2.5	ND	10,000	10	1,100	45	350	11	2,000	1.0	3	400	ND	1.8	40	2.3	3.6	ND
Pregnancy																				
≤18 y	ND	17	2.5	ND	8,000	10	900	45	350	9	1,700	1.0	3.5	400	ND	ND	34	2.3	3.6	ND
19–50 y	ND	20	2.5	ND	10,000	10	1,100	45	350	11	2,000	1.0	3.5	400	ND	ND	40	2.3	3.6	ND
Lactation																				
≤18 y	ND	17	2.5	ND	8,000	10	900	45	350	9	1,700	1.0	4	400	ND	ND	34	2.3	3.6	ND
19–50 y	ND	20	2.5	ND	10,000	10	1,100	45	350	11	2,000	1.0	4	400	ND	ND	40	2.3	3.6	ND

^aUL = the maximum level of daily nutrient intake that is likely to pose no risk of adverse effects. Unless otherwise specified, the UL represents total intake from food, water, and supplements. Due to lack of suitable data, ULs could not be established for arsenic, chromium, silicon, and potassium. In the absence of ULs, extra caution may be warranted in consuming levels above recommended intakes.

^bAlthough the UL was not determined for arsenic, there is no justification for adding arsenic to food or supplements.

^cThe ULs for magnesium represent intake from a pharmacological agent only and do not include intake from food and water.

^dAlthough silicon has not been n shown to cause adverse effects in humans, there is no justification for adding silicon to supplements.

^eAlthough vanadium in food has not been shown to cause adverse effects in humans, there is no justification for adding vanadium to food and vanadium supplements should be used with caution. The UL is based on adverse effects in laboratory animals and this data could be used to set a UL for adults but not children and adolescents.

^fND = Not determinable due to lack of data of adverse effects in this age group and concern with regard to lack of ability to handle excess amounts. Source of intake should be from food only to prevent high levels of intake.

Source: Dietary Reference Intake Tables: The Complete Set. Institute of Medicine, National Academy of Sciences. Available online at www.nap.edu. Reprinted with permission from *Dietary Reference Intakes: The Essential Guide to Nutrient Requirements,* 2006, by the National Academy of Sciences, Washington, D.C.

Dietary Reference Intake Values for Energy: Total Energy Expenditure (TEE) Equations for Overweight and Obese Individuals

Life Stage Group	TEE Prediction Equation (Cal/day)	PA Values
Overweight boys aged 3–18 years	$TEE = 114 - (50.9 \times \text{age in yrs}) + PA[(19.5 \times \text{weight in kg}) + (1161.4 \times \text{height in m})]$	Sedentary = 1.00 Low active = 1.12 Active = 1.24 Very active = 1.45
Overweight girls aged 3–18 years	$TEE = 389 - (41.2 \times \text{age in yrs}) + PA[(15.0 \times \text{weight in kg}) + (701.6 \times \text{height in m})]$	Sedentary = 1.00 Low active = 1.18 Active = 1.35 Very active = 1.60
Overweight and obese men aged 19 years and older	$TEE = 1086 - (10.1 \times \text{age in yrs}) + PA[(13.7 \times \text{weight in kg}) + (416 \times \text{height in m})]$	Sedentary = 1.00 Low active = 1.12 Active = 1.29 Very active = 1.59
Overweight and obese women aged 19 years and older	$TEE = 448 - (7.95 \times \text{age in yrs}) + PA[(11.4 \times \text{weight in kg}) + (619 \times \text{height in m})]$	Sedentary = 1.00 Low active = 1.16 Active = 1.27 Very active = 1.44

Source: Institute of Medicine, Food and Nutrition Board "Dietary Reference Intakes for Energy, Carbohydrates, Fiber, Fat, Protein and Amino Acids," Washington, DC: National Academy Press, 2002.

Appendix B
Standards for Body Size

Body Mass Index (BMI) and Associated Risk

Body mass index (BMI) is the measurement of choice for determining health risks associated with body weight. To use the table, find the appropriate height in the left-hand column. Move across the row to the given weight. The number at the top of the column is the BMI for that height and weight. Use the table above to determine the risks associated with BMI and waist circumference.

BMI (kg/m²)	19	20	21	22	23	24	25	26	27	28	29	30	35	40
Height (in.)	Weight (lb.)													
58	91	96	100	105	110	115	119	124	129	134	138	143	167	191
59	94	99	104	109	114	119	124	128	133	138	143	148	173	198
60	97	102	107	112	118	123	128	133	138	143	148	153	179	204
61	100	106	111	116	122	127	132	137	143	148	153	158	185	211
62	104	109	115	120	126	131	136	142	147	153	158	164	191	218
63	107	113	118	124	130	135	141	146	152	158	163	169	197	225
64	110	116	122	128	134	140	145	151	157	163	169	174	204	232
65	114	120	126	132	138	144	150	156	162	168	174	180	210	240
66	118	124	130	136	142	148	155	161	167	173	179	186	216	247
67	121	127	134	140	146	153	159	166	172	178	185	191	223	255
68	125	131	138	144	151	158	164	171	177	184	190	197	230	262
69	128	135	142	149	155	162	169	176	182	189	196	203	236	270
70	132	139	146	153	160	167	174	181	188	195	202	207	243	278
71	136	143	150	157	165	172	179	186	193	200	208	215	250	286
72	140	147	154	162	169	177	184	191	199	206	213	221	258	294
73	144	151	159	166	174	182	189	197	204	212	219	227	265	302
74	148	155	163	171	179	186	194	202	210	218	225	233	272	311
75	152	160	168	176	184	192	200	208	216	224	232	240	279	319
76	156	164	172	180	189	197	205	213	221	230	238	246	287	328

BMI (kg/m²)		Waist less than or equal to 40 in. (men) or 35 in. (women)	Waist greater than 40 in. (men) or 35 in. (women)
18.5 or less	Underweight	—	N/A
18.5–24.9	Normal	—	N/A
25.0–29.9	Overweight	Increased	High
30.0–34.9	Obese	High	Very High
35.0–39.9	Obese	Very High	Very High
40 or greater	Extremely Obese	Extremely High	Extremely High

Source: Adapted from Partnership for Healthy Weight Management http://www.consumer.gov/weightloss/bmi.htm

Birth to 36 months: Girls
Length-for-age and Weight-for-age percentiles

Published May 30, 2000 (modified 4/20/01).

Source: Developed by the National Center for Health Statistics in collaboration with the National Center for Chronic Disease Prevention and Health Promotion (2000). www.cdc.gov/growthcharts

SAFER · HEALTHIER · PEOPLE™

Published May 30, 2000 (modified 4/20/01).

Source: Developed by the National Center for Health Statistics in collaboration with the National Center for Chronic Disease Prevention and Health Promotion (2000). www.cdc.gov/growthcharts

SAFER · HEALTHIER · PEOPLE™

2 to 20 years: Girls
Body mass index-for-age percentiles

NAME _____

RECORD # _____

Date	Age	Weight	Stature	BMI*	Comments

*To Calculate BMI: Weight (kg) ÷ Stature (cm) ÷ Stature (cm) x 10,000
or Weight (lb) ÷ Stature (in) ÷ Stature (in) x 703

BMI

AGE (YEARS)

kg/m²

Published May 30, 2000 (modified 10/16/00).

Source: Developed by the National Center for Health Statistics in collaboration with the National
Center for Chronic Disease Prevention and Health Promotion (2000). www.cdc.gov/growthcharts

CDC

SAFER · HEALTHIER · PEOPLE™

509

2 to 20 years: Boys
Body mass index-for-age percentiles

Date	Age	Weight	Stature	BMI*	Comments

*To Calculate BMI: Weight (kg) ÷ Stature (cm) ÷ Stature (cm) x 10,000
or Weight (lb) ÷ Stature (in) ÷ Stature (in) x 703

AGE (YEARS)

Published May 30, 2000 (modified 10/16/00).

Source: Developed by the National Center for Health Statistics in collaboration with the National Center for Chronic Disease Prevention and Health Promotion (2000). www.cdc.gov/growthcharts

CDC
SAFER · HEALTHIER · PEOPLE™

Appendix C
Normal Blood Values of Nutritional Relevance

Red blood cells	
Men	4.6–6.2 million/mm^3
Women	4.2–5.2 million/mm^3
White blood cells	5,000–10,000/mm^3
Hematocrit	
Men	40–54 ml/100 ml
Women	36–47 ml/100 ml
Children	35–49 ml/100 ml
Hemoglobin	
Men	14–18 g/100 ml
Women	12–16 g/100 ml
Children	11.2–16.5 g/100 ml
Ferritin	
Men	20–300 ng/ml
Women	20–120 ng/ml
Calcium	9–11 mg/100 ml
Iodine	3.8–8 µg/100 ml
Iron	
Men	75–175 µg/100 ml
Women	65–165 µg/100 ml
Zinc	0.75–1.4 µg/ml
Magnesium	1.8–3.0 mg/100 ml
Potassium	3.5–5.0 mEq/liter
Sodium	136–145 mEq/liter
Chloride	100–108 mEq/liter
Vitamin A	20–80 µg/100 ml
Vitamin B$_{12}$	200–800 pg/100 ml
Vitamin C	0.6–2.0 mg/100 ml
Carotene	48–200 µg/liter
Folate	2–20 ng/ml
pH	7.35–7.45
Total protein	6.6–8.0 g/100 ml
Albumin	3.0–4.0 g/100 ml
Cholesterol	<200 mg/100 ml
Glucose	60–100 mg/100 ml blood, 70–120 mg/100 ml serum

Source: Handbook of Clinical Dietetics, American Dietetic Association, © 1981 by Yale University Press (New Haven, Conn.); and Committee on Dietetics of the Mayo Clinic, *Mayo Clinic Diet Manual* (Philadelphia: W. B. Saunders Company, 1981), pp. 275–277.

Guidelines for Determining Healthy Lipid Levels

Classification of LDL, Total, and HDL Cholesterol and Triglycerides (mg/dL)

LDL Cholesterol

<100	Optimal*
100–129	Near optimal/above optimal
130–159	Borderline high
160–189	High
≥190	Very high

Total Cholesterol

<200	Desirable
200–239	Borderline high
≥240	High

HDL Cholesterol

<40	Increases risk
≥60	Decreases risk

Triglycerides

<150	Normal
150–190	Borderline high
200–499	High
≥500	Very high

*For very high-risk people, LDL cholesterol should be <70.

Source: National Cholesterol Education Program, ATP III, Quick Reference Guide, 2004 update. Available online at http://www.nhlbi.nih.gov/fuidelines/cholesterol/atglance.pdf

High Blood Pressure (Hypertension) Guidelines

Classification

High	140/90 or above
Prehypertension	120–139 / 80–90
Normal	119/79 or below

Source: Joint National Committee on Prevention, Detection, Evaluation, and Treatment of High Blood Pressure (2003). *The seventh report of the Joint National Committee on Prevention, Detection, Evaluation, and Treatment of High Blood Pressure.* NIH Publication No. 03-5233. Bethesda, MD: U.S. Department of Health and Human Services.

Appendix D
U.S. Nutrition Recommendations and Guidelines

Dietary Guidelines for Americans, 2005

Key Recommendations of the 2005 Dietary Guidelines for Americans

ADEQUATE NUTRIENTS WITHIN CALORIE NEEDS

Key Recommendations

- Consume a variety of nutrient-dense foods and beverages within and among the basic food groups while choosing foods that limit the intake of saturated and *trans* fats, cholesterol, added sugars, salt, and alcohol.
- Meet recommended intakes within energy needs by adopting a balanced eating pattern, such as the USDA Food Guide or the DASH Eating Plan.

Key Recommendations for Specific Population Groups

- **People over age 50:** Consume vitamin B_{12} in its crystalline form (i.e., fortified foods or supplements).
- **Women of childbearing age who may become pregnant:** Eat foods high in heme-iron and/or consume iron-rich plant foods or iron-fortified foods with an enhancer of iron absorption, such as vitamin C-rich foods.
- **Women of childbearing age who may become pregnant and those in the first trimester of pregnancy:** Consume adequate synthetic folic acid daily (from fortified foods or supplements) in addition to food forms of folate from a varied diet.
- **Older adults, people with dark skin, and people exposed to insufficient ultraviolet band radiation (i.e., sunlight):** Consume extra vitamin D from vitamin D-fortified foods and/or supplements.

WEIGHT MANAGEMENT

Key Recommendations

- To maintain body weight in a healthy range, balance calories from foods and beverages with calories expended.
- To prevent gradual weight gain over time, make small decreases in food and beverage calories and increase physical activity.

Key Recommendations for Specific Population Groups

- **Those who need to lose weight:** Aim for a slow, steady weight loss by decreasing calorie intake while maintaining an adequate nutrient intake and increasing physical activity.
- **Overweight children:** Reduce the rate of body weight gain while allowing growth and development. Consult a healthcare provider before placing a child on a weight-reduction diet.
- **Pregnant women:** Ensure appropriate weight gain as specified by a healthcare provider.
- **Breastfeeding women:** Moderate weight reduction is safe and does not compromise weight gain of the nursing infant.
- **Overweight adults and overweight children with chronic diseases and/or on medication:** Consult a healthcare provider about weight loss strategies prior to starting a weight-reduction program to ensure appropriate management of other health conditions.

(continued)

PHYSICAL ACTIVITY

Key Recommendations

- Engage in regular physical activity and reduce sedentary activities to promote health, psychological well-being, and a healthy body weight.
  - To reduce the risk of chronic disease in adulthood engage in at least 30 minutes of moderate-intensity physical activity, above usual activity, at work or home on most days of the week.
  - For most people, greater health benefits can be obtained by engaging in physical activity of more vigorous intensity or longer duration.
  - To help manage body weight and prevent gradual, unhealthy body weight gain in adulthood engage in approximately 60 minutes of moderate- to vigorous-intensity activity on most days of the week while not exceeding caloric intake requirements.
  - To sustain weight loss in adulthood participate in at least 60 to 90 minutes of daily moderate-intensity physical activity while not exceeding caloric intake requirements. Some people may need to consult with a healthcare provider before participating in this level of activity.
- Achieve physical fitness by including cardiovascular conditioning, stretching exercises for flexibility, and resistance exercises or calisthenics for muscle strength and endurance.

Key Recommendations for Specific Population Groups

- **Children and adolescents:** Engage in at least 60 minutes of physical activity on most, preferably all, days of the week.
- **Pregnant women:** In the absence of medical or obstetric complications, incorporate 30 minutes or more of moderate-intensity physical activity on most, if not all, days of the week. Avoid activities with a high risk of falling or abdominal trauma.
- **Breastfeeding women:** Be aware that neither acute nor regular exercise adversely affects the mother's ability to breastfeed successfully.
- **Older adults:** Participate in regular physical activity to reduce functional declines associated with aging and to achieve the other benefits of physical activity identified for all adults.

FOOD GROUPS TO ENCOURAGE

Key Recommendations

- Consume a sufficient amount of fruits and vegetables while staying within energy needs. Two cups of fruit and 2½ cups of vegetables per day are recommended for a reference 2,000-Calorie intake, with higher or lower amounts depending on the calorie level.
- Choose a variety of fruits and vegetables each day. In particular, select from all five vegetable subgroups (dark green, orange, legumes, starchy vegetables, and other vegetables) several times a week.
- Consume 3 or more ounce-equivalents of whole-grain products per day, with the rest of the recommended grains coming from enriched or whole-grain products. In general, at least half the grains should come from whole grains.
- Consume 3 cups per day of fat-free or low-fat milk or equivalent milk products.

Key Recommendations for Specific Population Groups

- **Children and adolescents:** Consume whole-grain products often; at least half the grains should be whole grains. Children 2 to 8 years should consume 2 cups per day of fat-free or low-fat milk or equivalent milk products. Children 9 years of age and older should consume 3 cups per day of fat-free or low-fat milk or equivalent milk products.

FATS

Key Recommendations

- Consume less than 10 percent of calories from saturated fatty acids and less than 300 mg/day of cholesterol, and keep *trans* fatty acid consumption as low as possible.

(continued)

- Keep total fat intake between 20 to 35 percent of calories, with most fats coming from sources of polyunsaturated and monounsaturated fatty acids, such as fish, nuts, and vegetable oils.

- When selecting and preparing meat, poultry, dry beans, and milk or milk products, make choices that are lean, low-fat, or fat-free.

- Limit intake of fats and oils high in saturated and/or *trans* fatty acids, and choose products low in such fats and oils.

Key Recommendations for Specific Population Groups

- **Children and adolescents:** Keep total fat intake between 30 to 35 percent of calories for children 2 to 3 years of age and between 25 to 35 percent of calories for children and adolescents 4 to 18 years of age, with most fats coming from sources of polyunsaturated and monounsaturated fatty acids, such as fish, nuts, and vegetable oils.

CARBOHYDRATES

Key Recommendations

- Choose fiber-rich fruits, vegetables, and whole grains often.

- Choose and prepare foods and beverages with little added sugars or caloric sweeteners, such as amounts suggested by the USDA Food Guide and the DASH Eating Plan.

- Reduce the incidence of dental caries by practicing good oral hygiene and consuming sugar- and starch-containing foods and beverages less frequently.

SODIUM AND POTASSIUM

Key Recommendations

- Consume less than 2,300 mg (approximately 1 tsp of salt) of sodium per day.

- Choose and prepare foods with little salt. At the same time, consume potassium-rich foods, such as fruits and vegetables.

Key Recommendations for Specific Population Groups

- **Individuals with hypertension, blacks, and middle-aged and older adults:** Aim to consume no more than 1,500 mg of sodium per day, and meet the potassium recommendation (4,700 mg/day) with food.

ALCOHOLIC BEVERAGES

Key Recommendations

- Those who choose to drink alcoholic beverages should do so sensibly and in moderation—defined as the consumption of up to one drink per day for women and up to two drinks per day for men.

- Alcoholic beverages should not be consumed by some individuals, including those who cannot restrict their alcohol intake, women of childbearing age who may become pregnant, pregnant and lactating women, children and adolescents, individuals taking medications that can interact with alcohol, and those with specific medical conditions.

- Alcoholic beverages should be avoided by individuals engaging in activities that require attention, skill, or coordination, such as driving or operating machinery.

FOOD SAFETY

Key Recommendations

- To avoid microbial foodborne illness:
  - Clean hands, food contact surfaces, and fruits and vegetables. Meat and poultry should not be washed or rinsed.
  - Separate raw, cooked, and ready-to-eat foods while shopping, preparing, or storing foods.
  - Cook foods to a safe temperature to kill microorganisms.
  - Chill (refrigerate) perishable food promptly and defrost foods properly.
  - Avoid raw (unpasteurized) milk or any products made from unpasteurized milk, raw or partially cooked eggs or foods containing raw eggs, raw or undercooked meat and poultry, unpasteurized juices, and raw sprouts.

(continued)

Key Recommendations of the 2005 Dietary Guidelines for Americans (continued)

Key Recommendations for Specific Population Groups

- **Infants and young children, pregnant women, older adults, and those who are immunocompromised:** Do not eat or drink raw (unpasteurized) milk or any products made from unpasteurized milk, raw or partially cooked eggs or foods containing raw eggs, raw or undercooked meat and poultry, raw or undercooked fish or shellfish, unpasteurized juices, and raw sprouts.

- **Pregnant women, older adults, and those who are immunocompromised:** Only eat certain deli meats and frankfurters that have been reheated to steaming hot.

Source: Dietary Guidelines for Americans. Available on line at http://www.health.gov/dietaryguidelines/dga2005/document/html/executivesummary.htm

American Institute for Cancer Research Recommendations for Cancer Prevention

Ten recommendations for cancer prevention

1. Be as lean as possible without becoming underweight.
2. Be physically active for at least 30 minutes every day.
3. Avoid sugary drinks. Limit consumption of energy-dense foods (particularly processed foods high in added sugar, or low in fiber, or high in fat).
4. Eat more of a variety of vegetables, fruits, whole grains and legumes such as beans.
5. Limit consumption of red meats (such as beef, pork and lamb) and avoid processed meats.
6. If consumed at all, limit alcoholic drinks to 2 for men and 1 for women a day.
7. Limit consumption of salty foods and foods processed with salt (sodium).
8. Don't use supplements to protect against cancer.

Special Population Recommendations

9. It is best for mothers to breastfeed exclusively for up to 6 months and then add other liquids and foods.
10. After treatment, cancer survivors should follow the recommendations for cancer prevention.

And always remember—do not smoke or chew tobacco.

Source: American Institute of Cancer Research. Available online at http://www.aicr.org/site/PageServer?pagename=dc_home_guides. Reprinted with permission from the American Institute for Cancer Research.

Dietary Approaches to Stop Hypertension: DASH Diet Recommendations

Type of food	Daily servings for 1600–3100 Calorie diets	Daily servings for a 2000 Calorie diet
Grains and grain products (include at least 3 whole grain foods each day)	6–12	7–8
Fruits	4–6	4–5
Vegetables	4–6	4–5
Low fat or non fat dairy foods	2–4	2–3
Lean meats, fish, poultry	1.5–2.5	2 or less
Nuts, seeds, and legumes	3–6 per week	4–5 per week
Fats and sweets	2–4	limited

Source: The DASH Diet Eating Plan. Available online at http://dashdiet.org/

Nutrition and Physical Fitness Recommendations from the American Cancer Society

Maintain a healthy weight throughout life.
- Balance calorie intake with physical activity.
- Avoid excessive weight gain throughout life.
- Achieve and maintain a healthy weight if currently overweight or obese.

Adopt a physically active lifestyle.
- **Adults:** Engage in at least 30 minutes of moderate to vigorous physical activity, above usual activities, on 5 or more days of the week; 45 to 60 minutes of intentional physical activity are preferable.
- **Children and adolescents:** Engage in at least 60 minutes per day of moderate to vigorous physical activity at least 5 days per week.

Eat a healthy diet, with an emphasis on plant sources.
- Choose foods and drinks in amounts that help achieve and maintain a healthy weight.
- Eat 5 or more servings of a variety of vegetables and fruits every day.
- Choose whole grains over processed (refined) grains.
- Limit intake of processed and red meats.

If you drink alcoholic beverages, limit your intake.
- Drink no more than 1 drink per day for women or 2 per day for men.

Source: Some adapted from Complete Guide—Nutrition and Physical Activity for Cancer Prevention. Available online at http://www.cancer.org/docroot/PED/content/PED_3_2X_Diet_and_Activity_Factors_That_Affect_Risks.asp?sitearea=PED. Reprinted by the permission of the American Cancer Society, Inc. All rights reserved.

Healthy People 2010

Goals
1. Increase quality and years of healthy life.
2. Eliminate health disparities.

Leading Health Indicators
1. Physical activity
2. Overweight and obesity
3. Tobacco use
4. Substance abuse
5. Responsible sexual behavior
6. Mental health
7. Injury and violence
8. Environmental quality
9. Immunization
10. Access to health care

Focus Areas

Access to quality health services	*Injury and violence prevention*
Arthritis, osteoporosis, and chronic back conditions	*Maternal, infant, and child health*
Cancer	*Medical product safety*
Chronic kidney disease	*Mental health and mental disorders*
Diabetes	*Nutrition and overweight*
Disability and secondary conditions	*Occupational safety and health*
Educational and community-based programs	*Oral health*
Environmental health	*Physical activity and fitness*
Family planning	*Public health infrastructure*
Food safety	*Respiratory diseases*
Health communication	*Sexually transmitted diseases*
Heart disease and stroke	*Substance abuse*
HIV	*Tobacco use*
Immunization and infectious diseases	*Vision and hearing*

Source: Healthy People 2010. Available online at www.health.gov/healthy people.

Appendix E
Exchange Lists

Starch

Bread	
Food	*Serving Size*
Bagel, large (about 4 oz)	¼ (1 oz)
⚠ Biscuit, 2½ inches across	1
Bread	
☺ reduced-calorie	2 slices (1½ oz)
white, whole-grain, pumpernickel, rye, unfrosted raisin	1 slice (1 oz)
Chapatti, small, 6 inches across	1
⚠ Cornbread, 1¾ inch cube	1 (1½ oz)
English muffin	½
Hot dog bun or hamburger bun	½ (1 oz)
Naan, 8 inches by 2 inches	¼
Pancake, 4 inches across, ¼ inch thick	1
Pita, 6 inches across	½
Roll, plain, small	1 (1 oz)
⚠ Stuffing bread	⅓ cup
⚠ Taco shell, 5 inches across	2
Tortilla, corn, 6 inches across	1
Tortilla, corn, 6 inches across	1
Tortilla, flour, 10 inches across	⅓ tortilla
⚠ Waffle, 4-inch square or 4 inches across	1

☺ = More than 3 grams of dietary fiber per serving.

⚠ = Extra fat, or prepared with added fat. (Count as 1 starch + 1 fat.)

ⓢ = 480 milligrams or more of sodium per serving.

The Exchange Lists are the basis of a meal planning system designed by a committee of the American Diabetes Association and The American Dietetic Association. While designed primarily for people with diabetes and others who must follow special diets, the Exchange Lists are based on principles of good nutrition that apply to everyone. Copyright © 2008 by the American Diabetes Association and The American Dietetic Association.

Cereals and Grains

Food	Serving Size
Barley, cooked	⅓ cup
Bran, dry	
☺ oat	¼ cup
☺ wheat	½ cup
☺ Bulgur (cooked)	½ cup
Cereals	
☺ bran	½ cup
cooked (oats, oatmeal)	½ cup
puffed	1½ cups
shredded wheat, plain	½ cup
sugar-coated	½ cup
unsweetened, ready-to-eat	¾ cup
Couscous	⅓ cup
Granola	
low-fat	¼ cup
⚠ regular	¼ cup
Grits, cooked	½ cup
Kasha	½ cup
Millet, cooked	⅓ cup
Muesli	¼ cup
Pasta, cooked	⅓ cup
Polenta, cooked	⅓ cup
Quinoa, cooked	⅓ cup
Rice, white or brown, cooked	⅓ cup
Tabbouleh (tabouli), prepared	½ cup
Wheat, germ, dry	3 Tbsp
Wild rice, cooked	½ cup

Starchy Vegetables

Food	Serving Size
Cassava	⅓ cup
Corn	½ cup
on cob, large	½ cup (5 oz)
☺ Hominy, canned	¾ cup
☺ Mixed vegetables with corn, peas, or pasta	1 cup
☺ Parsnips	½ cup
☺ Peas, green	½ cup
Plantain, ripe	⅓ cup
Potato	
baked with skin	¼ large (3 oz)
boiled, all kinds	½ cup or ½ medium (3 oz)
⚠ mashed, with milk and fat	½ cup
French fried (oven-baked)	1 cup (2 oz)
☺ Pumpkin, canned, no sugar added	1 cup
Spaghetti/pasta sauce	½ cup
☺ Squash, winter (acorn, butternut)	1 cup
☺ Succotash	½ cup
Yam, sweet potato, plain	½ cup

Crackers and Snacks

Food	Serving Size
Animal crackers	8
Crackers	
⚠ round-butter type	6
saltine-type	6
⚠ sandwich-style, cheese or peanut butter filling	3
⚠ whole-wheat regular	2–5 (¾ oz)
☺ whole-wheat lower fat or crispbreads	2–5 (¾ oz)
Graham cracker, 2½-inch square	3
Matzoh	¾ oz
Melba toast, about 2-inch by 4-inch piece	4 pieces
Oyster crackers	20
Popcorn	3 cups
⚠ ☺ with butter	3 cups
☺ no fat added	3 cups
☺ lower fat	3 cups
Pretzels	¾ oz
Rice cakes, 4 inches across	2
Snack chips	
fat-free or baked (tortilla, potato), baked pita chips	15–20 (¾ oz)
⚠ regular (tortilla, potato)	9–13 (¾ oz)

Beans, Peas, and Lentils

The choices on this list count as 1 starch + 1 lean meat.

Food	Serving Size
☺ Baked beans	⅓ cup
☺ Beans, cooked (black, garbanzo, kidney, lima, navy, pinto, white)	½ cup
☺ Lentils, cooked (brown, green, yellow)	½ cup
☺ Peas, cooked (black-eyed, split)	½ cup
ⓢ ☺ Refried beans, canned	½ cup

Fruits

Fruit	
The weight listed includes skin, core, seeds, and rind.	
Food	**Serving Size**
Apple, unpeeled, small	1 (4 oz)
Apples, dried	4 rings
Applesauce, unsweetened	½ cup
Apricots	
canned	½ cup
dried	8 halves
☺ fresh	4 whole (5½ oz)
Banana, extra small	1 (4 oz)
☺ Blackberries	¾ cup
Blueberries	¾ cup
Cantaloupe, small	⅛ melon or 1 cup cubed (11 oz)
Cherries	
sweet, canned	½ cup
sweet fresh	12 (3 oz)
Dates	3
Dried fruits (blueberries, cherries, cranberries, mixed fruit, raisins)	2 Tbsp
Figs	
dried	1½
☺ fresh	1½ large or 2 medium (3½ oz)
Fruit cocktail	½ cup
Grapefruit	
large	½ (11 oz)
sections, canned	¾ cup
Grapes, small	17 (3 oz)
Honeydew melon	1 slice or 1 cup cubed (10 oz)
☺ Kiwi	1 (3½ oz)
Mandarin oranges, canned	¾ cup
Mango, small	1/2 fruit (5½ oz) or ½ cup
Nectarine, small	1 (5 oz)
☺ Orange, small	1 (6½ oz)
Papaya	½ fruit or 1 cup cubed (8 oz)
Peaches	
canned	½ cup
fresh, medium	1 (6 oz)
Pears	
canned	½ cup
fresh, large	½ (4 oz)
Pineapple	
canned	½ cup
fresh	¾ cup
Plums	
canned	½ cup
dried (prunes)	3
small	2 (5 oz)
☺ Raspberries	1 cup
☺ Strawberries	1¼ cup whole berries
☺ Tangerines, small	2 (8 oz)
Watermelon	1 slice or 1¼ cups cubes (13½ oz)

Fruit Juice

Food	Serving Size
Apple juice/cider	½ cup
Fruit juice blends, 100% juice	⅓ cup
Grape juice	⅓ cup
Grapefruit juice	½ cup
Orange juice	½ cup
Pineapple juice	½ cup
Prune juice	⅓ cup

Milk

Milk and Yogurts

Food	Serving Size	Count as
Fat-free or low-fat (1%)		
Milk, buttermilk, acidophilus milk, Lactaid	1 cup	1 fat-free milk
Evaporated milk	½ cup	1 fat-free milk
Yogurt, plain or flavored with an artificial sweetener	⅔ cup (6 oz)	1 fat-free milk
Reduced-fat (2%)		
Milk, acidophilus milk, kefir, Lactaid	1 cup	1 reduced-fat milk
Yogurt, plain	⅔ cup (6 oz)	1 reduced-fat milk
Whole		
Milk, buttermilk, goat's milk	1 cup	1 whole milk
Evaporated milk	½ cup	1 whole milk
Yogurt, plain	8 oz	1 whole milk

Dairy-Like Foods

Food	Serving Size	Count as
Chocolate milk		
fat-free	1 cup	1 fat-free milk + 1 carbohydrate
whole	1 cup	1 whole milk + 1 carbohydrate
Eggnog, whole milk	½ cup	1 carbohydrate + 2 fats
Rice drink		
flavored, low-fat	1 cup	2 carbohydrates
plain, fat-free	1 cup	1 carbohydrate
Smoothies, flavored, regular	10 oz	1 fat-free milk + 2½ carbohydrates
Soy milk		
light	1 cup	1 carbohydrate + ½ fat
regular, plain	1 cup	1 carbohydrate + 1 fat
Yogurt		
and juice blends	1 cup	1 fat-free milk + 1 carbohydrate
low carbohydrate (less than 6 grams carbohydrate per choice)	⅔ cup (6 oz)	½ fat-free milk
with fruit, low-fat	⅔ cup (6 oz)	1 fat-free milk + 1 carbohydrate

Sweets, Desserts, and Other Carbohydrates

Beverages, Soda, and Energy/Sports Drinks

Food	Serving Size	Count as
Cranberry juice cocktail	½ cup	1 carbohydrate
Energy drink	1 can (8.3 oz)	2 carbohydrates
Fruit drink or lemonade	1 cup (8 oz)	2 carbohydrates
Hot chocolate		
regular	1 envelope added to 8 oz water	1 carbohydrate + 1 fat
sugar-free or light	1 envelope added to 8 oz water	1 carbohydrate
Soft drink (soda), regular	1 can (12 oz)	2½ carbohydrates
Sports drink	1 cup (8 oz)	1 carbohydrate

Brownies, Cake, Cookies, Gelatin, Pie, and Pudding

Food	Serving Size	Count as
Brownie, small, unfrosted	1¼-inch square, ⅞ inch high (about 1 oz)	1 carbohydrate + 1 fat
Cake		
angel food, unfrosted	1/12 of cake (about 2 oz)	2 carbohydrates
frosted	2-inch square (about 2 oz)	2 carbohydrates + 1 fat
unfrosted	2-inch square (about 2 oz)	1 carbohydrate + 1 fat
Cookies		
chocolate chip	2 cookies (2¼ inches across)	1 carbohydrate + 2 fats
gingersnap	3 cookies	1 carbohydrate
sandwich, with crème filling	2 small (about ⅔ oz)	1 carbohydrate + 1 fat
sugar-free	3 small or 1 large (¾–1 oz)	1 carbohydrate + 1–2 fats
vanilla wafer	5 cookies	1 carbohydrate + 1 fat
Cupcake, frosted	1 small (about 1¾ oz)	2 carbohydrates + 1–1½ fats
Fruit cobbler	½ cup (3½ oz)	3 carbohydrates + 1 fat
Gelatin, regular	½ cup	1 carbohydrate
Pie		
commercially prepared fruit, 2 crusts	⅙ of 8-inch pie	3 carbohydrates + 2 fats
pumpkin or custard	⅛ of 8-inch pie	1½ carbohydrates + 1½ fats
Pudding		
regular (made with reduced-fat milk)	½ cup	2 carbohydrates
sugar-free or sugar-and fat-free (made with fat-free milk)	½ cup	1 carbohydrate

Candy, Spreads, Sweets, Sweeteners, Syrups, and Toppings

Food	Serving Size	Count as
Candy bar, chocolate/peanut	2 "fun size" bars (1 oz)	1½ carbohydrates + 1½ fats
Candy, hard	3 pieces	1 carbohydrate
Chocolate "kisses"	5 pieces	1 carbohydrate + 1 fat
Coffee creamer		
dry, flavored	4 tsp	½ carbohydrate + ½ fat
liquid, flavored	2 Tbsp	1 carbohydrate
Fruit snacks, chewy (pureed fruit concentrate)	1 roll (¾ oz)	1 carbohydrate
Fruit spreads, 100% fruit	1½ Tbsp	1 carbohydrate
Honey	1 Tbsp	1 carbohydrate
Jam or jelly, regular	1 Tbsp	1 carbohydrate
Sugar	1 Tbsp	1 carbohydrate
Syrup		
chocolate	2 Tbsp	2 carbohydrates
light (pancake type)	2 Tbsp	1 carbohydrate
regular (pancake type)	1 Tbsp	1 carbohydrate

Condiments and Sauces

Food	Serving Size	Count as
Barbeque sauce	3 Tbsp	1 carbohydrate
Cranberry sauce, jellied	¼ cup	1½ carbohydrates
Gravy, canned or bottled	½ cup	½ carbohydrate + ½ fat
Salad dressing, fat-free, low-fat, cream-based	3 Tbsp	1 carbohydrate
Sweet and sour sauce	3 Tbsp	1 carbohydrate

Frozen Bars, Frozen Desserts, Frozen Yogurt, and Ice Cream

Food	Serving Size	Count as
Frozen pops	1	½ carbohydrate
Fruit juice bars, frozen, 100% juice	1 bar (3 oz)	1 carbohydrate
Ice cream		
fat-free	½ cup	1½ carbohydrates
light	½ cup	1 carbohydrate + 1 fat
no sugar added	½ cup	1 carbohydrate + 1 fat
regular	½ cup	1 carbohydrate + 2 fats
Sherbet, sorbet	½ cup	2 carbohydrates
Yogurt, frozen		
fat-free	⅓ cup	1 carbohydrate
regular	½ cup	1 carbohydrate + 0–1 fat

Doughnuts, Muffins, Pastries, and Sweet Breads

Food	Serving Size	Count as
Banana nut bread	1-inch slice (1 oz)	2 carbohydrates + 1 fat
Doughnut		
cake, plain	1 medium (1½ oz)	1½ carbohydrates + 2 fats
yeast type, glazed	3¾ inches across (2 oz)	2 carbohydrates + 2 fats
Muffin (4 oz)	¼ muffin (1 oz)	1 carbohydrate + ½ fat
Sweet roll or Danish	1 (2½ oz)	2½ carbohydrates + 2 fats

Granola Bars, Meal Replacement Bars/Shakes, and Trail Mix

Food	Serving Size	Count as
Granola or snack bar, regular or low-fat	1 bar (1 oz)	1½ carbohydrates
Meal replacement bar	1 bar (1⅓ oz)	1½ carbohydrates + 0–1 fat
Meal replacement bar	1 bar (2 oz)	2 carbohydrates + 1 fat
Meal replacement shake, reduced calorie	1 can (10–11 oz)	1½ carbohydrates + 0–1 fat
Trail mix		
candy/nut-based	1 oz	1 carbohydrate + 2 fats
dried fruit-based	1 oz	1 carbohydrate + 1 fat

Nonstarchy Vegetables

Nonstarchy Vegetables

Amaranth or Chinese spinach
Artichoke
Artichoke hearts
Asparagus
Baby corn
Bamboo shoots
Beans (green, wax, Italian)
Bean sprouts
Beets
🧂 Borscht
Broccoli
♨ Brussels sprouts
Cabbage (green, bok choy, Chinese)
♨ Carrots
Cauliflower
Celery
♨ Chayote
Coleslaw, packaged, no dressing
Cucumber
Eggplant
Gourds (bitter, bottle, luffa, bitter melon)
Green onions or scallions
Greens (collard, kale, mustard, turnip)
Hearts of palm
Jicama
Kohlrabi

Leeks
Mixed vegetables (without corn, peas, or pasta)
Mung bean sprouts
Mushrooms, all kinds, fresh
Okra
Onions
Oriental radish or daikon
Pea pods
♨ Peppers (all varieties)
Radishes
Rutabaga
🧂 Sauerkraut
Soybean sprouts
Spinach
Squash (summer, crookneck, zucchini)
Sugar pea snaps
♨ Swiss chard
Tomato
Tomatoes, canned
🧂 Tomato sauce
🧂 Tomato/vegetable juice
Turnips
Water chestnuts
Yard-long beans

525

Meat and Meat Substitutes

Lean Meat and Meat Substitutes

Food	Amount
Beef: Select or Choice grades trimmed of fat: ground round, roast (chuck, rib, rump), round, sirloin, steak (cubed, flank, porterhouse, T-bone), tenderloin	1 oz
⑤ Beef jerky	1 oz
Cheeses with 3 grams of fat or less per oz	1 oz
Cottage cheese	¼ cup
Egg substitutes, plain	¼ cup
Egg whites	2
Fish, fresh or frozen, plain: catfish, cod, flounder, haddock, halibut, orange roughy, salmon, tilapia, trout, tuna	1 oz
⑤ Fish, smoked: herring or salmon (lox)	1 oz
Game: buffalo, ostrich, rabbit, venison	1 oz
⑤ Hot dog with 3 grams of fat or less per oz (8 dogs per 14 oz package) *Note: May be high in carbohydrate.*	1
Lamb: chop, leg, or roast	1 oz
Organ meats: heart, kidney, liver *Note: May be high in cholesterol.*	1 oz
Oysters, fresh or frozen	6 medium
Pork, lean	
⑤ Canadian bacon	1 oz
rib or loin chop/roast, ham, tenderloin	1 oz

Medium-Fat Meat and Meat Substitutes

Food	Amount
Beef: corned beef, ground beef, meatloaf, Prime grades trimmed of fat (prime rib), short ribs, tongue	1 oz
Cheeses with 4–7 grams of fat per oz: feta, mozzarella, pasteurized processed cheese spread, reduced-fat cheeses, string	1 oz
Egg *Note: High in cholesterol, so limit to 3 per week.*	1
Fish, any fried product	1 oz
Lamb: ground, rib roast	1 oz
Pork: cutlet, shoulder roast	1 oz
Poultry: chicken with skin; dove, pheasant, wild duck, or goose; fried chicken; ground turkey	1 oz
Ricotta cheese	2 oz or ¼ cup
⑤ Sausage with 4–7 grams of fat per oz	1 oz
Veal, cutlet (no breading)	1 oz
Poultry, without skin: Cornish hen, chicken, domestic duck or goose (well-drained of fat), turkey	1 oz
Processed sandwich meats with 3 grams of fat or less per oz: chipped beef, deli thin-sliced meats, turkey ham, turkey kielbasa, turkey pastrami	1 oz
Salmon, canned	1 oz
Sardines, canned	2 medium
⑤ Sausage with 3 grams of fat or less per oz	1 oz
Shellfish: clams, crab, imitation shellfish, lobster, scallops, shrimp	1 oz
Tuna, canned in water or oil, drained	1 oz
Veal, lean chop, roast	1 oz

High-Fat Meat and Meat Substitutes

These foods are high in saturated fat, cholesterol, and calories and may raise blood cholesterol levels if eaten on a regular basis. Try to eat 3 or fewer servings from this group per week.

Food	Amount
Bacon	
pork	2 slices (16 slices per lb or 1 oz each, before cooking)
turkey	3 slices (½ oz each before cooking)
Cheese, regular: American, bleu, brie, cheddar, hard goat, Monterey jack, queso, and Swiss	1 oz
Hot dog: beef, pork, or combination (10 per lb-sized package)	1
Hot dog: turkey or chicken (10 per lb-sized package)	1
Pork: ground, sausage, spareribs	1 oz
Processed sandwich meats with 8 grams of fat or more per oz: bologna, pastrami, hard salami	1 oz
Sausage with 8 grams fat or more per oz: bratwurst, chorizo: Italian, knockwurst, Polish, smoked, summer	1 oz

Plant-Based Proteins

Because carbohydrate content varies among plant-based proteins, you should read the food label.

Food	Amount	Count as
"Bacon" strips, soy-based	3 strips	1 medium-fat meat
Baked beans	⅓ cup	1 starch + 1 lean meat
Beans, cooked: black, garbanzo, kidney, lima, navy, pinto, white	½ cup	1 starch + 1 lean meat
"Beef" or "sausage" crumbles, soy-based	2 oz	½ carbohydrate + 1 lean meat
"Chicken" nuggets, soy-based	2 nuggets (1½ oz)	½ carbohydrate + 1 medium-fat meat
Edamame	½ cup	½ carbohydrate + 1 lean meat
Falafel (spiced chickpea and wheat patties)	3 patties (about 2 inches across)	1 carbohydrate + 1 high-fat meat
Hot dog, soy-based	1 (1½ oz)	½ carbohydrate + 1 lean meat
Hummus	⅓ cup	1 carbohydrate + 1 high-fat meat
Lentils, brown, green, or yellow	½ cup	1 carbohydrate + 1 lean meat
Meatless burger, soy-based	3 oz	½ carbohydrate + 2 lean meats
Meatless burger, vegetable- and starch-based	1 patty (about 2½ oz)	1 carbohydrate + 2 lean meats
Nut spreads: almond butter, cashew butter, peanut butter, soy nut butter	1 Tbsp	1 high-fat meat
Peas, cooked: black-eyed and split peas	½ cup	1 starch + 1 lean meat
Refried beans, canned	½ cup	1 starch + 1 lean meat
"Sausage" patties, soy-based	1 (1½ oz)	1 medium-fat meat
Soy nuts, unsalted	¾ oz	½ carbohydrate + 1 medium-fat meat
Tempeh	¼ cup	1 medium-fat meat
Tofu	4 oz (½ cup)	1 medium-fat meat
Tofu, light	4 oz (½ cup)	1 lean meat

Fats

Fats and oils have mixtures of unsaturated (polyunsaturated and monounsaturated) and saturated fats. Foods on the **Fats** list are grouped together based on the major type of fat they contain. In general, 1 fat choice equals:

- 1 teaspoon of regular margarine, vegetable oil, or butter
- 1 tablespoon of regular salad dressing

Unsaturated—Monounsaturated Fats

Food	Serving Size
Avocado, medium	2 Tbsp (1 oz)
Nut butters (*trans* fat-free): almond butter, cashew butter, peanut butter (smooth or crunchy)	1½ tsp
Nuts	
almonds	6 nuts
Brazil	2 nuts
cashews	6 nuts
filberts (hazelnuts)	5 nuts
macadamia	3 nuts
mixed (50% peanuts)	6 nuts
peanuts	10 nuts
pecans	4 halves
pistachios	16 nuts
Oil: canola, olive, peanut	1 tsp
Olives	
black (ripe)	8 large
green, stuffed	10 large

Polyunsaturated Fats

Food	Serving Size
Margarine: lower-fat spread (30%–50% vegetable oil, *trans* fat-free)	1 Tbsp
Margarine: stick, tub (*trans* fat-free), or squeeze (*trans* fat-free)	1 tsp
Mayonnaise	
reduced-fat	1 Tbsp
regular	1 tsp
Mayonnaise-style salad dressing	
reduced-fat	1 Tbsp
regular	2 tsp
Nuts	
Pignolia (pine nuts)	1 Tbsp
walnuts, English	4 halves
Oil: corn, cottonseed, flaxseed, grape seed, safflower, soybean, sunflower	1 tsp
Oil: made from soybean and canola oil—Enova	1 tsp
Plant stanol esters	
light	1 Tbsp
regular	2 tsp
Salad dressing	
⑤ reduced-fat *Note: May be high in carbohydrate.*	2 Tbsp
⑤ regular	1 Tbsp
Seeds	
flaxseed, whole	1 Tbsp
pumpkin, sunflower	1 Tbsp
sesame seeds	1 Tbsp
Tahini or sesame paste	2 tsp

Saturated Fats

Food	Serving Size
Bacon, cooked, regular or turkey	1 slice
Butter	
reduced-fat	1 Tbsp
stick	1 tsp
whipped	2 tsp
Butter blends made with oil	
reduced-fat or light	1 Tbsp
regular	1½ tsp
Chitterlings, boiled	2 Tbsp (½ oz)
Coconut, sweetened, shredded	2 Tbsp
Coconut milk	
light	⅓ cup
regular	1½ Tbsp
Cream	
half and half	2 Tbsp
heavy	1 Tbsp
light	1½ Tbsp
whipped	2 Tbsp
whipped, pressurized	¼ cup
Cream cheese	
reduced-fat	1½ Tbsp (¾ oz)
regular	1 Tbsp (½ oz)
Lard	1 tsp
Oil: coconut, palm, palm kernel	1 tsp
Salt pork	¼ oz
Shortening, solid	1 tsp
Sour cream	
reduced-fat or light	3 Tbsp
regular	2 Tbsp

Free Foods

A "free" food is any food or drink choice that has less than 20 calories and 5 grams or less of carbohydrate per serving.

Selection Tips

- Most foods on this list should be limited to 3 servings (as listed here) per day. Spread out the servings throughout the day. If you eat all 3 servings at once, it could raise your blood glucose level.
- Food and drink choices listed here without a serving size can be eaten whenever you like.

Low Carbohydrate Foods

Food	Serving Size
Cabbage, raw	½ cup
Candy, hard (regular or sugar-free)	1 piece
Carrots, cauliflower, or green beans, cooked	¼ cup
Cranberries, sweetened with sugar substitute	½ cup
Cucumber, sliced	½ cup
Gelatin	
dessert, sugar-free	
unflavored	
Gum	
Jam or jelly, light or no sugar added	2 tsp
Rhubarb, sweetened with sugar substitute	½ cup
Salad greens	
Sugar substitutes (artificial sweeteners)	
Syrup, sugar-free	2 Tbsp

Modified Fat Foods with Carbohydrate

Food	Serving Size
Cream cheese, fat-free	1 Tbsp (½ oz)
Creamers	
nondairy, liquid	1 Tbsp
nondairy, powdered	2 tsp
Margarine spread	
fat-free	1 Tbsp
reduced-fat	1 tsp
Mayonnaise	
fat-free	1 Tbsp
reduced-fat	1 tsp
Mayonnaise-style salad dressing	
fat-free	1 Tbsp
reduced-fat	1 tsp
Salad dressing	
fat-free or low-fat	1 Tbsp
fat-free, Italian	2 Tbsp
Sour cream, fat-free or reduced-fat	1 Tbsp
Whipped topping	
light or fat-free	2 Tbsp
regular	1 Tbsp

Condiments

Food	Serving Size
Barbecue sauce	2 tsp
Catsup (ketchup)	1 Tbsp
Honey mustard	1 Tbsp
Horseradish	
Lemon juice	
Miso	1½ tsp
Mustard	
Parmesan cheese, freshly grated	1 Tbsp
Pickle relish	1 Tbsp
Pickles	
dill	1½ medium
sweet, bread and butter	2 slices
sweet, gherkin	¾ oz
Salsa	¼ cup
Soy sauce, light or regular	1 Tbsp
Sweet and sour sauce	2 tsp
Sweet chili sauce	2 tsp
Taco sauce	1 Tbsp
Vinegar	
Yogurt, any type	2 Tbsp

Drinks/Mixes

Any food on this list—without a serving size listed—can be consumed in any moderate amount.

- Bouillon, broth, consomme
- Bouillon or broth, low-sodium
- Carbonated or mineral water
- Club soda
- Cocoa powder, unsweetened (1 Tbsp)
- Coffee, unsweetened or with sugar substitute
- Diet soft drinks, sugar-free
- Drink mixes, sugar-free
- Tea, unsweetened or with sugar substitute
- Tonic water, diet
- Water
- Water, flavored, carbohydrate free

Seasonings

Any food on this list can be consumed in any moderate amount.

- Flavoring extracts (for example, vanilla, almond, peppermint)
- Garlic
- Herbs, fresh or dried
- Nonstick cooking spray
- Pimento
- Spices
- Hot pepper sauce
- Wine, used in cooking
- Worcestershire sauce

531

Combination Foods

Many of the foods you eat are mixed together in various combinations, such as casseroles. These "combination" foods do not fit into any one choice list. This is a list of choices for some typical combination foods. This list will help you fit these foods into your meal plan. Ask your RD for nutrient information about other combination foods you would like to eat, including your own recipes.

Entrees

Food	Serving Size	Count as
Casserole type (tuna noodle, lasagna, spaghetti with meatballs, chili with beans, macaroni and cheese)	1 cup (8 oz)	2 carbohydrates + 2 medium-fat meats
Stews (beef/other meats and vegetables)	1 cup (8 oz)	1 carbohydrate + 1 medium-fat meat + 0–3 fats
Tuna salad or chicken salad	½ cup (3½ oz)	½ carbohydrate + 2 lean meats + 1 fat

Frozen Meals/Entrees

Food	Serving Size	Count as
Burrito (beef and bean)	1 (5 oz)	3 carbohydrates + 1 lean meat + 2 fats
Dinner-type meal	generally 14–17 oz	3 carbohydrates + 3 medium-fat meats + 3 fats
Entree or meal with less than 340 calories	about 8–11 oz	2–3 carbohydrates + 1–2 lean meats
Pizza		
cheese/vegetarian, thin crust	¼ of a 12 inch (4½–5 oz)	2 carbohydrates + 2 medium-fat meats
meat topping, thin crust	¼ of a 12 inch (5 oz)	2 carbohydrates + 2 medium-fat meats + 1½ fats
Pocket sandwich	1 (4½ oz)	3 carbohydrates + 1 lean meat + 1–2 fats
Pot pie	1 (7 oz)	2½ carbohydrates + 1 medium-fat meat + 3 fats

Salads (Deli-Style)

Food	Serving Size	Count as
Coleslaw	½ cup	1 carbohydrate + 1½ fats
Macaroni/pasta salad	½ cup	2 carbohydrates + 3 fats
Potato salad	½ cup	1½–2 carbohydrates + 1–2 fats

Soups

	Food	Serving Size	Count as
⑤	Bean, lentil, or split pea	1 cup	1 carbohydrate + 1 lean meat
⑤	Chowder (made with milk)	1 cup (8 oz)	1 carbohydrate + 1 lean meat + 1½ fats
⑤	Cream (made with water)	1 cup (8 oz)	1 carbohydrate + 1 fat
⑤	Instant	6 oz prepared	1 carbohydrate
⑤	with beans or lentils	8 oz prepared	2½ carbohydrates + 1 lean meat
⑤	Miso soup	1 cup	½ carbohydrate + 1 fat
⑤	Oriental noodle	1 cup	2 carbohydrates + 2 fats
	Rice (congee)	1 cup	1 carbohydrate
⑤	Tomato (made with water)	1 cup (8 oz)	1 carbohydrate
⑤	Vegetable beef, chicken noodle, or other broth-type	1 cup (8 oz)	1 carbohydrate

Fast Foods

The choices in the **Fast Foods** list are not specific fast food meals or items, but are estimates based on popular foods. You can get specific nutrition information for almost every fast food or restaurant chain. Ask the restaurant or check its website for nutrition information about your favorite fast foots.

Breakfast Sandwiches

	Food	Serving Size	Count as
⑤	Egg, cheese, meat, English muffin	1 sandwich	2 carbohydrates + 2 medium-fat meats
⑤	Sausage biscuit sandwich	1 sandwich	2 carbohydrates + 2 high-fat meats + 3½ fats

Main Dishes/Entrees

	Food	Serving Size	Count as
⑤ ☺	Burrito (beef and beans)	1 (about 8 oz)	3 carbohydrates + 3 medium-fat meats + 3 fats
⑤	Chicken breast, breaded and fried	1 (about 5 oz)	1 carbohydrate + 4 medium-fat meats
	Chicken drumstick, breaded and fried	1 (about 2 oz)	2 medium-fat meats
⑤	Chicken nuggets	6 (about 3½ oz)	1 carbohydrate + 2 medium-fat meats + 1 fat
⑤	Chicken thigh, breaded and fried	1 (about 4 oz)	½ carbohydrate + 3 medium-fat meats + 1½ fats
⑤	Chicken wings, hot	6 (5 oz)	5 medium-fat meats + 1½ fats

Oriental

Food	Serving Size	Count as
Beef/chicken/shrimp with vegetables in sauce	1 cup (about 5 oz)	1 carbohydrate + 1 lean meat + 1 fat
Egg roll, meat	1 (about 3 oz)	1 carbohydrate + 1 lean meat + 1 fat
Fried rice, meatless	½ cup	1½ carbohydrates + 1½ fats
Meat and sweet sauce (orange chicken)	1 cup	3 carbohydrates + 3 medium-fat meats + 2 fats
Noodles and vegetables in sauce (chow mein, lo mein)	1 cup	2 carbohydrates + 1 fat

Pizza

Food	Serving Size	Count as
Pizza		
cheese, pepperoni, regular crust	⅛ of a 14 inch (about 4 oz)	2½ carbohydrates + 1 medium-fat meat + 1½ fats
cheese/vegetarian, thin crust	¼ of a 12 inch (about 6 oz)	2½ carbohydrates + 2 medium-fat meats + 1½ fats

Sandwiches

Food	Serving Size	Count as
Chicken sandwich, grilled	1	3 carbohydrates + 4 lean meats
Chicken sandwich, crispy	1	3½ carbohydrates + 3 medium-fat meats + 1 fat
Fish sandwich with tartar sauce	1	2½ carbohydrates + 2 medium-fat meats + 2 fats
Hamburger		
large with cheese	1	2½ carbohydrates + 4 medium-fat meats + 1 fat
regular	1	2 carbohydrates + 1 medium-fat meat + 1 fat
Hot dog with bun	1	1 carbohydrate + 1 high-fat meat + 1 fat
Submarine sandwich		
less than 6 grams fat	6-inch sub	3 carbohydrates + 2 lean meats
regular	6-inch sub	3½ carbohydrates + 2 medium-fat meats + 1 fat
Taco, hard or soft shell (meat and cheese)	1 small	1 carbohydrate + 1 medium-fat meat + 1½ fats

Salads

Food	Serving Size	Count as
🧂 😋 Salad, main dish (grilled chicken type, no dressing or croutons)	Salad	1 carbohydrate + 4 lean meats
Salad, side, no dressing or cheese	Small (about 5 oz)	1 vegetable

Sides/Appetizers

Food	Serving Size	Count as
⚠️ French fries, restaurant style	small	3 carbohydrates + 3 fats
	medium	4 carbohydrates + 4 fats
	large	5 carbohydrates + 6 fats
🧂 Nachos with cheese	small (about 4⅛ oz)	2½ carbohydrates + 4 fats
🧂 Onion rings	1 serving (about 3 oz)	2½ carbohydrates + 3 fats

Desserts

Food	Serving Size	Count as
Milkshake, any flavor	12 oz	6 carbohydrates + 2 fats
Soft-serve ice cream cone	1 small	2½ carbohydrates + 1 fat

Alcohol

Nutrition Tips
- In general, 1 alcohol choice (½ oz absolute alcohol) has about 100 calories.

Selection Tips
- If you choose to drink alcohol, you should limit it to 1 drink or less per day for women, and 2 drinks or less per day for men.
- To reduce your risk of low blood glucose (hypoglycemia), especially if you take insulin or a diabetes pill that increases insulin, always drink alcohol with food.
- While alcohol, by itself, does not directly affect blood glucose, be aware of the carbohydrate (for example, in mixed drinks, beer, and wine) that may raise your blood glucose.
- Check with your RD if you would like to fit alcohol into your meal plan.

Alcoholic Beverage	Serving Size	Count as
Beer		
light (4.2%)	12 fl oz	1 alcohol equivalent + ½ carbohydrate
regular (4.9%)	12 fl oz	1 alcohol equivalent + 1 carbohydrate
Distilled spirits: vodka, rum, gin, whiskey 80 or 86 proof	1½ fl oz	1 alcohol equivalent
Liqueur, coffee (53 proof)	1 fl oz	1 alcohol equivalent + 1 carbohydrate
Sake	1 fl oz	½ alcohol equivalent
Wine		
dessert (sherry) dry,	3½ fl oz	1 alcohol equivalent + 1 carbohydrate
red or white (10%)	5 fl oz	1 alcohol equivalent

Appendix F
Food Labeling Information

Sample Label for a Granola Bar

Nutrition Facts

Serving Size 1 bar (24g)
Servings Per Container 12

Amount Per Serving

Calories 120   Calories from Fat 45

	% Daily Value*
Total Fat 5g	**8%**
Saturated Fat 1g	**5%**
Cholesterol 0mg	**0%**
Sodium 65mg	**3%**
Total Carbohydrate 17g	**6%**
Dietary Fiber 1g	**4%**
Sugars 6g	
Protein 2g	

Vitamin A 0%	•	Vitamin C 0%
Calcium 0%	•	Iron 4%

* Percent Daily Values are based on a 2,000 calorie diet. Your daily values may be higher or lower depending on your calorie needs:

	Calories:	2,000	2,500
Total Fat	Less than	65g	80g
Sat Fat	Less than	20g	25g
Cholesterol	Less than	300mg	300mg
Sodium	Less than	2,400mg	2,400mg
Total Carbohydrate		300g	375g
Dietary Fiber		25g	30g

Calories per gram:
Fat 9 • Carbohydrate 4 • Protein 4

Ingredients: Rolled oats, sugar, sunflower oil, brown sugar syrup, honey, salt, soy lecithin

Daily Reference Values Used to Establish Daily Values

Food Component	Daily Reference Value (2000 Kcal)
Total fat	Less than 65 g (30% of energy)
Saturated fat	Less than 20 g (10% of energy)
Cholesterol	Less than 300 mg
Total carbohydrate	300 g (60% of energy)
Dietary fiber	25 g (11.5 g/1000 Kcal)
Sodium	Less than 2400 mg
Potassium	3500 mg
Protein	50 g (10% of energy)

Source: USDA A Food Labeling Guide Appendix F. Available online at http://www.cfsan.fda.gov/~dms/2lg-xf.html

Statement of identity

Net quantity of contents

Structure-function claim

Directions

Supplement Facts panel

Other ingredients in descending order of predominance and by common name of proprietary blend

Name and place of business of manufacturer packer or distributor. This is the address to write for more product information

"When you need to perform your best, take ginseng." This statement has not been evaluated by the Food and Drug Administration. This product is not intended to diagnose, treat, cure, or prevent any disease.

DIRECTIONS FOR USE:
Take one capsule daily.

Supplement Facts

Serving Size 1 Capsule

Amount Per Capsule

Oriental Ginseng, powdered (root)   250 mcg*

*Daily Value not established.

Other ingredients: Gelatin, water, and glycerin.

ABC Company
Anywhere, MD 00001

GINSENG
A DIETARY SUPPLEMENT
60 CAPSULES

Recommended Dietary Intakes (RDIs)* Used to Establish Daily Values

Vitamins and Minerals	Units of Measurement	Adults and Children 4 or more Years of Age	Infants	Children Under 4 Years of Age	Pregnant or Lactating Women
Vitamin A	International Units†	5000 (1000 µg)	1500	2500	8000
Vitamin D	International Units†	400 (10 µg)	400	400	400
Vitamin E	International Units†	30 (10 µg)	5	10	30
Vitamin C	Milligrams	60	35	40	60
Folic acid	Micrograms	400	0.1	0.2	0.8
Thiamin	Milligrams	1.5	0.5	0.7	1.7
Riboflavin	Milligrams	1.7	0.6	0.8	2.0
Niacin	Milligrams	20	8	9	20
Vitamin B_6	Milligrams	2.0	0.4	0.7	2.5
Vitamin B_{12}	Micrograms	6.0	2	3	8
Biotin	Micrograms	300	0.05	0.15	0.30
Pantothenic acid	Milligrams	10	3	5	10
Calcium	Milligrams	1000	0.6	0.8	1.3
Phosphorous	Milligrams	1000	0.5	0.8	1.3
Iodine	Micrograms	150	45	70	150
Iron	Milligrams	18	15	10	18
Magnesium	Milligrams	400	70	200	450
Copper	Milligrams	2.0	0.6	1.0	2.0
Zinc	Milligrams	15	5	8	15
Vitamin K	Micrograms	80	—‡	—‡	—‡
Chromium	Micrograms	120	—	—	—
Selenium	Micrograms	70	—	—	—
Molybdenum	Micrograms	75	—	—	—
Manganese	Milligrams	2	—	—	—
Chloride	Milligrams	3400	—	—	—

*Based on National Academy of Sciences' 1968 Recommended Dietary Allowances.

†The RDIs for fat-soluble vitamins are expressed in International Units (IU). Values that are approximately equivalent in micrograms are given in parentheses.

‡No values yet established for vitamin K, chromium, selenium, molybdenum, manganese, or chloride for this population.

Source: USDA Food Labeling Guide. Available online at http://www.cfsan.fda.gov/~dms/2lg-xf.htm

Health Claims Permitted on Food or Supplement Labels

Health Claims That Meet Significant Scientific Agreement

These are authorized by the FDA based on an extensive review of the scientific literature or information from a scientific body of the U.S. government or the National Academy of Sciences that supports the nutrient/disease relationship.

- Calcium and osteoporosis
- Dietary fat and cancer
- Dietary saturated fat and cholesterol and risk of coronary heart disease
- Dietary non-carcinogenic carbohydrate sweeteners and dental caries
- Fiber-containing grain products, fruits, and vegetables and cancer
- Folic acid and neural tube defects
- Fluoridated water and reduced risk of dental caries
- Fruits, vegetables and grain products and cancer
- Fruits, vegetables, and grain products that contain fiber, particularly soluble fiber, and risk of coronary heart disease
- Plant sterol/stanol and coronary heart disease
- Potassium and the risk of high blood pressure and stroke
- Saturated fat, cholesterol and trans fat and reduced risk of heart disease
- Sodium and hypertension
- Soluble fiber from certain foods and risk of coronary heart disease
- Soy protein and risk of coronary heart disease
- Stanols/sterols and risk of coronary heart disease
- Whole grain foods and the risk of heart disease and certain cancers

Qualified Health Claims

These are used when there is emerging evidence for a relationship between a food, food component, or dietary supplement and reduced risk of a disease or health-related condition but there is not enough scientific support for the FDA to issue an authorizing regulation.

- Qualified claims about cancer risk: selenium and cancer, antioxidant vitamins and cancer, green tea and cancer, tomatoes and cancer.
- Qualified claims about cardiovascular disease risk: nuts and heart disease, walnuts and heart disease, omega-3 fatty acids and coronary heart disease, B vitamins and vascular disease, monounsaturated fatty acids from olive oil and reduced coronary heart disease risk, unsaturated fatty acids from canola oil and coronary heart disease risk, corn oil and coronary heart disease.
- Qualified claims about chromium picolinate and diabetes
- Qualified claims about calcium and colorectal cancer and colon/rectal polyps, calcium and hypertension and preeclampsia
- Qualified claims about cognitive function: phosphatidylserine and cognitive dysfunction and dementia
- Qualified claims about neural tube birth defects: 0.8 mg folic acid and neural tube birth defects

Source: U.S. Food and Drug Administration. Center for Food Safety and Applied Nutrition. Label Claims. Available online at http://www.cfsan.fda.gov/~dms/2lg-xc.html

Nutrient Content Descriptors Commonly Used on Food Labels

Free	Means that a product contains no amount of, or a trivial amount of, fat, saturated fat, cholesterol, sodium, sugars, or kcalories. For example, "sugar free" and "fat free" both mean less than 0.5 g per serving. Synonyms for "free" include "without," "no," and "zero."
Low	Used for foods that can be eaten frequently without exceeding the Daily Value for fat, saturated fat, cholesterol, sodium, or Calories. Specific definitions have been established for each of these nutrients. For example, "low fat" means that the food contains 3 g or less per serving, and "low cholesterol" means that the food contains less than 20 mg of cholesterol per serving. Synonyms for "low" include "little," "few," and "low source of."
Lean and extra lean	Used to describe the fat content of meat, poultry, seafood, and game meats. "Lean" means that the food contains less than 10 g fat, less than 4.5 g saturated fat, and less than 95 mg of cholesterol per serving and per 100 g. "Extra lean" means that the food contains less than 5 g fat, less than 2 g saturated fat, and less than 95 mg of cholesterol per serving and per 100 g.
High	Can be used if a food contains 20% or more of the Daily Value for a particular nutrient. Synonyms for "high" include "rich in" and "excellent source of."
Good source	Means that a food contains 10 to 19% of the Daily Value for a particular nutrient per serving.
Reduced	Means that a nutritionally altered product contains 25% less of a nutrient or of energy than the regular or reference product.
Less	Means that a food, whether altered or not, contains 25% less of a nutrient or of energy than the reference food. For example, pretzels may claim to have "less fat" than potato chips. "Fewer" may be used as a synonym for "less."
Light	May be used in different ways. First, it can be used on a nutritionally altered product that contains one-third fewer kcalories or half the fat of a reference food. Second, it can be used when the sodium content of a low-calorie, low-fat food has been reduced by 50%. The term "light" can be used to describe properties such as texture and color as long as the label explains the intent—for example, "light and fluffy."
More	Means that a serving of food, whether altered or not, contains a nutrient that is at least 10% of the Daily Value more than the reference food. This definition also applies to foods using the terms "fortified," "enriched," or "added."
Healthy	May be used to describe foods that are low in fat and saturated fat and contain no more than 360 mg of sodium and no more than 60 mg of cholesterol per serving and provide at least 10% of the Daily Value for vitamins A or C, or iron, calcium, protein, or fiber.
Fresh	May be used on foods that are raw and have never been frozen or heated and contain no preservatives.

Source: USDA. A food Labeling Guide Appendix A. Available online at
http://www.cfsan.fda.gov/~dms/2lg-xa.html

539

Appendix G
Canadian Nutrition Recommendations and Guidelines

Canada's Guidelines for Healthy Eating

- Enjoy a VARIETY of foods.
- Emphasize cereals, breads, other grain products, vegetables and fruits.
- Choose low-fat dairy products, lean meats, and foods prepared with little or no fat.
- Achieve and maintain a healthy body weight be enjoying regular physical activity and healthy eating.

Limit salt, alcohol and caffeine

Source: Health Canada. Available on line at http://www.hc-sc.gc.ca/fn-an/nutrition/pol/action_healthy_eating-action_saine_alimentation-02-eng.php#6

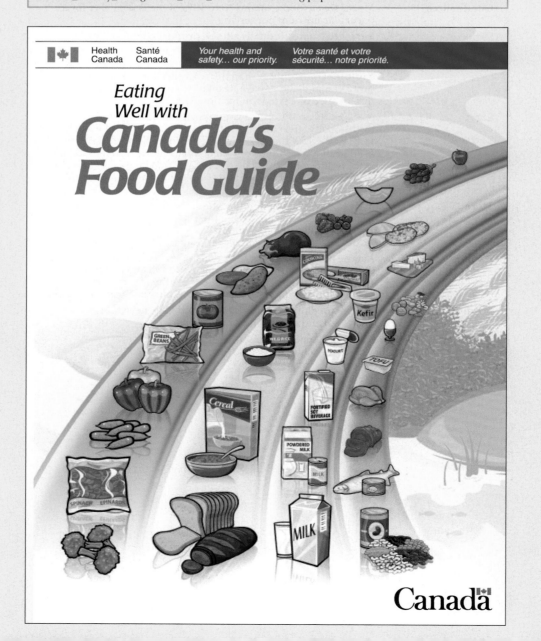

Advice for different ages and stages...

Children

Following *Canada's Food Guide* helps children grow and thrive.

Young children have small appetites and need calories for growth and development.

- Serve small nutritious meals and snacks each day.

- Do not restrict nutritious foods because of their fat content. Offer a variety of foods from the four food groups.

- Most of all... be a good role model.

Women of childbearing age

All women who could become pregnant and those who are pregnant or breastfeeding need a multivitamin containing **folic acid** every day. Pregnant women need to ensure that their multivitamin also contains **iron**. A health care professional can help you find the multivitamin that's right for you.

Pregnant and breastfeeding women need more calories. Include an extra 2 to 3 Food Guide Servings each day.

Here are two examples:
- Have fruit and yogurt for a snack, or
- Have an extra slice of toast at breakfast and an extra glass of milk at supper.

Men and women over 50

The need for **vitamin D** increases after the age of 50.

In addition to following *Canada's Food Guide*, everyone over the age of 50 should take a daily vitamin D supplement of 10 µg (400 IU).

How do I count Food Guide Servings in a meal?

Here is an example:

Vegetable and beef stir-fry with rice, a glass of milk and an apple for dessert		
250 mL (1 cup) mixed broccoli, carrot and sweet red pepper	=	2 **Vegetables and Fruit** Food Guide Servings
75 g (2 ½ oz.) lean beef	=	1 **Meat and Alternatives** Food Guide Serving
250 mL (1 cup) brown rice	=	2 **Grain Products** Food Guide Servings
5 mL (1 tsp) canola oil	=	part of your **Oils and Fats** intake for the day
250 mL (1 cup) 1% milk	=	1 **Milk and Alternatives** Food Guide Serving
1 apple	=	1 **Vegetables and Fruit** Food Guide Serving

Eat well and be active today and every day!

The benefits of eating well and being active include:

- Better overall health.
- Lower risk of disease.
- A healthy body weight.
- Feeling and looking better.
- More energy.
- Stronger muscles and bones.

Be active

To be active every day is a step towards better health and a healthy body weight.

Canada's Physical Activity Guide recommends building 30 to 60 minutes of moderate physical activity into daily life for adults and at least 90 minutes a day for children and youth. You don't have to do it all at once. Add it up in periods of at least 10 minutes at a time for adults and five minutes at a time for children and youth.

Start slowly and build up.

Eat well

Another important step towards better health and a healthy body weight is to follow *Canada's Food Guide* by:

- Eating the recommended amount and type of food each day.
- Limiting foods and beverages high in calories, fat, sugar or salt (sodium) such as cakes and pastries, chocolate and candies, cookies and granola bars, doughnuts and muffins, ice cream and frozen desserts, french fries, potato chips, nachos and other salty snacks, alcohol, fruit flavoured drinks, soft drinks, sports and energy drinks, and sweetened hot or cold drinks.

Read the label

- Compare the Nutrition Facts table on food labels to choose products that contain less fat, saturated fat, trans fat, sugar and sodium.
- Keep in mind that the calories and nutrients listed are for the amount of food found at the top of the Nutrition Facts table.

Limit trans fat

When a Nutrition Facts table is not available, ask for nutrition information to choose foods lower in trans and saturated fats.

Nutrition Facts
Per 0 mL (0 g)

Amount	% Daily Value
Calories 0	
Fat 0 g	0 %
Saturates 0 g	0 %
+ Trans 0 g	
Cholesterol 0 mg	
Sodium 0 mg	0 %
Carbohydrate 0 g	0 %
Fibre 0 g	0 %
Sugars 0 g	
Protein 0 g	

Vitamin A	0 %	Vitamin C	0 %
Calcium	0 %	Iron	0 %

Take a step today...

- ✓ Have breakfast every day. It may help control your hunger later in the day.
- ✓ Walk wherever you can – get off the bus early, use the stairs.
- ✓ Benefit from eating vegetables and fruit at all meals and as snacks.
- ✓ Spend less time being inactive such as watching TV or playing computer games.
- ✓ Request nutrition information about menu items when eating out to help you make healthier choices.
- ✓ Enjoy eating with family and friends!
- ✓ Take time to eat and savour every bite!

For more information, interactive tools, or additional copies visit Canada's Food Guide on-line at:
www.healthcanada.gc.ca/foodguide

or contact:
Publications
Health Canada
Ottawa, Ontario K1A 0K9
E-Mail: publications@hc-sc.gc.ca
Tel.: 1-866-225-0709
Fax: (613) 941-5366
TTY: 1-800-267-1245

Également disponible en français sous le titre :
Bien manger avec le Guide alimentaire canadien

This publication can be made available on request on diskette, large print, audio-cassette and braille.

Recommended Number of *Food Guide Servings* per Day

	Children			Teens		Adults			
Age in Years	2-3	4-8	9-13	14-18		19-50		51+	
Sex	Girls and Boys			Females	Males	Females	Males	Females	Males
Vegetables and Fruit	4	5	6	7	8	7-8	8-10	7	7
Grain Products	3	4	6	6	7	6-7	8	6	7
Milk and Alternatives	2	2	3-4	3-4	3-4	2	2	3	3
Meat and Alternatives	1	1	1-2	2	3	2	3	2	3

The chart above shows how many Food Guide Servings you need from each of the four food groups every day.

Having the amount and type of food recommended and following the tips in *Canada's Food Guide* will help:

• Meet your needs for vitamins, minerals and other nutrients.

• Reduce your risk of obesity, type 2 diabetes, heart disease, certain types of cancer and osteoporosis.

• Contribute to your overall health and vitality.

Appendix H
World Health Organization Nutrition Recommendations

Ranges of Population Nutrient Intake Goals

Dietary Factor	Goal (% of total energy, unless otherwise stated)
Total fat	15–30%
Saturated fatty acids	<10%
Polyunsaturated fatty acids (PUFAs)	6–10%
n-6 Polyunsaturated fatty acids (PUFAs)	5–8%
n-3 Polyunsaturated fatty acids (PUFAs)	1–2%
Trans fatty acids	<1%
Monounsaturated fatty acids (MUFAs)	By difference[a]
Total carbohydrate	55–75%[b]
Free sugars[c]	<10%
Protein	10–15%[d]
Cholesterol	<300 mg per day
Sodium chloride (sodium)[e]	<5 g per day (<2 g per day)
Fruits and vegetables	≥400 g per day
Total dietary fiber	From foods[f]
Non-starch polysaccharides (NSP)	From foods[f]

[a]This is calculated as: total fat − (saturated fatty acids + polyunsaturated fatty acids + trans fatty acids).

[b]The percentage of total energy available after taking into account that consumed as protein and fat, hence the wide range.

[c]The term "free sugars" refers to all monosaccharides and disaccharides added to foods by the manufacturer, cook or consumer, plus sugars naturally present in honey, syrups and fruit juices.

[d]The suggested range should be seen in the light of the Joint WHO/FAO/UNU Expert Consultation on Protein and Amino Acid Requirements in Human Nutrition, held in Geneva from 9 to 16 April 2002 (2).

[e]Salt should be iodized appropriately (6). The need to adjust salt iodization, depending on observed sodium intake and surveillance of iodine status of the population, should be recognized.

[f]See page 58 of the full report, under "Non-starch polysaccharides."

Source: Diet, nutrition and the prevention of chronic diseases. A report of a Joint WHO/FAO Expert Consultation. © World Health Organization 2003. Available online at http://www.who.int/hpr/NPH/docs/who_fao_expert_report.pdf. Reproduced with permission.

Appendix I
Energy Expenditure for Various Activities

Energy Expenditure for Various Activities

Type of Activity	Calories per Hour (by body weight)				
	100 lb	120 lb	150 lb	180 lb	200 lb
Aerobics (heavy)	363	435	544	653	726
Aerobics (medium)	227	272	340	408	454
Aerobics (light)	136	163	204	245	272
Archery	159	190	238	286	317
Backpacking	408	490	612	735	816
Badminton (doubles)	181	218	272	327	363
Badminton (singles)	231	278	347	416	463
Basketball (nonvigorous)	431	517	646	776	862
Basketball (vigorous)	499	599	748	898	998
Bicycling (6 mph)	159	190	238	286	317
Bicycling (10 mph)	249	299	374	449	499
Bicycling (11 mph)	295	354	442	531	590
Bicycling (12 mph)	340	408	510	612	680
Bicycling (13 mph)	385	463	578	694	771
Billiards	91	109	136	163	181
Bowling	177	212	265	318	354
Boxing—competition	603	724	905	1086	1206
Boxing—sparring	376	452	565	678	753
Calisthenics (heavy)	363	435	544	653	726
Calisthenics (light)	181	218	272	327	363
Canoeing (2.5 mph)	150	180	224	269	299
Canoeing (5 mph)	340	408	510	612	680
Carpentry	227	272	340	408	454
Climbing (mountain)	454	544	680	816	907
Disco dancing	272	327	408	490	544
Ditch digging (hand)	263	316	395	473	526
Fencing	340	408	510	612	680
Fishing (bank/boat)	159	190	238	286	317
Fishing (in waders)	249	299	374	449	499
Football (touch)	340	408	510	612	680
Gardening	145	174	218	261	290
Golf (carry clubs)	227	272	340	408	454
Golf (pull cart)	163	196	245	294	327
Golf (ride in cart)	113	136	170	204	227
Handball (vigorous)	454	544	680	816	907
Hiking (X-country)	249	299	374	449	499
Hiking (mountain)	340	408	510	612	680
Horseback trotting	231	278	347	416	463

(continued)

Energy Expenditure for Various Activities *(continued)*

Type of Activity	Calories per Hour (by body weight)				
	100 lb	120 lb	150 lb	180 lb	200 lb
Housework	181	218	272	327	363
Hunting (carry load)	272	327	408	490	544
Ice hockey (vigorous)	454	544	680	816	907
Ice skating (10 mph)	263	316	395	473	526
Jazzercise (heavy)	363	435	544	653	726
Jazzercise (medium)	227	272	340	408	454
Jazzercise (light)	136	163	204	245	272
Jog (9 min/mile)	499	599	748	898	998
Jog (10 min/mile)	454	544	680	816	907
Jog (12 min/mile)	385	463	578	694	771
Jog (13 min/mile)	317	381	476	571	635
Jog (14 min/mile)	272	327	408	490	544
Jog (15 min/mile)	227	272	340	408	454
Jog (17 min/mile)	181	218	272	327	363
Lawn mowing (hand)	295	354	442	531	590
Lawn mowing (power)	163	196	245	294	327
Musical instrument playing	113	136	170	204	227
Racquetball (social)	385	463	578	694	771
Racquetball (vigorous)	454	544	680	816	907
Roller skating	231	278	347	416	463
Rowboating (2.5 mph)	200	239	299	359	399
Rowing (11 mph)	590	707	884	1061	1179
Run (5 min/mile)	816	980	1224	1469	1633
Run (6 min/mile)	703	844	1054	1265	1406
Run (7 min/mile)	612	735	918	1102	1224
Run (8 min/mile)	544	653	816	980	1088
Sailing	159	190	238	286	317
Shuffleboard/skeet	136	163	204	245	272
Skiing (X-country)	454	544	680	816	907
Skiing (downhill)	363	435	544	653	726
Square dancing	272	327	407	490	544
Swimming (competitive)	680	816	1020	1224	1361
Swimming (fast)	426	512	639	767	853
Swimming (slow)	349	419	524	629	698
Table tennis	236	283	354	424	472
Tennis (doubles)	227	272	340	408	454
Tennis (singles)	295	354	442	531	590
Tennis (vigorous)	385	463	578	694	771
Volleyball	231	278	347	416	463
Walking (20 min/mile)	159	190	238	286	317
Walking (26 min/mile)	136	163	204	245	272
Water skiing	317	381	476	571	635
Weight lifting (heavy)	408	490	612	735	816
Weight lifting (light)	181	218	272	327	363
Wood chopping (sawing)	295	354	442	531	590

Source: Data reprinted with permission from N-Squared Computing. First Databank Division of the Hearst Corporation.

Appendix J
Calculations and Conversions

Weights and Measures		
Measure	*Abbreviation*	*Equivalent*
1 gram	g	1000 milligrams
1 milligram	mg	1000 micrograms
1 microgram	μg	1/1000000 of a gram
1 nanogram	ng	1/1000000000 of a gram
1 picogram	pg	1/1000000000000 of a gram
1 kilogram	kg	1000 grams
		2.2 lb
1 pound	lb	454 grams
		16 ounces
1 teaspoon	tsp	approximately 5 grams
1 tablespoon	Tbsp	3 teaspoons
1 ounce	oz	28.4 grams
1 cup	c	8 fluid ounces
		16 tablespoons
1 pint	pt	2 cups
		16 fluid ounces
1 quart	qt	2 pints
		32 fluid ounces
1 gallon	gal	128 fluid ounces
		4 quarts
1 liter	l	1.06 quarts
		1000 milliliters
1 milliliter	ml	1000 microliters
1 deciliter	dl	100 milliliters
1 kcalorie	kcal, Cal	1000 calories
		4.167 kilojoules
1 kilojoule	kJ	1000 joules

Converting Vitamin A Units

Form and Source	Amount Equal to 1 µg Retinol
Preformed vitamin A in food or supplements	1 µg
	1 RAE
	1 µg RE
	3.3 IU
β-carotene in foods*	12 µg
	1 RAE
	2 µg RE
	20 IU
α-carotene or β-cryptoxanthin in food	24 µg
	1 RAE
	2 µg RE
	40 IU

*β-carotene in supplements may be better absorbed than β-carotene in food and so provides more vitamin A activity. It is estimated that 2 µg of β-carotene dissolved in oil provides 1 µg of vitamin A activity.

Converting Vitamin E Values into mg α-Tocopherol

To estimate the α-tocopherol intake from foods:

- If values are given as mg α-TEs:
  $$\text{mg } \alpha\text{-TE} \times 0.8 = \text{mg } \alpha\text{-tocopherol}$$
- If values are given in IUs:
  First, determine if the source of the α-tocopherol is natural or synthetic.
- For natural α-tocopherol:
  $$\text{IU of natural } \alpha\text{-tocopherol} \times 0.67 = \text{mg } \alpha\text{-tocopherol}$$
- For synthetic α-tocopherol (dl-α-tocopherol):
  $$\text{IU of synthetic } \alpha\text{-tocopherol} \times 0.45 = \text{mg } \alpha\text{-tocopherol}$$

Source: Institute of Medicine, Food and Nutrition Board, http://www.nap.edu/catalog.php?record_id=9810 *Dietary Reference Intakes for Vitamin C, Vitamin E, Selenium, and Carotenoids* (2000). Available online at http://books.nap.edu/openbook.php?record_id=9810&page=192

Calculating Dietary Folate Equivalents in Fortified Foods

The folate listed on labels of fortified foods is primarily folic acid, which is more available than natural forms of folate. In order to compare the folate content of these foods to recommendations, the amount of folic acid must be converted to dietary folate equivalents, expressed as µg DFE. This calculation assumes that all of the folate in these foods is from added folic acid.

Determine the amount (µg) of folic acid in the fortified food:

- Multiply the Daily Value for folate by the % Daily Values listed on the label.
- Daily Value is 400 µg.

Convert the µg folic acid into µg DFE:

- Multiply the µg folic acid by 1.7.
- Folic acid added to a food in fortification provides 1.7 times more available folate per µg than folate naturally present in foods.

For example:

- A serving of English muffins provides 6% of the Daily Value for folate:
  To find the µg folic acid: 400 µg × 6% = 24 µg folic acid
  To convert to µg DFE: 24 µg folic acid × 1.7 = 41 µg DFE

Source: Institute of Medicine, food and Nutrition Board, http://www.nap.edu/catalog.php?record_id=6015 *Dietary Reference Intakes for Thiamin, Riboflavin, Niacin, Vitamin B6, Folate, Vitamin B12, Pantothenic Acid, Biotin, and Choline* (1998). Available online at http://books.nap.edu/openbook.php?record_id=6015&page=210

Appendix K
Answers to Case Studies

Chapter 1 What's Wrong with This Diet?

What's wrong with Helen's diet? Helen needs to increase the variety in her diet. Not only is she choosing the same foods every day, but she is not choosing foods from all of the food groups. She doesn't eat any fruit, and her only vegetable is lettuce. Increasing the variety of her diet will ensure she is meeting her nutrient needs as well as getting a variety of phytochemicals. She can still stick with a routine, but have different types of cereal every morning and top them with a variety of fresh and dried fruit. She can have sandwiches for lunch but make them using different types of breads and fillings. For dinner she can try different grains and a variety of vegetables rather than just rice and a salad. When she has a salad she can include a variety of greens, fruit, nuts, and seeds to add nutrients, texture, and taste.

Based on this photo, what might be wrong with Amy's diet? Amy's diet is varied, but based on this photograph, she is short on moderation. Her portions are large, and if the calories she consumes are not balanced with enough exercise, she will gain weight.

Chapter 2 Using Food Labels to Make Healthy Choices

Use the labels shown here to determine whether they are equivalent in terms of the amounts of saturated fat and added sugar. The old fashioned oats are much lower in saturated fat, providing only 0.5 gram per serving (3% of the Daily Value) compared to 3.5 grams of saturated fat (18% of the Daily Value) and a gram of *trans* fat in the granola. It is recommended that both saturated fat and *trans* fat be limited in the diet. The oats have no *trans* fat and only 0.5 gram saturated fat per serving (3% of the Daily Value). The granola is higher in sugars; 16 grams compared to 0 gram per serving in the oatmeal. The ingredient list tells us that no sugar has been added to the oats, but much of the sugar in the granola comes from added brown sugar, which is the third ingredient, with a small amount from honey.

Which choice provides more vitamin C? The orange juice provides more vitamin C: 120% of the Daily Value, compared to 100% of the Daily Value for the juice drink.

Other than water, what is the most abundant ingredient, by weight, in the juice drink? in the orange juice? High fructose corn syrup is the most abundant ingredient (other than water) in the juice drink. In the orange juice it is concentrated orange juice.

The added vitamin C increases the nutrient density of the juice drink, but does that make it a better choice than the orange juice? No. The juice drink provides less vitamin C than the orange juice, and it contains more total sugar, much of which is added sugar. The sugar in the orange juice is from the oranges used to make the juice and comes with the other nutrients and phytochemicals that are present in these oranges. These nutrients increase the nutrient density of the orange juice. The high fructose corn syrup used to sweeten the juice drink adds nothing but calories. Some of the sugar in the juice drink comes from fruit juice concentrates, which do add nutrients, but their placement on the ingredient list tells us that, by weight, they are present in smaller amounts than the high fructose corn syrup.

When Scott is choosing between more- and less-processed products, what advice would you give him? Choosing less-processed products usually means they are lower in added sugars (and salt – discussed in chapter 8) and contain more of the nutrients present in the original plant or animal product.

Chapter 3 How Do Changes in the GI Tract Affect Health?

What effect might this have on his nutrition and health? If he doesn't have enough saliva, he will have difficulty swallowing and tasting his food. This will decrease the appeal of food and may reduce his food intake. Also because saliva helps protect the teeth, the likelihood that he will develop cavities will increase.

How might this affect the digestion and absorption of nutrients contained in the carrots? If she can't chew the carrots well, the enzymes needed to digest them will not have access to all of the carrot. As a result, pieces will remain undigested and pass through the GI tract and the vitamins and minerals they contain will not be available for absorption.

How does this change affect the amount of fluid she needs to consume? Much of the water that enters the large intestine is absorbed there. If most of her large intestine is removed she will lose a lot more water and she will need to consume more fluid than before to prevent dehydration.

What type of foods should he avoid and why? He should avoid fatty foods. Bile is needed for fat absorption. Fat entering the small intestine causes the gallbladder to contract and release bile. A low-fat diet will minimize gallbladder contraction and the pain this causes.

Why can't she eat as much food as before or absorb all the nutrients from the food she eats? The surgery reduces the size of her stomach so she can only consume small amounts of food at any one time. Small meals are also important because the surgery bypasses the sphincter that regulates the entry of food into the small intestine. A large meal would allow too much material to enter the small intestine too rapidly and cause diarrhea. She does not absorb all the nutrients from her food because a section of the small intestine has been bypassed, reducing the area available for absorption. In addition, the smaller stomach may reduce the efficiency of both mechanical and chemical digestion in the stomach. Undigested food cannot be absorbed.

Chapter 4 Becoming Less Refined

How does her intake of grains, fruits, and vegetables compare with MyPyramid recommendations? MyPyramid recommends she consume 7 ounces of grains, half of which should be whole grains, 3 cups of vegetables, and 2 cups of fruit. She therefore consumes fewer grains than recommended and only about half as much fruit and vegetables.

Choose a combination of fruits and vegetables from this list that will add at least 13 grams of fiber to Guadalupe's diet. There are many possible answers. For example, a half-cup of beans, a cup of asparagus, and an apple will provide 14 grams of fiber. A cup of broccoli, 2 kiwis, and an orange provide almost 13 grams.

What are the carbohydrate pluses and minuses of these two choices? Neither the dried apricots not the granola bar is a good source of fiber, each providing only 8% of the Daily Value. The fiber in the granola bar comes from whole grain oats, the first ingredient in the list. Both choices are fairly high in sugar; 15 grams of sugars in the apricots and 11 in the granola bar. All of the sugar in the dried apricots comes from the fruit, whereas the sugar in the granola bar comes from added sugar (second ingredient in the ingredient list), with smaller amounts form honey and brown sugar syrup.

Chapter 5 Improving Heart Health

Which of the factors listed here increase Rafael's risk of developing cardiovascular disease? He has a family history of heart disease because his mother died of a heart attack before the age of 65. He is a smoker and is inactive, so his lifestyle further increases his risk. His blood pressure is elevated and his total blood cholesterol of 210 mg/100 mL is over the recommended maximum of 200 mg/100 mL. His LDL cholesterol of 160 mg/100 mL is also above the recommended maximum of 100 mg/100 mL and his HDL cholesterol is less than the recommended minimum 40 mg/100 mL. His triglycerides are in the healthy range.

What could he choose at his favorite fast-food restaurant to reduce his intake of saturated fat? A grilled chicken sandwich would be lower in saturated fat than a cheeseburger. A vegetarian pizza would be lower than a triple-meat option. A chicken taco would be lower in saturated fat than a burrito with beef and cheese.

Which of the following snack choices is the most heart healthy? Give two reasons. The fruit and nut mixture is the more heart healthy choice because nuts are a good source of heart healthy monounsaturated fatty acids. A serving provides 3.5 grams of monounsaturated fat, only one gram of saturated fat, and no *trans* fat. The cheese crackers have 14 grams of total fat per serving of which 3.5 grams is saturated, 4 grams is *trans* fat, and only 1 gram is monounsaturated fat. The cheese crackers are low in cholesterol, with only 5 mg, but the fruit and nut mix has no cholesterol. The fruit and nut mix is also a better choice when it comes to fiber. It provides 2 grams per serving compared to less than one gram in the cheese crackers.

Chapter 6 Is a Vegetarian Diet Always Healthy?

What is the RDA for protein for someone of Simon's age and weight? The RDA is 0.8 grams per kilogram of body weight. Simon weighs 154 pounds, which is 70 kilograms (154 lbs ÷ 2.2 lbs/kg = 70 kg). Therefore his recommended protein intake is 56 g per day (70 kg × 0.8 g/kg = 56 g).

This is a photo of Simon's typical lunch. Why is it high in saturated fat? Whole fat dairy products are high in total fat and saturated fat. The cheese provides about 4 grams of saturated fat per ounce. The 2 ounces of cheese on this sandwich would have about 8 grams of saturated fat. If butter was used to grill the sandwich it adds about 7 grams of saturated fat per tablespoon.

Is this diet providing all the health benefits of a vegetarian diet? No. Simon may not be eating meat, but he is consuming lots of high fat dairy products. Since these are animal products they can be high in saturated fat and cholesterol. His diet is also low in fruits and vegetables. He has cereal for breakfast, which might be a whole grain, but the pizza or lasagna he has for dinner is probably not made with whole grain. So he is not benefiting from the high intake of whole grains, fruits, and vegetables, and the low saturated fat and cholesterol content typical of a healthy vegetarian diet.

What could be included in Simon's vegan diet to meet his needs for calcium and vitamin D? To increase his calcium intake he could eat more leafy green vegetables and legumes, which are a good source of calcium and use calcium fortified products like orange juice, soymilk, and breakfast cereal. To make sure he gets enough vitamin D he could spend plenty of time outdoors in the sun to boost vitamin D synthesis in his skin and use vitamin D-fortified breakfast cereal and soymilk to boost his vitamin D intake.

Suggest a sandwich Simon could have for lunch that makes use of complementary plant proteins. Peanut butter (legumes) and bread (grain) provide complimentary proteins. Another option is hummus, which is made from chickpeas (legume), with bread.

Chapter 7 How Much Vitamin A Is in Your Fast-Food Meal?

Which of the meals shown here is higher in vitamin A? Which ingredients are sources of vitamin A? The pizza is higher in vitamin A because it has cheese, which is a source of preformed vitamin A and tomato sauce, tomatoes, and peppers, which provide provitamin A. The beef, bun, and fries in the other meal are all poor sources of vitamin A.

What could John add to his breakfast and lunch to provide some good sources of vitamin A? He could boost his provitamin A intake by adding a carotenoid-rich fruit such as cantaloupe, mango, or apricots to his breakfast. He could increase his intake of preformed vitamin A by replacing the soda he has at lunch with a glass of milk. He could add some high-carotenoid vegetables to his lunch. For example, he could put some sweet red peppers and spinach on his sandwich and bring a bag of baby carrots to crunch on.

John's meals are also low in vitamin C. What could he add to his breakfast and lunch to increase his intake of vitamin C? The key to increasing vitamin C intake is increasing fruit and vegetable intake. Adding fruits such as strawberries or a glass of orange juice at breakfast and an orange or kiwis at lunch will add vitamin C. Including some sliced sweet peppers or raw broccoli florets with his lunch will provide vegetable source of vitamin C.

Chapter 8 Avoiding Anemia

What puts Hanna at risk for iron deficiency anemia? She is a lacto-ovo vegetarian so she does not consume highly absorbable heme iron. She is a menstruating female so her iron losses are high.

What does the blood test reveal about Hanna's iron status? Is her tiredness due to iron deficiency anemia? Why or why not? No, her iron stores are depleted and iron levels in her plasma are low, but the amount of iron in her red blood cells is still normal so her symptoms are not due to iron deficiency anemia.

Name three dietary factors that put Hanna at risk for iron deficiency. Her overall iron intake is low and she consumes only nonheme iron, which is poorly absorbed. Her diet is high whole grains, which reduce iron absorption because they are high in phytates. She drinks a lot if tea, which is high in tannins, which inhibit iron absorption.

What could Hanna do to increase the absorption of the nonheme iron in her diet? Include a source of vitamin C, such as an orange, with meals that contain iron.

Chapter 9 Balancing Energy: Genetics and Lifestyle

What is her BMI? Is it in the healthy range? Ashya is 64 inches tall and weighs 155 lbs:

Her BMI is equal to 155 lbs $\div$ (64 in)^2 = 26.6 kg/m^2, which is in the overweight range.

What is her EER?
Ashya is 64 inches tall and weighs 155 lbs:

$$64 \text{ in.} \times 0.0254 \text{ m/in.} = 1.63 \text{ m}$$
$$155 \text{ lbs} \div 2.2 \text{ lbs/kg} = 70.4 \text{ kg}$$

Ashya is in the low active activity category, so PA = 1.12

Using the equation in table 9.1 Aysha's EER is equal to:

$$\text{EER} = 354 - (6.91 \times 23 \text{ yrs}) + 1.12[(9.36 \times 70.4 \text{ kg}) + (726 \times 1.63 \text{ m}) = 2259 \text{ Calories}$$

Note: This answer uses the EER equations in Table 9.1. Because Ashya is overweight, it is more accurate to use the equations in Appendix A for calculating the total energy expenditure of individuals who are overweight or obese:

$$\text{TEE} = 448 - (7.95 \times 23 \text{ yrs}) + 1.16[(11.4 \times 70.4 \text{ kg}) + (619 \times 1.63 \text{ m}) = 2367 \text{ Calories}$$

How does Aysha's EER compare with her intake? Is she in energy balance? She consumes about 2450 Calories per day but is expending only 2259 Calories per day, so she is not in energy balance. She is consuming 191 Calories per day more than she is expending.

How can Meal B have fewer calories even though it looks like more food? The meal on the left is much higher is fat (9 Calories/gram), making it more energy dense. The vegetables in the sandwich and the fruit in the meal on the right are high in fiber and water, which add bulk and volume to the meal, but provide few calories.

Why might Meal B satisfy hunger just as well as or better than Meal A? The high fat content of the meal on the left provides satiety. In the meal on the right, the fiber in the whole grain bread and the fiber and fluid in the apple and vegetables help fill up your stomach and provide satiety.

If Aysha adds an additional 30 minutes of moderate-intensity exercise every day, by how much will her EER increase? This will boost Ashya into the active physical activity category and her EER will increase to:

$$\text{EER} = 354 - (6.91 \times 23 \text{ yrs}) + 1.27[(9.36 \times 70.4 \text{ kg}) + (726 \times 1.63 \text{ m}) = 2535 \text{ Calories}$$

If the equation from Appendix A for calculating the total energy expenditure of individuals who are overweight or obese is used:

$$\text{TEE} = 448 - (7.95 \times 23 \text{ yrs}) + 1.27[(11.4 \times 70.4 \text{ kg}) + (619 \times 1.63 \text{ m}) = 2566 \text{ Calories}$$

Do you think Aysha is destined to be overweight? Explain your answer. Ashya is not destined to be overweight, but to maintain her weight in a healthy range she probably needs to monitor her energy intake more carefully and exercise more than an individual with no genetic tendency to store excess body fat. If she makes small changes in her diet and exercise patterns that she can stick with, she is more likely to succeed.

Chapter 10 What Are You Getting from That Sports Bar?

What are the advantages and disadvantages of sports bars? The biggest advantage of sports bars is their convenience. They are pre-portioned, ready to eat, and transportable. They may also provide a psychological edge if the consumer believes they will enhance performance. A disadvantage is that they are expensive and do not provide everything you get from food. If they take the place of the whole grains, fresh vegetables and fruits, low-fat dairy products, and lean meats or meat substitutes that make up a healthy diet, the overall quality of the diet may suffer. They also don't provide fluid – an essential during any activity. If you choose to use these bars, wash them down with plenty of water. They do provide calories, generally about 200 to 300 per bar. Even though they are eaten to support activity they still add to your overall energy intake and can contribute to weight gain if consumed in excess.

Based on the labels shown here, how do sports bars differ from candy bars? Typically sports bars are lower in total fat, saturated fat, cholesterol, and sugar; higher in fiber and protein; and contain more vitamins and minerals than candy bars.

Suggest a snack for Mark that is nutritionally comparable to a sports bar but less expensive. Granola or cereal bars, fruit filled cookies, and fresh or dried fruit, sandwich, bagel, trail mix.

Chapter 11 Nutrient Needs for a Successful Pregnancy

Based on the graph below, how much weight would you recommend that Tina gain? Why would gaining only 20 pounds or gaining 50 pounds put the baby at risk? The graph illustrates that the incidence of low-birth-weight babies increases as maternal weight gain decreases, but as maternal weight gain increases the incidence of large-for-gestational age babies increases. Based on this graph, to minimize having a high- or low-birth-weight baby, Tina should gain between 20 and 35 pounds.

How should the amounts of food from each food group be changed in order for Tina to meet her needs during the second trimester of her pregnancy? Based on Tina's MyPyramid Plan for Moms, she should consume 8 ounces of grains, 3 cups of vegetables, 2 cups of fruit, 3 cups of milk, and 6.5 ounces from the meat and beans group. She would therefore need to add 1.5 cups of vegetables, 1 cup of fruit, 1 cup of milk, and 0.5 ounce of meat and beans to her current diet.

Suggest some foods that Tina could include in her diet in order to obtain an additional 13.5 mg of iron. Red meat is the best source of absorbable heme iron. Fortified breakfast cereals, legumes, and leafy greens are good sources of nonheme iron.

Do you think it is reasonable for Tina to consume 27 mg of iron each day from her diet alone? Why or why not? No. Even if she chose all of the foods listed above in one day she would still not consume enough.

Chapter 12 Under- and Overnutrition

Based on this growth chart, how has Sam's BMI percentile changed over the past year? Sam's BMI has gone from about the 65th percentile to the 87th percentile in just a few months. The increase in BMI indicates that his weight gain was not accompanied by a corresponding increase in height. This weight gain moves Sam from the healthy weight range into the overweight range.

What nutrients are likely to be excessive or deficient in this dietary pattern? The diet is high in added sugar and fat from the doughnuts, candy, and chips. The whole milk Sam drinks adds calcium, total fat, saturated fat, and cholesterol. His intake from all the food groups except milk and possibly grains is low so he is likely to consume less than the recommended amounts of vitamin C, vitamin A, and iron.

Why might excessive consumption of dairy products contribute to Sam's anemia? Calcium interferes with iron absorption. Sam seems to have milk with every meal so he is probably consuming calcium with the iron in his meals and the calcium is reducing iron absorption.

How might Sam's iron deficiency have contributed to his weight gain? Iron deficiency causes fatigue and lethargy, which would have caused a decrease in his activity level, shifting his energy balance toward weight gain.

Chapter 13 Food Detectives

Based on the graph, which food is the most likely cause of the illness? Why? The frozen custard is most likely to be the cause because a greater number of people who ate the custard because ill than for any of the other foods.

How can eggs become contaminated with *Salmonella*? The outside of the eggs can become contaminated with *Salmonella* when they come in contact with fecal material in the chicken coop. The inside of the egg can be contaminated with *Salmonella* before the shell is formed if the hen is infected with *Salmonella*. Therefore, raw eggs can cause *Salmonella* food-borne illness even if the shell is clean.

The cookie and cupcake recipes also called for eggs. Why are these unlikely to be the cause of the problem? Both of these foods were cooked after the eggs were added. The cooking temperature was high enough to kill the bacteria.

Suggest a reason why 20 children who consumed the frozen custard did not get ill. They may have consumed smaller amounts of custard. They may have been larger children. It take more bacteria to make a larger person ill than a smaller person.

What could the fourth-graders have done to avoid the risk of *Salmonella* in their frozen custard? They could have used an ice cream recipe that did not call for eggs or used pasteurized liquid eggs instead of whole eggs from the shell.

Chapter 14 What Can You Do?

What are the advantages and disadvantages of these salad options in terms of convenience, food safety, and environmental impact? The prepackaged lettuce in the grocery store is more convenient. It is pre-washed and just needs to be poured into a bowl. The disadvantage is that once open it has goes bad more quickly, it uses more energy to produce and it generates plastic waste from the bags. The unpackaged produce requires more washing and cutting to make your salad but uses fewer of the earth's resources.

The following are some inexpensive changes Keesha can make to reduce her impact on the environment. What are the advantages and disadvantages of each?

Action	Advantages	Disadvantages
Bike instead of drive on short trips around town.	Uses no gas so saves money, reduces fossil fuel use, and reduces pollution, as well as increases your fitness level.	Difficult to carry heavy or bulky items, and requires more time for each errand.
Buy a canvas bag to carry groceries.	Reduces the number of plastic grocery bags that must be disposed of.	Small monetary cost of the bags.
Bring juice in a thermos instead of buying a nonrecyclable bottle.	Reduces the amount of material that ends up in landfills.	Must be washed after each use. This takes time and uses energy to heat water and generates waste water.
Compost vegetable scraps.	Reduces the amount of material that ends up in landfills and generates fertile material that can be added to a garden.	Cost and time needed to set up and maintain a composting bin.
Buy locally grown produce.	Contains fewer pesticides. Likely to be fresher because it is purchased soon after harvest.	Less variety. Not everything is available at all times of the year.
Buy organically grown produce.	Reduces the pesticides on food. Reduces the environmental damage associated with food production.	Costs more. Occasionally has more insect damage.

Appendix L
Answers to Self-Tests

Chapter 1: 1b; 2d; 3a; 4b; 5c; 6c; 7d; 8a; 9d; 10d; 11a; 12c; 13c; 14b; 15a

Chapter 2: 1d; 2c; 3d; 4a; 5b; 6a; 7a; 8d; 9c; 10c; 11e; 12e; 13a; 14b; 15d

Chapter 3: 1c; 2e; 3a; 4d; 5c; 6c; 7b; 8a; 9c; 10b; 11c; 12b; 13c; 14a; 15b

Chapter 4: 1c; 2b; 3b; 4a; 5d; 6c; 7b; 8d; 9c; 10c; 11b; 12a; 13a; 14a; 15d

Chapter 5: 1d; 2a; 3e; 4d; 5b; 6b; 7c; 8e; 9e; 10c; 11a; 12c; 13a; 14c; 15a

Chapter 6: 1d; 2a; 3c; 4e; 5a; 6b; 7c; 8a; 9b; 10d; 11c; 12b; 13d; 14b; 15a

Chapter 7: 1d; 2a; 3b; 4c; 5d; 6d; 7c; 8e; 9a; 10c; 11b; 12c; 13e; 14b; 15c

Chapter 8: 1d; 2e; 3b; 4e; 5d; 6a; 7b; 8a; 9c; 10e; 11b; 12e; 13b; 14a; 15c

Chapter 9: 1c; 2e; 3a; 4d; 5a; 6c; 7d; 8c; 9b; 10c; 11a; 12b; 13b; 14e; 15d

Chapter 10: 1a; 2e; 3d; 4a; 5a; 6b; 7c; 8b; 9a; 10d; 11a; 12c; 13c; 14a; 15b

Chapter 11: 1b; 2b; 3d; 4d; 5c; 6b; 7a; 8a; 9b; 10d; 11b; 12c; 13a; 14c; 15c

Chapter 12: 1d; 2b; 3a; 4c; 5d; 6b; 7e; 8c; 9a; 10b; 11c; 12a; 13c; 14a; 15b

Chapter 13: 1b; 2e; 3b; 4a; 5c; 6b; 7b; 8c; 9a; 10c; 11b; 12d; 13c; 14a; 15b

Chapter 14: 1d; 2c; 3a; 4d; 5c; 6c; 7b; 8b; 9c; 10b; 11a; 12b; 13d; 14d; 15a

GLOSSARY

absorption   The process of taking substances from the gastrointestinal tract into the interior of the body.

acceptable daily intake (ADI)   The amount of food additive that can be consumed daily over a lifetime without appreciable health risk to a person on the basis of all the known facts at the time of the evaluation.

Acceptable Macronutrient Distribution Ranges (AMDRs)   Healthy ranges of intake for carbohydrate, fat, and protein, expressed as percentages of total energy intake.

accidental contaminants   Substances not regulated by the FDA that unexpectedly enter the food supply.

acrylamide   A chemical created in foods when starches and other carbohydrates are overheated (over 120°C or 250°F) during cooking, that may be a carcinogen.

active transport   The transport of substances across a cell membrane with the aid of a carrier molecule and the expenditure of energy.

Adequate Intakes (AIs)   Nutrient intakes that should be used as a goal when no RDA exists. AI values are an approximation of the nutrient intake that sustains health.

adipocytes   Cells that store fat.

adipose tissue   Tissue found under the skin and around body organs that is composed of fat-storing cells.

adjustable gastric banding   A surgical procedure in which an adjustable band is placed around the upper portion of the stomach to limit the volume that the stomach can hold and the rate of stomach emptying.

adolescent growth spurt   An 18- to 24-month period of peak growth velocity that begins at about ages 10 to 13 in girls and 12 to 15 in boys.

aerobic capacity   The maximum amount of oxygen that can be consumed by the tissues during exercise. Also called maximal oxygen consumption, or VO_2 max.

aerobic exercise   Endurance exercise that increases heart rate and uses oxygen to produce energy as ATP.

aerobic metabolism   Metabolism in the presence of oxygen. It can completely break down glucose to yield carbon dioxide, water, and energy in the form of ATP.

aerobic zone   A rate of activity that raises the heart rate to between 60 and 85% of maximum heart rate.

age-related bone loss   The bone loss that occurs in both men and women as they advance in age.

aging   The inevitable accumulation of changes associated with and responsible for an ever-increasing susceptibility to disease and death.

alcohol   An energy-containing molecule that contains 7 Calories per gram and is made by the fermentation of carbohydrates from plant products; the type of alcohol that is consumed in the diet is called ethanol.

alcohol poisoning   Potentially fatal mental confusion, stupor, vomiting, seizures, slow irregular breathing, and/or hypothermia caused by depression of the central nervous system due to excessive alcohol consumption.

alcoholic hepatitis   Inflammation of the liver caused by alcohol consumption.

alcoholism   A chronic disorder characterized by dependence on alcohol, with repeated excessive use of alcoholic beverages and development of withdrawal symptoms when alcohol intake is reduced.

alcohol-related birth defects (ARBD)   Malformations in the skeleton or major organ systems that are linked to prenatal alcohol exposure.

alcohol-related neurodevelopmental disorders (ARND)   Functional or mental impairments linked to prenatal alcohol exposure.

aldosterone   A hormone secreted by the adrenal glands that increases sodium reabsorption and therefore enhances water reabsorption by the kidney.

allergen   A substance that causes an allergic reaction.

alpha-carotene (α-carotene)   A carotenoid, some of which can be converted into vitamin A, that is found in leafy green vegetables, carrots, and squash.

alpha-linolenic acid (α-linolenic acid)   An 18-carbon omega-3 polyunsaturated fatty acid known to be essential in humans.

alpha-tocopherol (α-tocopherol)   The form of tocopherol (vitamin E) active in humans.

Alzheimer's disease   A disease that results in a relentless and irreversible loss of mental function.

amenorrhea   Delayed onset of menstruation or the absence of three or more consecutive menstrual cycles.

amino acid pool   All the amino acids in body tissues and fluids that are available for use by the body.

amino acids   The building blocks of proteins. Each contains an amino group, an acid group, and a unique side chain.

anabolic steroids   Synthetic fat-soluble hormones that mimic testosterone and are used to increase muscle strength and mass.

anaerobic metabolism   Metabolism in the absence of oxygen.

anorexia nervosa   An eating disorder characterized by self-starvation, a distorted body image, and abnormally low body weight.

antibodies   Proteins, released by a type of lymphocyte, that interact with and deactivate specific antigens.

antidiuretic hormone (ADH)   A hormone secreted by the pituitary gland that increases the amount of water reabsorbed by the kidney and therefore retained in the body.

antigen   A foreign substance that, when introduced into the body, stimulates an immune response.

antioxidant   A substance that is able to neutralize reactive oxygen molecules and thereby prevent cell damage.

appetite   A desire to consume specific foods that is independent of hunger.

arachidonic acid   A 20-carbon omega-6 polyunsaturated fatty acid that can be synthesized from linoleic acid.

arteries   Blood vessels that carry blood away from the heart.

arterioles   Small arteries that carry blood to capillaries.

arthritis   A disease characterized by inflammation of the joints, pain, and sometimes changes in structure.

ascorbic acid   The chemical term for vitamin C.

556

aseptic processing The placement of sterilized food in a sterilized package using a sterile process.

atherosclerosis A type of cardiovascular disease that involves the buildup of fatty material in the artery walls.

atherosclerotic plaque Cholesterol-rich material that is deposited in the arteries of individuals with atherosclerosis. It consists of cholesterol, smooth muscle cells, fibrous tissue, and eventually calcium.

atoms The smallest units of an element that retain the properties of the element.

ATP (adenosine triphosphate) A high-energy molecule that the body uses to power activities that require energy.

atrophic gastritis An inflammation of the stomach lining that results in reduced secretion of stomach acid, microbial overgrowth, and, in severe cases, a reduction in the production of intrinsic factor.

atrophy Wasting or decrease in the size of a muscle or other tissue caused by lack of use.

attention-deficit/hyperactivity disorder (ADHD) A condition characterized by a short attention span and a high level of activity, excitability, and distractibility.

autoimmune disease A disease that results from immune reactions that destroy normal body cells.

basal metabolic rate (BMR) The rate of energy expenditure under resting conditions. It is measured after 12 hours without food or exercise.

basal metabolism The energy expended to maintain an awake, resting body that is not digesting food.

behavior modification A process that is used to gradually and permanently change habitual behaviors.

beriberi A thiamin deficiency disease that causes weakness, nerve degeneration, and, in some cases, heart changes.

beta-carotene (β-carotene) A pigment found in many yellow and red-orange fruits and vegetables that is a precursor of vitamin A. It is also an antioxidant.

beta-cryptoxanthin (β-cryptoxanthin) A carotenoid found in corn, green peppers, and lemons that can provide some vitamin A activity.

bicarbonate A chemical released by the pancreas into the small intestine that neutralizes stomach acid.

bile A digestive fluid made in the liver and stored in the gallbladder that is released into the small intestine, where it aids in fat digestion and absorption.

binge drinking The consumption of five or more drinks in a row for males or four or more for females.

binge-eating disorder An eating disorder characterized by recurrent episodes of binge eating in the absence of purging behavior.

bioaccumulation The process by which compounds accumulate or build up in an organism faster than they can be broken down or excreted.

bioavailability The extent to which the body can absorb and use a nutrient.

biotechnology The process of manipulating life forms via genetic engineering in order to provide desirable products for human use.

biotin One of the B vitamins, needed in energy production.

blackout drinking Amnesia following a period of excessive alcohol consumption.

blood pressure The amount of force exerted by the blood against the walls of arteries.

body composition The term used to describe the different components **(lean versus fat tissues)** that when taken together make up an individual's body weight.

body image The way a person perceives and imagines his or her body.

body mass index (BMI) A measure of body weight relative to height that is used to compare body size with a standard.

bolus A ball of chewed food mixed with saliva.

bone remodeling A continuous process in which small amounts of bone are removed and replaced by new bone.

bone resorption The process by which bone is broken down by osteoclasts releasing calcium from bone to the blood.

botulism A severe food-borne intoxication that results from consuming the toxin produced by *Clostridium botulinum*.

bovine somatotropin (bST) A hormone naturally produced by cows that stimulates the production of milk. A synthetic version of this hormone is now being produced by genetic engineering.

bovine spongiform encephalopathy (BSE) A fatal neurological disease that affects cattle (mad cow disease) and may be transmitted to humans by consuming contaminated beef by-products.

bran The protective outer layers of whole grains. It is a concentrated source of dietary fiber.

brush border The microvilli surface of the intestinal mucosa, which contains some digestive enzymes.

bulimia nervosa An eating disorder characterized by the consumption of a large amount of food at one time (binge eating) followed by purging behaviors such as self-induced vomiting to prevent weight gain.

calcitonin A hormone produced by the thyroid gland that stimulates bone mineralization and inhibits bone breakdown, thus lowering blood calcium levels.

calorie A unit of measure used to express the amount of energy provided by different kinds of food.

capillaries Small, thin-walled blood vessels through which blood and the body's cells exchange gases and nutrients.

carbohydrate loading or **glycogen supercompensation** A regimen designed to increase muscle glycogen stores beyond their usual capacity.

carbohydrates A class of nutrients that includes sugars, starches, and fibers. Chemically, they all contain carbon, along with hydrogen and oxygen, in the same proportions as in water (H_2O).

cardiorespiratory endurance The efficiency with which the body delivers to cells the oxygen and nutrients needed for muscular activity and transports waste products from cells.

cardiovascular disease Any disease affecting the heart and blood vessels.

cardiovascular system The system of heart and blood vessels that circulate blood throughout the body.

carotenoids Natural pigments synthesized by plants and many microorganisms.

They give yellow and red-orange fruits and vegetables their color.

cash crops   Crops that are grown to be sold for monetary return rather than as food for the local population.

cataracts   A disease of the eye that results in cloudy spots on the lens (and sometimes the cornea), which obscure vision.

celiac disease   A disorder that causes damage to the intestines when the protein gluten is eaten.

cell differentiation   Structural and functional changes that cause cells to mature into specialized cells.

cells   The basic structural and functional units of living things.

cellular respiration   The reactions that break down carbohydrates, fats, and proteins to produce carbon dioxide, water, and energy in the form of ATP.

cellulose   An insoluble fiber that is the most prevalent structural material of plant cell walls.

cesarean section   The surgical removal of the fetus from the uterus.

cholesterol   A sterol, produced by the liver and consumed in the diet, that is needed to build cell membranes and make hormones and other essential molecules. High blood levels increase the risk of heart disease.

choline   A compound needed for the synthesis of the phospholipid phosphatidylcholine and neurotransmitter acetylcholine. It is important for a number of biochemical reactions, and there is evidence that it is essential in the diet during certain stages of life.

chylomicrons   Lipoproteins that transport lipids from the mucosal cells of the small intestine and deliver triglycerides to other body cells.

chyme   A mixture of partially digested food and stomach secretions.

cirrhosis   Chronic and irreversible liver disease characterized by loss of functioning liver cells and accumulation of fibrous connective tissue.

cobalamin   The chemical term for vitamin B_{12}.

coenzymes   Organic nonprotein substances that bind to enzymes to promote their activity.

cofactor   An inorganic ion or coenzyme that is required for enzyme activity.

collagen   The major protein in connective tissue.

colostrum   The first milk, produced by the breast late in pregnancy and for up to a week after delivery. Compared to mature milk, it contains more water, protein, immune factors, minerals, and vitamins and less fat.

complex carbohydrates   Carbohydrates composed of sugar molecules linked together in straight or branching chains. They include oligosaccharides, starches, and fibers.

conditionally essential amino acids   Amino acids that are essential in the diet only under certain conditions or at certain times of life; also called semiessential amino acids.

constipation   Infrequent or difficult defecation.

control group   In a scientific experiment, the group of participants used as a basis of comparison. They are similar to the participants in the experimental group but do not receive the treatment being tested.

creatine   A compound that can be converted into creatine phosphate, which replenishes muscle ATP during short bursts of activity. Creatine is a dietary supplement used by athletes to increase muscle mass and delay fatigue during short intense exercise.

creatine phosphate   A compound stored in muscle that can be broken down quickly to make ATP.

cretinism   A condition resulting from poor maternal iodine intake during pregnancy that impairs mental development and growth in the offspring.

critical control points   Possible points in food production, manufacturing, and transportation where contamination could occur or be prevented or eliminated.

critical period   Time in growth and development when an organism is more susceptible to harm from poor nutrition or other environmental factors.

cross-contamination   The transfer of contaminants from one food or object to another.

cycle of malnutrition   A cycle in which malnutrition is perpetuated by an inability to meet nutrient needs at all life stages.

Daily Value   A reference value for the intake of nutrients used on food labels to help consumers see how a given food fits into their overall diet.

DASH (Dietary Approaches to Stop Hypertension) diet   A dietary pattern recommended to lower blood pressure. It is abundant in fruits and vegetables; includes low-fat dairy products, whole grains, legumes, and nuts; and incorporates moderate amounts of lean meat.

deamination   The removal of the amino group from an amino acid

dehydration   A state that occurs when not enough water is present to meet the body's needs.

Delaney Clause   A clause added to the 1958 Food Additives Amendment of the Pure Food and Drug Act that prohibits the intentional addition to foods of any compound that has been shown to induce cancer in animals or humans at any dose.

dementia   A deterioration of mental state that results in impaired memory, thinking, and/or judgment.

denaturation   Alteration of a protein's three-dimensional structure.

dental caries   Cavities, or decay of the tooth enamel caused by acid produced when bacteria growing on the teeth metabolize carbohydrate.

designer foods or **nutraceuticals**   Foods or supplements thought to have health benefits in addition to their nutritive value.

diabetes mellitus   A disease characterized by elevated blood glucose due to either insufficient production of insulin or decreased sensitivity of cells to insulin.

diarrhea   An intestinal disorder characterized by frequent or watery stools.

dietary folate equivalents (*DFEs*)   The amount of folate equivalent to 1 μg of folate naturally occurring in food, 0.6 μg of synthetic folic acid from fortified food or supplements consumed with food, or 0.5 μg synthetic folic acid consumed on an empty stomach.

Dietary Guidelines for Americans   A set of nutrition recommendations designed to promote population-wide dietary changes to reduce the incidence of nutrition-related chronic disease.

Dietary Reference Intakes *(DRIs)* A set of four reference values for the intake of nutrients and food components that can be used for planning and assessing the diets of healthy people in the United States and Canada.

dietary supplements Products sold to supplement the diet; may include nutrients (vitamins, minerals, amino acids, fatty acids), enzymes, herbs, or other substances.

diffusion The movement of molecules from an area of higher concentration to an area of lower concentration without the expenditure of energy.

digestion The process by which food is broken down into components small enough to be absorbed into the body.

dipeptide Two amino acids linked by a peptide bond.

direct food additives Substances intentionally added to foods. They are regulated by the FDA.

disaccharide A carbohydrate made up of two sugar units.

discretionary calories The calories remaining after an individual has met recommended intake levels with healthy choices from all the food groups.

diuretic A substance that increases the amount of urine passed from the body.

diverticula Sacs or pouches that protrude from the wall of the large intestine.

diverticulitis A condition in which diverticula in the large intestine become inflamed.

diverticulosis A condition in which outpouches (or sacs) form in the wall of the large intestine.

docosahexaenoic acid (DHA) A 22-carbon omega-3 polyunsaturated fatty acid found in fish that may be needed in the diet of newborns. It can be synthesized from α-linolenic acid.

Down syndrome A disorder caused by extra genetic material that results in distinctive facial characteristics, mental impairment, and other abnormalities.

eating disorder A psychological illness characterized by specific abnormal eating behaviors, often intended to control weight.

eating disorders not otherwise specified (EDNOS) A category of eating disorders that do not fit the exact definition of anorexia nervosa or bulimia nervosa.

eclampsia Convulsions or seizures brought on by seriously high blood pressure during pregnancy (preeclampsia). Untreated, it can lead to coma or death.

edema Swelling due to the buildup of extracellular fluid in the tissues.

eicosanoids Regulatory molecules that can be synthesized from omega-3 and omega-6 fatty acids.

eicosapentaenoic acid *(EPA)* A 20-carbon-omega-3 polyunsaturated fatty acid found in fish that can be synthesized from α-linolenic acid but may be essential in humans under some conditions.

electrolytes Positively and negatively charged ions that conduct an electrical current in solution. Commonly refers to sodium, potassium, and chloride.

elements Substances that cannot be broken down into products with different properties.

embryo The developing human from two through eight weeks after fertilization.

empty calories Energy with few additional nutrients.

emulsifiers Substances with both water-soluble and fat-soluble portions that can break fat into tiny droplets and suspend it in a watery fluid.

endorphins Compounds that cause a natural euphoria and reduce the perception of pain under certain stressful conditions.

endosperm The largest portion of a kernel of grain. It is primarily starch and serves as a food supply for the sprouting seed.

energy balance The amount of energy consumed in the diet compared with the amount expended by the body over a given period.

energy-yielding nutrients Nutrients that can be metabolized to produce energy in the body. They include carbohydrates, fats, and proteins.

enrichment The addition of specific amounts of thiamin, riboflavin, niacin, and iron to refined grains. Since 1998 folic acid has also been added to enriched grains.

enzymes Protein molecules that accelerate the rate of specific chemical reactions without themselves being changed.

epidemiology The branch of science that studies health and disease trends and patterns in populations.

epiglottis A piece of elastic connective tissue that covers the opening to the lungs during swallowing.

ergogenic aid A substance, appliance, or procedure that improves athletic performance.

essential amino acids (also called **indispensable amino acids**) Amino acids that cannot be synthesized by the body in sufficient amounts to meet its needs and therefore must be included in the diet.

essential fatty acid deficiency A condition characterized by dry, scaly skin and poor growth that results when the diet does not supply sufficient amounts of linoleic acid and α-linolenic acid.

essential fatty acids Fatty acids that must be consumed in the diet because they cannot be made by the body or cannot be made in sufficient quantities to meet needs.

essential nutrients Nutrients that a person must consume in order to maintain health.

Estimated Average Requirements (EARs) Nutrient intakes estimated to meet the needs of 50% of the healthy individuals in a given gender and life-stage group.

Estimated Energy Requirements (EERs) Average energy intake values predicted to maintain body weight in healthy individuals.

ethanol The alcohol in alcoholic beverages; it is produced by yeast fermentation of sugar.

Exchange Lists A system of grouping foods based on their carbohydrate, protein, fat, and energy content.

experimental group In a scientific experiment, the group of participants who undergo the treatment being tested.

extreme obesity or morbid obesity A body mass index is greater than 40.

facilitated diffusion Assisted diffusion of a substance across the cell membrane.

failure to thrive   Inability of a child's growth to keep up with normal growth curves.

famine   A widespread lack of access to food due to a disaster that causes a collapse in the food production and marketing systems.

fasting hypoglycemia   Low blood sugar that is not related to food intake; often caused by an insulin-secreting tumor.

fatigue   Inability to continue an activity at an optimal level.

fat-soluble vitamins   Vitamins that do not dissolve in water; includes vitamins A, D, E, and K.

fatty acids   Molecules made up of a chain of carbons linked to hydrogens, with an acid group at one end of the chain.

fatty liver   The accumulation of fat in the liver.

feces   Body waste, including unabsorbed food residue, bacteria, mucus, and dead cells, which is eliminated from the gastrointestinal tract by way of the anus.

female athlete triad   The combination of disordered eating, amenorrhea, and osteoporosis that occurs in some female athletes, particularly those involved in sports in which low body weight and appearance are important.

fertilization   The union of a sperm and an egg.

fetal alcohol syndrome (FAS)   A characteristic group of physical and mental abnormalities in an infant resulting from maternal alcohol consumption during pregnancy.

fetus   A developing human from the ninth week after fertilization to birth.

fiber   A type of carbohydrate that cannot be digested by humans.

fibrin   The protein formed during normal blood clotting that is the essence of the clot.

fitness   A set of attributes related to the ability to perform routine physical activities without undue fatigue.

fluorosis   A condition caused by chronic overconsumption of fluoride, characterized by black and brown stains and cracking and pitting of the teeth.

foam cells   Cholesterol-filled white blood cells.

folate   A general term that refers to the many forms of this B vitamin, which is needed for the synthesis of DNA and the metabolism of some amino acids.

folic acid   An easily absorbed form of the vitamin folate that is present in dietary supplements and fortified foods.

food additive   A substance that is intentionally added to or can reasonably be expected to become a component of a food during processing.

food allergy   An adverse immune response to a specific food protein.

food-borne illness   An illness caused by consumption of contaminated food.

food-borne infection   Illness produced by the ingestion of food containing microorganisms that can multiply inside the body and produce effects that are injurious.

food-borne intoxication   Illness caused by consuming a food containing a toxin.

food guides   Food group systems that suggest amounts of different types of foods needed to meet nutrient intake recommendations.

food insecurity   A situation in which people lack adequate physical, social, or economic access to sufficient, safe, nutritious food that meets their dietary needs and food preferences for an active and healthy life.

food intolerance, or **food sensitivity**   An adverse reaction to a food that does not involve the production of antibodies by the immune system.

food recovery   The collection of wholesome food for distribution to the poor and hungry, including collection of crops from farmers' fields that have already been mechanically harvested or on fields where it is not economically profitable to harvest.

fortification   The addition of nutrients to foods.

fortified foods   Foods to which one or more nutrients have been added.

free radicals   One type of highly reactive atom or molecule that causes oxidative damage.

fructose   A monosaccharide found in fruits and honey that is composed of six carbon atoms arranged in a ring structure; commonly called fruit sugar.

functional foods   Foods that have health-promoting and/or disease-preventing properties beyond basic nutritional functions.

galactose   A monosaccharide composed of six carbon atoms arranged in a ring structure; when combined with glucose, it forms the disaccharide lactose.

gallstones   Stones formed in the gallbladder or biliary passages that form when substances in the bile harden.

gastric bypass   A surgical procedure that reduces the size of the stomach and bypasses a portion of the small intestine.

gastric juice   A substance produced by the gastric glands of the stomach that contains an inactive form of pepsin and hydrochloric acid.

gastrin   A hormone secreted by the mucosa of the stomach that stimulates the secretion of enzymes and acid in the stomach.

gastroesophageal reflux disease (GERD)   A chronic condition in which acidic stomach contents leak into the esophagus, causing pain and damaging the esophagus.

gastrointestinal tract   A hollow tube consisting of the mouth, pharynx, esophagus, stomach, small intestine, and large intestine in which digestion of food and absorption of nutrients occur; also called the alimentary canal, GI tract or digestive tract.

gene   A length of DNA that contains the information needed to synthesize a polypeptide chain.

gene expression   The events of protein synthesis in which the information coded in a gene is used to synthesize a protein.

generally recognized as safe (GRAS)   A group of chemical additives that are considered safe, based on their long-standing presence in the food supply without harmful effects.

genes   Units of a larger molecule called DNA that are responsible for inherited traits.

genetically modified (GM)   An organism whose genetic material has been altered using genetic engineering techniques, a product containing or produced by genetic modification.

genetic engineering   A set of techniques used to manipulate DNA for the purpose of changing the characteristics of an organism or creating a new product.

germ The embryo or sprouting portion of a kernel of grain. It contains vegetable oil, vitamins, and minerals.

gestational diabetes A condition characterized by high blood glucose levels that develop during pregnancy.

gestational hypertension High blood pressure that develops after the 20th week of pregnancy and returns to normal after delivery. It may be an early sign of preeclampsia.

ghrelin A hormone produced by the stomach that affects food intake.

glucagon A hormone made in the pancreas that raises blood glucose levels by stimulating the breakdown of liver glycogen and the synthesis of glucose.

glucose A 6-carbon monosaccharide that is the primary form of carbohydrate used to produce energy in the body.

glutathione peroxidase A selenium-containing enzyme that protects cells from oxidative damage by neutralizing peroxides.

glycemic index A ranking of the effect that the consumption of a single carbohydrate-containing food has on blood glucose in relation to consumption of a reference carbohydrate such as white bread or glucose.

glycemic load An index of the glycemic response that occurs after eating specific foods. It is calculated by multiplying a food's glycemic index by the amount of available carbohydrate in a serving of the food.

glycemic response The rate, magnitude, and duration of the rise in blood glucose that occurs after food is consumed.

glycogen The storage form of carbohydrate in animals, made up of many glucose molecules linked together in a highly branched structure.

glycogen super-compensation or **carbohydrate loading** A regimen designed to increase muscle glycogen stores beyond their usual capacity.

glycolysis An anaerobic metabolic pathway that splits glucose into two three-carbon pyruvate molecules; the energy released from one glucose molecule is used to make two molecules of ATP.

goiter An enlargement of the thyroid gland caused by a deficiency of iodine.

goitrogens Substances that interfere with the utilization of iodine or the function of the thyroid gland.

Hazard Analysis Critical Control Point (HACCP) A food safety system that focuses on identifying and preventing hazards that could cause food-borne illness.

health claims Claims on food labels that describe the relationship between a nutrient or food and a disease or health condition. Only approved health claims may appear on food labels.

healthy life expectancy The amount of time a human can expect to stay healthy.

Healthy People A set of national health promotion and disease prevention objectives for the U.S. population.

heartburn A burning sensation in the chest or throat caused when acidic stomach contents leak back into the esophagus.

heat cramps Muscle cramps caused by an imbalance of sodium and potassium; may result from excessive exercise without adequate fluid and electrolyte replacement.

heat exhaustion Low blood pressure, rapid pulse, fainting, and sweating caused when dehydration decreases blood volume so much that blood can no longer both cool the body and provide oxygen to the muscles.

heat-related illnesses Conditions, including heat cramps, heat exhaustion, and heat stroke, that can occur due to an unfavorable combination of exercise, hydration status, and climatic conditions.

heat stroke Elevated body temperature as a result of fluid loss and the failure of the temperature regulatory center of the brain.

heme iron A readily absorbable form of iron found in meat, fish, and poultry that is chemically associated with certain proteins.

hemochromatosis An inherited disorder that results in increased iron absorption.

hemoglobin An iron-containing protein in red blood cells that binds and transports oxygen through the bloodstream to cells.

hemolytic anemia A condition in which there is an insufficient number of red blood cells because many have burst.

hemolytic-uremic syndrome A disorder, usually in children, that occurs when an infection in the digestive system produces toxic substances that destroy red blood cells causing them to block capillaries, eventually resulting in kidney failure.

hemorrhoids Swollen veins in the anal or rectal area.

hepatic portal vein The vein that transports blood from the gastrointestinal tract to the liver.

heterocyclic amines (HAs) A class of mutagenic substances produced when there is incomplete combustion of amino acids during the cooking of meats—for example, when meat is charred.

high-density lipoproteins (HDL) Lipoproteins that pick up cholesterol from cells and transport it to the liver so that it can be eliminated from the body.

high quality protein or **complete dietary protein** An easily digestible protein that contains all of the amino acids needed for protein synthesis in amounts similar to those found in body proteins.

hormones Chemical messengers that are produced in one location in the body, released into the blood, and travel to other locations, where they elicit responses.

hunger A desire to consume food that is triggered by internal physiological signals or the recurrent involuntary lack of food that over time may lead to malnutrition.

hydrogenation A process whereby hydrogen atoms are added to the carbon–carbon double bonds of unsaturated fatty acids, making them more saturated.

hydrolyzed protein, or **protein hydrolysates** A mixture of amino acids or amino acids and polypeptides that results when a protein is completely or partially broken down by treatment with acid or enzymes.

hypercarotenemia A condition caused by the accumulation of carotenoids in the adipose tissue, causing the skin to appear yellow-orange.

hypertension   Blood pressure that is consistently elevated to 140/90 mm mercury or greater.

hypertensive disorders of pregnancy, or **pregnancy-induced hypertension**   A spectrum of conditions involving a rise in blood pressure during pregnancy.

hypertrophy   An increase in the size of a muscle or organ.

hypoglycemia   Abnormally low blood glucose levels.

hyponatremia   Abnormally low concentration of sodium in the blood.

hypothesis   A proposed explanation for an observation or a scientific problem that can be tested through experimentation.

implantation   The process through which a developing embryo embeds itself in the uterine lining.

incomplete dietary protein   A protein that is deficient in one or more of the amino acids required for protein synthesis in humans.

indirect food additives   Substances that are expected to unintentionally enter foods during manufacturing or from packaging. They are regulated by the FDA.

infancy   The period of early childhood, generally from birth to 2 years of age.

infant botulism   A potentially life-threatening disease in which the bacteria *Clostridium botulinum* grows within the baby's gastrointestinal tract.

infant mortality rate   The number of deaths during the first year of life per 1000 live births.

inflammation   A protective response to injury or destruction of tissues; signs of acute inflammation include pain, heat, redness, swelling and loss of function.

insoluble fiber   Fiber that, for the most part, does not dissolve in water and cannot be broken down by bacteria in the large intestine. It includes cellulose, some hemicelluloses, and lignin.

insulin   A hormone made in the pancreas that allows glucose to enter cells and stimulates the synthesis of protein, fat, and liver and muscle glycogen.

insulin resistance   A condition in which the normal amount of insulin produces a subnormal effect in the body.

integrated pest management (IPM)   A method of agricultural pest control that integrates nonchemical and chemical techniques.

intestinal microflora   Microorganisms that inhabit the large intestine.

intrinsic factor   A protein produced in the stomach that is needed for the absorption of adequate amounts of vitamin B_{12}.

iodized salt   Table salt to which a small amount of sodium iodide or potassium iodide has been added in order to supplement the iodine content of the diet.

ion   An atom or a group of atoms that carries an electrical charge.

iron deficiency anemia   An iron deficiency disease that occurs when the oxygen-carrying capacity of the blood is decreased because there is insufficient iron to make hemoglobin.

iron overload   A condition in which iron accumulates in the tissues; characterized by bronzed skin and enlarged liver and diabetes mellitus and abnormalities of the pancreas and the joints.

irradiation   A process that exposes foods to radiation in order to kill contaminating organisms and retard the ripening and spoilage of fruits and vegetables.

keshan disease   A heart disease that occurs in an area of China where the soil is very low in selenium.

ketones or **ketone bodies**   Acidic molecules formed when there is not sufficient carbohydrate to completely metabolize the acetyl-CoA produced from fatty acid breakdown.

ketosis   High levels of ketones in the blood.

kilocalories *(kcal)*   Units of heat that are used to express the amount of energy provided by foods. It is the amount of heat required to raise the temperature of 1 kilogram of water 1 degree Celsius (1 kcalorie = 1000 calories. When Calorie is spelled with a capital C it denotes kilocalorie).

kwashiorkor   A form of protein-energy malnutrition in which only protein is deficient.

lactation   Production and secretion of milk.

lacteals   Lymph vessels in the villi of the small intestine that pick up particles containing the products of fat digestion.

lactic acid   An end product of anaerobic metabolism and an additive used in food to maintain acidity or form curds.

lactose   A disaccharide made of glucose linked to galactose that is found in milk.

lactose intolerance   The inability to digest lactose due to a reduction in the levels of the enzyme lactase.

large for gestational age   Weighing more than 4 kg (8.8 lbs) at birth.

LDL receptor   *See* Low-density lipoprotein receptor.

lean body mass   Body mass attributed to nonfat body components such as bone, muscle, and internal organs; also called *fat-free mass.*

lecithin   A phosphoglyceride composed of a glycerol backbone, two fatty acids, a phosphate group, and a molecule of choline; often used as an emulsifier in foods.

legumes   The starchy seeds of plants that produce bean pods; include peas, peanuts, beans, soybeans, and lentils.

leptin   A protein hormone produced by adipocytes that signals information about the amount of body fat.

let-down   The release of milk from the milk-producing glands and its movement through the ducts and storage sinuses.

life expectancy   The average length of life for a particular population of individuals.

life span   The maximum age to which members of a species can live.

limiting amino acid   The essential amino acid that is available in the lowest concentration relative to the body's needs.

linoleic acid   An omega-6 essential fatty acid with 18 carbons and 2 double bonds.

lipases   Fat-digesting enzymes.

lipid bilayer   Two layers of phosphoglyceride molecules oriented so that the fat-soluble fatty acid tails are sandwiched between the water soluble phosphate-containing heads.

lipids   A class of nutrients that is commonly called fats. Chemically, they contain carbon, hydrogen, and oxygen, and most of them do not dissolve in water. They include fatty acids, triglycerides, phospholipids, and sterols.

lipoprotein lipase   An enzyme that breaks down triglycerides into free fatty acids and glycerol; attached to the outside of the cells that line the blood vessels.

lipoproteins   Particles that transport lipids in the blood.

liposuction   A procedure that suctions out adipose tissue from under the skin; used to decrease the size of local fat deposits such as on the abdomen or hips.

low birth weight   A birth weight less than 2.5 kg (5.5 lbs).

low-density lipoproteins (LDLs) Lipoproteins that transport cholesterol to cells.

Low-density lipoprotein receptor   A protein on the surface of cells that binds to LDL particles and allows their contents to be taken up for use by the cell.

lumen   The inside cavity of a tube, such as the gastrointestinal tract.

lymphatic system   The system of lymph vessels and other lymph organs and tissues that drains excess fluid from the space between cells and provides immune function.

lymphocytes   Small white blood cells (leukocytes) that play a large role in defending the body against disease.

macrocytic anemia, or megaloblastic anemia   A reduction in the blood's capacity to carry oxygen that is characterized by abnormally large immature and mature red blood cells.

macronutrients   Nutrients needed by the body in large amounts. These include water and the energy-yielding nutrients carbohydrates, lipids, and proteins.

macrophages   A type of white blood that ingests foreign material as part of the immune response to foreign invaders such as infectious microorganisms.

macula   an irregularly oval, yellow-pigmented area on the central retina, that is the central point of sharpest vision.

macular degeneration   Degeneration of a portion of the retina that results in loss of visual detail and eventually in blindness.

major minerals   Minerals needed in the diet in amounts greater than 100 mg/day

or present in the body in amounts greater than 0.01% of body weight.

malnutrition   A condition resulting from an energy or nutrient intake either above or below that which is optimal.

maltose   A disaccharide made of two glucose molecules linked together.

marasmus   A form of protein-energy malnutrition in which a deficiency of energy in the diet causes severe body wasting.

maximum heart rate   The maximum number of beats per minute that the heart can attain.

menopause   The time in a woman's life when the menstrual cycle ends.

metabolic pathways   Series of chemical reactions inside of a living organism that result in the transformation of one molecule into another.

metabolism   The sum of all the chemical reactions that take place in a living organism.

micelles   Particles that are formed in the small intestine when the products of fat digestion are surrounded by bile. They facilitate the absorption of lipids.

microbes   Microscopic organisms, or microorganisms, including bacteria, viruses, and fungi.

micronutrients   Nutrients needed by the body in small amounts. These include vitamins and minerals.

microvilli   Minute projections on the mucosal cell membrane that increase the absorptive surface area in the small intestine.

minerals   In nutrition, elements needed by the body in small amounts to maintain structure and regulate chemical reactions and body processes.

mitochondria (plural, *mitochondria*)   The cellular organelles that are responsible for generating energy in the form of ATP via aerobic metabolism; the citric acid cycle and electron transport chain are located here.

modified atmosphere packaging (MAP)   A preservation technique used to prolong the shelf life of processed or fresh food by changing the gases surrounding the food in the package.

mold   Multicellular fungi that form filamentous branching growths.

molecules   Units of two or more atoms of the same or different elements bonded together.

monosaccharide   A carbohydrate made up of a single sugar unit.

monosodium glutamate (MSG)   An additive used as a flavor enhancer, commonly used in Chinese food; made up of the amino acid glutamate bound to sodium.

monounsaturated fatty acid   A fatty acid containing one carbon–carbon double bond.

morning sickness   Nausea and vomiting that affects many women during the first few months of pregnancy and that in some women can continue throughout the pregnancy.

MSG symptom complex, or Chinese restaurant syndrome   A group of symptoms including headache, flushing, tingling, burning sensations, and chest pain reported by some individuals after consuming monosodium glutamate (MSG).

mucosa   The layer of tissue lining the gastrointestinal tract and other body cavities.

mucosal cells   A type of epithelial cells that make up the lining of the gastrointestinal tract and other body cavities.

mucus   A viscous fluid secreted by glands in the digestive tract and other parts of the body. It lubricates, moistens, and protects cells from harsh environments.

muscle endurance   The ability of a muscle group to continue muscle movement over time.

muscle strength   The amount of force that can be produced by a single contraction of a muscle.

myelin   A soft, white fatty substance that covers nerve fibers and aids in nerve transmission.

myoglobin   An iron-containing protein in muscle cells that binds oxygen.

MyPyramid: Steps to a Healthier You A food group system developed by the USDA as a guide to the amounts of different types of foods needed to provide an adequate diet and comply with current nutrition recommendations.

National School Lunch Program   A federally funded program designed to provide free or reduced costs lunches to school age children.

neural tube defects   Abnormalities in the brain or spinal cord that result from errors that occur during prenatal development.

neurotransmitter   A chemical substance produced by a nerve cell that can stimulate or inhibit another cell.

niacin   Vitamin B_3 needed in energy production.

niacin equivalents *(NEs)*   Units used to express the amount of niacin present in food including that which can be made from its precursor, tryptophan. One NE is equal to 1 mg of niacin or 60 mg of tryptophan.

night blindness   Inability to see clearly in dim light.

nitrogen balance   The amount of nitrogen consumed in the diet compared with the amount excreted over a given period.

nitrosamines   Carcinogenic compounds produced by reactions between nitrites and amino acids.

nonessential or **dispensable amino acids**   Amino acids that can be synthesized by the human body in sufficient amounts to meet needs.

nonexercise activity thermogenesis (NEAT)   The energy expended for everything we do other than sleeping, eating, or sports-like exercise.

nonnutritive sweetener or **artificial sweetener**   A substance used to sweeten food that provide few or no kcalories

nursing bottle syndrome   Extreme tooth decay in the upper teeth resulting from putting a child to bed with a bottle containing milk or other sweetened liquids.

nutrient content claims   Claims on food labels used to describe the level of a nutrient in a food. The Nutrition Labeling and Education Act of 1990 defines there terms and regulates the circumstances under which they can be used.

nutrient density   A measure of the nutrients provided by a food relative to its calorie content.

nutrients   Substances in food that provide energy and structure to the body and regulate body processes.

Nutrition Facts   The portion of a food label that provides information about the nutritional composition of a food and how that food fits into the overall diet.

nutrition transition   A series of changes in diet, physical activity, health, and nutrition that occurs as poor countries become more prosperous.

nutritional genomics or **nutrigenomics**   The study of how diet affects our genes and how individual genetic variation can affect the impact of nutrients or other food components on health.

nutritional status   An individual's health, as it is influenced by the intake and utilization of nutrients.

obese   Having excess body fat. Obesity is defined as having a body mass index (ratio of weight to height squared) of 30 kg/m^2 or greater.

obesity genes   Genes that code for proteins involved in the regulation of body fat. When they are abnormal, the result is abnormal amounts of body fat.

oldest old   Individuals over 85 years of age.

oligosaccharides   Short carbohydrate chains containing 3 to 10 sugar units.

omega-3 *(ω-3)* **fatty acid**   A fatty acid containing a carbon–carbon double bond between the third and fourth carbons from the omega end; includes α-linolenic acid found in vegetable oils and eicosapentaenoic acid (EPA) and docosahexaenoic acid found in fish oils.

omega-6 *(ω-6)* **fatty acid**   A fatty acid containing a carbon–carbon double bond between the sixth and seventh carbons from the omega end; includes linoleic and arachidonic acid.

organ systems   Groups of cooperative organs.

organic compounds   Substances that contain carbon bonded to hydrogen.

organic food   Food that is produced, processed, and handled in accordance with the standards of the USDA National Organic Program.

organs   Discrete structures composed of more than one tissue that perform a specialized function.

osmosis   The unassisted diffusion of water across the cell membrane.

osteomalacia   A vitamin D deficiency disease in adults, characterized by loss of minerals from bone, bone pain, muscle aches, and an increase in bone fractures.

osteopenia   A reduction in bone density to below normal levels.

osteoporosis   A bone disorder characterized by reduced bone mass, increased bone fragility, and increased risk of fractures.

overload principle   The concept that the body adapts to the stresses placed on it.

overnutrition   Poor nutritional status resulting from a dietary intake in excess of that which is optimal for health.

overtraining syndrome   A collection of emotional, behavioral, and physical symptoms that occurs when the amount and intensity of exercise exceeds an athlete's capacity to recover.

overweight   Being too heavy for one's height, usually due to an excess of body fat. Overweight is defined as having a body mass index of 25 to 29.9 kilograms/meter^2 (kg/m^2).

oxidative damage   Damage caused by highly reactive oxygen molecules that steal electrons from other compounds, causing changes in structure and function.

oxidized LDL cholesterol   A substance formed when the cholesterol in LDL particles is oxidized by reactive oxygen molecules. It is key in the development of atherosclerosis because it is taken up by scavenger receptors on white blood cells.

oxytocin   A hormone released by the posterior pituitary that stimulates the ejection or let-down of milk during lactation.

pancreatic amylase   A starch-digesting enzyme found in pancreatic juice.

pancreatic juice   The secretion of the pancreas containing bicarbonate to neutralize acid and enzymes for the digestion of carbohydrates, fats, and proteins.

pantothenic acid   One of the B vitamins, needed in energy production.

parasites   Organisms that live at the expense of others.

parathyroid hormone (PTH) A hormone released by the parathyroid gland that acts to increase blood calcium levels.

pasteurization The process of heating food products in order to kill disease-causing organisms.

pathogen An organism or a substance that causes disease.

peak bone mass The maximum bone density attained at any time in life, usually occurring in young adulthood.

peer-review process The review of the design and validity of a research experiment by experts in the field of study who did not participate in the research.

pellagra A disease resulting from niacin deficiency, which causes dermatitis, diarrhea, dementia, and, if not treated, death.

pepsin A protein-digesting enzyme produced by the stomach. It is secreted in the gastric juice in an inactive form (pepsinogen) and activated by acid in the stomach.

peptic ulcers Open sores in the lining of the stomach, esophagus, or upper small intestine.

peptide bonds Chemical linkages between the amino group of one amino acid and the acid group of another.

peptides Two or more amino acids joined by peptide bonds.

peristalsis Coordinated muscular contractions that move material through the GI tract.

pernicious anemia A macrocytic anemia resulting from vitamin B12 deficiency that occurs when dietary vitamin B12 cannot be absorbed due to a lack of intrinsic factor.

phagocytes The type of white blood cells that engulfs and consumes foreign particles such as bacteria.

pharynx A funnel-shaped opening that connects the nasal passages and mouth to the respiratory passages and esophagus. It is a common passageway for food and air and is responsible for swallowing.

phenylketonuria (PKU) A genetic disease in which the amino acid phenylalanine cannot be metabolized normally, causing it to build up in the blood. If untreated, the condition results in brain damage.

phosphate group A chemical group consisting of one phosphorus atom and four oxygen atoms.

phospholipids Types of lipids whose structure includes a phosphorus atom.

photosynthesis The metabolic process by which plants trap energy from the sun and use it to make sugars from carbon dioxide and water.

physical frailty Impairment in function and reduction in physiologic reserves severe enough to cause limitations in the basic activities of daily living.

phytochemicals Substances found in plant foods that are not essential nutrients but may have health-promoting properties.

pica An abnormal craving for and ingestion of nonfood substances that have little or no nutritional value.

placebo A fake medicine or supplement that is indistinguishable in appearance from the real thing. It is used to disguise the control and experimental groups in an experiment.

placenta An organ produced from maternal and embryonic tissues. It secretes hormones, transfers nutrients and oxygen from the mother's blood to the fetus, and removes metabolic wastes.

plant sterols Compounds found in plant cell membranes that resemble cholesterol in structure. They can lower blood cholesterol by competing with cholesterol for absorption in the gastrointestinal tract.

platelets Cell fragments found in blood that are involved in blood clotting.

polychlorinated biphenyls (PCBs) Carcinogenic industrial compounds that have found their way into the environment and, subsequently, the food supply. Repeated exposure causes them to accumulate in biological tissues over time.

polycyclic aromatic hydrocarbons (PAHs) A class of mutagenic substances produced during cooking when there is incomplete combustion of organic materials—for example, when fat drips on a grill.

polypeptide A chain of amino acids linked by peptide bonds that is part of the structure of a protein.

polysaccharide A carbohydrate made up of many sugar units linked together.

polyunsaturated fatty acid A fatty acid that contains two or more carbon–carbon double bonds.

postmenopausal bone loss The accelerated bone loss that occurs in women for about five years after the menstrual cycle stops.

prebiotics Substances that pass undigested into the colon and stimulate the growth and/or activity of certain types of bacteria.

prediabetes A consistent elevation of blood glucose levels to between 100 and 125 mg/dl of blood, a level above normal but not high enough to be diagnostic of diabetes but thought to increase the risk of developing diabetes.

preeclampsia A condition characterized by elevated blood pressure, a rapid increase in body weight, protein in the urine, and edema. Also called *toxemia.*

prehypertension Blood pressures of 120 to 139 millimeters of mercury systolic (top number) or 80 to 90 diastolic (bottom number). It increases the risk of developing hypertension as well as the risk of artery damage and heart disease.

preterm or **premature** An infant born before 37 weeks of gestation.

prion A pathogenic protein that is the cause of degenerative brain diseases called spongiform encephalopathies. *Prion* is short for *proteinaceous infectious particle.*

prior-sanctioned substances Substances that the FDA or the USDA had determined were safe for use in a specific food prior to the 1958 Food Additives Amendment.

probiotics Products that contain live bacteria, which when consumed temporarily live in the colon and confer health benefits on the host.

prolactin A hormone released from the anterior pituitary that stimulates the mammary glands to produce milk.

proteases Protein-digesting enzymes.

protein A class of nutrients that includes molecules made up of one or more intertwining chains of amino acids. They contain carbon, hydrogen, oxygen, and nitrogen.

protein complementation   The process of combining proteins from different sources so that they collectively provide the proportions of amino acids required to meet the body's needs.

protein-energy malnutrition (PEM)   A condition characterized by loss of muscle and fat mass and an increased susceptibility to infection that results from the long-term consumption of insufficient amounts of energy and/or protein to meet the body's needs.

protein quality   A measure of how efficiently a protein in the diet can be used to make body proteins.

prothrombin   A blood protein required for blood clotting.

provitamin or **vitamin precursor**   A compound that can be converted into the active form of a vitamin in the body.

puberty   A period of rapid growth and physical changes that ends in the attainment of sexual maturity.

pyridoxal phosphate   The major coenzyme form of vitamin B_6 that functions in more than 100 enzymatic reactions, many of which involve amino acid metabolism.

qualified health claims   Health claims on food labels that have been approved based on emerging but not well-established evidence of a relationship between a food, food component, or dietary supplement and reduced risk of a disease or health-related condition.

reactive hypoglycemia   Low blood sugar that occurs an hour or so after the consumption of high-carbohydrate foods; results from an overproduction of insulin.

recombinant DNA   DNA that has been formed by joining DNA from different sources.

Recommended Dietary Allowances (RDAs)   Intakes that are sufficient to meet the needs of almost all healthy people in a specific gender and life-stage group.

refined   Refers to foods that have undergone processing to remove the coarse parts of the original food.

renewable resources   Resources that are restored and replaced by natural processes and can therefore be used forever.

resistance-training exercise or **strength-training exercise**   Activities that are specifically designed to increase muscle strength, endurance, and size.

resistant starch   Starch that escapes digestion in the small intestine of healthy people.

resting heart rate   The number of times that the heart beats per minute while a person is at rest.

resting metabolic rate (RMR)   The rate of energy expenditure at rest. It is measured after 5 to 6 hours without food or exercise.

retinoids   The chemical forms of preformed vitamin A: retinol, retinal, and retinoic acid.

retinol activity equivalents (RAEs)   The amounts of retinol, α-carotene, β-carotene, or β-crytoxanthin that must be consumed to equal the vitamin A activity of 1 μg of retinol.

retinol-binding protein   A protein that is necessary to transport vitamin A from the liver to tissues in need.

rhodopsin   A light-sensitive compound found in the retina of the eye that is composed of the protein opsin loosely bound to retinal.

riboflavin   Vitamin B_2 needed in energy production.

rickets   A vitamin D deficiency disease in children, characterized by poor bone development because of inadequate calcium absorption.

saliva   A watery fluid that is produced and secreted into the mouth by the salivary glands. It contains lubricants, enzymes, and other substances.

salivary amylase   An enzyme secreted by the salivary glands that breaks down starch into smaller units.

satiety   The feeling of fullness and satisfaction caused by food consumption that eliminates the desire to eat.

saturated fats   Lipids that are most abundant in solid animal fats and are associated with an increased risk of heart disease.

saturated fatty acid   A fatty acid in which the carbon atoms are bonded to as many hydrogen atoms as possible; it therefore contains no carbon–carbon double bonds.

scavenger receptors   Proteins on the surface of macrophages that bind to oxidized LDL cholesterol and allow it to be taken up by the cell.

scientific method   The general approach of science that is used to explain observations about the world around us.

scurvy   A vitamin C deficiency disease characterized by bleeding gums, tooth loss, joint pain, bleeding into the skin and mucous membranes, and fatigue.

set point   A level at which body fat or body weight seems to resist change despite changes in energy intake or output.

simple carbohydrates   Carbohydrates known as sugars that include monosaccharides and disaccharides.

simple diffusion   The unassisted diffusion of a substance across the cell membrane.

small-for-gestational-age   An infant born at term weighing less than 2.5 kg (5.5 lb).

sodium chloride   The chemical formula of table salt.

soluble fiber   Fiber that dissolves in water or absorbs water and can be broken down by intestinal microflora. It includes pectins, gums, and some hemicelluloses.

solvent   A fluid in which one or more substances dissolve.

Special Supplemental Nutrition Program for Women, Infants, and Children (WIC)   A program funded by the federal government that provides nutrition education and food vouchers to pregnant and lactating women and their young children.

sphincter   A muscular valve that helps control the flow of materials in the gastrointestinal tract.

spina bifida   A neural tube defect in which part of the spinal cord is exposed through a gap in the backbone, causing varying degrees of disability.

spores   Dormant states of some bacteria that are resistant to heat but can germinate and produce a new organism when environmental conditions are favorable.

sports anemia   A temporary decrease in hemoglobin concentration that occurs during exercise training. It occurs as an adaptation to training and does not impair delivery of oxygen to tissues.

starch   A carbohydrate found in plants, made up of many glucose molecules linked in straight or branching chains.

starvation A severe reduction in nutrient and energy intake that impairs health and eventually causes death. It is the most extreme form of malnutrition.

steroid precursors Androgenic hormones produced primarily by the adrenal glands and gonads that act as precursors in the production of testosterone and estrogen. They can be taken as nutritional supplements.

sterols Types of lipids with a structure composed of multiple chemical rings.

strength-training exercise or **resistance-training exercise** Activities that are specifically designed to increase muscle strength, endurance, and size.

structure/function claims Claims on food labels that describe the role of a nutrient or dietary ingredient in maintaining normal structure or function in humans.

stunting A decrease in linear growth rate.

subcutaneous fat Adipose tissue located under the skin which is not associated with a great increase in the risk of chronic diseases.

subsistence crops Crops that are grown as food for the local population.

sucrose A disaccharide commonly known as table sugar that is made of glucose linked to fructose.

sudden infant death syndrome (SIDS, or crib death) The unexplained death of an infant, usually during sleep.

sugar unit A sugar molecule that cannot be broken down to yield other sugars.

Supplement Facts Portion of a dietary supplement label that includes information about, serving size, ingredients, amount per serving size (by weight), and percent of Daily Value, if established.

sustainable agriculture Agricultural methods that maintain soil productivity and a healthy ecological balance while having minimal long-term impacts.

teratogen A chemical, biological, or physical agent that causes birth defects.

theory A formal explanation of an observed phenomenon made after a hypothesis has been supported and tested through experimentation.

thermic effect of food (TEF) or **diet-induced thermogenesis** The energy required for the digestion of food and absorption, metabolism, and storage of nutrients.

thiamin Vitamin B_1 needed in energy production.

thirst A sensation of dryness in the mouth and throat associated with a desire for liquids.

thyroid gland A gland located in the neck that produces thyroid hormones and calcitonin.

thyroid hormones Hormones produced by the thyroid gland that regulate metabolic rate.

thyroid-stimulating hormone A hormone that stimulates the synthesis and secretion of thyroid hormones from the thyroid gland.

tissues A collection of similar cells that together carry out a specific function.

tocopherol The chemical name for vitamin E.

Tolerable Upper Intake Levels (ULs) Maximum daily intake levels that are unlikely to pose risks of adverse health effects to almost all individuals in a given gender and life-stage group.

tolerances The maximum amount of pesticide residues that may legally remain in food, set by the EPA.

total energy expenditure The sum of basal energy expenditure, the thermic effect of food, and the energy used in physical activity, regulation of body temperature, deposition of new tissue, and production of milk.

trace minerals Minerals required in the diet in amounts of 100 mg or less/day or present in the body in amounts of 0.01% of body weight or less.

***trans* fatty acids** Unsaturated fatty acids in which the hydrogens are on opposite sides of the carbon–carbon double bond.

transamination The process by which an amino group from one amino acid is transferred to a carbon compound to form a new amino acid.

transcription The process of copying the information in DNA to a molecule of mRNA.

transgenic An organism with a gene or group of genes intentionally transferred from another species or breed.

transit time The time between the ingestion of food and the elimination of the solid waste from that food.

translation The process of translating the mRNA code into the amino acid sequence of a protein.

triglycerides The major form of lipid in food and the body; consist of three fatty acids attached to a glycerol molecule.

trimester A term used to describe each third or three-month period of a pregnancy.

tripeptide Three amino acids linked together by peptide bonds.

tropical oils A term used in the popular press to refer to the saturated plant oils—coconut, palm, and palm kernel oil—that are derived from plants grown in tropical regions.

type 1 diabetes The form of diabetes caused by autoimmune destruction of insulin-producing cells in the pancreas, usually leading to absolute insulin deficiency.

type 2 diabetes The form of diabetes characterized by insulin resistance and relative (rather than absolute) insulin deficiency.

undernutrition Poor nutritional status resulting from a dietary intake below that which meets nutritional needs.

underweight A body mass index of less than 18.5 kg/m², or a body weight 10% or more below the desirable body weight standard.

unrefined foods Foods eaten either just as they are found in nature or with only minimal processing.

unsaturated fats Lipids that are most abundant in plant oils and are associated with a reduced risk of heart disease.

unsaturated fatty acid A fatty acid that contains one or more carbon–carbon double bonds; may be either monounsaturated or polyunsaturated.

urea A nitrogen-containing waste product from the breakdown of proteins that is excreted in the urine.

variable A factor or condition that is changed in an experimental setting.

variant Creutzfeldt-Jakob Disease (vCJD) A rare, degenerative, fatal brain disorder in humans. It is believed that the persons who have developed vCJD became infected through their consumption of cattle products contaminated with BSE.

vegan diets Plant-based diets that eliminate all animal products.

vegetarian diets Diets that include plant-based foods and eliminate some or all foods of animal origin.

veins Vessels that carry blood toward the heart.

venules Small veins that drain blood from capillaries and pass it to larger veins for return to the heart.

very low birth weight A birth weight less than 1.5 kg (3.3 lbs).

very-low-density lipoproteins *(VLDLs)* Lipoproteins assembled by the liver that carry lipid from the liver and deliver triglycerides to body cells.

villi *(singular, villus)* Fingerlike protrusions of the lining of the small intestine that participate in the digestion and absorption of foodstuffs.

visceral fat Adipose tissue deposited in the abdominal cavity around the internal organs. High levels are associated with an increased risk of heart disease, high blood pressure, stroke, diabetes, and breast cancer.

vitamin A A fat soluble vitamin needed in cell differentiation, reproduction and vision.

vitamin B$_{12}$ One of the B vitamins, only found in animal foods.

vitamin B$_6$ One of the B vitamins, needed in protein metabolism.

vitamin C A water soluble vitamin needed for the maintenance of collagen.

vitamin D A fat soluble vitamin, that can be made in the body in response to sunlight, that is needed for calcium absorption.

vitamin E A fat soluble vitamin that functions as an antioxidant.

vitamin K A fat soluble vitamin needed for blood clotting.

vitamins Organic compounds needed in the diet in small amounts to promote and regulate the chemical reactions and processes needed for growth, reproduction, and the maintenance of health.

water intoxication A condition that occurs when a person drinks enough water to significantly lower the concentration of sodium in the blood.

water-soluble vitamins Vitamins that dissolve in water; includes the B vitamins and vitamin C.

Wernicke-Korsakoff syndrome A form of thiamin deficiency associated with alcohol abuse that is characterized by mental confusion, disorientation, loss of memory, and a staggering gait.

whole-grain product Products made from the entire kernel of a grain including the bran, endosperm and germ.

xerophthalmia A spectrum of eye conditions resulting from vitamin A deficiency that may lead to blindness.

zoochemicals Substances found in animal foods (zoo means animal) that are not essential nutrients but may have health-promoting properties.

REFERENCES

Chapter 1

1 American Dietetic Association. Position of the American Dietetic Association: Fortification and nutritional supplements. *J Am Diet Assoc* 105:1300–1311, 2005.

2 Rao, A.V., and Rao, L.G. Carotenoids and human health. *Pharmacol Res* 5:207–216, 2007.

3 Erdman, J.W., Balentine, D., and Arab, L. Flavonoids and heart health: Proceedings of the ILSI North America Flavonoids Workshop, May 31–June 1, 2005, Washington, DC. *J Nutr* 137:718S–737S, 2007.

4 Rice, S., and Whitehead, S.A. Phytoestrogens oestrogen synthesis and breast cancer. *J. Steroid Biochem Mol Biol* 108:186–195, 2008.

5 Sacks, F.M., Lichtenstein, A., Van Horn, L., et al. Soy protein, isoflavones, and cardiovascular health: An American Heart Association science advisory for professionals from the nutrition committee. *Circulation* 113:1034–1044, 2006.

6 Cassidy, A., and Hooper, L. Phytoestrogens and cardiovascular disease. *J Br Menopause Soc* 12:49–56, 2006.

7 Galeone, C., Pelucchi, C., Levi, F., et al. Onion and garlic use and human cancer. *Am J Clin Nutr* 84:1027–1032, 2006.

8 Stan, S.D., Kar, S., Stoner, G.D., and Singh, S.V. Bioactive food components and cancer risk reduction. *J Cell Biochem* 104:339–356, 2008.

9 Schatzkin A., Mouw, T., Park Y., et al. Dietary fiber and whole-grain consumption in relation to colorectal cancer in the NIH-AARP Diet and Health Study. *Am J Clin Nutr.* 85:1353–1360, 2007.

10 Van Horn, L., McCoin, M. Kris-Etherton, P.M., et al. The evidence for dietary prevention and treatment of cardiovascular disease. *J. Am. Diet. Assoc.* 108:287–331, 2008.

11 Shukla, Y. Tea and cancer chemoprevention: A comprehensive review. *Asian Pac J Cancer Prev* 8:155–166, 2007.

12 Trumbo, P.R., and Ellwood, K.C. Lutein and zeaxanthin intakes and risk of age-related macular degeneration and cataracts: An evaluation using the Food and Drug Administration's evidence-based review system for health claims. *Am J Clin Nutr* 84:971–974, 2006.

13 Centers for Disease Control and Prevention. *Prevalence of Overweight and Obesity Among Adults: United States, 2003–2004.* Available online at www.cdc.gov/nchs/products/pubs/pubd/hestats/overweight/overwght_adult_03.htm. Accessed February 12, 2008.

14 World Health Organization. *Diet, Nutrition and the Prevention of Chronic Diseases* (Technical Report Series no. 916). Available online at www.who.int/dietphysicalactivity/publications/trs916/download/en/index.html. Accessed January 14, 2008.

15 Mokdad, A.H., Marks, J.S., Stroup, D.F., and Gerberding, J.L. Actual causes of death in the United States, 2000. *JAMA* 291:1238–1245, 2004.

16 Ogden, C.L., Carroll, M.D., and Flegal, K.M. High body mass index for age among U.S. children and adolescents, 2003–2006. *JAMA* 299:2401–2405, 2008.

17 Center for Disease Control and Prevention. Deaths: Final Data for 2006 *National Vital Statistics Reports*, Vol. 57, No. 14, April, 2009. Available online at http://www.cdc.gov/nchs/data/nvsr/nvsr57/nvsr57_14.pdf Accessed May 23, 2009.

18 Kaput, J. Nutrigenomics—2006 update. *Clin Chem Lab Med* 45:279–287, 2007.

Chapter 2

1 Davis, C., and Saltos, E. Dietary recommendations and how they have changed over time. Chapter 2 in *America's Eating Habits: Changes and Consequences.* Available online at www.ers.usda.gov/publications/aib750/aib750.pdf. Accessed December 7, 2008.

2 National Cholesterol Education Program. *Adult Treatment Panel III Report, 2001, 2004.* Available online at www.nhlbi.nih.gov/guidelines/cholesterol/atglance.pdf. Accessed May 13, 2009.

3 U.S. Department of Health and Human Services. *Healthy People 2020: The Road Ahead.* Available online at www.healthypeople.gov/hp2020/. Accessed October 28, 2008.

4 Institute of Medicine, Food and Nutrition Board. *Dietary Reference Intakes for Energy, Carbohydrate, Fiber, Fat, Fatty Acids, Cholesterol, Protein, and Amino Acids.* Washington, DC: National Academies Press, 2002.

5 U.S. Department of Health and Human Services, U.S. Department of Agriculture. *Dietary Guidelines for Americans 2005.* Available online at www.healthierus.gov/dietaryguidelines. Accessed December 7. 2008.

6 U.S. Food and Drug Administration, *A Key to Choosing Healthful Foods: Using the Nutrition Facts on the Food Label.* Available online at www.fda.gov/Food/ResourcesForYou/Consumers/ucm079449.htm. Accessed June 16, 2009.

7 U.S. Food and Drug Administration, Center for Food Safety and Applied Nutrition. *A Labeling Guide for Restaurants and Other Retail Establishments Selling Away-from-Home Foods,* April 2008. Available online at www.cfsan.fda.gov/~dms/labrguid.html. Accessed December 7, 2008.

8 U.S. Food and Drug Administration, Center for Food Safety and Applied Nutrition /Office of Nutrition, Labeling, and Dietary Supplements. April, 2008. Guidance for food industry, *A Food Labeling Guide.* Available at http://www.cfsan.fda.gov/~dms/2lg-toc.html. Accessed January 24, 2009.

9 U.S. Food and Drug Administration, Center for Food Safety and Applied Nutrition /Office of Nutrition, Labeling, and Dietary Supplements. April, 2005. Guidance for food industry, *A Dietary Supplement Labeling Guide.* Available at http://www.cfsan.fda.gov/~dms/dslg-toc.html. Accessed January 24, 2009.

Chapter 3

1 Guarner, F., and Malagelada, J. R. Gut flora in health and disease. *Lancet* 361:512–519, 2003.

2 Johnston, B.C., Supina, A.L., Ospina, M., and Vohra, S. Probiotics for the prevention of pediatric antibiotic-associated diarrhea. *Cochrane Database Syst Rev* 18:CD004827, 2007.

3 Gill, H., and Prasad, J. Probiotics, immunomodulation, and health benefits. *Adv Exp Med Biol* 606:423–454, 2008.

4 Isolauri, E., and Salminen, S. Nutrition, Allergy, Mucosal Immunology, and Intestinal Microbiota (NAMI) Research Group Report: Probiotics: Use in allergic disorders: A Nutrition, Allergy, Mucosal Immunology, and Intestinal Microbiota (NAMI) Research Group Report. *J Clin Gastroenterol* 42(Suppl 2):S91–S96, 2008.

5 Rescigno, M. The pathogenic role of intestinal flora in IBD and colon cancer. *Curr Drug Targets* 9:395–403, 2008.

6 Bäckhed, F., Ding, H., Wang, T., et al. The gut microbiota as an environmental factor that regulates fat storage. *Proc Natl Acad Sci USA* 101:18–23, 2004.

7 Centers for Disease Control and Prevention. Food Allergies. Available online at www.cdc.gov/HealthyYouth/foodallergies/ Accessed May 29, 2009.

8 Konturek, S.J., Konturek, P.C., Konturek, J.W., et al. *Helicobacter pylori* and its involvement in gastritis and peptic ulcer formation. *J Physiol Pharmacol* 57(Suppl 3):29–50, 2006.

9 Lynch, N.A. *Helicobacter pylori* and ulcers: A paradigm revisited. Available online at http://opa.faseb.org/pdf/pylori.pdf. Accessed December 20, 2008.

10 Marieb, E.N., and Hoehn, K. *Human Anatomy and Physiology,* 7th ed. Menlo Park, CA: Benjamin Cummings, 2007.

Chapter 4

1. The National Digestive Diseases Information Clearinghouse (NDDIC), National Institute of Diabetes and Digestive and Kidney Diseases (NIDDK), and National Institutes of Health of the U.S. Department of Health and Human Services. *Lactose Intolerance.* Available online at http://digestive.niddk.nih.gov/ddiseases/pubs/lactoseintolerance/. Accessed March 18, 2008.

2. Blaut, M. Relationship of prebiotics and food to intestinal microflora. *Eur J Nutr* 41 (Suppl 1):111–116, 2002.

3. Topping, D.L., Fukushima, M., and Bird, A.R. Resistant starch as a prebiotic and synbiotic: State of the art. *Proc Nutr Soc* 62:171–176, 2003.

4. Andoh, A., Tsujikawa, T., Fujiyama, Y. Role of dietary fiber and short-chain fatty acids in the colon. *Curr Pharm Des* 9:347–358, 2003.

5. National Institute of Diabetes and Digestive and Kidney Diseases. *National Diabetes Statistics fact sheet: General information and national estimates on diabetes in the United States, 2007.* Bethesda, MD: U.S. Department of Health and Human Services, National Institute of Health, 2007. Available online at http://diabetes.niddk.nih.gov/dm/pubs/statistics/#7. Accessed January 10, 2009.

6. American Diabetes Association. Standards of Medical Care in Diabetes—2008. *Diabetes Care* 31:S12–S54, 2008.

7. American Diabetes Association. Nutrition Recommendations and Interventions for Diabetes. A position statement of the American Diabetes Association. *Diabetes Care* 31:S61–S78, 2008.

8. Hayes, C., and Kriska, A. Role of physical activity in diabetes management and prevention. *J Am Diet Assoc* 108(4 Suppl 1):S19–S23, 2008.

9. Gross, L.S., Li, L., Ford, E.S., and Liu, S. Increased consumption of refined carbohydrates and the epidemic of type 2 diabetes in the United States: An ecologic assessment. *Am J Clin Nutr* 79:774–779, 2004.

10. Riccardi, G., Rivellese, A.A., and Giacco, R. Role of glycemic index and glycemic load in the healthy state, in prediabetes, and in diabetes. *Am J Clin Nutr* 87:269S–274S, 2008.

11. Villegas, R., Liu, S., Gao, Y.T., et. al. Prospective study of dietary carbohydrates, glycemic index, glycemic load, and incidence of type 2 diabetes mellitus in middle-aged Chinese women. *Arch Intern Med* 167:2310–2316, 2007.

12. Krishnan, S., Rosenberg, L., Singer, M., et al. Glycemic index, glycemic load, and cereal fiber intake and risk of type 2 diabetes in US black women. *Arch Intern Med* 167:2304–2309, 2007.

13. van Dam, R.M., and Seidell, J.C. Carbohydrate intake and obesity. *Eur J Clin Nutr* 61 (Suppl 1):S75–S99, 2007.

14. Westman, E.C., Feinman, R.D., and Mavropoulos, J.C. Low-carbohydrate nutrition and metabolism. *Am J Clin Nutr* 86:276–284, 2007.

15. American Dietetic Association. Position of the American Dietetic Association: Use of nutritive and non-nutritive sweeteners. *J Am Diet Assoc* 104:255–275, 2004.

16. Stevia sweetener gets US FDA go-ahead, December 18, 2008. Available online at www.foodnavigator-usa.com/Legislation/Stevia-sweetener-gets-US-FDA-go-ahead. Accessed January 12, 2009.

17. Fried, S.K., and Rao, S.P. Sugars, hypertriglyceridemia, and cardiovascular disease. *Am J Clin Nutr* 78:873S–880S, 2003.

18. Van Horn, L., McCoin, M., Kris-Etherton, P.M., et al. The evidence for dietary prevention and treatment of cardiovascular disease. *J Am Diet Assoc* 108:287–331, 2008.

19. Marlett, J.A. Dietary fiber and cardiovascular disease. In Cho, S.S., Dreher, L.L. (eds.). *Handbook of Dietary Fiber.* New York: Marcel Dekker, 2001, pp. 17–25.

20. Anderson, J.W. Whole grains protect against atherosclerotic cardiovascular disease. *Proc Nutr Soc* 62:135–142, 2003.

21. Peters, U., Sinha, R., Chatterjee, N., et al. Dietary fibre and colorectal adenoma in a colorectal cancer early detection programme. *Lancet* 361:1491–1495, 2003.

22. Bingham, S.A., Day, N.E., Luben, R., et al. Dietary fibre in food and protection against colorectal cancer in the European Prospective Investigation into Cancer and Nutrition (EPIC): An observational study. *Lancet* 361:1496–1501, 2003.

23. Schatzkin, A., Mouw, T., Park, Y., et al. Dietary fiber and whole-grain consumption in relation to colorectal cancer in the NIH-AARP Diet and Health Study. *Am J Clin Nutr* 85:1353–1360, 2007.

24. Park, Y., Hunter, D.J., Spiegelman, D., et al. Dietary fiber intake and colorectal cancer: A pooled analysis of prospective cohort studies. *JAMA* 294:2849–2857, 2005.

25. Institute of Medicine, Food and Nutrition Board. *Dietary Reference Intakes for Energy, Carbohydrates, Fiber, Fat, Protein and Amino Acids.* Washington, DC: National Academies Press, 2002.

26. U.S. Department of Agriculture. Agriculture Fact Book 2001-2001, Chapter 2, Profiling Food Consumption in America. Available online at www.usda.gov/factbook/chapter2.htm Accessed April 17, 2009.

Chapter 5

1. Popkin, B.M., Siega-Riz, A.M., Haines, P.S., and Jahns, L. Where's the fat? Trends in U.S. diets 1965–1996. *Prev Med* 32:245–254, 2001.

2. Centers for Disease Control and Prevention. Trends in intake of energy and macronutrients—United States, 1971–2000. *MMWR Morb Mortal Wkly Rep* 53:80–82, 2004.

3. Simopoulos, A.P. The importance of the ratio of omega-6/omega-3 essential fatty acids. *Biomed Pharmacother* 56:365–379, 2002.

4. American Heart Association. *Diet and Lifestyle Recommendations.* Available online at www.americanheart.org/presenter.jhtml?identifier=851. Accessed February 16, 2009.

5. American Heart Association. *Heart Disease and Stroke Statistics: 2008 Update.* Available online at www.americanheart.org/downloadable/heart/1200082005246HS_Stats%202008.final.pdf. Accessed March 10, 2008.

6. Institute of Medicine, Food and Nutrition Board. *Dietary Reference Intakes for Energy, Carbohydrates, Fiber, Fat, Protein, and Amino Acids.* Washington, DC: National Academies Press, 2002.

7. Libby, P. Inflammation and cardiovascular disease mechanisms. *Am J Clin Nutr* 83:456S–460S, 2006.

8. Kher, N., and Marsh, J.D. Pathobiology of atherosclerosis—A brief review. *Semin Thromb Hemost* 30:665–672, 2004.

9. American Heart Association. *Statistical Fact Sheet –Populations, 2008 Update: African American and Cardivascular Disease –Statistics.* Available online at www.americanheart.org/downloadable/heart/1197933296813FS01AF08.pdf. Accessed February 17, 2009.

10. National Cholesterol Education Program. *Adult Treatment Panel III Report, 2001, 2004.* Available online at www.nhlbi.nih.gov/guidelines/cholesterol/atglance.pdf. Accessed April 21, 2008.

11. Hibbeln, J.R., Nieminen,L.R., Blasbalg, T.L., et al. Healthy intakes of n-3 and n-6 fatty acids: estimations considering worldwide diversity. *Am J Clin Nutr* 83 (6 Suppl):1483S–1493S, 2006.

12. Kuriyama, S., Shimazu, T., Ohmori, K., et al. Green tea consumption and mortality due to cardiovascular disease, cancer, and all causes in Japan: The Ohsaki study. *JAMA* 296:1255–1265, 2006.

13. Van Horn, L., McCoin, M., Kris-Etherton, P.M., et al. The evidence for dietary prevention and treatment of cardiovascular disease. *J Am Diet Assoc* 108:287–331, 2008.

14. Breslow, J.L. n-3 fatty acids and cardiovascular disease. *Am J Clin Nutr* 83(6 Suppl): 1477S–1482S, 2006.

[15] Griel, A.E., Cao, Y., Bagshaw, D.D., et al. A macadamia nut–rich diet reduces total and LDL-cholesterol in mildly hypercholesterolemic men and women. *J Nutr* 138:761–767, 2008.

[16] Ros, E., Nunez, I., Perez-Heras, A., et al. A walnut diet improves endothelial function in hypercholesterolemic subjects: a randomized crossover trial. *Circulation* 109:1609–1614, 2004.

[17] Fung, T.T., Chiuve, S.E., McCullough. M,L, et al. Adherence to a DASH-style diet and risk of coronary heart disease and stroke in women. *Arch Intern Med* 168:713–720, 2008.

[18] Bruckdorfer, K.R. Antioxidants and CVD. *Proc Nutr Soc* 67:214–222, 2008.

[19] Humphrey, L.L., Fu, R., Rogers, K., et al. Homocysteine level and coronary heart disease incidence: A systematic review and meta-analysis. *Mayo Clin Proc* 83:1203–1212, 2008.

[20] World Cancer Research Fund/American Institute for Cancer Research (AICR). *Food, Nutrition, Physical Activity, and the Prevention of Cancer: A Global Perspective.* Washington DC: AICR, 2007.

[21] Schulz, M., Hoffmann, K., Weikert, C., et al. Identification of a dietary pattern characterized by high-fat food choices associated with increased risk of breast cancer: The European Prospective Investigation into Cancer and Nutrition (EPIC)-Potsdam Study. *Br J Nutr* 100:942–946, 2008.

[22] Voorrips, L. E., Brants, H. A., Kardinaal, A. F., et al. Intake of conjugated linoleic acid, fat and other fatty acids in relation to post menopausal breast cancer: the The Netherlands Study on Diet and Cancer. *Am J Clin Nutr* 76:873–882, 2002.

[23] Hall, M.N., Chavarro, J.E., Lee, I.M., et al. A 22-year prospective study of fish, n-3 fatty acid intake, and colorectal cancer risk in men. *Cancer Epidemiol Biomarkers Prev.* 17:1136–1143, 2008.

[24] Devitt, A.A., and Mattes, R.D. Effects of food unit size and energy density on intake in humans. *Appetite* 42:213–220, 2004.

[25] Ledikwe, J.H., Blanck, H.M., Kettel Khan, L., et al. Dietary energy density is associated with energy intake and weight status in US adults. *Am J Clin Nutr* 83:1362–1368, 2006.

[26] Willett, W.C., and Leibel, R.L. Dietary fat is not a major determinant of body fat. *Am J Med* 113:47S–59S, 2002.

[27] Hill, J.O. Understanding and addressing the epidemic of obesity: An energy balance perspective. *Endocr Rev* 27:750–761, 2006.

[28] Gidding, S.S., Dennison, B.A., Birch, L.L., et al. Dietary recommendations for children and adolescents: a guide for practitioners:

Consensus statement from the American Heart Association. *Circulation* 112:2061–2075, 2005.

[29] Kris-Etherton, P.M., Harris, W.S., and Appel, L.J. Fish consumption, fish oil, omega-3 fatty acids, and cardiovascular disease. *Circulation* 106:2747–2752, 2002.

[30] Revealing trans fats. *FDA Consum* 37:20–26, September/October 2003.

[31] American Dietetic Association. Position of the American Dietetic Association: Fat replacers. *J Am Diet Assoc* 105:266–275, 2005.

Chapter 6

[1] Williams, C.D. Kwashiorkor: Nutritional disease of children associated with maize diet. *Lancet* 2:1151–1154, 1935.

[2] Alebiosu, C.O. An update on "progression promoters" in renal diseases. *J Natl Med Assoc* 95:30–42, 2003.

[3] Institute of Medicine, Food and Nutrition Board. *Dietary Reference Intakes for Energy, Carbohydrates, Fiber, Fat, Protein and Amino Acids.* Washington, DC: National Academies Press, 2002.

[4] Heaney, R.P., and Layman, D.K. Amount and type of protein influences bone health. *Am J Clin Nutr* 87:1567S–1570S, 2008.

[5] Kerstetter, J., O'Brien, K., and Insogna, K. Dietary protein, calcium metabolism, and skeletal homeostasis revisited. *Am J Clin Nutr* 78(Suppl):S584–S592, 2003.

[6] Weikert, C., Walter, D., Hoffmann, K., et al. The relation between dietary protein, calcium and bone health in women: Results from the EPIC-Potsdam cohort. *Ann Nutr Metab* 49:312–318, 2005.

[7] Siener, R. Impact of dietary habits on stone incidence. *Urol Res* 34:131–133, 2006.

[8] van't Veer, P., Jansen, M.C., Klerk, M., and Kok, F.J. Fruits and vegetables in the prevention of cancer and cardiovascular disease. *Public Health Nutr* 3:103–107, 2000.

[9] U.S. Department of Health and Human Services, U.S. Food and Drug Administration. *FDA and Monosodium Glutamate (MSG) FDA Backgrounder,* August 31, 1995. Available online at http://vm.cfsan.fda.gov/~lrd/msg.html. Accessed December 20. Accessed February 16, 2009.

[10] Fasano, A., Berti, I., Gerarduzzi, T., et al. Prevalence of celiac disease in at-risk and not-at-risk groups in the United States. *Arch Intern Med* 163:268–292, 2003.

[11] Fulgoni, V.L. Current protein intake in America: Analysis of the National Health and Nutrition Examination Survey, 2003–2004. *Am J Clin Nutr* 87:1554S–1557S, 2008.

[12] American Dietetic Association. Position of the American Dietetic Association, Dietitians of

Canada, and American College of Sports Medicine: Nutrition and athletic performance. *J Am Diet Assoc* 109:509–527, 2009.

[13] Stipanuk, M.H. Protein and amino acid requirements. In Stipanuk, M.H. (ed.) *Biochemical, Physiological and Molecular Aspects of Human Nutrition,* 2nd ed. St. Louis: Saunders Elsevier, 2006, pp. 419–448.

[14] American Dietetic Association. Position of the American Dietetic Association and Dietitians of Canada: Vegetarian diets. *J Am Diet Assoc* 103:748–765, 2003.

[15] Leitzmann, C. Vegetarian diets: What are the advantages? *Forum Nutr* 57:147–156, 2005.

[16] Berkow, S.E., and Barnard, N. Vegetarian diets and weight status. *Nutr Rev* 64:175–188, 2006.

[17] Sacks, F.M., Lichtenstein, A., Van Horn L, et al. Soy protein, isoflavones, and cardiovascular health: An American Heart Association Science Advisory for professionals from the Nutrition Committee. *Circulation* 113:1034–1044, 2006.

Chapter 7

[1] Miller, D.F. Enrichment programs: Helping mother nature along. *Food Product Development* 12:30–38, 1978.

[2] Briefel, R., Hanson, C., Fox, M.K., et al. Feeding Infants and Toddlers Study: Do vitamin and mineral supplements contribute to nutrient adequacy or excess among US infants and toddlers? *J Am Diet Assoc* 106:S52–S65, 2006.

[3] Arsenault, J.E., and Brown, K.H. Zinc intake of US preschool children exceeds new dietary reference intakes. *Am J Clin Nutr* 78:1011–1017, 2003.

[4] Food and Nutrition Board, Institute of Medicine. *Dietary Reference Intakes for Vitamin C, Vitamin E, Selenium, and Carotenoids.* Washington, DC: National Academies Press, 2000.

[5] Food and Drug Administration. Food labeling; guidelines for voluntary nutrition labeling of raw fruits, vegetables, and fish. *Fed Regist* 71(142):42031–42047, July 25, 2006. Available online at www.cfsan.fda.gov/~lrd/fr060725.html. Accessed January 4, 2009.

[6] Institute of Medicine, Food and Nutrition Board. *Dietary Reference Intakes for Thiamin, Riboflavin, Niacin, Vitamin B-6, Folate, Vitamin B-12, Pantothenic Acid, Biotin, and Choline.* Washington, DC: National Academies Press, 1998.

[7] Saffert, A., Pieper, G., and Jetten, J. Effect of package light transmittance on vitamin content of milk. *Technology and Science* 21:47–55, 2008.

[8] Seal, A.J., Creeke, P.I., Dibari, F, et al. Low and deficient niacin status and pellagra are endemic in postwar Angola. *Am J Clin Nutr* 85:218–242, 2007.

9 Ford, E. S., Smith, S. J., Stroup, D. F., et al. Homocyst(e)ine and cardiovascular disease: A systematic review of the evidence with special emphasis on case-control studies and nested case-control studies. *Int J Epidemiol* 31:59–70, 2002.

10 USDA Agricultural Research Service. *Results from USDA's 1994–1996 Continuing Survey of Food Intakes by Individuals and 1994–1996 Health Knowledge Survey*, 1997. Available online at www.barc.usda.gov/bhnrc/foodsurvey/home/htm/. Accessed March 6, 2008.

11 Aufiero, E., Stitik, T.P., Foye, P.M., and Chen, B. Pyridoxine hydrochloride treatment of carpal tunnel syndrome: A review. *Nutr Rev* 62:96–104, 2004.

12 Bendich, A. The potential for dietary supplements to reduce premenstrual syndrome (PMS) symptoms. *J Am Coll Nutr* 19:3–12, 2000.

13 Centers for Disease Control and Prevention. Spina bifida and anencephaly before and after folic acid mandate—United States, 1995–1996 and 1999–2000. *MMWR Morb Mortal Wkly Rep* 17:362–365, 2004. Available online at www.cdc.gov/MMWR/preview/mmwrhtml/mm5317a3.htm. Accessed April 17, 2008.

14 De Wals, P., Tiarou, F., Van Allen, M.I., et al. Reduction in neural-tube defects after folic acid fortification in Canada. *N Engl J Med* 357:135–142, 2007.

15 Hubner, R.A., and Houlston, R.S. Folate and colorectal cancer prevention. *Br J Cancer* 100:233–239, 2009.

16 Larsson, S.C., Bergkvist, L., and Wolk, A. Folate intake and risk of breast cancer by estrogen and progesterone receptor status in a Swedish cohort. *Cancer Epidemiol Biomarkers Prev* 17:3444–3449, 2008.

17 Larsson, S.C., Håkansson, N., Giovannucci, E., and Wolk, A. Folate intake and pancreatic cancer incidence: A prospective study of Swedish women and men. *J Natl Cancer Inst* 98:407–413, 2006.

18 American Dietetic Association. Position of the American Dietetic Association: Vegetarian diets. *J Am Diet Assoc* 103:748–765, 2003.

19 Douglas, R.M., Hemilä, H., Chalker, E., and Treacy, B. Vitamin C for preventing and treating the common cold. *Cochrane Database Syst Rev* 4:CD000980, 2004.

20 Fischer, L. M., daCasta, K.A., Kwock, L., et al. Sex and menopausal status influence human dietary requirements for the nutrient choline. *Am J Clin Nutr* 85:1275–1285, 2007.

21 Food and Nutrition Board, Institute of Medicine. *Dietary Reference Intakes: Vitamin A, Vitamin K, Arsenic, Boron, Chromium, Copper, Iodine, Iron, Manganese, Molybdenum, Nickel, Silicon, Vanadium, and Zinc.* Washington, DC: National Academies Press, 2001.

22 World Health Organization. *Micronutrient Deficiencies. Vitamin A Deficiency: The Challenge.* Available online at www.who.int/nutrition/topics/vad/en/index.html. Accessed April 23, 2008.

23 Michaelsson, K., Lithell, H., Vessby, B., and Melhus, H. Serum retinol levels and the risk of fracture. *N Engl J Med* 348:287–294, 2003.

24 Pryor, W.A., Stahl, W., and Rock, C.L. Beta-carotene: From biochemistry to clinical trials. *Nutr Rev* 58(2 Pt. I):39–53, 2000.

25 Nagpal, S., Na, S., and Rathnachalam, R. Non-calcemic actions of vitamin D receptor ligands. *Endocr Rev* 26:62–68, 2005.

26 Garland, C.F., Garland, F.C., Gorham, E.D., et al. The role of vitamin D in cancer prevention. *Am J Public Health* 96:252–261, 2006.

27 Holick, M.F., and Chen, T.C. Vitamin D deficiency: A worldwide problem with health consequences. *Am J Clin Nutr* 87(Suppl.):1080S–1086S, 2008.

28 Holick, M.F. Resurrection of vitamin D deficiency and rickets. *J Clin Invest* 116:2062–2072, 2006.

29 Holick, M.F. Vitamin D deficiency: What a pain it is. *Mayo Clin Proc* 78:1457–1459, 2003.

30 Food and Nutrition Board, Institute of Medicine. *Dietary Reference Intakes: Calcium, Phosphorus, Magnesium, Vitamin D, and Fluoride.* Washington, DC: National Academies Press, 1997.

31 Vieth, R. Vitamin D toxicity, policy, and science. *J Bone Miner Res* 22(Suppl. 2):V64–V68, 2007.

32 Sabat, R., Guthmann, F., and Rüstow, B. Formation of reactive oxygen species in lung alveolar cells: Effect of vitamin E deficiency. *Lung* 186:115–122, 2008.

33 Harris, A., Devaraj, S., and Jailal, I. Oxidative stress, alpha-tocopherol therapy, and atherosclerosis. *Curr Atheroscler Rep* 4:373–380, 2002.

34 Singh, U., Devaraj, S., and Jialal, I. Vitamin E, oxidative stress, and inflammation. *Annu Rev Nutr* 25:151–174, 2005.

35 Traber, M.G., Frei, B., and Beckman, J.S. Vitamin E revisited: Do new data validate benefits for chronic disease prevention? *Curr Opin Lipidol* 19:30–38, 2008.

36 Jialal, I., and Devaraj, S. Scientific evidence to support a vitamin E and heart disease health claim: Research needs. *J Nutr* 135:348–353, 2005.

37 Bjelakovic, G., Nikolova, D., Gluud, L.L., et al. Mortality in randomized trials of antioxidant supplements for primary and secondary prevention: Systematic review and meta-analysis. *JAMA* 297:842–857, 2007.

38 Maras, J.E., Bermudez, O.I., Qiao, N., et al. Intake of alpha-tocopherol is limited among US adults. *J Am Diet Assoc* 104:567–575, 2004.

39 Bügel, S. Vitamin K and bone health in adult humans. *Vitam Horm* 78:393–416, 2008.

40 Cashman, K.D. Diet, nutrition, and bone health. *J Nutr* 137:2507S–2512S, 2007.

41 American Dietetic Association. *America's Food and Nutrition Attitudes and Behaviors—Nutrition and You: Trends 2000.* Available online at www.eatright.org/cps/rde/xchg/ada/hs.xsl/media_3854_ENU_HTML.htm. Accessed January 27, 2008.

42 Sarubin, A. *The Health Professional's Guide to Popular Dietary Supplements.* Chicago: American Dietetic Association, 2000.

43 American Dietetic Association. Position of the American Dietetic Association: Fortification and nutritional supplements. *J Am Diet Assoc* 105:1300–1311, 2005.

44 Bruno, R.S., and Traber, M.G. Cigarette smoke alters human vitamin E requirements. *J Nutr* 135:671–674, 2005.

45 Ernst, E. The risk–benefit profile of commonly used herbal therapies: *Ginkgo*, St. John's wort, ginseng, Echinacea, saw palmetto, and kava. *Ann Intern Med* 136:42–53, 2002.

46 Smith, J.V., and Luo, Y. Studies on molecular mechanisms of *Ginkgo biloba* extract. *Appl Microbiol Biotechnol* 64:465–472, 2004.

47 Solomon, P.R., Adams, F., Silver, A., et al. *Ginkgo* for memory enhancement: A randomized controlled trial. *JAMA* 288:835–840, 2002.

48 Hu, Z., Yang, X., Ho, P.C., et al. Herb—drug interactions: A literature review. *Drugs* 65:1239–1282, 2005.

49 National Center for Complimentary and Alternative Medicine. *Herbs at a Glance: St. John's Wort.* Available online at http://nccam.nih.gov/health/stjohnswort/ataglance.htm. Accessed January 12, 2008.

50 Mills, E., Montori, V., Perri, D., et al. Natural health product–HIV drug interactions: A systematic review. *Int J STD AIDS* 16:181–186, 2005.

51 Zhou, W., Chai, H., Lin, P.H., et al. Molecular mechanisms and clinical applications of ginseng root for cardiovascular disease. *Med Sci Monit* 10:RA187–192, 2004.

52 Helms, S. Cancer prevention and therapeutics: Panax ginseng. *Altern Med Rev* 9:259–274, 2004.

53 Hermansen, K., Dinesen, B., Hoie, L.H.,et al. Effects of soy and other natural products on LDL:HDL ratio and other lipid parameters: A literature review. *Adv Ther* 20:50–78, 2003.

54 Caruso, T.J., and Gwaltney, J.M., Treatment of the common cold with echinacea: A structured review. *Clin Infect Dis* 40:807–810, 2005.

55 Food and Drug Administration. Current good manufacturing practice in manufacturing, packaging, labeling, or holding operations for dietary supplements; final rule. *Fed Regist* 72(121):34751–34958, June 25, 2007. Available online at www.cfsan.fda.gov/~lrd/ fr07625a.html Accessed May 27, 2008.

Chapter 8

1 Shen, H.-P. Body fluids and water balance. In Stipanuk, M.H. (ed.) *Biochemical, Physiological, and Molecular Aspects of Human Nutrition*, 2nd ed. St. Louis: Saunders Elsevier, 2006, pp. 973–1000.

2 Murray, B. Hydration and physical performance. *J Am Coll Nutr* 26:542S–548S, 2007.

3 Coyle, E.F. Fluid and fuel intake during exercise. *J Sports Sci* 22:39–55, 2004.

4 Institute of Medicine, Food and Nutrition Board. *Dietary Reference Intakes for Water, Potassium, Sodium, Chloride, and Sulfate*. Washington, DC: National Academies Press, 2004.

5 Christiansen Bullers, A. Bottled Water: Better Than the Tap? *FDA Consumer* Jul–Aug 2002. Available online at www.fda.gov/FDAC/ features/2002/402_h2o.html. Accessed August 24, 2008

6 Chobanian, A.V., Bakris, G.L., Black, H.R., et al. Seventh report of the Joint National Committee on Prevention, Detection, Evaluation, and Treatment of High Blood Pressure. Joint National Committee on Prevention, Detection, Evaluation, and Treatment of High Blood Pressure. National Heart, Lung, and Blood Institute. *Hypertension* 42:1206–1252, 2003.

7 Ostchega, Y., Yoon, S.S., Hughes, J., and Louis, T. *Hypertension Awareness, Treatment, and Control—Continued Disparities in Adults: United States, 2005–2006*. Available online at www.cdc.gov/nchs/data/databriefs/ db03.pdf. Accessed August 25, 2008.

8 American Heart Association. Am I at Risk? Factors That Contribute to High Blood Pressure. Available online at www.americanheart.org/ presenter.jhtml?identifier=2142. Accessed August 25, 2008.

9 Carvalho, J.J., Baruzzi, R.G., Howard, P.F., et al. Blood pressure in four remote populations in the Intersalt study. *Hypertension* 14:238–246, 1989.

10 Houston, M.C., and Harper, K.J. Potassium, magnesium, and calcium: Their role in both the cause and treatment of hypertension. *J Clin Hypertens (Greenwich)* 10(7 Suppl 2): 3–11, 2008.

11 Greenland, P. Beating high blood pressure with low sodium DASH. *N Engl J Med* 344:53–55, 2001.

12 Sacks, F.M., Svetkey, L.P., Vollmer, W.M., et al. Effects on blood pressure of reduced dietary sodium and the Dietary Approaches to Stop Hypertension (DASH) diet. DASH-Sodium Collaborative Research Group. *N Engl J Med* 344:3–10, 2001.

13 Appel, L.J., Moore, T.J., Obarzanek, E., et al. A clinical trial of the effects of dietary patterns on blood pressure. *N Engl J Med* 336:1117–1124, 1997.

14 U.S. Department of Health and Human Services, U.S. Department of Agriculture. *Dietary Guidelines for Americans 2005*. Available online at www.healthierus.gov/dietaryguidelines. Accessed May 19, 2005.

15 Bügel, S. Vitamin K and bone health in adult humans. *Vitam Horm* 78:393–416, 2008.

16 United States Department of Health and Human Services. *Bone Health and Osteoporosis: A Report of the Surgeon General*. Rockville, MD: US Department of Health and Human Services, Office of the Surgeon General, 2004.

17 Center for Science in the Public Interest. *Liquid Candy: How Soft Drinks Are Harming America's Health*. Available online at www.cspinet.org/sodapop/liquid_candy.htm. Accessed March 19, 2009.

18 Reid, I.R. Relationships between fat and bone. *Osteoporos Int* 19:595–606, 2008.

19 New, S.A., Robins, S.P., Campbell, M.K., et al. Dietary influences on bone mass and bone metabolism: Further evidence of a positive link between fruit and vegetable consumption and bone health. *Am J Clin Nutr* 71:142–151, 2000.

20 Teucher, B., and Fairweather-Tait, S. Dietary sodium as a risk factor for osteoporosis: Where is the evidence? *Proc Nutr Soc* 62:859–866, 2003.

21 Kerstetter, J.E., O'Brien, K.O., Caseria, D.M., et al. The impact of dietary protein on calcium absorption and kinetic measures of bone turnover in women. *J Clin Endocrinol Metab* 90:26–31, 2005.

22 Institute of Medicine, Food and Nutrition Board. *Dietary Reference Intakes for Calcium, Phosphorus, Magnesium, Vitamin D, and Fluoride*. Washington, DC: National Academies Press, 1997.

23 Nordin, B.E.C., Need, A.G., Morris, H.A., et al. Effect of age on calcium absorption in postmenopausal women. *Am J Clin Nutr* 80:998–1002, 2004.

24 Heaney, R.P., Weaver, C.M., and Recker, R.R. Calcium absorption from spinach. *Am J Clin Nutr* 47:707–709, 1988.

25 Tucker, K.L., Morita, K., Qiao, N., et al. Colas, but not other carbonated beverages, are associated with low bone mineral density in older women: The Framingham Osteoporosis Study. *Am J Clin Nutr* 84: 936–942, 2006.

26 Rude, R.K., and Gruber, H.E. Magnesium deficiency and osteoporosis: Animal and human observations. *J Nutr Biochem*12: 710–716, 2004.

27 Al-Delaimy, W.K., Rimm, E.B., Willett, W.C., et al. Magnesium intake and risk of coronary heart disease among men. *J Am Coll Nutr* 23:63–70, 2004.

28 Food and Nutrition Board, Institute of Medicine. *Dietary Reference Intakes: Vitamin A, Vitamin K, Arsenic, Boron, Chromium, Copper, Iodine, Iron, Manganese, Molybdenum, Nickel, Silicon, Vanadium, and Zinc*. Washington, DC: National Academies Press, 2001.

29 Centers for Disease Control and Prevention. Iron deficiency—United States, 1999–2000. *MMWR Morb Mortal Wkly Rep* 51:897–899, 2002. Available online at www.cdc.gov/ mmwr/preview/mmwrhtml/mm5140a1. htm. Accessed January 21, 2009.

30 World Health Organization. *Micronutrient Deficiencies: Iron Deficiency Anemia*. Available online at www.who.int/nutrition/topics/ida/en/ index.html. Accessed January 21, 2009.

31 Killip, S., Bennett, J.M., and Chambers, M.D. Iron deficiency anemia. *Am Fam Phys* 75:671–678, 2007.

32 Food and Drug Administration. Iron-containing supplements and drugs: Label warning statements and unit-dose packaging requirements. *Fed Regist* 68(201):59714–59715, January, 1997.

33 Siah, C.W., Trinder, D., and Olynyk, J.K. Iron overload. *Clin Chim Acta* 358:24–36, 2005.

34 Centers for Disease Control and Prevention. *Iron Overload and Hemochromatosis: Hereditary Hemochromatosis*. Available online at www.cdc.gov/ncbddd/hemochromatosis/. Accessed June 21, 2005.

35 Tapiero, H., and Tew, K.D. Trace elements in human physiology and pathology: Zinc and metallothioneins. *Biomed Pharmacother* 57:399–411, 2003.

36 Caruso, T.J., Prober, C.G., and Gwaltney, J.M., Jr. Treatment of naturally acquired common colds with zinc: a structured review. *Clin Infect Dis* 45:569–574, 2007.

37 Haase, H., Mocchegiani, E., and Rink, L. Correlation between zinc status and immune function in the elderly. *Biogerontology* 7:421–428, 2006.

38 Beck, M.A., Levander, O., and Handy, J. Selenium deficiency and viral infection. *J Nutr* 133:1463S–1467S, 2003.

39 Food and Nutrition Board, Institute of Medicine. *Dietary Reference Intakes for Vitamin C, Vitamin E, Selenium, and Carotenoids*. Washington, DC: National Academies Press, 2000.

40 Clark, L.C., Combs, G.F., Jr., Turnbull, B.W., et al. Effect of selenium supplementation for

[40] cancer prevention in patients with carcinoma of the skin. *JAMA* 276:1957–1968, 1996.

[41] Greenwald, P., Anderson, D., Nelson, S.A., and Taylor, P.R. Clinical trials of vitamin and mineral supplements for cancer prevention. *Am J Clin Nutr* 85(Suppl):314S–317S, 2007.

[42] World Health Organization. *Micronutrient Deficiencies: Iodine Deficiency Disorders.* Available online at www.who.int/nutrition/topics/idd/en/index.html. Accessed May 20, 2008.

[43] Vincent, J.B. Recent advances in the nutritional biochemistry of trivalent chromium. *Proc Nutr Soc* 63:41–47, 2004.

[44] Di Luigi, L. Supplements and the endocrine system in athletes. *Clin Sports Med* 27:131–151, 2008.

[45] Rubin, C.D., Pak, C.Y., Adams-Huet, B., et al. Sustained-release sodium fluoride in the treatment of the elderly with established osteoporosis. *Arch Intern Med* 161:2325–2333, 2001.

[46] Populations receiving optimally fluoridated public drinking water—United States, 2000. *MMWR Morb Mortal Wkly Rep* 51;144–147, 2002. Available online at www.cdc.gov/mmwr/preview/mmwrhtml/mm5107a2.htm. Accessed March 6, 2009.

[47] Palmer, C., and Wolfe, S.H. Position of the American Dietetic Association: The impact of fluoride on health. *J Am Diet Assoc* 105:1620–1628, 2005.

Chapter 9

[1] Ogden, C.L., Carroll, M.D., Curtin, L.R., et al. Prevalence of overweight and obesity in the United States 1999–2004, *JAMA* 295:1549–1555, 2006.

[2] World Health Organization. *Obesity and Overweight,* September 2006. Fact sheet no. 311. Available online at www.who.int/mediacentre/factsheets/fs311/en/print.html. Accessed July 2, 2008.

[3] Onyike, C.U., Crum, R.M., Lee, H.B., et al. Is obesity associated with major depression? Results from the third NHANES. *Am J Epidemiol* 158:1139–1147, 2003.

[4] National Institutes of Diabetes and Digestive and Kidney Diseases, Weight Control Information Network. *Statistics Related to Overweight and Obesity.* Available online at www.win.niddk.nih.gov/statistics. Accessed January 12, 2009.

[5] U.S. Department of Health and Human Services, U.S. Department of Agriculture. *Dietary Guidelines for Americans, 2005.* Available online at www.health.gov/DietaryGuidelines/dga2005/document. Accessed March 24, 2009.

[6] National Institutes of Health, National Heart, Lung, and Blood Institute. *The Practical Guide:*

Identification, Evaluation and Treatment of Overweight and Obesity in Adults. NIH publication no. 02-4084. Bethesda, MD: National Institutes of Health, 2000.

[7] Flegal, K.M., Graubard, B.I., Williamson, D.F., and Gail, M.H. Excess deaths associated with underweight, overweight, and obesity. *JAMA* 293:1861–1867, 2005.

[8] Gallagher, D., Heymsfield, S., Heo, M., et al. Healthy percentage body fat ranges: an approach for developing guidelines based on body mass index. *Am J Clin Nutr* 72:694–701, 2000.

[9] Redinger, R.N. The physiology of adiposity. *J Ky Med Assoc* 106:53–62, 2008.

[10] Bouchard, C., Tremblay, A., Després, J.-P., et al. The response to long term feeding in identical twins. *N Engl J Med* 322:1477–1482, 1990.

[11] Albu, J., Allison, D., Boozer, C. N., et al. Obesity solutions: Report of a meeting. *Nutr Rev* 55:150–156, 1997.

[12] Wright, J.D., Kennedy-Stephenson, J., Wang, C. Y., et al. Trends in intake of energy and macronutrients—United States, 1971–2000. *MMWR Morb Mortal Wkly Rep* 6:80–82, 2004. Available online at www.cdc.gov/mmwr/preview/mmwrhtml/mm5304a3.htm. Accessed March 7, 2005.

[13] Hill, J.O., and Peters, J.C. Environmental contributions to the obesity epidemic. *Science* 280:1371–1374, 1998.

[14] Young, L.R., and Nestle, M. The contribution of expanding portion size to the obesity epidemic. *Am J Public Health* 92:246–249, 2002.

[15] Rolls, B.J., Morris, E.L., and Roe, L.S. Portion size of food affects energy intake in normal-weight and overweight men and women. *Am J Clin Nutr* 76:1207–1213, 2002.

[16] Bassett, D.R., Schneider P.L., and Huntington, G.E. Physical activity in an Old Order Amish community. *Med Sci Sports Exerc* 36:79–85, 2004.

[17] Ogden, C.L., Carroll, M.D., and Flegal, K.M. High body mass index for age among US children and adolescents, 2003—2006. *JAMA* 299:2401–2405, 2008.

[18] Institute of Medicine, Food and Nutrition Board. *Dietary Reference Intakes for Energy, Carbohydrate, Fiber, Fat, Protein and Amino Acids.* Washington, DC: National Academies Press, 2002.

[19] Kriketos, A.D., Peters, J.C., and Hill, J.O. Cellular and whole-animal energetics. In Stipanuk, M.H. (ed.) *Physiological and Physiological Aspects of Human Nutrition.* Philadelphia: W.B. Saunders Company, 2000, pp. 411–424.

[20] Weinsier, R.L., Nagy, T.R., Hunter, G.R., et al. Do adaptive changes in metabolic rate favor

weight regain in weight-reduced individuals? An examination of the set-point theory. *Am J Clin Nutr* 72:1088–1094, 2000.

[21] Chagnon, Y.C., Rankinen, T., Snyder, E.E., et al. The human obesity gene map: The 2002 update. *Obes Research* 11:313–367, 2003.

[22] Wardle, J., Carnell, S., Haworth, C.M., and Plomin, R. Evidence for a strong genetic influence on childhood adiposity despite the force of the obesogenic environment. *Am J Clin Nutr* 87:398–404, 2008.

[23] Stunkard, A.J., Harris, J.R., Pedersen, N.L., and McClearn, G.E. The body-mass index of twins who have been reared apart. *N Engl J Med* 322:1483–1487, 1990.

[24] Ravussin, E., Valencia, M.E., Esparza, J., et al. Effects of a traditional lifestyle on obesity in Pima Indians. *Diabetes Care* 17:1067–1074, 1994.

[25] Norman, R.A., Thompson, D.B., Foroud, T., et al. Genomewide search for genes influencing percent body fat in Pima Indians: Suggestive linkage at chromosome 11q21-q22. *Am J Human Genet* 60:166–173, 1997.

[26] Esparza, J., Fox, C., Harper, I.T., et al. Daily energy expenditure in Mexican and USA Pima Indians: Low physical activity as a possible cause of obesity. *Int. J.Obes. Relat. Metab. Disord.* 24:55–59, 2000.

[27] Major, G.C., Doucet, E., Trayhurn, P., et al. Clinical significance of adaptive thermogenesis. *Int J Obes (Lond)* 31:204–212, 2007.

[28] Wynne, K., Stanley, S., McGowan, B., and Bloom, S. Appetite control. *J Endocrinol* 184:291–318, 2005.

[29] Batterham, R.L., Cowley, M.A., Small, C.J., et al. Gut hormone PYY(3-36) physiologically inhibits food intake. *Nature* 418:650–654, 2002.

[30] Enriori, P.J., Evans, A.E., Sinnayah, P., and Cowley, M.A. Leptin resistance and obesity. *Obesity* 14:254S–258S, 2006.

[31] Peters, J.C. Control of energy balance. In Stipanuk, M.H. (ed.). *Biochemical and Physiological Aspects of Human Nutrition,* 2nd ed. Philadelphia: W.B. Saunders, 2006, pp. 618–639.

[32] Tsigos, C., Kyrou, I., and Raptis, S.A. Monogenic forms of obesity and diabetes mellitus. *J Pediatr Endocrinol Metab* 15:241–253, 2002.

[33] Levine, J.A., Lanningham-Foster, L.M., McCrady, S.K., et al. Interindividual variation in posture allocation: Possible role in human obesity. *Science* 307:584–586, 2005.

[34] Kroke, A., Liese, A.D., Schulz, M., et al. Recent weight changes and weight cycling as predictors of subsequent two year weight change in a middle-aged cohort. *Int. J.Obes. Relat. Metab. Disord.* 26:403–409, 2002.

35. U.S. Department of Health and Human Services, Office of the Surgeon General. *The Surgeon General's Call to Action to Prevent and Decrease Overweight and Obesity.* Available online at www.surgeongeneral.gov/topics/obesity. Accessed January 10, 2009.

36. Hill, J.O., Wyatt, H.R., Reed, G.W., and Peters, J.C. Obesity and the environment: Where do we go from here? *Science* 299:853–855, 2003.

37. Westman, E.C., Feinman, R.D., Mavropoulos, J.C., et al. Low-carbohydrate nutrition and metabolism. *Am J Clin Nutr* 86:276–284, 2007.

38. Pittler, M.H., and Ernst, E. Dietary supplements for body-weight reduction: A systematic review. *Am J Clin Nutr* 79:529–536, 2004.

39. Li, J.J., Huang, C.J., and Xie, D. Anti-obesity effects of conjugated linoleic acid, docosahexaenoic acid, and eicosapentaenoic acid. *Mol Nutr Food Res* 52:631–645, 2008.

40. Saper, R.B., Eisenberg, D.M., and Phillips, R.S. Common dietary supplements for weight loss. *Am Fam Physician* 70:1731–1738, 2004.

41. Vincent, J.B. The potential value and toxicity of chromium picolinate as a nutritional supplement, weight loss agent and muscle development agent. *Sports Med* 33:213–230, 2003.

42. Hess, A.M., and Sullivan, D.L. Potential for toxicity with use of bitter orange extract and guarana for weight loss. *Ann Pharmacother* 39:574–575, 2005.

43. Sarma, D.N., Barrett, M.L., Chavez, M.L., et al. Safety of green tea extracts: A systematic review by the U.S. Pharmacopeia. *Drug Saf* 31:469–484, 2008.

44. Hsu, C.H., Tsai, T.H., Kao, Y.H., et al. Effect of green tea extract on obese women: A randomized, double-blind, placebo-controlled clinical trial. *Clin Nutr* 27:363–370, 2008.

45. Bent, S., Tiedt, T.N., Odden, M.C., and Shlipak, M.G. The relative safety of ephedra compared with other herbal products. *Ann Intern Med* 138:468–471, 2003.

46. U.S. Food and Drug Administration. *Sales of Supplements Containing Ephedrine Alkaloids (Ephedra) Prohibited.* Available online at www.fda.gov/oc/initiatives/ephedra/february2004/. Accessed January 11, 2009.

47. Kurtzweil, P. Dieter's brews make tea time a dangerous affair. *FDA Consumer* July–August 1997. Available online at www.fda.gov/fdac/features/1997/597_tea.html/. Accessed February 18, 2001.

48. National Institute of Diabetes and Digestive and Kidney Diseases, Weight-Control Information Network. *Gastrointestinal Surgery for Severe Obesity.* Available online at http://win.niddk.nih.gov/publications/gastric.htm. Accessed November 29, 2005.

49. American Dietetic Association. Position of the American Dietetic Association: Nutrition intervention in the treatment of anorexia nervosa, bulimia nervosa, and other eating disorders. *J Am Diet Assoc* 106:2073–2082, 2006.

50. Stice, E. Sociocultural influences on body weight and eating disturbance. In Fairburn, C.G., and Brownell, K.D. (eds.). *Eating Disorders and Obesity: A Comprehensive Handbook,* 2nd ed. New York: The Guilford Press, 2002, pp. 103–107.

51. Body image worries hit Zulu women. BBC News, April 16, 2004. Available online at http://news.bbc.co.uk/2/hi/health/3631359.stm. Accessed April 2, 2009.

52. Mediascope. *Body Image and Advertising.* Available online at www.mediascope.org/pubs/ibriefs/bia.htm. Accessed April 20, 2005.

53. Spann, N., and Pritchard, M. Disordered eating in men: A look at perceived stress and excessive exercise. *Eat Weight Disord* 13:e25–e27, 2008.

54. Tozzi, F., Thornton, L.M., Klump, K.L., et al. Symptom fluctuation in eating disorders: Correlates of diagnostic crossover. *Am J Psychiatry* 162:732–740, 2005.

55. Vandereycken, W. History of anorexia nervosa and bulimia nervosa. In Fairburn, C.G., and Brownell, K.D. (eds.). *Eating Disorders and Obesity: A Comprehensive Handbook,* 2nd ed. New York: The Guilford Press, 2002, pp.151–154.

56. Ebeling, H., Tapanainen, P., and Joutsenoja, A. A practice guideline for treatment of eating disorders in children and adolescents. *Ann Med* 35:488–501, 2003.

57. CME Binge Eating Disorder. Available online at www.healthieryou.com/binge.html. Accessed April 20, 2005.

58. Sundgot-Borgen, J., and Torstveit, M.K. Prevalence of eating disorders in elite athletes is higher than in the general population. *Clin J Sport Med* 14:25–32, 2004.

59. Goebel-Fabbri, A.E., Fikkan, J., Connell, A., et al. Identification and treatment of eating disorders in women with type 1 diabetes mellitus. *Treat Endocrinol* 1:155–162, 2002.

Chapter 10

1. Gallagher, D., Heymsfield, S., Heo, M., et al. Healthy percentage body fat ranges: An approach for developing guidelines based on body mass index. *Am J Clin Nutr* 72:694–701, 2000.

2. The President's Council on Physical Fitness and Sports. *Physical Activity Protects Against the Health Risks of Obesity.* Available online at www.fitness.gov/digest_dec2000.htm. Accessed June 12, 2008.

3. Fontaine, K.R. *Physical Activity Improves Mental Health.* Available online at www.physsportsmed.com/index.php?art=psm_10_2000?article=1256. Accessed April 7, 2009.

4. Antunes, H.K., Stella, S.G., Santos, R.F., et al. Depression, anxiety and quality of life scores in seniors after an endurance exercise program. *Rev Bras Psiquiatr* 27:266–271, 2005.

5. Institute of Medicine, Food and Nutrition Board. *Dietary Reference Intakes for Energy, Carbohydrates, Fiber, Fat, Protein and Amino Acids.* Washington, DC: National Academies Press, 2002.

6. Centers for Disease Control and Prevention. *Physical Activity and Health: A Report of the Surgeon General.* Available online at www.cdc.gov/nccdphp/sgr/adults.htm/. Accessed February 3, 2009.

7. U.S. Department of Health and Human Services, U.S. Department of Agriculture. *Dietary Guidelines for Americans, 2005.* Available online at www.healthierus.gov/dietaryguidelines. Accessed May 19, 2005.

8. United States Department of Health and Human Services. *2008 Physical Activity Guidelines for Americans.* Available online at www.health.gov/paguidelines/ Accessed June 16, 2009.

9. Haskell, W.L., Lee, I.-M., Pate, R.R., et al. Physical activity and public health: Updated recommendations for adults from the American College of Sports Medicine and the American Heart Association. *Circulation* 116:1081–1093, 2007.

10. Manore, M., and Thompson, J. *Sport Nutrition for Health and Performance.* Champaign, IL: Human Kinetics, 2000.

11. Cairns, S.P. Lactic acid and exercise performance: Culprit or friend? *Sports Med* 36:279–291, 2006.

12. Sundgot-Borgen, J., and Torstveit, M.K. Prevalence of eating disorders in elite athletes is higher than in the general population. *Clin J Sport Med* 14:25–32, 2004.

13. Kazis, K., and Iglesias, E. The female athlete triad. *Adolescent Medicine* 14:87–95, 2003.

14. Remick, D., Chancellor, K., Pederson, J., et al. Hyperthermia and dehydration-related deaths associated with intentional rapid weight loss in three collegiate wrestlers—North Carolina, Wisconsin, and Michigan, November–December, 1997. *MMWR Morb Mortal Wkly Rep* 47:105–108, 1998. Available online at www.cdc.gov/mmwr/preview/mmwrhtml/00051388.htm. Accessed March 25, 2009.

15. American Dietetic Association. Position of the American Dietetic Association, Dietitians of Canada, and American College of Sports Medicine: Nutrition and athletic performance. *J Am Diet Assoc* 109:509–527, 2009.

16 Tipton, K.D., and Wolfe, R.R. Protein and amino acids for athletes. *J Sports Sci* 22:65–79, 2004.

17 Jackson, M.J., Khassaf, M., Vasilaki, F., et al. Vitamin E and the oxidative stress of exercise. *Ann N Y Acad Sci* 1031:158–168, 2004.

18 Finaud, J., Lac, G., and Filaire, E. Oxidative stress: Relationship with exercise and training. *Sports Med* 36:327–358, 2006.

19 Margaritis, I., and Rousseau, A.S. Does physical exercise modify antioxidant requirements? *Nutrition Research Reviews* 21:3–12, 2008.

20 Suedekum, N.A., and Dimeff, R.J. Iron and the athlete. *Curr Sports Med Rep* 4:199–202, 2005.

21 Di Santolo, M., Stel, G., Banfi, G., et al. Anemia and iron status in young fertile non-professional female athletes. *Eur J Appl Physiol* 102:703–709, 2008.

22 Food and Nutrition Board, Institute of Medicine. *Dietary Reference Intakes: Vitamin A, Vitamin K, Arsenic, Boron, Chromium, Copper, Iodine, Iron, Manganese, Molybdenum, Nickel, Silicon, Vanadium, and Zinc*. Washington, DC: National Academies Press, 2001.

23 NOAA's National Weather Service: *Heat Index*. Available online at www.weather.gov/os/heat/index.shtml. Accessed March 10, 2009.

24 Almond, C.S.D., Shin, A.Y., Fortescue, E.B., et al. Hyponatremia among runners in the Boston Marathon., *N Engl J Med* 352:1550–1556, 2005.

25 Senay, L.C. Water and electrolytes during physical activity. In Wolinski, I. (ed.). *Nutrition in Exercise and Sport*, 3rd ed. Boca Raton, FL: CRC Press, 1998, pp. 257–276.

26 Bergstrom, J., Hermansen, L., Hultman, E., and Saltin, B. Diet, muscle glycogen and physical performance. *Acta Physiologica Scandinavica* 71:140–150, 1967.

27 Burke, L.M. Nutrition strategies for the marathon: Fuel for training and racing. *Sports Med* 37:344–347, 2007.

28 Bussau, V.A., Fairchild, T.J., Rao, A., et al. Carbohydrate loading in human muscle: An improved 1 day protocol. *Eur J Appl Physiol* 87:290–295, 2002.

29 Karp, J.R., Johnston, J.D., Tecklenburg, T.D., et al. Chocolate milk as a post-exercise recovery aid. *Int J Sport Nutr Exerc Metab* 16:78–91, 2006.

30 Berardi, J.M., Price, T.B., Noreen, E.E., and Lemon, P.W. Postexercise muscle glycogen recovery enhanced with a carbohydrate-protein supplement. *Med Sci Sports Exerc* 38:1106–1113, 2006.

31 Di Luigi, L. Supplements and the endocrine system in athletes. *Clin Sports Med* 27:131–151, 2008.

32 Nissen, S.L., and Sharp, R.L. Effect of dietary supplements on lean mass and strength gains with resistance exercise: A meta-analysis. *J Appl Physiol* 94:651–659, 2003.

33 Liu, H., Bravata, D.M., Olkin, I., et al. Systematic review: The effects of growth hormone on athletic performance. *Ann Intern Med* 148:747–758, 2008.

34 Kanaley, J.A. Growth hormone, arginine and exercise. *Curr Opin Clin Nutr Metab Care* 11:50–54, 2008.

35 Chromiak, J.A., and Antonio, J. Use of amino acids as growth hormone-releasing agents by athletes. *Nutrition* 18:657–661, 2002.

36 NutraBio.com. *Congress Passes Steroid Control Act*. Available online at www.nutrabio.com/News/news.steroid_control_act_2.htm. Accessed June 25, 2008.

37 Brown, G.A., Vukovich, M., and King, D.S. Testosterone prohormone supplements. *Med Sci Sports Exerc* 38:1451–1461, 2006.

38 Tokish, J.M., Kocher, M.S., and Hawkins, R.J. Ergogenic aids: A review of basic science, performance, side effects, and status in sports. *Am J Sports Med* 32:1543–1553, 2004.

39 Sjöqvist, F., Garle, M., and Rane, A. Use of doping agents, particularly anabolic steroids, in sports and society. *Lancet* 371:1872–1882, 2008.

40 Nissen, S., Sharp, R., Ray, M., et al. Effect of leucine metabolite beta-hydroxy-beta-methyl-butyrate on muscle metabolism during resistance-exercise training. *J Appl Physiol* 81:2095–2104, 1996.

41 O'Connor, D.M., and Crowe, M.J. Effects of six weeks of beta-hydroxy-beta-methylbutyrate (HMB) and HMB/creatine supplementation on strength, power, and anthropometry of highly trained athletes. *J Strength Cond Res* 21:419–423, 2007.

42 Raymer, G.H., Marsh, G.D., Kowalchuk, J.M., and Thompson, R.T. Metabolic effects of induced alkalosis during progressive forearm exercise to fatigue. *J Appl Physiol* 96:2050–2056, 2004.

43 Paddon-Jones, D., Borsheim, E., and Wolfe, R.R. Potential ergogenic effects of arginine and creatine supplementation. *J Nutr* 134 (10 Suppl):2888S–2894S, 2004.

44 Bemben, M.G., and Lamont, H.S. Creatine supplementation and exercise performance: Recent findings. *Sports Med* 35:107–125, 2005.

45 Terjung, R. L., Clarkson, P., Eichner, E. R., et al. American College of Sports Medicine roundtable: The physiological and health effects of oral creatine supplementation. *Med Sci Sports Exerc* 32:706–717, 2000.

46 Volek, J.S., and Rawson, E.S. Scientific basis and practical aspects of creatine supplementation for athletes. *Nutrition* 20:609–614, 2004.

47 Shao, A., and Hathcock, J.N. Risk assessment for creatine monohydrate. *Regul Toxicol Pharmacol* 45:242–251, 2006.

48 Brass, E.P. Carnitine and sports medicine: Use or abuse? *Ann N Y Acad Sci* 1033:67–78, 2004.

49 Jeukendrup, A.E., and Aldred, S. Fat supplementation, health, and endurance performance. *Nutrition* 20:678–688, 2004.

50 Horowitz, J.F., Mora-Rodriguez, R., Byerley, L.O., and Coyle, E.F. Preexercise medium-chain triglyceride ingestion does not alter muscle glycogen use during exercise. *J Appl Physiol* 88:219–225, 2000.

51 Sökmen, B., Armstrong, L.E., Kraemer, W.J., et al. Caffeine use in sports: Considerations for the athlete. *J Strength Cond Res* 22:978–986, 2008.

52 Birkeland, K.I., Stray-Gundersen, J., Hemmersbach, P., et al. Effect of rhEPO administration on serum levels of sTfR and cycling performance. *Med Sci Sports Exerc* 32:1238–1243, 2000.

Chapter 11

1 Committee to Reexamine IOM Pregnancy Weight Guidelines, Institute of Medicine, National Research Council. *Weight Gain During Pregnancy: Reexamining the Guidelines*. Washington, DC: National Acadamies Press, 2009.

2 Bryson, S.R., Theriot, L., Ryan, N. J., et al. Primary follow-up care in a multidisciplinary setting enhances catch-up growth of very-low-birth-weight infants. *J Am Diet Assoc* 97:386–390, 1997.

3 National Women's Health Information Center, U.S. Department of Health and Human Services. *Healthy Pregnancy*. Available online at www.womenshealth.gov/pregnancy/you-are-pregnant/staying-healthy-safe.cfm#a. Accessed June 19, 2009.

4 Kaiser, L., and Allen, L.A. Position of the American Dietetic Association: Nutrition and lifestyle for a healthy pregnancy outcome. *J Am Diet Assoc* 108:553–561, 2008.

5 American College of Obstetricians and Gynecologists. ACOG Committee Opinion number 315, September 2005. Obesity in pregnancy. *Obstet Gynecol* 106:671–675, 2005.

6 Linne, Y., Dye, L., Barkeling, B., and Rossner, S. Long-term weight development in women: A 15-year follow-up of the effects of pregnancy. *Obes Res* 12:1166–1178, 2004.

7 Oken, E., Taveras, E.M., Kleinman, K.P., et al. Gestational weight gain and child adiposity at age 3 years. *Am J Obstet Gynecol* 196:322.e1–322.e8, 2007.

8 United States Department of Health and Human Services. *2008 Physical Activity*

Guidelines for Americans. Available online at www.health.gov/paguidelines. Accessed June 19, 2009.

9 National Center for Health Statistics, Centers for Disease Control and Prevention. *FastStats: Infant Health.* Available online at www.cdc.gov/nchs/fastats/infant_health.htm. Accessed July 3, 2009.

10 National Center for Health Statistics, Centers for Disease Control and Prevention. *Deaths: Final Data for 2004.* Available online at www.cdc.gov/nchs/products/pubs/pubd/hestats/finaldeaths04/finaldeaths04.htm. Accessed July 30, 2008.

11 Chang, J., Elam-Evans, L.D., Berg, C.J., et al. Pregnancy-related mortality surveillance—United States, 1991–1999. *MMWR Morb Mortal Wkly Rep* 52:1–8, 2003.

12 Food and Nutrition Board, Institute of Medicine. *Dietary Reference Intakes: Water, Potassium, Sodium, Chloride, and Sulfate.* Washington, DC: National Academies Press, 2004.

13 Kumar, A., Devi, S.G., Batra, S., et al. Calcium supplementation for the prevention of pre-eclampsia. *Int J Gynaecol Obstet* 104:32–36, 2009.

14 Hofmeyr, G.J., Roodt, A., Atallah, A.N., and Duley, L. Calcium supplementation to prevent pre-eclampsia—A systematic review. *S Afr Med J* 93:224–228, 2003.

15 Office of Minority Health and Health Disparities, Centers for Disease Control and Prevention. *Eliminate Disparities in Diabetes.* Available online at www.cdc.gov/omhd/AMH/factsheets/diabetes.htm. Accessed February 23, 2009.

16 Damm, P. Future risk of diabetes in mother and child after gestational diabetes mellitus. *Int J Gynaecol Obstet* 104(Suppl. 1):S25–S26, 2009.

17 Food and Nutrition Board, Institute of Medicine. *Dietary Reference Intakes for Energy, Carbohydrates, Fiber, Fat, Protein and Amino Acids.* Washington, DC: National Academies Press, 2002.

18 Koletzko, B., Lien, E., Agostoni, C., et al. The roles of long-chain polyunsaturated fatty acids in pregnancy, lactation and infancy: Review of current knowledge and consensus recommendations. *J Perinat Med* 36:5–14, 2008.

19 Food and Nutrition Board, Institute of Medicine. *Dietary Reference Intakes for Water, Potassium, Sodium, Chloride, and Sulfate.* Washington, DC: National Academies Press, 2004.

20 Food and Nutrition Board, Institute of Medicine. *Dietary Reference Intakes for Calcium, Phosphorus, Magnesium, Vitamin D, and Fluoride.*

Washington, DC: National Academies Press, 1997.

21 Hollis, B.W., and Wagner, C.L. Assessment of dietary vitamin D requirements during pregnancy and lactation. *Am J Clin Nutr* 79:717–726, 2004.

22 Holick, M.F. Vitamin D deficiency: What a pain it is. *Mayo Clin Proc* 78:1457–1459, 2003.

23 Scholl, T.O., and Johnson, W.G. Folic acid: Influence on the outcome of pregnancy. *Am J Clin Nutr* 71 (Suppl.):1295S–1303S, 2000.

24 Food and Nutrition Board, Institute of Medicine. *Dietary Reference Intakes for Thiamin, Riboflavin, Niacin, Vitamin B-6, Folate, Vitamin B-12, Pantothenic Acid, Biotin, and Choline.* Washington, DC: National Academies Press, 1998.

25 Centers for Disease Control and Prevention. Spina bifida and anencephaly before and after folic acid mandate—United States, 1995–1996 and 1999–2000, *MMWR Morb Mortal Wkly Rep* 17:362–365, 2004. Available online at www.cdc.gov/MMWR/preview/mmwrhtml/mm5317a3.htm. Accessed April 17, 2008.

26 De Wals, P., Tiarou, F., Van Allen, M.I., et al. Reduction in neural-tube defects after folic acid fortification in Canada. *N Engl J Med* 357:135–142, 2007.

27 Food and Nutrition Board, Institute of Medicine. *Dietary Reference Intakes for Vitamin A, Vitamin K, Arsenic, Boron, Chromium, Copper, Iodine, Iron, Manganese, Molybdenum, Nickel, Silicon, Vanadium, and Zinc.* Washington, DC: National Academies Press, 2001.

28 Scholl, T.O. Iron status during pregnancy: Setting the stage for mother and infant. *Am J Clin Nutr* 81:1218S–1222S, 2005.

29 King, J.C. Determinants of maternal zinc status during pregnancy. *Am J Clin Nutr* 71 (Suppl.):1334S–1343S, 2000.

30 Mills, M.E. Craving more than food: The implications of pica in pregnancy. *Nurs Womens Health* 11:266–273, 2007.

31 Centers for Disease Control and Prevention. *Birth Defects.* Available online at www.cdc.gov/ncbddd/bd/. Accessed February 3, 2009.

32 Stein, A.D., Zybert, P.A., van de Bor, M., and Lumey, L.H. Intrauterine famine exposure and body proportions at birth: The Dutch Hunger Winter. *Int J Epidemiol* 33:831–836, 2004.

33 Gluckman, P.D., Hanson, M.A., Cooper, C., and Thornburg, K.L. Effect of in utero and early-life conditions on adult health and disease. *N Engl J Med* 359:61–73, 2008.

34 Roseboom, T., de Rooij, S., and Painter, R. The Dutch famine and its long-term consequences for adult health. *Early Hum Dev* 82:485–491, 2006.

35 Kramer, M.S., Seguin, L., Lydon, J., and Goulet, L. Socio-economic disparities in pregnancy outcome: Why do the poor fare so poorly? *Paediatr Perinat Epidemiol* 14:194–210, 2000.

36 Casanueva, E., Roselló-Soberón, M.E., and De-Regil, L.M. Adolescents with adequate birth weight newborns diminish energy expenditure and cease growth. *J Nutr* 136:2498–2501, 2006.

37 National Center for Health Statistics, Centers for Disease Control and Prevention. *FastStats: Teen Births.* Available online at www.cdc.gov/nchs/fastats/teenbrth.htm. Accessed July 12, 2009.

38 National Down Syndrome Congress. *Facts About Down Syndrome.* Available online at www.ndsccenter.org/resources/package3.php. Accessed February 4, 2009.

39 Pediatric and Pregnancy Nutrition Surveillance System, Centers for Disease Control and Prevention. *Maternal Health Indicators.* Available online at www.cdc.gov/pednss/what_is/pnss_health_indicators.htm#Maternal%20Health%20Indicators. Accessed January 12, 2008.

40 Weng, X., Odouli, R., and Li, D.K. Maternal caffeine consumption during pregnancy and the risk of miscarriage: A prospective cohort study. *Am J Obstet Gynecol* 198: 279e1–279e8. Epub 2008.

41 U.S. Food and Drug Administration, Center for Food Safety and Applied Nutrition. Food Safety for Moms-to-Be. Available online at www.cfsan.fda.gov/~pregnant/safeats.html. Accessed April 19, 2009.

42 Delgado, A.R. Listeriosis in pregnancy. *J Midwifery Womens Health* 53:255–259, 2008.

43 Center for the Evaluation of Risks to Human Reproduction (CERHR). *Toxoplasmosis.* Available online at http://cerhr.niehs.nih.gov/common/toxoplasmosis.html. Accessed July 16, 2008.

44 Goodlett, C.R., and Horn, K.H. Mechanisms of alcohol-induced damage to the developing nervous system. *Alcohol Res Health* 25:175–184, 2001. Available online at http://pubs.niaaa.nih.gov/publications/arh25-3/175-184.pdf. Accessed April 20, 2009.

45 Rogers, J.M. Tobacco and pregnancy: Overview of exposures and effects. *Birth Defects Res C Embryo Today* 84:1–15, 2008.

46 Xiao, D., Huang, X., Yang, S., and Zhang, L. Direct effects of nicotine on contractility of the uterine artery in pregnancy. *J Pharmacol Exp Ther* 322:180–185, 2007.

47 National Center for Chronic Disease Prevention and Health Promotion. *Women and Smoking:*

A Report of the Surgeon General, March 2001. Available online at www.surgeongeneral.gov/library/womenandtobacco/. Accessed April 20, 2009.

48 The National Council on Alcoholism and Drug Dependence. *Alcohol- and Other Drug-Related Birth Defects, Facts and Information.* Available online at www.ncadd.org/facts/defects.html. Accessed July 14, 2008.

49 Schempf, A.H. Illicit drug use and neonatal outcomes: A critical review. *Obstet Gynecol Surv* 62:749–757, 2007.

50 Fajemirokun-Odudeyi, O., and Lindow, S.W. Obstetric implications of cocaine use in pregnancy: A literature review. *Eur J Obstet Gynecol Reprod Biol* 112:2–8, 2004.

51 Schiller, C., and Allen, P.J. Follow-up of infants prenatally exposed to cocaine. *Pediatr Nurs* 31:427–436, 2005.

52 Prentice, A. Calcium requirements of breast-feeding mothers. *Nutr Rev* 56:124–130, 1998.

53 National Center for Health Statistics, Centers for Disease Control and Prevention. *2000 CDC Growth Charts: United States.* Available online at www.cdc.gov/growthcharts/. Accessed August 25, 2004.

54 Gartner, L.M., and Greer, F.R. Prevention of rickets and vitamin D deficiency: New guidelines for vitamin D intake. *Pediatrics* 111:908–910, 2003.

55 American Academy of Pediatrics, policy statement, Committee on Fetus and Newborn. Controversies concerning vitamin K and the newborn. *Pediatrics* 112:191–192, 2003.

56 American Dietetic Association. Position of the American Dietetic Association: Promoting and supporting breastfeeding. *J Am Diet Assoc* 105:810–818, 2005.

57 Gartner, L.M. Breastfeeding and the use of human milk. *Pediatrics* 115:496–506, 2005.

58 World Health Organization, United Nations Children's Fund. *Global Strategy for Infant and Young Child Feeding.* Geneva, Switzerland: World Health Organization, 2003.

59 Lawrence, R.M., and Lawrence, R.A. Breast milk and infection. *Clin Perinatol* 31:501–528, 2004.

60 Ip, S., Chung, M., Raman, G., et al. Breastfeeding and maternal and infant health outcomes in developed countries. *Evid Rep Technol Assess (Full Rep)* 153:1–186, 2007.

61 Hamprecht, K., Maschmann, J., Jahn, G., et al. Cytomegalovirus transmission to preterm infants during lactation. *J Clin Virol* 41:198–205, 2008.

62 Greer, F.R., Sicherer, S.H., and Burks, A.W. Effects of early nutritional interventions on the development of atopic disease in infants and children: the role of maternal dietary

restriction, breastfeeding, timing of introduction of complementary foods, and hydrolyzed formulas. *Pediatrics* 121:183–191, 2008.

63 Ziegler, E.E. Adverse effects of cow's milk in infants. *Nestle Nutr Workshop Ser Pediatr Program* 60:185–196, 2007.

64 American Academy of Pediatrics. The use and misuse of fruit juice in pediatrics. *Pediatrics* 107:1210–1213, 2001.

Chapter 12

1 Institute of Medicine, Food and Nutrition Board. *Dietary Reference Intakes for Energy, Carbohydrate, Fiber, Fat, Protein, and Amino Acids.* Washington, DC: National Academies Press, 2002.

2 Institute of Medicine, Food and Nutrition Board. *Dietary Reference Intakes for Water, Potassium, Sodium, Chloride, and Sulfate.* Washington, DC: National Academies Press, 2004.

3 Nicklas, T.A., and Hayes, D. Position of the American Dietetic Association: Nutrition guidance for healthy children ages 2 to 11 years. *J Am Diet Assoc* 108:1038–1047, 2008.

4 Institute of Medicine, Food and Nutrition Board. *Dietary Reference Intakes for Calcium, Phosphorus, Magnesium, Vitamin D, and Fluoride.* Washington, DC: National Academies Press, 1997.

5 Rovner, A.J., and O'Brien, K.O. Hypovitaminosis D among healthy children in the United States: A review of the current evidence. *Arch Pediatr Adolesc Med* 162:513–519, 2008.

6 Haas, J.D., and Brownlie, T. IV. Iron deficiency and reduced work capacity: A critical review of the research to determine a causal relationship. *J Nutr* 131:676S–690S, 2001.

7 Grantham-McGregor, S., and Ani, C. A review of studies on the effect of iron deficiency on cognitive development in children. *J Nutr* 131:649S–668S, 2001.

8 Slatter, E. *Secrets of Feeding a Healthy Family.* Madison, WI: Kelsey Press, 1999.

9 American Academy of Pediatrics. The use and misuse of fruit juice in pediatrics. *Pediatrics* 107:1210–1213, 2001.

10 Patrick, H., and Nicklas, T.A. A review of family and social determinants of children's eating patterns and diet quality. *J Am Coll Nutr* 24:83–92, 2005.

11 U.S. Department of Health and Human Services, Centers for Disease Control and Prevention, National Center for Health Statistics. *CDC Growth Charts: United States.* Advance Data, No. 314, June 8, 2000 (revised). Available online at www.cdc.gov/growthcharts/. Accessed August 28, 2008.

12 Rampersaud, G.C., Pereira, M.A., Girard, B.L., et al. Breakfast habits, nutritional status, body weight, and academic performance in children and adolescents. *J Am Diet Assoc* 105:743–760, 2005.

13 Alaimo, K., Olson, C., and Frongillo, E. Food insufficiency and American school-aged children's cognitive, academic, and psychosocial development. *Pediatrics* 108:44–53, 2001.

14 Kleinman, R.E., Hall, S., Green, H., et al. Diet, breakfast, and academic performance in children. *Ann Nutr Metab* 46(Suppl. 1):24–30, 2002.

15 Gillman, M.W., Rifas-Shiman, S.L., Frazier, A.L., et al. Family dinner and diet quality among older children and adolescents. *Archives of Family Medicine* 9:235–240, 2000.

16 U.S. Department of Agriculture, Food and Nutrition Service. *National School Lunch Program.* Available online at www.fns.usda.gov/cnd/Lunch/AboutLunch/NSLPFactSheet.pdf. Accessed February 20, 2009.

17 U.S. Department of Agriculture, Food and Nutrition Service. *Children's Diets in the Mid-1990s: Dietary Intake and Its Relationship with School Meal Participation.* Special Nutrition Programs Report No. CN-01-CD1, January 2001. Available online at www.fns.usda.gov/OANE/menu/Published/CNP/FILES/ChilDiet.pdf. Accessed April 20, 2009.

18 Ogden, C.L., Carroll, M.D., and Flegal, K.M. High body mass index for age among U.S. children and adolescents, 2003–2006. *JAMA* 299:2401–2405, 2008.

19 National Diabetes Information Clearinghouse. *National Diabetes Statistics, 2007.* Available online at http://diabetes.niddk.nih.gov/dm/pubs/statistics/index.htm#13. Accessed September 4, 2008.

20 Mayer-Davis, E.J. Type 2 diabetes in youth: Epidemiology and current research toward prevention and treatment. *J Am Diet Assoc* 108:S45–S51, 2008.

21 Centers for Disease Control and Prevention. *About BMI for Children and Teens.* Available online at www.cdc.gov/nccdphp/dnpa/healthyweight/assessing/bmi/childrens_BMI/about_childrens_BMI.htm. Accessed September 8, 2008.

22 Ogden, C.L., Flegal, K.M., Carroll, M.D., and Johnson, C.L. Prevalence and trends among US children and adolescents, 1999–2000. *JAMA* 288:1728–1732, 2002.

23 Hedley, A.A., Ogden, C.L., Johnson, C.L., et al. Prevalence of overweight and obesity among US children, adolescents, and adults, 1999–2002. *JAMA* 291:2847–2850, 2004.

24 Academy of Pediatrics, Committee on Nutrition. *Cholesterol in Childhood.* Available

online at http://aappolicy.aappublications.org/cgi/reprint/pediatrics;101/1/141.pdf. Accessed September 4, 2008.

[25] Coon, K.A., and Tucker, K.L. Television and children's consumption patterns. A review of the literature. *Minerva Pediatr* 54:423–436, 2002.

[26] Eisenmann, J.C., Bartee, R.T., and Wang, M.Q. Physical activity, TV viewing, and weight in U.S. youth: 1999 Youth Risk Behavior Survey. *Obes Res* 10:379–385, 2002.

[27] Batada, A., Seitz, M., Wotan, M., et al. Nine out of ten food advertisements shown during Saturday morning children's television programming are for food high in fat, sodium, or added sugars, or low in nutrients. *J Am Diet Assoc* 108:673–678, 2008.

[28] Cormier, E., and Elder, J.H. Diet and child behavior problems: Fact or fiction? *Pediatr Nurs* 33:138–143, 2007.

[29] Rojas, N.L., and Chan, E. Old and new controversies in the alternative treatment of attention-deficit hyperactivity disorder. *Ment Retard Dev Disabil Res Rev* 11:116–30, 2005.

[30] Farley, D. Dangers of lead still linger. *FDA Consum* 32:16–21, 1998.

[31] Centers for Disease Control and Prevention. Blood lead levels—United States, 1999–2002. *MMWR Morb Mortal Wkly Rep* 54:513–516, 2005. Available online at www.cdc.gov/mmwr/preview/mmwrhtml/mm5420a5.htm. Accessed April 20, 2009.

[32] Jusko, T.A., Henderson, C.R. Jr, Lanphear, B.P., et al. Blood lead concentrations below 10 microg/dL and child intelligence at 6 years of age. *Environ Health Perspect* 116:243–248, 2008.

[33] American Academy of Pediatrics Policy Statement. Lead Exposure in Children: Prevention, Detection, and Management. *Pediatrics* 116:1036–1046, 2005.

[34] Weng, F.L., Shults, J., Leonard, M.B., et al. Risk factors for low serum 25-hydroxyvitamin D concentrations in otherwise healthy children and adolescents. *Am J Clin Nutr*, 86: 150–158, 2007.

[35] Centers for Disease Control and Prevention. Iron Deficiency—United States, 1999–2000. *MMWR Morb Mortal Wkly Rep* 51:897–899, 2002. Available online at www.cdc.gov/MMWR/preview/mmwrhtml/mm5140a1. htm. Accessed September 11, 2008.

[36] National Institute of Child Health and Human Development. *Milk Matters. About milk matters* Available online at www.nichd.nih.gov/milk/about/index.cfm. Accessed April 27, 2009.

[37] Nielsen, S.J., and Popkin, B.M. Changes in beverage intake between 1977 and 2000. *Am J Prev Med* 27:205–210, 2004.

[38] USDA/ARC Children's Nutrition Research Center at Baylor College of Medicine. *Survey Tracks Trends in Children's Dietary Habits.* Available online at www.bcm.edu/cnrc/consumer/archives/mealtime.htm . Accessed April 27, 2009.

[39] Beals, K.A., and Manore, M.M. Nutritional status of female athletes with subclinical eating disorders. *J Am Diet Assoc* 98:419–425, 1998.

[40] Kazis, K., and Iglesiasl, E. The female athlete triad. *Adolescent Medicine* 14:87–95, 2003.

[41] Palmersheim, K.A. Trends in cigarette smoking among high school youth in Wisconsin and the United States, 1993–2004. *WMJ* 104:23–27, 2005.

[42] Facchini, M., Rozensztejn, R., and Gonzalez, C. Smoking and weight control behaviors. *Eat Weight Disord* 10:1–7, 2005.

[43] Palaniappan, U., Jacobs Starkey, L., O'Loughlin, J., and Gray-Donald, K. Fruit and vegetable consumption is lower and saturated fat intake is higher among Canadians reporting smoking. *J Nutr* 131:1952–1958, 2001.

[44] YRBSS, 2007 National Youth Risk Behavior Survey Overview. Available online at www.cdc.gov/HealthyYouth/yrbs/pdf/yrbs07_us_overview.pdf Accessed April 26, 2009.

[45] National Council on Alcohol and Drug Dependence. *Youth, Alcohol and Other Drugs.* Available online at www.ncadd.org/facts/youthalc.html. Accessed July 20, 2009.

[46] Centers for Disease Control and Prevention. Deaths: Final data for 2005. *Natl Vital Stat Rep* 56:1–124, 2008. Available online at www.cdc.gov/nchs/data/nvsr/nvsr56/nvsr56_10.pdf. Accessed April 1, 2009.

[47] World Health Organization. *The World Health Report, 2003. Healthy Life Expectancy. Annex Table 4 Healthy Life Expectancy (HALE) in All Member States, Estimates for 2002.* Available online at www.who.int/whr/2003/en/Annex4-en.pdf. Accessed September 12, 2008.

[48] Federal Interagency Forum on Aging-Related Statistics. *Older Americans 2008: Key Indicators of Wellbeing, Population.* Available online at www.agingstats.gov/agingstatsdotnet/Main_Site/Data/Data_2008.aspx. Accessed September 12, 2008.

[49] U.S. Department of Health and Human Services, Administration on Aging. *1997 Census Estimates of the Older Population.* Available online at www.aoa.gov/AoARoot/Aging_Statistics/Census_Population/Population/1997/rankxpercent.aspx . Accessed February 17, 2001.

[50] Cohn, S.H., Vartsky, D., Yasumura, A., et al. Compartmental body composition based on total-body nitrogen, potassium, and calcium. *Am J Physiol* 239 (*Endocrinol Metabol* 2): E524–E530, 1980.

[51] American Dietetic Association. Position of the American Dietetic Association: Nutrition across the spectrum of aging. *J Am Diet Assoc* 105:616–633, 2005.

[52] Institute of Medicine, Food and Nutrition Board. *Dietary Reference Intakes for Thiamin, Riboflavin, Niacin, Vitamin B$_6$, Folate, Vitamin B$_{12}$, Pantothenic Acid, Biotin, and Choline.* Washington, DC: National Academies Press, 1998.

[53] National Institutes of Health, Office of Dietary Supplements. *Dietary Supplement Fact Sheet: Vitamin B12.* Available online at http://ods.od.nih.gov/factsheets/vitaminb12.asp. Accessed August 21, 2008.

[54] Holick, M.F., and Chen, T.C. Vitamin D deficiency: A worldwide problem with health consequences. *Am J Clin Nutr* 87(Suppl.):1080S–1086S, 2008.

[55] U.S. Department of Health and Human Services. Securing the Benefits of Medical Innovation for Seniors: The Role of Prescription Drugs and Drug Coverage. July 2002. Available online at http://aspe.hhs.gov/health/Reports/medicalinnovation/ Accessed July 20, 2009.

[56] Blumberg, J. Nutritional needs of seniors. *J Am Coll Nutr* 16:517–523, 1997.

[57] Proctor, D.N., Balagopal, P., and Nair, K.S. Age-related sarcopenia in humans is associated with reduced synthetic rates of specific muscle proteins. *J Nutr* 128:351S–355S, 1998.

[58] Chandra, R.K. Impact of nutritional status and nutrient supplements on immune responses and incidence of infection in older individuals. *Ageing Res Rev* 3:91–104, 2004.

[59] Centers for Disease Control and Prevention. Health Information for Older Adults. Available online at www.cdc.gov/Aging/info.htm#2. Accessed July 21, 2009.

[60] Centers for Disease Control and Prevention. *Arthritis.* Available online at www.cdc.gov/nchs/fastats/arthrits.htm. Accessed September 14, 2008.

[61] Gregory, P.J., Sperry, M., and Wilson, A.F. Dietary supplements for osteoarthritis. *Am Fam Physician* 77:177–184, 2008.

[62] Christen, W.G. Antioxidant vitamins and age-related eye disease. *Proceedings of the Association of American Physicians* 111:16–21, 1999.

[63] Hajjar, E.R., Cafiero, A.C., and Hanlon, J.T. Polypharmacy in elderly patients. *Am J Geriatr Pharmacother* 5:314–316, 2007.

[64] Administration on Aging. *A Profile of Older Americans: 2007.* Available online at www.agingcarefl.org/aging/AOA-2007profile.pdf. Accessed September 14, 2008.

[65] Nord, M., Andrews, M., and Carlson, S. *Household Food Security in the United States,*

2007. November 2008. Available online at www.ers.usda.gov/Publications/ERR66/. Accessed April 20, 2009.

[66] Willcox, B.J., Willcox, D.C., Todoriki, H., et al. Caloric restriction, the traditional Okinawan diet, and healthy aging: The diet of the world's longest-lived people and its potential impact on morbidity and life span. *Ann N Y Acad Sci* 1114:434–455, 2007.

[67] U.S. Department of Health and Human Services. *2008 Physical Activity Guidelines for Americans.* Available online at www.health.gov/paguidelines/ Accessed June 16, 2009.

[68] American Dietetic Association. Position paper of the American Dietetic Association: Nutrition across the spectrum of aging. *J Am Diet Assoc* 105:1203–1210, 2005.

[69] Dorner, B., Niedert, K.C., and Welch, P.K. Position of the American Dietetic Association: Liberalized diets for older adults in long-term care. *J Am Diet Assoc* 102:1316–1323, 2002.

[70] American Medical Association. *Harmful Consequences of Alcohol Use on the Brains of Children, Adolescents and College Students, 2002.* Fact Sheet. Available online at www.ama-assn.org/ama1/pub/upload/mm/388/harmful_consequences.pdf . Accessed April 27, 2009.

[71] Bode, C., and Bode, J.C. Effect of alcohol consumption on the gut. *Best Pract Res Clin Gastroenterol* 17:575–592, 2003.

[72] Lieber, C.S. Relationships between nutrition, alcohol use, and liver disease. *Alcohol Res and Health* 27:220–231, 2003.

[73] Yi, H., Chen, C.M. and Williams, G.D. *Surveillance Report #76: Trends in Alcohol-Related Fatal Traffic Crashes, United States, 1982–2004.* Bethesda, MD: National Institute on Alcohol Abuse and Alcoholism, Division of Epidemiology and Prevention Research (August 2006). Available online at http://pubs.niaaa.nih.gov/publications/surveillance76/FARS04.pdf . Accessed April 16, 2004.

[74] Whitfield, J.B. Alcohol and gene interactions. *Clin Chem Lab Med* 43:480–487, 2005.

[75] Bagnardi, V., Blangiardo, M., La Vecchia, C., and Corrao, G. A meta-analysis of alcohol drinking and cancer risk. *Br J Cancer* 85:1700–1705, 2001.

[76] Dumitrescu, R.G., and Shields, P.G. The etiology of alcohol-induced breast cancer. *Alcohol* 35:213–225, 2005.

[77] Allen, N.E., Beral, V., and Casabonne, D. Moderate alcohol intake and cancer incidence in women. *J Natl Cancer Inst* 101:296–305, 2009.

[78] Lucas, D.L., Brown, R.A., Wassef, M., and Giles, T.D. Alcohol and the cardiovascular system: Research challenges and opportunities. *J Am Coll Cardiol* 45:1916–1924, 2005.

[79] Saremi, A., and Arora, R. The cardiovascular implications of alcohol and red wine. *Am J Ther* 15:265–277, 2008.

Chapter 13

[1] Mead, P.S., Slutsker, L., Dietz, V., et al. *Food-Related Illness and Death in the United States.* Available online at www.cdc.gov/ncidod/eid/vol5no5/mead.htm. Accessed August 1, 2008.

[2] Centers for Disease Control and Prevention. *Foodborne Illness.* Available online at www.cdc.gov/ncidod/dbmd/diseaseinfo/foodborneinfections_g.htm. Accessed March 23, 2009.

[3] U.S. Food and Drug Administration, Center for Food Safety and Nutrition. *Foodborne Pathogenic Microorganisms and Natural Toxins Handbook: The "Bad Bug Book."* Available online at www.foodsafety.gov/~mow/intro.html. Accessed July 22, 2009.

[4] Samuel, M.C., Vugia, D.J., Shallow, S., et al. Epidemiology of sporadic *Campylobacter* infection in the United States and declining trend in incidence, FoodNet 1996–1999. *Clin Infect Dis* 38(Suppl. 3):S165–S174, 2004.

[5] Centers for Disease Control and Prevention. *CDC Health Update: Multi-State Outbreak of E-coli 0157 Infections, November–December 2006.* Available online at www2a.cdc.gov/HAN/ArchiveSys/ViewMsgV.asp?AlertNum=00255. Accessed August 7, 2008.

[6] Centers for Disease Control and Prevention, Division of Foodborne, Bacterial, and Mycotic Disease. *Listeriosis.* Available online at www.cdc.gov/nczved/dfbmd/disease_listing/listeriosis_gi.html. Accessed August 6, 2008.

[7] Koepke, R., Sobel, J., and Arnon, S.S. Global occurrence of infant botulism, 1976–2006. *Pediatrics* 122:73–82, 2008.

[8] Widdowson, M.A., Sulka, A., Bulens, S.N., et al. Norovirus and foodborne disease, United States, 1991–2000. *Emerg Infect Dis* 11:95–102, 2005.

[9] National Institute of Environmental Health Sciences, National Institutes of Health. Aflatoxin and liver cancer. Available online at www.niehs.nih.gov/health/impacts/aflatoxin.cfm. Accessed April 30, 2009.

[10] Centers for Disease Control and Prevention. Cryptosporidium *Infection.* Available online at www.cdc.gov/ncidod/dpd/parasites/cryptosporidiosis/factsht_cryptosporidiosis.htm. Accessed August 1, 2008.

[11] Centers for Disease Control and Prevention. *vCJD (Variant Creutzfeldt-Jakob Disease).* Available online at www.cdc.gov/ncidod/dvrd/vcjd/. Accessed August 7, 2008.

[12] Food and Drug Administration. *Bovine Spongiform Encephalopathy (BSE).* Available online at www.fda.gov/oc/opacom/hottopics/bse.html. Accessed August 8, 2008.

[13] Preliminary Foodnet Data on the Incidence of Infection with Pathogens Transmitted Commonly Through Food—10 States, 2008. *MMWR* 58:333–337, 2009.

[14] Partnership for Food Safety Education. *Cook to Safe Temperature.* Available online at www.fightbac.org/images/pdfs/cook.pdf. Accessed March 19, 2009.

[15] U.S. Environmental Protection Agency. *Assessing Health Risks from Pesticides.* Available online at www.epa.gov/pesticides/factsheets/riskassess.htm. Accessed August 1, 2008.

[16] U.S. Environmental Protection Agency. *Setting Tolerances for Pesticide Residues in Foods.* Available online at www.epa.gov/pesticides/factsheets/stprf.htm. Accessed August 1, 2008.

[17] U.S. Food and Drug Administration, Center for Food Safety and Applied Nutrition. *Pesticide Program Residue Monitoring, 2004–2006.* Available online at www.cfsan.fda.gov/~dms/pes04-06.html. Accessed August 8, 2008.

[18] U.S. Food and Drug Administration, Center for Food Safety and Applied Nutrition. *Pesticide Program Residue Monitoring 2002.* Available online at www.cfsan.fda.gov/~dms/pes02rep.html. Accessed August 8, 2008.

[19] U.S. Department of Agriculture, Agricultural Marketing Service. *National Organic Program.* Available online at www.ams.usda.gov/AMSv1.0/ams.fetchTemplateData.do?template=TemplateA&navID=NationalOrganicProgram&leftNav=NationalOrganicProgram&page=NOPNationalOrganicProgramHome&acct=nop. Accessed August 1, 2008.

[20] U.S. Department of Health and Human Services and U.S. Environmental Protection Agency. *What You Need to Know About Mercury in Fish and Shellfish.* EPA-823-R-04-005, March 2004. Available online at www.cfsan.fda.gov/~dms/admehg3.html. Accessed August 1, 2008.

[21] International Food Information Council. *Fact Sheet: FDA's Approval Process for Food Animal Antibiotics—A Focus on Human Food Safety.* May 2008. Available online at www.ific.org/publications/factsheets/fdaanimalantifs.cfm. Accessed August 9, 2008.

[22] Pew Commission on Industrial Farm Animal Production. *Final Report: Putting Meat on The Table: Industrial Farm Animal Production in America.* Available online at www.ncifap.org/_images/PCIFAPFin.pdf. Accessed August 11, 2008.

[23] U.S. Food and Drug Administration, Center for Veterinary Medicine. *Report on the Food and Drug Administration's Review of the Safety of Recombinant Bovine Somatotropin.* Available

online at www.fda.gov/cvm/RBRPTFNL.htm. Accessed August 1, 2008.

24 Exon, J.H. A review of the toxicology of acrylamide. *J Toxicol Environ Health B Crit Rev* 9:397–412, 2006.

25 Friedman, M., and Levin, C.E. Review of methods for the reduction of dietary content and toxicity of acrylamide. *J Agric Food Chem* 56:6113–6140, 2008.

26 Morehouse, K.M. *Food Irradiation: The Treatment of Foods with Ionizing Radiation.* Available online at www.cfsan.fda.gov/~dms/opa-fdir.html. Accessed August 1, 2008.

27 U.S. Food and Drug Administration. *Food Irradiation: A Safe Measure.* January 2000. Available online at www.fda.gov/opacom/catalog/irradbro.html. Accessed July 31, 2008.

28 Osterholm, M.T., and Norgan, A.P. The role of irradiation in food safety. *N Engl J Med* 350:1898–1901, 2004.

29 National Toxicology Program, Center for the Evaluation of Risks to Human Reproduction. *NTP-CERHR Monograph on the Potential Human Reproductive and Developmental Effects of Bisphenol A.* National Institutes of Health publication number 08-5994, September 2008. Available online at http://cerhr.niehs.nih.gov/chemicals/bisphenol/bisphenol.pdf. Accessed February 6, 2009.

30 Eichholzer, M., and Gutzwiller, F. Dietary nitrates, nitrites, and N-nitroso compounds and cancer risk: A review of the epidemiologic evidence. *Nutr Rev* 56:95–105, 1998.

31 U.S. Food and Drug Administration, Center for Food Safety and Applied Nutrition. *EAFUS: A Food Additives Database.* Available online at www.foodsafety.gov/~dms/eafus.html. Accessed August 19, 2008.

32 International Food Information Council (IFIC) and U.S. Food and Drug Administration. *Types of Food Ingredients.* Available online at www.cfsan.fda.gov/~dms/foodic.html#types. Accessed August 19, 2008.

33 Margawati, E.T. *Transgenic Animals: Their Benefits to Human Welfare.* Available online at www.actionbioscience.org/biotech/margawati.html. Accessed March 21, 2009.

34 Gonsalves, D., and Ferreira, S. *Transgenic Papaya: A Case for Managing Risks of Papaya Ringspot Virus in Hawaii.* Available online at www.plantmanagementnetwork.org/pub/php/review/2003/papaya/. Accessed August 21, 2008.

35 Smith, N. *Seeds of Opportunity: An Assessment of the Benefits, Safety and Oversight of Plant Genomics and Agricultural Biotechnology.* U.S. House of Representatives report, April 13, 2000. Available online at www.house.gov/

science/documents.htm/. Accessed September 3, 2004.

36 Paine, J.A., Shipton, C.A., Chaggar, S., et al. Improving the nutritional value of golden rice through increased pro-vitamin A content. *Nat Biotechnol* 23:482–7, 2005.

37 Sautter, C., Poletti, S., Zhang, P., and Gruissem, W. Biofortification of essential nutritional compounds and trace elements in rice and cassava. *Proc Nutr Soc* 65:153–159, 2006.

38 Ye, X., Al-Babili, S., Kloti, A., et al. Engineering the provitamin A (beta-carotene) biosynthetic pathway into (carotenoid-free) rice endosperm. *Science* 287:303–305, 2000.

39 National Academy of Sciences, National Research Council. *Genetically Modified Pest-Protected Plants: Science and Regulation.* Washington, DC: National Academies Press, 2000.

40 Shewry, P.R., Tatham, A.S., and Halford, N.G. Genetic modification and plant food allergens: Risks and benefits. *Journal of Chromatography. B, Biomedical Sciences and Applications* 756:327–335, 2001.

41 Nordlee, J.A., Taylor, S. L., Townsend, J. A., et al. Identification of a Brazil-nut allergen in transgenic soybeans. *N Engl J Med* 334:688–692, 1996.

42 Bren, L. Genetic engineering: The future of foods? *FDA Consum* November/December 2003. Available online at www.fda.gov/fdac/features/2003/603_food.html/. Accessed September 17, 2004.

43 U.S. Food and Drug Administration. *FDA Talk Paper: FDA Proposes Draft Guidance for Industry for New Plant Varieties Intended for Food Use.* November 19, 2004 Available online at www.fda.gov/bbs/topics/ANSWERS/2004/ANS01327.html. Accessed October 6, 2005.

44 Caporael, L.R. Ergotism: The Satan loosed in Salem? *Science* 192:21–26, 1976.

Chapter 14

1 Food and Agriculture Organization of the United Nations. *The State of Food Insecurity in the World 2008.* Available online at www.fao.org/docrep/011/i0291e/i0291e00.htm. Accessed July 23, 2009.

2 Caulfield, L. E., de Onis, M. Blössner, M., and Black, R. E. Undernutrition as an underlying cause of child deaths associated with diarrhea, pneumonia, malaria, and measles. *Am J Clin Nutr* 80:193–198, 2004.

3 Black, R.E., Allen, L.H., Bhutta, Z.A., et al. Maternal and child undernutrition: Global and regional exposures and health consequences. *Lancet* 371:243–260, 2008.

4 World Health Organization. *The Global Burden of Disease: 2004 update, 2008.* Available online at

www.who.int/healthinfo/global_burden_disease/2004_report_update/en/index.html Accessed May 4, 2009.

5 Infant Mortality Rates. Available online at www.geographyiq.com/ranking/ranking_Infant_Mortality_Rate_aall.htm Accessed August 28, 2008.

6 World Health Organization. *Low Birth Weight: Country, regional and global estimates, 2005.* Available online at http://who.int/reproductive-health/publications/low_birthweight/index.html Accessed May 4, 2009.

7 UNICEF Progress for Children. *A World Fit for Children. Statistical Review.* Available online at www.unicef.org/progressforchildren/2007n6/index_41401.htm Accessed May 4, 2009.

8 James, P.T., Leach, R., Kalamara, E., and Shayeghi, M. The worldwide obesity epidemic. *Obes Res* 9:228S–233S, 2001.

9 World Health Organization. *Global Strategy on Diet Physical Activity and Health: Obesity and Overweight.* Available online at www.who.int/dietphysicalactivity/publications/facts/obesity/en/. Accessed August 27, 2008.

10 Food and Agricultural Organization of the United Nations. *The Nutrition Transition and Obesity.* Available Online at www.fao.org/FOCUS/E/obesity/obes2.htm Accessed March 26, 2009.

11 Kelly, T., Yang, W., Chen, C-S., et al. Global burden of obesity in 2005 and projections to 2030. *Int J Obes (Lond)* 32:1431–1437, 2008.

12 Wang, Y., and Lobstein, T. Worldwide trends in childhood overweight and obesity. *Int J Pediatr Obes* 1:11–25, 2006.

13 Lobstein, T., Baur, L., and Uauy, R. Obesity in children and young people: A crisis in public health. *Obes Rev* 5:4–104, 2004.

14 De Onis, M., and Blössner, M. Prevalence and trends of overweight among preschoolchildren in developing countries. *Am J Clin Nutr* 72,1032–1039, 2000.

15 Vorster, H. H., Bourne, L. T., Venter, C. S., and Oosthuizen, W. Contribution of nutrition to the health transition in developing countries: A framework for research and intervention. *Nutr Rev* 57:341–349, 1999.

16 Eberwine, D. Globesity: A crisis of growing proportions. *Perspectives in Health* 7:12–16, 2002. Available online at www.paho.org/English/DPI/Number15_article2_2.htm. Accessed February 12, 2006.

17 Chen, C.M. Overview of obesity in mainland China. *Obes Rev* 9:14–21, 2008.

18 Subramanian, S.V., and Smith, G.D. Patterns, distribution, and determinants of under- and overnutrition: A population-based study of

women in India. *Am J Clin Nutr* 84:633–640, 2006.

[19] Kennedy, E.T. The global face of nutrition: What can governments and industry do? *J Nutr* 135:913–915, 2005.

[20] Popkin, B.M. The nutrition transition: An overview of world patterns of change. *Nutr Rev* 62:S140–S143, 2004.

[21] The World Bank. *Global Purchasing Power Parities and Real Expenditures: 2005 International Comparison Program*. Available online at http://siteresources.worldbank.org/ICPINT/ Resources/icp-final.pdf. Accessed April 23, 2009.

[22] Food and Agriculture Organization of the United Nations. *The State of Food Insecurity in the World 2006*. Available online at www.fao.org/docrep/009/a0750e/ a0750e00.htm Accessed May 4, 2009.

[23] Bread for the World. *Are We On Track to End Hunger?* 2004. Available online at www.bread.org/learn/hunger-reports/ are-we-on-track-to-end.html. Accessed May 7, 2004.

[24] Population Reference Bureau. World population highlights: Key findings from PRB's 2008 world population data sheet, *Population Bulletin* 63(3):1–16, 2008. Available online at www.prb.org/pdf08/63.3highlights.pdf. Accessed August 30, 2008.

[25] Brown, L.R. *World Facing Huge New Challenge on Food Front—Business-as-Usual Not a Viable Option*. April 16, 2008. Available online at www.earthpolicy.org/Updates/2008/ Update72.htm. Accessed August 30, 2008.

[26] Rosen, S., and Shapouri, S. Rising food prices intensify food insecurity in developing countries. *Amber Waves* 6(1):16–21, February 2008. Available online at www.ers.usda.gov/ AmberWaves/February08/PDF/RisingFood. pdf. Accessed August 30, 2008.

[27] Reijnders, L., and Soret, S. Quantification of the environmental impact of different dietary protein choices. *Am J Clin Nutr* 78:664S–668S, 2003.

[28] Steinfeld, H., Gerber, P., Wassenaar, T., et al. *Livestock's Long Shadow: Environmental Issues and Options*. 2006. Available online at http://meteo.lcd.lu/globalwarming/FAO/ livestocks_long_shadow.pdf. Accessed March 17, 2009.

[29] World Health Organization. *Micronutrient Deficiencies: Iron Deficiency Anemia*. September 3, 2003. Available online at www.who.int/ nutrition/topics/ida/en/index.html. Accessed April 24, 2009.

[30] World Health Organization. *Micronutrient Deficiencies: Iodine Deficiency Disorders*. Available online at www.who.int/nutrition/topics/ idd/en/index.html. Accessed May 20, 2008.

[31] World Health Organization. *Micronutrient Deficiencies: Vitamin A Deficiency*. Available online at www.who.int/nutrition/topics/vad/en/ index.html. Accessed April 23, 2008.

[32] World Health Organization. *The World Health Report, 1998: Life in the 21st Century—A Vision for All*. Geneva: World Health Organization, 1998. Available online at www.who.int/whr/1998/ en/index.html. Accessed April 24, 2009.

[33] Lopez, A. Malnutrition and the burden of disease. *Asia Pac J Clin Nutr* 13:S7, 2004.

[34] Centers for Disease Control and Prevention. *Prevalence of Overweight and Obesity Among Adults: United States 2003–2004*. Available online at www.cdc.gov/nchs/products/ pubs/pubd/hestats/overweight/overwght_ adult_03.htm. Accessed February 12, 2008.

[35] Nord, M., Andrews, M., and Carlson, S. *Household Food Security in the United States, 2007*. ERR-66, U.S. Department of Agriculture Economic Research Service, November 2008.

[36] DeNavas-Walt, C., Proctor, B.D., and Smith, J.C. *Current Population Reports, P. 60–235, Income, Poverty, and Health Insurance Coverage in the United States: 2007*. Washington, DC: U.S. Government Printing Office, 2008.

[37] Jetter, K.M., and Cassady, D.L. The availability and cost of healthier food items. *Am J Prev Med* 30:38–44, January 2006.

[38] Native Edge. *Economic Development Guidance and Empowerment*. Available online at www.occ.treas.gov/cdd/edge.pdf. Accessed February 16, 2006.

[39] Hampton, T. Food insecurity harms health, well-being of millions in the United States. *JAMA* 298:1851–1853, 2007.

[40] MacDorman, M. F., and Mathews, T. J. Recent trends in infant mortality in the United States. *NCHS data brief*, no. 9. Hyattsville, MD: National Center for Health Statistics, 2008.

[41] U.S. Census Bureau. The 2009 Statistical Abstract. Table 670: Money income of households—distribution by income level and selected characteristics: 2006. Available online at www.census.gov/compendia/statab/ tables/09s0670.pdf Accessed May 7, 2009.

[42] McCarty, M. *Homelessness: Recent Statistics, Targeted Federal Programs, and Recent Legislation*. May 2005. Available online at www.fas.org/ sgp/crs/misc/RL30442.pdf. Accessed March 17, 2009.

[43] Federal Interagency Forum on Aging Related Statistics. *Older Americans 2004: Key Indicators of Well Being*. Available online at http://permanent.access.gpo.gov/lps58292/ OA_2004.pdf. Accessed April 24, 2009.

[44] United Nations. *End Poverty: Millennium Development Goals 2015*. Available online at www.un.org/millenniumgoals/ Accessed May 7, 2009.

[45] United Nations. *World Population to Increase by 2.6 Billion over Next 45 Years*. February 24, 2005. Available online at www.un.org/News/ Press/docs/2005/pop918.doc.htm Accessed September 4, 2008.

[46] Central Intelligence Agency. *The World Fact Book*. Available online at www.cia.gov/library/ publications/the-world-factbook/index.html. Accessed July 23, 2009.

[47] Berg, L.R., and Hager, M.C. *Visualizing Environmental Science*. Hoboken: John Wiley & Sons, 2007.

[48] Association of American Geographers. Population Module: Lesson 3, Page 2 - How does education affect fertility rates in different places. Available online at www.aag.org/ Education/center/cgge-aag%20site/ Population/lesson3_page2.html Accessed May 5, 2009.

[49] World Health Organization. *Infant and Young Child Nutrition: Global Strategy on Infant and Young Child Feeding*. April 16, 2002. Available online at http://ftp.who.int/gb/archive/ pdf_files/WHA55/ea5515.pdf. Accessed March 18, 2009.

[50] Kuhn, L., Aldrovandi, G.M., Sinkala, M., et al. Effects of early, abrupt weaning on HIV-free survival of children in Zambia. *N Engl J Med* 359:130–141, 2008.

[51] U.S. Department of Agriculture. Food and Nutrition Service. *The National Nutrition Safety Net: Tools for Community Food Security*. FNS-314, January, 2000.

[52] Economic Research Service, U.S. Department of Agriculture. *The Food Assistance Landscape: FY 2007 Annual Report*. Economic Bulletin 6-5, May 2008. Available online at www.ers.usda.gov/ Publications/EIB6-5/EIB6-5.pdf. Accessed September 5, 2008.

[53] Feeding America. *How We Work*. Available online at http://feedingamerica.org/ our-network/how-we-work.aspx. Accessed March 30, 2009.

[54] U.S. Department of Agriculture, Food Recovery and Gleaning Initiative. *A Citizen's Guide to Food Recovery*. Available online at www.usda.gov/news/pubs/gleaning/ content.htm. Accessed September 5, 2008.

[55] World Health Organization. Initiative for Vaccine Research. Hookworm disease. Available online at www.who.int/ vaccine_research/diseases/soa_parasitic/ en/index2.html Accessed July 23, 2009.

TABLE AND LINE ART CREDITS

Chapter 1

Figures 1.6b, 1.8B: From *Nutrition: Science and Applications* by Lori A. Smolin and Mary B. Grosvenor, John Wiley & Sons, Inc., copyright © 2008. Reprinted with permission of John Wiley & Sons, Inc. Figure 1.11: From *Nutrition: Everyday Choices* by Mary B. Grosvenor and Lori A. Smolin, John Wiley & Sons, Inc., Copyright © 2006. Reprinted with permission of John Wiley & Sons, Inc. Figure 1.12a: Reprinted by permission of the publisher from SEVEN COUNTRIES: A MULTIVARIATE ANALYSIS OF DEATH AND CORONARY HEART DISEASE by Ancel Keys, p. 253, Cambridge, Mass.: Harvard University Press, copyright © 1980 by the President and Fellows of Harvard College. *What A Scientist Sees* (page 20): From *Nutrition: Everyday Choices* by Mary B. Grosvenor and Lori A. Smolin, John Wiley & Sons, Inc., copyright © 2006. Reprinted with permission of John Wiley & Sons, Inc.

Chapter 2

Figure 2.2 Step 1: From *Nutrition: Science and Applications, Fourth Edition* by Lori A. Smolin and Mary B. Grosvenor, John Wiley & Sons, Inc., copyright © 2003. Reprinted with permission of John Wiley & Sons, Inc. Figures 2.4, 2.8a. 2.9, 2.10a: From *Nutrition: Science and Applications* by Lori A. Smolin and Mary B. Grosvenor, John Wiley & Sons, Inc., copyright © 2008. Reprinted with permission of John Wiley & Sons, Inc. Figures 2.12a: From *Nutrition: Everyday Choices* by Mary B. Grosvenor and Lori A. Smolin, John Wiley & Sons, Inc., copyright © 2006. Reprinted with permission of John Wiley & Sons, Inc. *Case Study* (page 47): From *Nutrition: Everyday Choices* by Mary B. Grosvenor and Lori A. Smolin, John Wiley & Sons, Inc., copyright © 2006. Reprinted with permission of John Wiley & Sons, Inc. Figure 2.13: From *Nutrition: Everyday Choices* by Mary B. Grosvenor and Lori A. Smolin, John Wiley & Sons, Inc., copyright © 2006. Reprinted with permission of John Wiley & Sons, Inc. Figure 2.14: From *Nutrition: Science and Applications* by Lori A. Smolin and Mary B. Grosvenor, John Wiley & Sons, Inc., copyright © 2008. Reprinted with permission of John Wiley & Sons, Inc.

Chapter 3

Figure 3.1: From *Nutrition: Everyday Choices* by Mary B. Grosvenor and Lori A. Smolin, John Wiley & Sons, Inc., copyright © 2006. Reprinted with permission of John Wiley & Sons, Inc. Figure 3.2: From *Principles of Anatomy and Physiology, 12e* by Gerard J. and Bryan H. Derrickson, John Wiley & Sons, Inc., copyright © 2009. Reprinted with permission of John Wiley & Sons, Inc. Figures 3.3a–b: From *Nutrition: Everyday Choices* by Mary B. Grosvenor and Lori A. Smolin, John Wiley & Sons, Inc., copyright © 2006. Reprinted with permission of John Wiley & Sons, Inc. Figure 3.4: From *Nutrition: Science and Applications* by Lori A. Smolin and Mary B. Grosvenor, John Wiley & Sons, Inc., copyright © 2008. Reprinted with permission of John Wiley & Sons, Inc. Figures 3.5a–b: From *Nutrition: Everyday Choices* by Mary B. Grosvenor and Lori A. Smolin, John Wiley & Sons, Inc., copyright © 2006. Reprinted with permission of John Wiley & Sons, Inc. Figures 3.6, 3.7a–b: From *Nutrition: Science and Applications* by Lori A. Smolin and Mary B. Grosvenor, John Wiley & Sons, Inc., copyright © 2008. Reprinted with permission of John Wiley & Sons, Inc. Figures 3.8, 3.10a–c: From *Nutrition: Everyday Choices* by Mary B. Grosvenor and Lori A. Smolin, John Wiley & Sons, Inc., copyright © 2006. Reprinted with permission of John Wiley & Sons, Inc. Figures 3.12a–d: From *Nutrition: Science and Applications* by Lori A. Smolin and Mary B. Grosvenor, John Wiley & Sons, Inc., copyright © 2008. Reprinted with permission of John Wiley & Sons, Inc. *Case Study* (page 75): From *Nutrition: Science and Applications* by Lori A. Smolin and Mary B. Grosvenor, John Wiley & Sons, Inc., copyright © 2008. Reprinted with permission of John Wiley & Sons, Inc. Figures 3.16, 3.18: *Nutrition:*

Everyday Choices by Mary B. Grosvenor and Lori A. Smolin, John Wiley & Sons, Inc., copyright © 2006. Reprinted with permission of John Wiley & Sons, Inc. Figure 3.19: From *Nutrition: Science and Applications* by Lori A. Smolin and Mary B. Grosvenor, John Wiley & Sons, Inc., copyright © 2008. Reprinted with permission of John Wiley & Sons, Inc. Figure 3.20: From *Nutrition: Everyday Choices* by Mary B. Grosvenor and Lori A. Smolin, John Wiley & Sons, Inc., copyright © 2006. Reprinted with permission of John Wiley & Sons, Inc.

Chapter 4

Figure 4.2a From *Nutrition: Everyday Choices* by Mary B. Grosvenor and Lori A. Smolin, John Wiley & Sons, Inc., copyright © 2006. Reprinted with permission of John Wiley & Sons, Inc. Figure 4.2b: Courtesy of Oldways Preservation Trust and the Whole Grains Council www.wholegrainscouncil.org. Figures 4.4a–c, 4.5, 4.7 left: From *Nutrition: Everyday Choices* by Mary B. Grosvenor and Lori A. Smolin, John Wiley & Sons, Inc., copyright © 2006. Reprinted with permission of John Wiley & Sons, Inc. Figure 4.7 right: From *Nutrition: From Science to Life* by Mary B. Grosvenor and Lori A. Smolin, John Wiley & Sons, Inc., copyright © 2002. Reprinted with permission of John Wiley & Sons, Inc. Figures 4.9a–b: From *Nutrition: Science and Applications* by Lori A. Smolin and Mary B. Grosvenor, John Wiley & Sons, Inc., copyright © 2008. Reprinted with permission of John Wiley & Sons, Inc. Figures 4.10, 4.11, 4.12, 4.13, 4.18a–b, 4.22a–b: From *Nutrition: Everyday Choices* by Mary B. Grosvenor and Lori A. Smolin, John Wiley & Sons, Inc., copyright © 2006.

Chapter 5

Figures 5.3a–b: From *Nutrition: Science and Applications* by Lori A. Smolin and Mary B. Grosvenor, John Wiley & Sons, Inc., copyright © 2008. Reprinted with permission of John Wiley & Sons, Inc. Figure 5.4: From *Nutrition: Everyday Choices* by Mary B. Grosvenor and Lori A. Smolin, John Wiley & Sons, Inc., copyright © 2006. Reprinted with permission of John Wiley & Sons, Inc. Figures 5.5, 5.6, 5.7a, 5.7c, 5.8a–b: From *Nutrition: Science and Applications* by Lori A. Smolin and Mary B. Grosvenor, John Wiley & Sons, Inc., copyright © 2008. Reprinted with permission of John Wiley & Sons, Inc. Figure 5.9: From *Nutrition: Everyday Choices* by Mary B. Grosvenor and Lori A. Smolin, John Wiley & Sons, Inc., copyright © 2006. Reprinted with permission of John Wiley & Sons, Inc. Figures 5.10, 5.11: From *Nutrition: Science and Applications* by Lori A. Smolin and Mary B. Grosvenor, John Wiley & Sons, Inc., copyright © 2008. Reprinted with permission of John Wiley & Sons, Inc. Figures 5.13, 5.14: From *Nutrition: Everyday Choices* by Mary B. Grosvenor and Lori A. Smolin, John Wiley & Sons, Inc., copyright © 2006. Reprinted with permission of John Wiley & Sons, Inc. Figure 5.15: From *Visualizing Human Biology, 2e* by Kathleen Anne Ireland, John Wiley & Sons, Inc., copyright © 2010 and *Nutrition: Science and Applications* by Lori A. Smolin and Mary B. Grosvenor, John Wiley & Sons, Inc., copyright © 2008. Reprinted with permission of John Wiley & Sons, Inc. Figure 5.16a: © 2000 Oldways Preservation & Exchange Trust, www.oldwayspt.org/med_pyramid.html. Figure 5.16b: © 2000 Oldways Preservation & Exchange Trust, www.oldwayspt.org/asian_pyramid.html. *Case Study* (page 140): From *Nutrition: Science and Applications* by Lori A. Smolin and Mary B. Grosvenor, John Wiley & Sons, Inc., copyright © 2008. Reprinted with permission of John Wiley & Sons, Inc.

Chapter 6

Figure 6.2: From *Nutrition: Everyday Choices* by Mary B. Grosvenor and Lori A. Smolin, John Wiley & Sons, Inc., copyright © 2006. Reprinted with permission of John Wiley & Sons, Inc. *What a Scientist Sees* (page 157), Figure

6.4: *Nutrition: Science and Applications* by Lori A. Smolin and Mary B. Grosvenor, John Wiley & Sons, Inc., copyright © 2008. Reprinted with permission of John Wiley & Sons, Inc. Figures 6.5, 6.6a–b: From *Nutrition: Everyday Choices* by Mary B. Grosvenor and Lori A. Smolin, John Wiley & Sons, Inc., copyright © 2006. Reprinted with permission of John Wiley & Sons, Inc. Figure 6.7a: From *Principles of Anatomy and Physiology, 12e* by Gerard J. and Bryan H. Derrickson, John Wiley & Sons, Inc., copyright © 2009. Reprinted with permission of John Wiley & Sons, Inc. Figure 6.7b: From *Nutrition: Science and Applications* by Lori A. Smolin and Mary B. Grosvenor, John Wiley & Sons, Inc., copyright © 2008. Reprinted with permission of John Wiley & Sons, Inc. Figure 6.8: From *Nutrition: Everyday Choices* by Mary B. Grosvenor and Lori A. Smolin, John Wiley & Sons, Inc., copyright © 2006. Reprinted with permission of John Wiley & Sons, Inc. Figure 6.9c: From *Visualizing Environmental Science, 2e* by Linda R. Berg and Mary Catherine Hager, John Wiley & Sons, Inc., copyright © 2009. Reprinted with permission of John Wiley & Sons, Inc. Figure 6.10: From *Nutrition: Everyday Choices* by Mary B. Grosvenor and Lori A. Smolin, John Wiley & Sons, Inc., copyright © 2006. Reprinted with permission of John Wiley & Sons, Inc. Figure 6.11: From *Nutrition: Science and Applications* by Lori A. Smolin and Mary B. Grosvenor, John Wiley & Sons, Inc., copyright © 2008. Reprinted with permission of John Wiley & Sons, Inc. Figure 6.14a: From *Nutrition: Everyday Choices* by Mary B. Grosvenor and Lori A. Smolin, John Wiley & Sons, Inc., copyright © 2006. Reprinted with permission of John Wiley & Sons, Inc.

Chapter 7

Figure 7.1: From *Nutrition: Science and Applications* by Lori A. Smolin and Mary B. Grosvenor, John Wiley & Sons, Inc., copyright © 2008. Reprinted with permission of John Wiley & Sons, Inc. *What a Scientist Sees,* left (page 187): From *Nutrition: Science and Applications* by Lori A. Smolin and Mary B. Grosvenor, John Wiley & Sons, Inc., copyright © 2008. Reprinted with permission of John Wiley & Sons, Inc. *What a Scientist Sees,* right (page 187): Reproduced with permission of United Nations University Press. Figure 7.3 left: From *Nutrition: Science and Applications* by Lori A. Smolin and Mary B. Grosvenor, John Wiley & Sons, Inc., copyright © 2008. Reprinted with permission of John Wiley & Sons, Inc. Figure 7.3 right: From *Nutrition: Everyday Choices* by Mary B. Grosvenor and Lori A. Smolin, John Wiley & Sons, Inc., copyright © 2006. Reprinted with permission of John Wiley & Sons, Inc. Figures 7.5, 7.6, 7.7, 7.8, 7.10b, 7.11, 7.12: From *Nutrition: Science and Applications* by Lori A. Smolin and Mary B. Grosvenor, John Wiley & Sons, Inc., copyright © 2008. Reprinted with permission of John Wiley & Sons, Inc. Figure 7.13a: From *Nutrition: Everyday Choices* by Mary B. Grosvenor and Lori A. Smolin, John Wiley & Sons, Inc., copyright © 2006. Reprinted with permission of John Wiley & Sons, Inc. Figure 7.13b: From *Visualizing Human Biology, 2e* by Kathleen Anne Ireland, John Wiley & Sons, Inc., copyright © 2010. Reprinted with permission of John Wiley & Sons, Inc. Figures 7.13d, 7.14. 7.15, 7.16, 7.17, 7.18, 7.19, 7.20. 7.21a, 7.22, 7.23b, 7.24: From *Nutrition: Science and Applications* by Lori A. Smolin and Mary B. Grosvenor, John Wiley & Sons, Inc., copyright © 2008. Figure 7.25 bottom: World Health Organization, http://www.who.int/vmnis/vitamina/prevalence/mn_vitamina_map_1995.pdf. Figure 7.27: From *Nutrition: Everyday Choices* by Mary B. Grosvenor and Lori A. Smolin, John Wiley & Sons, Inc., copyright © 2006. Reprinted with permission of John Wiley & Sons, Inc. Figures 7.29a, 7.30, 7.31, 7.32, 7.33, 7.35: From *Nutrition: Science and Applications* by Lori A. Smolin and Mary B. Grosvenor, John Wiley & Sons, Inc., copyright © 2008. Reprinted with permission of John Wiley & Sons, Inc.

Chapter 8

Figure 8.2a: From *Nutrition: Everyday Choices* by Mary B. Grosvenor and Lori A. Smolin, John Wiley & Sons, Inc., copyright © 2006. Reprinted with permission of John Wiley & Sons, Inc. Figures 8.3, 8.4, 8.8, 8.9, 8.12: From *Nutrition: Science and Applications* by Lori A. Smolin and Mary B. Grosvenor, John Wiley & Sons, Inc., copyright © 2008. Reprinted with permission of John Wiley & Sons, Inc. Figure 8.14: From *Nutrition: Everyday Choices* by Mary B. Grosvenor and Lori A. Smolin, John Wiley & Sons, Inc., copyright © 2006. Reprinted with permission of John Wiley & Sons, Inc. Figures 8.15 middle, bottom: From *Nutrition: Science and Applications* by Lori A. Smolin and Mary B. Grosvenor, John Wiley & Sons, Inc., copyright © 2008. Reprinted with permission of John Wiley & Sons, Inc. Figure 8.16a: From Mattes, R.D. and D. Donnelly, 1991. Relative Contributions of Dietary Sodium Sources. *Journal of the American College of Nutrition.* American College of Nutrition. Figure 8.16b: From *Nutrition: Science and Applications* by Lori A. Smolin and Mary B. Grosvenor, John Wiley & Sons, Inc., copyright © 2008. Reprinted with permission of John Wiley & Sons, Inc. Figure 8.17: From *Nutrition: Everyday Choices* by Mary B. Grosvenor and Lori A. Smolin, John Wiley & Sons, Inc., copyright © 2006. Reprinted with permission of John Wiley & Sons, Inc. Figure 8.18a, *What a Scientist Sees* (page 261): From *Nutrition: Science and Applications* by Lori A. Smolin and Mary B. Grosvenor, John Wiley & Sons, Inc., copyright © 2008. Reprinted with permission of John Wiley & Sons, Inc. Figure 8.19: From *Nutrition: Everyday Choices* by Mary B. Grosvenor and Lori A. Smolin, John Wiley & Sons, Inc., copyright © 2006. Reprinted with permission of John Wiley & Sons, Inc. Figure 8.20: From *Nutrition: Science and Applications* by Lori A. Smolin and Mary B. Grosvenor, John Wiley & Sons, Inc., copyright © 2008. Reprinted with permission of John Wiley & Sons, Inc. Figure 8.22: From *Nutrition: Everyday Choices* by Mary B. Grosvenor and Lori A. Smolin, John Wiley & Sons, Inc., copyright © 2006. Reprinted with permission of John Wiley & Sons, Inc. Figures 8.23, 8.25, 8.26b, Case Study (page 271), 8.27, 8.28, 8.29: From *Nutrition: Science and Applications* by Lori A. Smolin and Mary B. Grosvenor, John Wiley & Sons, Inc., copyright © 2008. Reprinted with permission of John Wiley & Sons, Inc. Figure 8.30: Yang, X.E., W.R. Chen, Y. Feng. Improving human micronutrient nutrition through biofortification in the soil-plant system: China as a case study. *Environmental Geochemistry and Health.* 2007 Oct; 29(5):413–28. Epub 2007 Mar 24 © Springer Science+Business Media B.V. 2007. With kind permission of Springer Science and Business Media. There are instances where we have been unable to trace or contact the copyright holder. If notified the publisher will be pleased to rectify any errors or omissions at the earliest opportunity. Figures 8.31, 8.32 top: From *Nutrition: Science and Applications* by Lori A. Smolin and Mary B. Grosvenor, John Wiley & Sons, Inc., copyright © 2008. Reprinted with permission of John Wiley & Sons, Inc. Figures 8.32 bottom: de Benoist, B., et al., eds. Iodine status worldwide. WHO Global Database on Iodine Deficiency. Geneva, World Health Organization, 2004. Figure 8.35: Reprinted with permission from Dietary Reference Intakes for Calcium, Phosphorus, Magnesium, Vitamin D and Fluoride. © 1997 by the National Academy of Sciences, Courtesy of the National Academies Press, Washington, D.C.

Chapter 9

Figure 9.2: From *Nutrition: Science and Applications* by Lori A. Smolin and Mary B. Grosvenor, John Wiley & Sons, Inc., copyright © 2008. Reprinted with permission of John Wiley & Sons, Inc. Figure 9.6 Adapted from Nielsen, S.J. and Popkin, B.M. Patterns and trends in food portion sizes, 1977–1998. *JAMA 289:*450–453, 2003. Figure 9.8b: From *Nutrition: Science and Applications* by Lori A. Smolin and Mary B. Grosvenor, John Wiley &

Sons, Inc., copyright © 2008. Reprinted with permission of John Wiley & Sons, Inc. Figures 9.9, 9.13, *What a Scientist Sees* (page 306): From *Nutrition: Everyday Choices* by Mary B. Grosvenor and Lori A. Smolin, John Wiley & Sons, Inc., copyright © 2006. Reprinted with permission of John Wiley & Sons, Inc. Figure 9.14: From Levine, James A., Lorraine M. Lanningham-Foster, Shelly K. McCrady, Alisa C. Krizan, Leslie R. Olson, Paul H. Kane, Michael D. Jensen, Matthew M. Clark (2005). Interindividual Variation in Posture Allocation: Possible Role in Human Obesity. Science 307(5709):584–6. Reprinted with permission from AAAS. Figure 9.16: From *Nutrition: Everyday Choices* by Mary B. Grosvenor and Lori A. Smolin, John Wiley & Sons, Inc., copyright © 2006. Reprinted with permission of John Wiley & Sons, Inc. Figures 9.20a, 9.21, 9.22b: From *Nutrition: Science and Applications* by Lori A. Smolin and Mary B. Grosvenor, John Wiley & Sons, Inc., copyright © 2008. Reprinted with permission of John Wiley & Sons, Inc. Figures 9.23, 9.24, 9.25: From *Nutrition: Everyday Choices* by Mary B. Grosvenor and Lori A. Smolin, John Wiley & Sons, Inc., copyright © 2006. Reprinted with permission of John Wiley & Sons, Inc.

Chapter 10

Figures 10.1d, 10.3, 10.5a: From *Nutrition: Science and Applications* by Lori A. Smolin and Mary B. Grosvenor, John Wiley & Sons, Inc., copyright © 2008. Reprinted with permission of John Wiley & Sons, Inc. Figure 10.7: From *Nutrition: Everyday Choices* by Mary B. Grosvenor and Lori A. Smolin, John Wiley & Sons, Inc., copyright © 2006. Reprinted with permission of John Wiley & Sons, Inc. Figures 10.8, 10.9, 10.11, 10.15: From *Nutrition: Science and Applications* by Lori A. Smolin and Mary B. Grosvenor, John Wiley & Sons, Inc., copyright © 2008. Reprinted with permission of John Wiley & Sons, Inc. Figure 10.19: Adapted from Saltin, B., and Castill, D. I. Fluid and electrolyte balance during prolonged exercise. In *Exercise, Nutrition, and Energy Metabolism.* E. S. Horton, and R. I. Tergung, eds. New York: Macmillan, 1988. Reprinted by permission of The McGraw-Hill Companies. Figure 10.22: From Bergstrom, J., L. Hermansen, E. Hultman, and B. Saltin. Diet, muscle glycogen and physical performance. Acta Physiologica Scandinavica 71:140–150, 1967. Wiley-Blackwell Publishers. *Case Study* (page 353).

Chapter 11

Figure 11.1: From *Visualizing Human Biology, 2e* by Kathleen Anne Ireland, John Wiley & Sons, Inc., copyright © 2010. Reprinted with permission of John Wiley & Sons, Inc. Figures 11.2, 11.4: From *Nutrition: Science and Applications* by Lori A. Smolin and Mary B. Grosvenor, John Wiley & Sons, Inc., copyright © 2008. Reprinted with permission of John Wiley & Sons, Inc. Figure 11.5: From *Visualizing Human Biology, 2e* by Kathleen Anne Ireland, John Wiley & Sons, Inc., copyright © 2010. Reprinted with permission of John Wiley & Sons, Inc. Figures 11.7, 11.9, *Case Study* (page 377): From *Nutrition: Science and Applications* by Lori A. Smolin and Mary B. Grosvenor, John Wiley & Sons, Inc., copyright © 2008. Reprinted with permission of John Wiley & Sons, Inc. Figure 11.11: This figure was published in The Developing Human, 5e, by K. Moore and T. Persaud, copyright Elsevier (1993). Figure 11.13: From *Nutrition: Science and Applications* by Lori A. Smolin and Mary B. Grosvenor, John Wiley & Sons, Inc., copyright © 2008. Reprinted with permission of John Wiley & Sons, Inc. Figure 11.14: Reprinted with permission from 'Down Syndrome: Prenatal Risk Assessment and Diagnosis,' August 15, 2000, American Family Physician. copyright © 2000 American Academy of Family Physicians. All Rights Reserved. Figures 11.16, 11.18: From *Nutrition: Science and Applications* by Lori A. Smolin and Mary B. Grosvenor, John Wiley & Sons, Inc., copyright © 2008. Reprinted with permission of John Wiley & Sons, Inc. Figure 11.21b: From

Nutrition: Everyday Choices by Mary B. Grosvenor and Lori A. Smolin, John Wiley & Sons, Inc., copyright © 2006. Reprinted with permission of John Wiley & Sons, Inc.

Chapter 12

Figure 12.6b: Reprinted from the Journal of the American Dietetic Association, Vol. 4, Issue 6. Ameena Batada, Maia Dock Seitz, Margo G. Wootan, and Mary Story. Nine out of 10 Food Advertisements Shown During Saturday Morning Children's Television Programming are for Foods High in Fat, Sodium, or Added Sugars, or Low in Nutrients. Pages 673–678, copyright 2008, with permission from Elsevier. *Case Study* (page 409): From *Nutrition: Science and Applications* by Lori A. Smolin and Mary B. Grosvenor, John Wiley & Sons, Inc., copyright © 2008. Reprinted with permission of John Wiley & Sons, Inc. Figure 12.9: Reprinted from American Journal of Preventive Medicine, Vol. 27/3, Samara J. Nielsen and Barry M. Popkin, Changes in beverage intake between 1977 and 2001, copyright 2004, with permission from Elsevier. Figures 12.13, 12.14, 12.15, 12.16a, 12.17: From *Nutrition: Science and Applications* by Lori A. Smolin and Mary B. Grosvenor, John Wiley & Sons, Inc., copyright © 2008. Reprinted with permission of John Wiley & Sons, Inc. *What a Scientist Sees* (page 423): Willcox BJ, Willcox DC, Todoriki H, et al. Caloric restriction, the traditional Okinawan diet, and healthy aging: the diet of the world's longest-lived people and its potential impact on morbidity and life span. *Ann N Y Acad Sci.* 1114:434–455, 2007. Figure 5. Wiley-Blackwell Publishers. Figures 12.19, 12.21, 12.22a, 12.23: From *Nutrition: Science and Applications* by Lori A. Smolin and Mary B. Grosvenor, John Wiley & Sons, Inc., copyright © 2008. Reprinted with permission of John Wiley & Sons, Inc.

Chapter 13

Figure 13.6b: National Institute of Environmental Health Sciences. The liver cancer data is from the GLOBOCAN 2002 database, and the aflatoxin data is from Williams et al., Human Aflatoxicosis in Developing Countries, *American Journal of Clinical Nutrition* 80:1106–22, 2004. Figure 13.9 left: From *Nutrition: Everyday Choices* by Mary B. Grosvenor and Lori A. Smolin, John Wiley & Sons, Inc., copyright © 2006. Reprinted with permission of John Wiley & Sons, Inc. Figure 13.9 right, *What a Scientist Sees* (page 452), Figure 13.12: From *Nutrition: Science and Applications* by Lori A. Smolin and Mary B. Grosvenor, John Wiley & Sons, Inc., copyright © 2008. Reprinted with permission of John Wiley & Sons, Inc. Figures 13.17a, 13.20: From *Nutrition: Everyday Choices* by Mary B. Grosvenor and Lori A. Smolin, John Wiley & Sons, Inc., copyright © 2006. Reprinted with permission of John Wiley & Sons, Inc. Figure 13.22: James, Clive. 2008. Global Status of Commercialized Biotech/GM Crops: 2008. ISAAA Brief No. 39. ISAAA: Ithaca, NY.

Chapter 14

Figure 14.1a: From *Nutrition: Science and Applications* by Lori A. Smolin and Mary B. Grosvenor, John Wiley & Sons, Inc., copyright © 2008. Reprinted with permission of John Wiley & Sons, Inc. Figure 14.1c: World Health Organization. The Global Burden of Disease: 2004 update, 2008. Figure 14.2a: Adapted from Vorster, H.H., Bourne, L.T., Venter, C.S., and Oosthuizen, W. Contribution of nutrition to the health transition in developing countries: A framework for research and intervention. *Nutr. Rev.* 57:341–349, 1999. Wiley-Blackwell Publishers. Figure 14.2b: World Health Organization, 2000. Figures 14.5, 14.9b: From *Nutrition: Science and Applications* by Lori A. Smolin and Mary B. Grosvenor, John Wiley & Sons, Inc., copyright © 2008. Reprinted with permission of John Wiley & Sons, Inc. Figure 14.10: United Nations Development Programme (UNDP)/Brazil. *What a Scientist Sees* (page 488): United Nations

Population Fund. 2003. State of World Population. Available on-line from http://www.unfpa.org/publicationsd/index.cfm?filterPub_Type=5. Accessed 7/5/04. Figure 14.13: From *Visualizing Environmental Science, 2e* by Linda R. Berg and Mary Catherine Hager, John Wiley & Sons, Inc., copyright © 2009. Reprinted with permission of John Wiley & Sons, Inc. Figure 14.15: From *Nutrition: Science and Applications* by Lori A. Smolin and Mary B. Grosvenor, John Wiley & Sons, Inc., copyright © 2008. Reprinted with permission of John Wiley & Sons, Inc.

Inside front and back covers

Reprinted with permission from *Dietary Reference Intake: The Essential Guide to Nutrient Requirements, 2006,* by the National Academy of Sciences, Washington, DC.

Appendices

Appendix A Pages 503–504: Reprinted with permission from *Dietary Reference Intake: The Essential Guide to Nutrient Requirements, 2006,* by the National Academy of Sciences, Washington, DC. **Appendix C** Page 511 *Handbook of Clinical Dietetics,* American Dietetic Association, © 1981 by Yale University Press (New Haven, Conn.); and Committee on Dietetics of the Mayo Clinic, *Mayo Clinic Diet Manual* (Philadelphia: W.B. Saunders Company, 1981), pp. 275–277. Reprinted by the permission of Yale University Press. **Appendix D** Page 516, middle: Reprinted with permission from the American Institute for Cancer Research. Page 516, bottom: The DASH Diet Action Plan, Pub. 2007, Amidon Press, Northbrook, IL. Page 517: Reprinted by the permission of the American Cancer Society, Inc. All rights reserved. **Appendix E** The Exchange Lists are the basis of a meal planning system designed by a committee of the American Diabetes Association and The American Dietetic Association. While designed primarily for people with diabetes and others who must follow special diets, the Exchange Lists are based on principles of good nutrition that apply to everyone, copyright © 2008 by the American Diabetes Association and The American Dietetic Association. **Appendix F** Page 536: From *Nutrition: Science and Applications* by Lori A. Smolin and Mary B. Grosvenor, John Wiley & Sons, Inc., copyright © 2008. Reprinted with permission of John Wiley & Sons, Inc. **Appendix H** Page 544: Diet, nutrition and the prevention of chronic diseases. A report of a Joint WHO/FAO Expert Consultation. © World Health Organization 2003. Available online at http://www.who.int/hpr/NPH/docs/who_fao_expert_report.pdf. Reproduced with permission. **Appendix I** Axxya Systems-Nutritionist Pro.

PHOTO CREDITS

Chapter 1

Pages 2–3: Justin Guariglia/NG Image Collection; Page 4: (center left) Sisse Brimberg & Cotton Coulson/NG Image Collection, (center right) iStockphoto, (bottom left) iStockphoto, (bottom right) Joel Sartore/NG Image Collection, (top left) iStockphoto, (top right) iStockphoto; Page 5: Todd Gipstein/NG Image Collection; Page 6: Andy Washnik; Page 7: (top right) Justin Guariglia/NG Image Collection, (top left) Tim Laman/NG Image Collection, (center left) B. Anthony Stewart/NG Image Collection, (center right) Mark Moffett/Minden Pictures/NG Image Collection, (bottom left) Spencer Grant/PhotoEdit, (bottom right) David Hoffman/Alamy; Page 9: (top) Jeffrey Coolidge/Getty Images, Inc., (bottom left) Charles D. Winters, (bottom right) Jeffrey Coolidge/Getty Images, Inc.; Page 10: Skip Brown/NG Image Collection; Page 11: Wendy Hope/Stockbyte/Getty Images, Inc.; Page 12: (bottom left) Rich Reid/NG Image Collection, (bottom right) W.E. Garrett/NG Image Collection; Page 13: Karen Kasmauski/NG Image Collection; Page 14: Evan Sklar/Getty Images, Inc.; Page 15: (top right) Picturenet/Blend Images/Getty Images, Inc., (center right) Kate Thompson/NG Image Collection, (top left) Andy Washnik, (center left) Andy Washnik; Page 19: (center right) Greg Ceo/Getty Images, Inc., (center left) iStockphoto, (bottom right) Yoav Levy/Phototake; Page 20: Lawrence Migdale/Photo Researchers, Inc.; Page 21: (left) Jose Luis Pelaez/Getty Images, Inc., (right) Gazimal/Getty Images, Inc.; Page 22: Joel Sartore/NG Image Collection; Page 23: (top) Todd Gipstein/NG Image Collection, (bottom) W.E. Garrett/NG Image Collection; Page 24: Andy Washnik; Page 25: Lori Smolin.

Chapter 2

Pages 28–29: Aude GUERRUCCI/AFP/Getty Images, Inc.; Page 30: U.S. National Archives; Page 31: Scott Camazine/Photo Researchers, Inc.; Page 32: Blair Seitz/Photo Researchers, Inc.; Page 34: David Young-Wolff/Getty Images, Inc.; Page 36: (top left) Raul Touzon/NG Image Collection, (center left) Photodisc/Getty Images, (center right) iStockphoto; Page 38: (left) Jose Luis Pelaez/Getty Images, Inc., (right) Alaska Stock Images/NG Image Collection; Page 39: Stephen Alvarez/NG Image Collection; Page 42: Todd Gipstein/NG Image Collection; Page 45: (left) iStockphoto, (right) Justin Guariglia/NG Image Collection; Page 50: Photodisc/Getty Images; Page 51: imagebroker/Alamy.

Chapter 3

Pages 54–55: David McLain/NG Image Collection; Page 57: Brian Bailey/Getty Images, Inc., Page 66: iStockphoto; Page 67: (top) David M. Martin/Photo Researchers, Inc., (bottom) SPL/Photo Researchers, Inc., (center right) S. Ito and D.W. Fawcett/Visuals Unlimited; Page 70: Andy Washnik; Page 71: (bottom left) George Wilder/Visuals Unlimited, (bottom right) Dennis Kunkel/Visuals Unlimited; Page 72: iStockphoto; Page 73: (top left) Yoray Liberman/Getty Images, (center) CNRI/SPL/Photo Researchers, (bottom left) Simon Fraser/Photo Researchers, Inc.; Page 82: (center left) CNRI/SPL/Photo Researchers, (top right) S. Ito and D.W. Fawcett/Visuals Unlimited.

Chapter 4

Pages 86–87: Rosenfeld/Age Fotostock America, Inc.; Page 88: (bottom left) Robert Clark/NG Image Collection, (center) Raul Touzon/NG Image Collection, (bottom right) iStockphoto, (center right) Image Source/Getty Images, Inc.; Page 89: (left) Jason Edwards/NG Image Collection, (center) Courtesy Oldways and the Whole Grains Council, wholegrainscouncil.org, (bottom left) Tui de Roy/Minden Pictures/NG Image Collection, (bottom right) iStockphoto; Page 90: (bottom left)

Taylor S. Kennedy/NG Image Collection, (center left and bottom right) iStockphoto, (top right) Image Source/Getty Images, Inc.; Page 92: (left) StockFood/Getty Images, (right) Gina Martin/NG Image Collection; Page 95: Scimat/Photo Researchers, Inc.; Page 96: Todd Gipstein/NG Image Collection; Page 104: (top) SPL/Photo Researchers, Inc., (bottom left) iStockphoto, (bottom right) ©IPN Stock; Page 105: Andy Washnik; Page 107: L.V. Bergman/Project Masters, Inc.; Page 108: Karen Kasmauski/NG Image Collection; Page 109: (top) iStockphoto, (bottom) iStockphoto; Page 111: (top) Andy Washnik, (center right) Andy Washnik; Page 114: Andy Washnik; Page 115: Andy Washnik photo and composition. Background corn photo from iStockphoto.com.

Chapter 5

Pages 118–119: Eric Futran—Chefshots/Getty Images, Inc.; Page 120: iStockphoto; Page 121: (left) iStockphoto, (right) Michael Newman/PhotoEdit; Page 122: (left) iStockphoto, (right) John Kernick/NG Image Collection; Page 125: (left) Rachel Epstein/PhotoEdit, (right) iStockphoto; Page 126: Science Photo Library/Photo Researchers, Inc.; Page 131: (bottom right) Karen Kasmauski/NG Image Collection, (bottom right inset) Ed Reschke/Peter Arnold, Inc.; Page 137: (top left) ©2000 Oldways Preservation & Exchange Trust, (center right) ©2000 Oldways Preservation & Exchange Trust, (bottom) Eriko Sugita/Reuters; Page 138: (top left) Todd Gipstein/NG Image Collection, (top right) Phil Schermeister/NG Image Collection, (center left) Gina Martin/NG Image Collection, (center right) Sisse Brimberg and Cotton Coulson/NG Image Collection; Page 142: Andy Washnik; Page 143: Andy Washnik; Page 144: Andy Washnik; Page 146: iStockphoto; Page 148: Andy Washnik; Page 149: Bart's Medical Library/Phototake.

Chapter 6

Pages 152–153: James P. Blair/NG Image Collection; Page 154: (left) Pixtal/SUPERSTOCK, (right) Michael Newman/PhotoEdit; Page 157: (top) Urbano Delvalle/Time Life Pictures/Getty Images, Inc., (bottom) Charles D. Winters; Page 162: David Phillips/Visuals Unlimited; Page 163: (left) Karen Kasmauski/NG Image Collection, (center) Gordon Wiltsie/NG Image Collection, (right) SPL/Photo Researchers, Inc.; Page 166: (left) Stephen Alvarez/NG Image Collection, (right) Bruce Brander/Photo Researchers, Inc.; Page 169: (left) Cameron Lawson/NG Image Collection, (center) Brian Yarvin/Photo Researchers, Inc., (right) Roy Toft/NG Image Collection; Page 170: (left) Jimmy Chin/NG Image Collection, (right) Michael Nichols/NG Image Collection; Page 171: Charles D. Winters/Photo Researchers, Inc.; Page 172: Melanie Acevedo/FoodPix/Jupiter Images Corp; Page 176: Teri Stratford; Page 177: iStockphoto; Page 178: Michael Newman/PhotoEdit; Page 179: (top) Gordon Wiltsie/NG Image Collection, (bottom) Stephen Alvarez/NG Image Collection; Page 180: Melanie Acevedo/FoodPix/Jupiter Images Corp; Page 181: Dr. Stanley Flegler/Visuals Unlimited/Getty Images/Getty Images, Inc.

Chapter 7

Pages 184–185: Fred Nicklen/NG Image Collection; Page 188: George Semple; Page 190: (center) iStockphoto, (bottom right) Michelle Del Guercio/The Medical File/Peter Arnold, Inc., (bottom left) Dennis Kunkel/Visuals Unlimited, (top right) Michael Krasowitz/Getty Images, Inc., (top left) Pritt Vesilind/NG Image Collection; Page 193: Foodcollection/Getty Images, Inc.; Page 195: U.S. Library of Medicine/Photo Researchers, Inc.; Page 196: Charles D. Winters; Page 197: Dr. M.A. Ansary/SPL/Photo Researchers; Page 201: Biophoto Associates/Photo Researchers, Inc.; Page 203: Wellcome Trust/Custom Medical Stock Photo, Inc.; Page 208:

Science Photo Library/Photo Researchers, Inc.; Page 212: Skip Brown/ NG Image Collection; Page 214: (left) iStockphoto, (right) iStockphoto; Page 216: ISM/Phototake; Page 217: (left) Ralph Lee Hopkins/NG Image Collection, (right) Science Photo Library/Photo Researchers, Inc.; Page 219: Rafiqur Rahman/REUTERS/Landov; Page 220: NG Maps; Page 221: (top left) Melissa Farlow/NG Image Collection, (top right) Alaska Stock Images/NG Image Collection, (bottom) Abraham Nowitz/NG Image Collection; Page 225: (top) Amethyst/Custom Medical Stock Photo, Inc., (center) Science Photo Library/Custom Medical Stock Photo, Inc., (bottom) Robert Mecea/AP/Wide World Photos; Page 229: (top left) Joel Sartore/NG Image Collection, (top right) iStockphoto, (center left) Lynn Johnson/NG Image Collection, (center) Abraham Nowitz/NG Image Collection, (center right) Konrad Wothe/Minden Pictures/NG Image Collection; Page 234: Abraham Nowitz/NG Image Collection; Page 235: Dean Conger/NG Image Collection; Page 237: ISM/Phototake.

Chapter 8

Pages 238–239: Jason Edwards/NG Image Collection; Page 241: James P. Blair/NG Image Collection; Page 244: Justin Guariglia/NG Image Collection; Page 245: Stacy Gold/NG Image Collection; Page 247: Michael Newman/PhotoEdit; Page 249: Charles D. Winters; Page 250: (center) iStockphoto, (bottom right) Michelle Del Guercio/The Medical File/ Peter Arnold, Inc., (bottom left) Dennis Kunkel/Visuals Unlimited, (top right) iStockphoto, (top left) Pritt Vesilind/NG Image Collection; Page 255: (top left) Michael Nichols/NG Image Collection, (top right) Andy Washnik; Page 259: (center) Dr. Michael Klein/Peter Arnold, Inc., (bottom) Larry Mulvehill/Photo Researchers, Inc.; Page 261: Tim Boyle/Getty Images, Inc.; Page 264: George Semple; Page 270: (left) B&B Photos/ Custom Medical Stock Photo, Inc., (right) Custom Medical Stock Photo, Inc.; Page 276: (right) John Paul Kay/Peter Arnold, Inc., (left) John Paul Kay/Peter Arnold, Inc., (bottom) ©World Health Organization; Page 277: George Semple; Page 278: George Semple; Page 279: (top) Medicimage/ The Medical File/Peter Arnold, Inc., (center) Science Photo Library/ Photo Researchers, Inc.; Page 282: (center) Charles D. Winters, (bottom) Michael Nichols/NG Image Collection; Page 283: (left) B&B Photos/ Custom Medical Stock Photo, Inc., (right) Custom Medical Stock Photo, Inc.; Page 285: NASA/NG Image Collection; Page 287: (top) John Paul Kay/Peter Arnold, Inc., (bottom) Science Photo Library/Photo Researchers, Inc.

Chapter 9

Pages 288–289: James P. Blair/NG Image Collection; Page 292: (top) Photolibrary Group Limited, (bottom left) Alamy, (center) Jodi Cobb/NG Image Collection, (bottom right) Joel Sartore/NG Image Collection; Page 293: (top left) David Young-Wolff/PhotoEdit, (top right) W. Jim Olive/ Peter Arnold, Inc., (center) David Young-Wolff/PhotoEdit, (bottom left) Yoav Levy/Phototake/Alamy, (bottom right) NewsCom; Page 294: (left) ©Corbis, (right) Tom McHugh/Photo Researchers, Inc.; Page 296: (top) Andy Washnik, (bottom right) Volkmar K. Wentzel/NG Image Collection; Page 298: PhotoDisc, Inc./Getty Images; Page 299: (left) St. Bartholomew's Hospital/Science/Custom Medical Stock Photo, (right) Tim Laman/NG Image Collection; Page 302: (left) Courtesy Lori Smolin, (right) Bruce Ayres/Getty Images, Inc.; Page 303: (bottom left) Andy Washnik, (bottom right) Andy Washnik; Page 304: Matt York/AP/Wide World Photos; Page 306: ©AP/Wide World Photos; Page 313: (top right) Alamy, (bottom left) Joel Sartore/NG Image Collection, (bottom right) iStockphoto; Page 314: Bill Aron/PhotoEdit; Page 315: Mark Goldman/Icon SMI/NewsCom; Page 317: (left) Nick Elgar/Getty Images News and Sport Services, (right) Gregory Pace/©Corbis; Page 320: (top right) SCPhotos/Alamy, (center

photos) © Corbis, (bottom left) Michael Nichols/NG Image Collection, (bottom right) Andy Washnick; Page 321: David Young-Wolff/PhotoEdit; Page 322: David Young-Wolff/PhotoEdit; Page 323: Richard Nowitz/NG Image Collection; Page 325: (center right) David Young-Wolff/PhotoEdit, (bottom left) Andy Washnik; Page 326: (top) Courtesy Lori Smolin, (bottom) David Young-Wolff/PhotoEdit; Page 327: Michael S. Yamashita/NG Image Collection; Page 328: W. Jim Olive/Peter Arnold, Inc.

Chapter 10

Pages 330–331: Richard Nowitz/NG Image Collection; Page 332: (left) Tim Laman/NG Image Collection, (right) Corbis/Alamy; Page 333: James Forte/NG Image Collection; Page 334: Cameron Lawon/NG Image Collection; Page 337: Michael Newman/PhotoEdit; Page 338: Bruce Dale/NG Image Collection; Page 342: Alamy; Page 343: (top left) Yva Momatiuk and John Eastcott/Minden Pictures/NG Image Collection, (top center) Alaska Stock Images/NG Image Collection, (top right) Rich Reid/NG Image Collection, (bottom) Fred Ernst/AP/Wide World Photos; Page 344: (left) Alaska Stock Images/NG Image Collection, (top right) Ed Reschke/Peter Arnold, Inc., (center right) Don W. Fawcett/Visuals Unlimited; Page 345: Carolyn Kaster/©AP/Wide World Photos; Page 350: Sven Kaestner/©AP/Wide World Photos; Page 351: Jignesh Jhaveri/ StockFood/Getty Images, Inc.; Page 352: iStockphoto; Page 353: (bottom left) George Semple, (bottom right) Andy Washnik; Page 355: Andy Washnik; Page 356: iStockphoto; Page 359: Corbis/Alamy; Page 361: Doug Pensinger/Getty Images, Inc.

Chapter 11

Pages 364–365: Paul Damien/NG Image Collection; Page 366: (center) Biophoto Associates/Photo Researchers, (bottom right) ©Meitchik/ Custom Medical Stock Photo, Inc.; Page 368: Sarah Leen/NG Image Collection; Page 369: Tracy Frankel/Getty Images, Inc.; Page 376: Andy Washnik; Page 378: ©Michael DiBari, Jr./AP/Wide World Photos; Page 380: Keystone Features/Getty Images, Inc.; Page 383: George Steinmetz/NG Image Collection; Page 388: (left) Raul Touzon/NG Image Collection, (center) Laura Dwight/PhotoEdit, (far right) iStockphoto; Page 390: Sean Sprague/The Image Works; Page 391: (left) Joel Sartore/NG Image Collection, (right) K.L. Boyd, D.D.S./Custom Medical Stock Photo, Inc.; Page 393: (bottom left) Alamy, (bottom right) Myrleen Ferguson Cate/ PhotoEdit; Page 394: Tracy Frankel/Getty Images, Inc.; Page 395: George Steinmetz/NG Image Collection; Page 396: Alamy; Page 397: Alamy.

Chapter 12

Pages 400–401: David McLain/NG Image Collection; Page 404: Tim Laman/NG Image Collection; Page 405: iStockphoto; Page 407: (bottom left) Science Photo Library/Photo Researchers, Inc., (center right) Katja Heinemann/Aurora/Getty Images, Inc.; Page 408: Donna Day/Stone/ Getty Images, Inc.; Page 411: Tom Carter/PhotoEdit; Page 415: (left) Bill Aron/PhotoEdit, (right) iStockphoto; Page 416: Purestock/Getty Images, Inc.; Page 420: (top right) Courtesy S.A. Jubias and K.E. Conley, University of Washington Medical Center, (bottom right) Joel Sartore/NG Image Collection; Page 422: ©Science Vu/Visuals Unlimited; Page 423: David McLain/NG Image Collection; Page 425: Ira Block/NG Image Collection; Page 427: Andy Washnik; Page 428: Science Photo Library/Photo Researchers, Inc.; Page 430: (left) Martin M. Rotker/Photo Researchers, Inc., (right) Biophoto Associates/Photo Researchers, Inc.; Page 432: (top) Ira Block/NG Image Collection, (bottom right) Biophoto Associates/ Photo Researchers, Inc.; Page 433: Mark Baker/©AP/Wide World Photos.

Chapter 13

Pages 436–437: Todd Gipstein/NG Image Collection; Page 439: (top left) Manoocher/NG Image Collection, (center left) Thinkstock Images/Getty Images, Inc., (bottom left) iStockphoto, (bottom right) Digital Vision/Getty Images, Inc., (center right) Joel Sartore/NG Image Collection; Page 440: Keen Press/NG Image Collection; Page 441: (left) Science Photo Library/Photo Researchers, Inc., (right) Dorling Kindersley/Getty Images, Inc.; Page 442: (left) Pete Ryan/NG Image Collection, (right) Jim Richardson/NG Image Collection; Page 443: David Arnold/NG Image Collection; Page 444: Howell Walker/NG Image Collection; Page 446: Manfred Kage/Peter Arnold, Inc.; Page 447: Image from http://en.wikipedia.org/wiki/File:Anisakids.jpg; Page 449: Michael P. Gadomski/Photo Researchers, Inc.; Page 450: Alamy; Page 452: James Shaffer/PhotoEdit; Page 456: (top) James L. Stanfield/NG Image Collection, (bottom) Courtesy Lori Smolin; Page 457: (top right) Jim Richardson/NG Image Collection, (center left) George F. Mobley/NG Image Collection; Page 459: Annie Griffiths Belt/NG Image Collection; Page 460: Council for Agricultural Science and Technology (CAST), 1989. Ionizing Energy in Food Processing and Pest Control: II. Applications; Page 461: Alaska Stock Images/NG Image Collection; Page 462: Joel Sartore/NG Image Collection; Page 467: (center left) Courtesy Marlin E. Rice, (bottom left) Courtesy Golden Rice Humanitarian Board, www.goldenrice.org; Page 469: Digital Vision/Getty Images, Inc.; Page 470: Council for Agricultural Science and Technology (CAST), 1989. Ionizing Energy in Food Processing and Pest Control: II. Applications; Page 471: ©H. Reinhard/Peter Arnold, Inc.

Chapter 14

Pages 474–475: Fritz Hoffmann/NG Image Collection; Page 476: Karen Kasmauski/NG Image Collection; Page 477: Steve Raymer/NG Image Collection; Page 479: Steve Raymer/NG Image Collection; Page 480: (top) Paula Bronstein/Getty Images, Inc., (center) Adiran Brooks/Getty Images, Inc., (bottom) W.E. Garrett/NG Image Collection; Page 482: Alaska Stock Images/NG Image Collection; Page 483: (top left) Bruce Brander/Photo Researchers, Inc., (top right) Stephen Alvarez/NG Image Collection, (center left) B&B Photos/Custom Medical Stock Photo, Inc., (center left) Custom Medical Stock Photo, Inc., (bottom left) John Paul Kay/Peter Arnold, Inc., (bottom right) ISM/Phototake; Page 487: Steve Raymer/NG Image Collection; Page 488: (top) Lynn Johnson/NG Image Collection, (bottom) Karen Kasmauski/NG Image Collection; Page 489: (left) iStockphoto, (right) Justin Sullivan/Getty Images, Inc.; Page 491: Robert Harding Picture LIbrary/Alamy; Page 494: ©Damian Dovarganes/©AP/Wide World Photos; Page 496: (top right) Steve Raymer/NG Image Collection, (bottom left) Robert Harding Picture Library/Alamy; Page 497: David Scharf/Peter Arnold, Inc.

Appendix G

Pages 540–543: Source ©Her Majesty the Queen in Right of Canada, represented by the Minister of Health Canada, 2007. This publication may be reproduced without permission. No changes permitted. HC Pub.: 4651 Cat.: H164-38/1-2007E ISBN: 0-662-44467-1.

INDEX

A

Absorption, 60
  carbohydrates, 96–97
  iron, 268f, 269
  mechanisms of, 60, 69, 69f
  minerals, 249, 249f
  proteins, 158f, 159
  vitamins, 189f
Acceptable daily intake (ADI), 105
Acceptable Macronutrient Distribution
  Ranges (AMRDs), 36, 36f, 108
Acesulfame K, 105f, 106
Acetaldehyde, 429f
Acetylcholine, 195f
Acetyl-CoA, 80f, 99f, 100f, 132f, 133, 133f,
  339f
Acrylamide, 459
Actin, 163f
Active lifestyle creation, 338, 338t
Active transport, 69, 69f
Activity level, calorie needs and, 300, 301f
Acute illness, older adults and, 421–422
Additives. See Food additives
Adenosine diphosphate (ADP), 80f, 81
Adenosine triphosphate (ATP)
  anaerobic vs. aerobic metabolism and,
    339–340, 339f
  exercise and, 343, 343f
  producing from amino acids, 164f
  source changes over time, 340, 341f
Adequate intakes (AIs), 34–35
ADI (Acceptable daily intake), 105
Adipex, 314
Adipocytes, 300
Adipose tissue, 131, 131f
Adjustable gastric binding, 316, 316f
Adolescents
  alcohol use and, 415
  athletics impact and, 414–415
  binge drinking and, 415
  calcium intake and, 412, 412f
  eating disorders and, 414
  energy and nutrient needs and, 412
  fast-food meals and, 414
  growth spurts and, 411f
  iron intake and, 412
  making healthier choices and, 414t
  milk and soft drink consumption and,
    412f
  MyPyramid and, 413–414, 413f
  puberty and, 411
  tobacco use and, 415
  vegetarian choices and, 414, 415f
  vitamins and, 412

Adolescent growth spurt, 411
Adult years. See also Older adults
  aging process and, 417, 417f
  energy needs and, 418, 418f
  energy-yielding nutrient
    recommendations, 418
  keeping healthy throughout, 423–426
  life expectancy and, 416, 416f
  malnutrition and, 420f
  mineral deficiencies and, 418–419
  nutrition and health concerns and,
    417–420
  secrets of longevity, 423
  vitamin deficiencies and, 418–419
  water needs and, 418
Advertising claims, 20, 22
Aerobic capacity, 333
Aerobic exercise, 332f, 333, 344f
Aerobic metabolism, 99, 99f, 132f, 299f,
  339, 339f, 342
Aerobic zone, 337, 337f
Age. See also Adolescents; Adult years;
  Children; Older adults
  bone loss and, 260, 260t
  dehydration risks and, 245f
  heart disease and, 136t
  hypertension and, 254
Age-related bone loss, 260
Aging process, 417, 417f
Agricultural chemicals. See Chemicals in
  food
Agroforestry, 490
Air displacement, body composition
  measurement and, 293f
Alcohol consumption
  absorption, transport, and excretion,
    427–428
  adolescents and, 415
  alcohol dehydrogenase (ADH), 429f
  alcohol metabolism, 428, 429f
  alcohol poisoning, 428–429
  alcoholic hepatitis, 430
  alcoholic liver disease, 430
  alcoholic mothers, 392
  alcoholism, 429
  benefits of, 430–431
  blackout drinking, 429
  blood alcohol levels, 427, 427f
  cancer and, 430
  cardiovascular disease and, 430
  cirrhosis and, 430, 430f
  fatty liver and, 430
  health risks and, 38–39, 39f
  heart disease risks and, 138f

  inflammation and, 430
  malnutrition and, 430
  nutrient absorption and, 430
  pregnancy and, 383, 383f
  risks and, 426–427
  short-term effects of, 428–429
  thiamin deficiency and, 195
Alcohol dehydrogenase (ADH), 429f
Alcoholism, 429
Alcohol poisoning, 428
Alcohol-related birth defects (ARBD), 383
Alcohol-related neurodevelopmental
  disorders (ARND), 383
Aldosterone, 253f
Allergens, 72
Allergic reactions, food, 72, 72f
Alli, 314
Alpha-carotene (α-carotene), 213
Alpha-linoleic acid (α-linolenic acid), 125
Alpha-tocopherol (α-tocopherol), 224
Alzheimer's disease, 422
AMDR, See Acceptable Macronutrient
  Distribution Ranges, 36, 36f, 108
Amenorrhea, 321
American Dietetic Association, 21
American Medical Association, 21
Amino acid pool, 160, 160f
Amino acids, 154 (See also Proteins)
  conditionally essential, 155
  energy use and, 165
  essential, 155
  functions of, 8
  limiting amino acids, 162
  nonessential, 155
  producing ATP from, 164f
  proteins and, 154
  structure of, 155, 156f
  supplements, 171, 171f, 356
  transamination and, 160, 161f
Amish community, obesity incidence and,
  296f
Anabolic steroids, 356–357
Anaerobic metabolism, 99, 99f, 339, 339f,
  340, 341f
Androstenedione (andro), 357
Anemia
  children and, 403
  hemolytic, 223
  iron deficiency, 270f, 271–272
  macrocytic, 203
  megaloblastic, 203–204, 204f
  physical activity and, 348, 348f
  vitamin B_6 and, 201f
Angiotensin, 253f

Erythropoietin, 358
Escherichia coli, 443, 443*f*, 448*t*
Esophagus, digestion and, 64
Essential amino acids, 155
Essential fatty acids, 125, 125*f*, 132, 134–135
Essential fatty acid deficiency, 134
Essential nutrients, 4
Estimated average requirements (EARs), 34, 35*f*
Estimated energy requirements (EERs), 35–36, 36*f*, 300–301, 301*f*
Estrogen, 261
Ethanol, 427
Exchange Lists, 43
Exercise. *See also* Fitness; Physical activity
    active lifestyle and, 338, 338*t*
    aerobic zone and, 337, 337*f*
    anaerobic *vs.* aerobic metabolism, 339, 339*f*, 340–342
    balancing calories and, 15*f*
    blood flow during, 77, 77*f*
    body weight management and, 335
    bone loss and, 261
    chronic disease risk and, 334, 334*f*
    dehydration and, 348–349, 349*f*
    duration and fuel use, 340–342
    eating after, 354
    eating before, 352, 352*f*
    eating during, 352
    energy balance and, 296, 296*f*
    fat-burning zone and, 342
    fatigue and, 343, 343*f*
    female athlete triad, 346, 346*f*
    fitness programs, 336–337
    fluid recommendations for, 350–351
    food intake balance and, 38, 38*f*
    fueling of, 339–344
    glycogen stores and, 351–352
    heat-related illness and, 348–349
    hypertension and, 254
    intensity and fuel use, 343–344, 343*f*
    making weight and, 346, 346*f*
    maximum heart rate and, 337
    older adults and, 425–426
    overtraining syndrome, 338
    oxidative damage and, 347
    oxygen delivery and, 340, 340*f*
    protein as fuel for, 342
    recommendations regarding, 335–338, 336*f*
    suggestions for starting and maintaining, 338*t*
    water loss and, 242
    water needs and, 348–351
    weight-loss guidelines and, 309
Expanded Food and Nutrition Education Program (EFNEP), 493*t*
Experimental groups, scientific testing and, 18
Extreme obesity, 292*f*

F

Facilitated diffusion, 69, 69*f*
Failure to thrive, 388
Family history
    food choices and, 7*f*
    heart disease and, 136*t*
Family planning efforts, hunger elimination and, 488
Famine, 479, 479*f*
Fashion models, body image and, 319, 320*f*
Fast-food meals, 414
Fasting hypoglycemia, 103
Fat burners, 315, 315*f*
Fat-burning zone, 342
Fat-free mass, 291
Fat-soluble vitamins, 186
    absorption and, 129, 189*f*, 212–227
    summary of, 227*t*
    vitamin A, 212–217
    vitamin D, 218–222
    vitamin E, 222–224
    vitamin K, 224–226
Fat stores, 133, 133*f*
Fatigue, exercise and, 343, 343*f*
Fats
    absorption of, 128–129, 314
    breakdown of, 100, 100*f*
    choosing wisely, 139–141
    consumption and obesity, 139
    as energy source, 133, 133*f*
    fat replacers, 144–145, 144*f*
    food sources, 120
    intake of, 139, 145
    metabolism of, 132*f*, 133
    physical activity and, 347, 347*f*
    U.S. changing fat intake, 120–121, 121*f*
    visible and hidden fats, 120, 120*f*
Fatty acids, 60, 123–126, 123*f*
    cis and *trans* fatty acids, 123–124, 125*f*
    composition of foods and, 124*f*
    digestion and, 60
    essential fatty acids, 125, 125*f*
    hydrogenation and, 124
    monosaturated fatty acids, 123*f*
    omega-3 fatty acids, 123*f*
    omega-6 fatty acids, 123*f*
    polyunsaturated fatty acids, 123*f*
    saturated fatty acids, 124
    types of, 124
    unsaturated fatty acids, 124
Fatty liver, 430
Feces, 60
Female athlete triad, 324*t*, 346, 346*f*
Ferritin, 160
Fertilization, 366, 366*f*
Fetal nourishment, 367–368
Fetus, 367
Fiber, 8
    blood cholesterol levels and, 106, 106*f*
    bowel health and, 107, 107*f*
    composition of, 91*f*
    effects of, 94, 95*f*
    functions of, 8
    insoluble, 92
    soluble, 92, 92*f*
Fibrin, 225*f*
Field gleaning, 494, 494*f*
Fight Bac!, 450*f*
Fitness. *See also* Exercise
    body composition and, 333*f*, 334
    cardiorespiratory endurance, 332–333, 332*f*
    components of, 332–334, 332*f*
    definition of, 332
    flexibility and, 333*f*, 334
    muscle strength and endurance, 332*f*, 333
    overload principle and, 332
    programs, 336–337
Fitness training, fuel use and, 344, 344*f*
Flexibility, 333*f*, 334
Fluid balance
    electrolytes and, 252
    proteins and, 163, 163*f*
Fluid requirements
    exercise and, 350–351
    infants and, 389
    pregnancy and, 373
Fluoride, 278–279
    bone formation and, 278
    dental caries and, 278
    fluoridation of water, 279
    fluorosis and, 279
    infants and, 390
    informational summary for, 281*f*
    meeting needs and, 278–279
    recommended intake for, 279, 279*f*
Fluorosis, 279
Foam cells, 134

Genetics
  nutritional status assessment and, 33*f*
  obesity and, 302–304, 302*f*
Germ, 88
Gestational diabetes, 102, 371
Gestational hypertension, 371
Ghrelin, 305
Giardia lamblia, 446, 448*t*
Ginkgo biloba, 229*f*
Ginseng, 229*f*
Globesity, 290
Glucagon, 98, 98*f*
Glucose, 91
  diabetes and, 101, 101*f*
  energy production and, 98–99, 99*f*
  production of, 90*f*, 91, 92*f*
  regulation of, 97–98, 98*f*
  stored, 300
Glucose tolerance factor, 277
Glutathione peroxidase, 275, 275*f*
Gluten intolerance, 168
Glycemic index, 96
Glycemic load, 96
Glycemic response, 96–97
Glycogen, 91, 91*f*
Glycogen stores, 351–352, 351*f*
Glycogen supercompensation, 351–352
Glycolysis, 98–99, 99*f*
Goiters, 276*f*, 277
Goitrogens, 277
Government policies, hunger elimination and, 488
Government programs preventing undernutrition, 493*t*
Grain enrichment, 187, 199
Grains, 141, 141*f*
Growth charts, 387–388, 387*f*
Growth hormone supplements, 356
Growth patterns, children, 404
Growth spurts, adolescents and, 411*f*

H
Hazard Analysis Critical Control Point (HACCP) system, 440, 440*f*–441*f*
Head Start, 493*t*
Health claims, food labels and, 46–48, 46*f*
Healthy diet
  balance and, 14–15, 15*f*
  example of, 16
  practicing moderation and, 16
  variety and, 15
Healthy life expectancy, 416
Healthy People 2010, 33, 493*t*

Heart
  improving heart health, 140
  role of, 76*f*, 77
Heart disease, 135–138
  atherosclerosis and, 134–136, 134*f*–135*f*
  carbohydrates and, 106
  diet and, 136–138
  eating to reduce risk of, 138, 138*f*
  folate and, 204
  risk factors for, 136, 136*t*
Heartburn, 72, 73*f*, 370*f*, 379
Heat cramps, 349
Heat exhaustion, 349
Heat index, 349, 349*f*
Heat-related illness, physical activity and, 348–349
Heat stroke, 349
Helicobacter pylori, 74
Heme iron, 269
Hemochromatosis, 272
Hemoglobin, 201*f*, 268
Hemolytic anemia, 223
Hemolytic-uremic syndrome, 443
Hemorrhoids, 107
  indigestible carbohydrates and, 107
  pregnancy and, 377
Hepatic portal vein, 78, 78*f*
Hepatitis A, 445, 448*t*
Herbal laxatives, 315
Herbal supplements, 229–231, 229*f*, 230*t*
Herring worm, 447*f*
Heterocyclic amines (HCAs), 459
High blood pressure. *See* Hypertension
High-carbohydrate foods, 9*f*
High-density lipoproteins (HDLs), 131
High-fat plant foods, 9*f*
High-fiber diets, 107
High-protein diets, 167
High quality protein or complete dietary protein, 172
HMB supplements, 357
Homeless Children Nutrition Program, 493*t*
Homelessness, 486
Homocysteine levels, 201*f*
Hormones, 11, 57
  administered to animals, 456
  organization of life and, 57
  role of, 11
Hunger, 486–494 (*See also* World hunger)
  appetite and, 295–296
  birth control as factor in, 488*f*
  controlling population growth and, 487–488

  defined, 476
  economic development and trade and, 490–491
  emergency food relief and, 487, 487*f*
  family planning and, 488
  food availability and, 490–491
  food supply fortification and, 492
  government policies and, 488
  increasing food production and, 489–490
  meal composition and, 66, 66*f*
  millennium development goals and, 486–487, 486*f*
  nutritional education and, 491
  providing short-term food aid, 487
  sustainable agriculture and, 489–490, 490*f*
Hydrogenation, 124
Hydrolyzed protein, or protein hydrolysates, 168
Hyperactivity, children and, 408–410
Hypercarotenemia, 217, 217*f*
Hypertension, 243, 407*f*
Hypertensive disorders of pregnancy (or pregnancy induced hypertension), 371
Hypoglycemia, 103
  carbohydrates and, 103
  fasting hypoglycemia, 103
  reactive hypoglycemia, 103
Hyponatremia, 246, 246*f*, 350, 350*f*
Hypothesis, scientific method and, 17

I
Indispensable amino acids (*See* essential amino acids)
Immune function, small intestine and, 71, 71*f*
Immunity
  and breast feeding, 392
  vitamin A in, 217
  and vitamin B$_6$, 202
Implantation, 367
Inactivity, energy balance and, 296, 296*f*
Incomplete dietary protein, 172
Indigestible carbohydrates, 94, 95*f*
Indirect food additives, 462
Indispensable amino acids, 155
Industrial chemicals. *See* Chemicals in food
Industrial contaminants, 455–456
Infancy, 387
Infant botulism, 444
Infant mortality rate, 477, 477*f*

Sodium chloride, 252
Soil selenium, 274, 274*f*
Soluble fiber, 92
    blood cholesterol levels and, 106, 106*f*
    polysaccharides and, 144*f*
    role of, 92, 92*f*
Solutes, 241
Solvents, 244
Soy products, 176, 176*f*
Special Milk Program, 493*t*
Special Supplemental Nutrition Program
        for Women, Infants, and Children
        (WIC), 380, 493*t*
Sphincter, 64
Spina bifida, 203*f*
Spores, food-borne, 444
Sports anemia, 348, 348*f*
Sports bars, 353
St. Johns wort, 229*f*
Staphylococcus aureus, 444, 448*t*
Starches, 91, 91*f*, 97
Starvation, 476
Steroid precursors, 357
Sterols, 123, 127, 127*f*
Stomach
    digestion and, 65–66
    gastric juices and, 65
    regulation of activity and, 66, 66*f*
    structure and function of, 65, 65*f*
Stomach flu, 444
Stored glucose, 300
Strength-training exercises, 332*f*, 333
Strontium-90, 455
Structure, protein, 162–163
Structure/function claims, dietary labels
        and, 49
Stunting, 477, 477*f*
Subcutaneous fat, 294–295
Subsistence crops, 491
Substance abuse, pregnancy and, 384
Sucrose, 90*f*, 91
Sudden infant death syndrome (SIDS), 383
Sugar units, 90
Sugars, refined, 89
Sulfites, 463
Sulfur, 267, 267*f*
Summer Food Service Program, 493*t*
Sun exposure, vitamin D and, 219–222,
        220*f*–221*f*
Superweeds, 467
Supplement Facts, dietary labels and,
        48–49, 48*f*
Supplemental Nutrition Assistance
        Program (SNAP), 493*t*, 494

Supplements
    amino acid, 171, 171*f*
    calcium, 263–264, 364*f*
    chromium picolinate, 278, 278*f*
    DNA and RNA, 358
    to enhance endurance, 358
    herbal products, 358
    muscle-building, 356–357
    for performance in short, intense
        activities, 357–358, 357*f*
    prenatal, 376*f*
    protein, 171, 171*f*
    vitamin and mineral, 355
    zinc, 274
Sustainable agriculture, 489–490, 490*f*
Swallowing, 63, 63f
Sweat, water loss and, 242

T

Tannins, 249, 249*f*
Team Nutrition, 493*t*
Technology for food safety. *See* Food safety
Teenagers, pregnant, 380–381, 381*f*
Television viewing, children and, 408,
        408*f*
Temperature
    food-borne illness and, 450*f*
    keeping food safe and, 458–460
Temporary Assistance for Needy Families
        (TANF), 493*t*
Teratogens, 379
Testosterone, 11*f*
Theory, scientific method and, 17
Thermic effect of food (TEF), 297, 299*f*
Thiamin, 194–195, 194*f*
    beriberi and, 194–195, 195*f*
    functioning of, 195*f*
    nerve function and, 194
    Wernicke-Korsakoff syndrome and, 195
Thirst, 242
Thyroid gland, iodine and, 275
Thyroid hormones, 275
Thyroid hormone synthesis, 275
Thyroid-stimulating hormone, 275–277
Tissues, organization of life and, 56–57,
        56*f*
Tobacco use, adolescents and, 415
Tocopherol, 224 (*See* Vitamin E)
Tolerable Upper Intake Levels (ULs), 35,
        35*f*
Tolerances, 454
Toothpaste, fluoride and, 278–279
Total energy expenditure, 297
Toxic substances, pregnancy and, 382–384

Toxoplasma gondii, 448*t*
Toxoplasmosis, 383
Trace minerals, 268–281
    chromium, 277–278
    copper, 272
    fluoride, 278–279
    iodine, 275–277
    iron, 268–272
    manganese, 280
    molybdenum, 280
    selenium, 274–275
    zinc, 273–274
trans fatty acids, 123, 124, 125*f*
Transamination, 160, 161*f*, 200*f*
Transcription process, 161*f*
Transgenic organisms, 466
Transit time, digestion and, 60
Translation, 161*f*
Transport, iron, 268*f*, 269
Trichinella spiralis, 446, 448*t*
Triglycerides, 122–123, 122*f*, 133, 133*f*
Trimester, 368
Tripeptides, 156*f*
Tropical oils, 124
Type 1 diabetes, 102
Type 2 diabetes, 102, 407*f*

U

Undernutrition, 12, 12*f*, 476–478, 493*t*
Underwater weighing, 293*f*
Underweight, 292
Underweight classification, 292*f*
United States
    eliminating food insecurity in, 492–494
    nutrition safety net and, 492–494, 493*t*
    poverty and food insecurity, 484–486,
        484*f*
Unrefined foods, 88, 88*f*
Unsaturated fats, 8
Unsaturated fatty acids, 124
Urea, 164*f*
Urinary system
    diagram of, 59*f*
    waste elimination and, 78, 79*f*
U.S. Department of Agriculture (USDA),
        30, 438*t*
U.S. Environmental Protection Agency
        (EPA), 438*t*
U.S. Food and Drug Administration
        (FDA), 438*t*

V

Vanadium, 355
Variable, 18